Systemic Sclerosis

Systemic Sclerosis

EDITORS

Philip J. Clements, M.D.

Professor of Medicine
Division of Rheumatology
Department of Medicine
University of California, Los Angeles
 School of Medicine
Los Angeles, California

Daniel E. Furst, M.D.

Clinical Professor of Medicine and Rheumatology
University of Washington
Seattle, Washington
Director, Arthritis Clinical Research Unit
Virginia Mason Research Center
Seattle, Washington

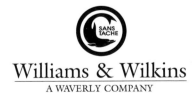

Williams & Wilkins
A WAVERLY COMPANY

BALTIMORE • PHILADELPHIA • LONDON • PARIS • BANGKOK
BUENOS AIRES • HONG KONG • MUNICH • SYDNEY • TOKYO • WROCLAW

Editor: Jonathan W. Pine, Jr.
Managing Editor: Molly L. Mullen
Production Coordinator: Raymond E. Reter
Copy Editor: James Morash
Designer: Martha W. Tenney/Textbook Writers Associates
Illustration Planner: Martha W. Tenney
Cover Design: Linda Dana Willis

Copyright © 1996 Williams & Wilkins

351 West Camden Street
Baltimore, Maryland 21201-2436 USA

Rose Tree Corporate Center
1400 North Providence Road
Building II, Suite 5025
Media, Pennsylvania 19063-2043 USA

Printed in the United States of America

Library of Congress Cataloging in Publication Data

Systemic sclerosis / editors, Philip J. Clements, Daniel E. Furst.
    p.   cm.
  Includes bibliographical references and index.
  ISBN 0-683-01740-3
  1. Systemic scleroderma.   I. Clements, Philip J.   II. Furst,
Daniel E., 1942–   .
    [DNLM: 1. Scleroderma, Systemic.   WR 260 S9942 1996]
  RC924.5.S34S95 1996
  616.797—dc20
  DNLM/DLC
  for Library of Congress   95-15204
                                                    CIP

95 96 97 98 99
1 2 3 4 5 6 7 8 9 10

We dedicate this book to the patients from whom we have learned all we know, to the telephone and express companies and postal service who made this book possible, and to our wives, Elaine and Ellie (plus our five children, two cats, and two dogs), to whom we owe so much.

Foreword

Systemic sclerosis resembles the proverbial elephant which, when examined by 6 blind men, was perceived to be a distinct and different structure by each, depending on which part of the elephant each examined. The manifestations, clinical courses, and outcomes of patients with systemic sclerosis differ greatly from patient to patient, depending on the pattern of organ system involvement, the rate of disease progression in the dominant organ system, and other intangible factors such as treatment.

This textbook, *Systemic Sclerosis*, utilizes the separate strengths of its authors for in-depth expositions on important aspects of the pathogenesis, clinical manifestations, and organ system involvements of systemic sclerosis, and then integrates the many parts into a coherent whole. Its international authorship includes most of the recognized experts on this disease. Conditions that are similar to systemic sclerosis are discussed in sufficient detail to assist the differential diagnostic efforts of clinicians.

An entire section of the book is devoted to treatment of this difficult disease, which is of great importance to physicians who care for systemic sclerosis patients. A surprisingly large number of interventions have been proposed to retard disease progression; methods are presented to design and conduct appropriate clinical trials to prospectively evaluate these treatments in patients. For day-to-day patient management, the extensive clinical experience of the world's experts is distilled in discussions of the practical approaches that they use to deal with and compensate for the often intractable problems encountered in the management of this chronic disease. These suggestions for optimal management often can make the difference between misery and an acceptable quality of life for patients trying to cope with their unique combination of disease manifestations. In addition, the section on *Resources* provides practical nursing tips for patients and their families as well as leads for the use of therapists and community resources.

The major strengths of the book are the breadth and depth of its authors, who include a large proportion of the still relatively small community of dedicated systemic sclerosis investigators. In addition to their aggregate clinical and encyclopedic knowledge base and skills, they are fully informed about ongoing research and the probable directions of future research. We already look forward to the next edition of this book to keep us informed about advances in this rapidly developing area.

Harold E. Paulus, M.D.
Professor of Medicine
University of California at Los Angeles

Preface

Over the past twenty years, longitudinal studies have provided significant improvements in our understanding of systemic sclerosis including its pathogenesis, its clinical manifestations, and even its treatment. As in other areas of medicine, the advent of molecular biological techniques has moved us ahead in understanding the causes and pathogenesis of systemic sclerosis.

Longitudinal studies, the application of good epidemiologic, genetic, and observational techniques, and consensus on clinical definitions has led to a better appreciation of the natural history of this illness. This appreciation, along with the use of better study methodology, has led to therapeutic advances of some import. Beyond that, the "art of medicine" has produced some relatively systematic approaches to therapeutics, both medicinal and supportive.

This book aims to provide *both* academically oriented physicians and practicing clinicians with an up-to-date, in-depth review of the background, pathogenesis, manifestations, and therapy of systemic sclerosis. The text can also serve as a resource for patient support and ancillary services.

An attempt has been made to integrate and interdigitate many of the related chapters. At the same time, the sections are separated into coherent, individual chapters. The following several examples may illustrate these characteristics: (*a*) different aspects of environmentally induced scleroderma are discussed in three separate chapters (Chapter 2 on epidemiology, Chapter 5 on clinical manifestations, and Chapter 10 on pathogenesis); (*b*) various aspects of systemic sclerosis pathogenesis are initially discussed separately and are then integrated into one chapter that attempts a unifying hypothesis of systemic sclerosis pathogenesis (Chapter 13); (*c*) literature-based reviews of treatment are discussed in the separate "organ" chapters but the practical aspects of treatment are integrated into one chapter that presents the personal approaches of experts to the treatment of this disease (Chapter 28).

The first section of the book (*I. General*) presents a general description of scleroderma and systemic sclerosis, including its detailed history, a background of its epidemiology and genetics, and a description of its classification and differential diagnosis. The second section (*II. Pathogenesis*) describes the state-of-the-art evidence supporting the various hypotheses about the pathogenesis of systemic sclerosis. This section's final chapter attempts a unifying hypothesis. The third section (*III. Organ Involvement*) includes separate chapters that describe, in detail, the organs affected by systemic sclerosis. Each of these chapters includes an analysis of the literature relating to systemic sclerosis treatment of the described organ system. The fourth section (*IV. Treatment*) opens with a chapter describing the problems involved in, and some suggested solutions for, designing trials of therapeutic interventions in systemic sclerosis. This is followed by chapters that deal with the overall treatment of systemic sclerosis and with *practical* approaches to treatment as used by experts in scleroderma therapy, including occupational and physical therapy and surgical therapy for hand involvement. The final section (*V. Resources*) is devoted to the often under-emphasized area of ancillary and supportive care, including extensive listings of resources available to patients and physicians for care of systemic sclerosis patients.

We hope that this book will encourage further interest in systemic sclerosis and that it will, at the same time, bring together information that can be useful to the physician faced with the treatment of a patient with this complex disease.

P.J.C.
D.E.F.

Contributing Authors

Roy D. Altman, M.D.
Professor of Medicine and Chief (Acting)
Arthritis, University of Miami School of Medicine
    and Director Clinical Research
GRECO
Miami Veterans Affairs Medical Center
Miami, Florida

Alfred J. Barnett, M.D., F.R.A.C.P.,
    FRCP(Lon)
Doctor
Consultant Physician
Alfred Hospital
Melbourne, AUSTRALIA

Carol M. Black, M.D. F.R.C.P.
Professor of Rheumatology
Department of Rheumatology
University College London Medical School
  and Royal Free Hospital School of Medicine
London, UNITED KINGDOM

Maria Blaszczyk, M.D.
Professor of Dermatology
Department of Dermatology
Warsaw School of Medicine
Warsaw, POLAND

Ken Blocka, M.D., F.R.C.P.(C)
Professor of Medicine
Department of Medicine, Royal University
    Hospital
University of Saskatchewan
Saskatoon, Saskatchewan
CANADA

James E. Bredfeldt, M.D., F.A.C.P.
Gastroenterologist/Hepatologist
Section of Gastroenterology
Virginia Mason Medical Center
Seattle, Washington

Philip J. Clements, M.D.
Professor of Medicine
Department of Medicine, Division
    of Rheumatology
UCLA School of Medicine
Los Angeles, California

Marie A. Coyle
President, Scleroderma Foundation
Peabody, Massachusetts

Angeline Douvas, M.D., Ph.D.
Department of Medicine/Rheumatology
    and Immunology
University of Southern California
Los Angeles, California

Ron M. du Bois, M.A., M.D., F.R.C.P.
Consultant Physician
Department of Occupational and Environmental
    Medicine
Royal Brompton Hospital
London, ENGLAND

William P. Follansbee, M.D.
Professor of Medicine
University of Pittsburgh School of Medicine
Pittsburgh, Pennsylvania

Daniel E. Furst, M.D.
Director of Arthritis Clinical Research
Virginia Mason Research Center
Clinical Professor of Medicine/Rheumatology
Department of Medicine
University of Washington
Seattle, Washington

M. Eric Gershwin, M.D.
Jack and Donal Chia Professor of Medicine
Internal Medicine
Division of Rheumatology/Allergy
University of California, Davis
Davis, California

Joan Guitart, M.D.
Assistant Professor
Department of Dermatology
Northwestern University
Chicago, Illinois

Ariane L. Herrick, M.D., M.R.C.P.
Senior Lecturer & Consultant in Rheumatology
Rheumatic Diseases Centre
University of Manchester
Hope Hospital
Salford, UNITED KINGDOM

Stephania Jabłońska, M.D.
Professor of Dermatology
Department of Dermatology
Warsaw School of Medicine
Warsaw, POLAND

Malcolm I.V. Jayson, M.D., F.R.C.P.
Professor of Rheumatology
Rheumatic Diseases Centre
University of Manchester
Hope Hospital
Salford, UNITED KINGDOM

Sergio A. Jimenez, M.D.
Professor of Medicine, Professor of Biochemistry
   and Molecular Biology
Departments of Medicine; Biochemistry
 and Molecular Biology
Jefferson Medical College
Thomas Jefferson University
Philadelphia, Pennsylvania

Geoffrey C. Jiranek, M.D.
Clinical Professor of Medicine
University of Washington
Department of Gastroenterology
Virginia Mason Medical Center
Seattle, Washington

Neil F. Jones, M.D., F.R.C.S., F.A.C.S.
Professor
Department of Orthopedic Surgery
Division of Plastic and Reconstructive Hand Surgery
Chief of Hand Surgery
University of California, Los Angeles
Los Angeles, California

M. Bashar Kahaleh, M.D.
Professor of Medicine
Chief, Division of Rheumatology
Department of Medicine
Medical College of Ohio
Toledo, Ohio

Peter A. Lachenbruch, Ph.D.
Branch Chief
Division of Biostatistics and Epidemiology
Food and Drug Administration
Rockville, Maryland

E. Carwile LeRoy, M.D.
Professor of Medicine
Rheumatology Department
Medical University of South Carolina
Charleston, South Carolina

Hildegard R. Maricq, M.D.
Professor of Research Medicine
Department of Medicine
Medical University of South Carolina
Charleston, South Carolina

Marco Matucci-Cerinic, M.D., Ph.D.
Associate Professor of Medicine
Institute of Internal Medicine
University of Cagliari
Cagliari, ITALY

Thomas A. Medsger, Jr., M.D.
Professor of Medicine
Department of Medicine
University of Pittsburgh School of Medicine
Pittsburgh, Pennsylvania

Giuseppe Micali, M.D.
Associate Professor of Dermatology
Department of Clinical Dermatology
University of Catania
Catania, ITALY

Yvon-Louis Pennec, M.D.
Professor of Internal Medicine
Department of Internal Medicine
Brest University Medical School Hospital
Brest Cedex, FRANCE

Janet L. Poole, Ph.D., O.T.R./L.
Lecturer III
Department of Occupational Therapy
University of New Mexico
Albuquerque, New Mexico

Robert P. Roca, M.D., M.P.H.
Director
Geriatrics Services
Sheppard and Enoch Pratt Hospital
Baltimore, Maryland

James R. Seibold, M.D.
Director, Scleroderma Program
Department of Medicine
UMDNJ-Robert Wood Johnson Medical School
New Brunswick, New Jersey

**Alan Jonathan Silman, M.D., M.S.C.,
    F.R.C.D., F.F.P.H.M.**
ARC Professor of Rheumatic Disease Epidemiology
ARC Epidemiology Research Unit
University of Manchester
Manchester, UNITED KINGDOM

Richard M. Silver, M.D.
Professor of Medicine and Pediatrics
Division of Rheumatology & Immunology
Medical University of South Carolina
Charleston, South Carolina

Lawrence M. Solomon, M.D.
Professor and Chairman of Dermatology
Department of Dermatology
University of Illinois
Chicago, Illinois

Virginia D. Steen, M.D.
Professor of Medicine
Department of Medicine
Georgetown University
Washington, D.C.

Esther M. Sternberg, M.D.
Chief, Section of Neuroendocrine Immunology
    and Behavior
Clinical Neuroendocrinology Branch
National Institute of Mental Health
National Institute of Health
Bethesda, Maryland

Mildred Goeke Sterz, R.N.
Clinic Coordinator
Department of Medicine/Rheumatology
UCLA
Los Angeles, California

John Varga, M.D.
Professor of Medicine
Head, Section of Rheumatology
University of Illinois School of Medicine
Chicago, Illinois

Steven R. Weiner, M.D.
Associate Clinical Professor
Department of Medicine/Rheumatology
UCLA School of Medicine
Van Nuy, California

Ken I. Welsh, Ph.D.
Oxford Transplant Centre
Churchill Hospital
Oxford, UNITED KINGDOM

Barbara White, M.D.
Associate Professor
Department of Medicine
University of Maryland
Baltimore, Maryland

Fredrick M. Wigley, M.D.
Associate Professor
Director, Division of Rheumatology
Department of Medicine/Rheumatology
The Johns Hopkins University
Baltimore, Maryland

Diane Williams
Founder
United Scleroderma Foundation, Inc.
Watsonville, California

Pierre Youinou, M.D., Ph.D.
Professor
Department of Immunology
Brest University Medical School
Brest, FRANCE

Farrukh Zaidi, M.D.
Senior Fellow in Rheumatology
University of Miami School of Medicine
Miami, Florida

Contents

II
Pathogenesis

III
Organ Involvement

IV
Treatment

V
Resources

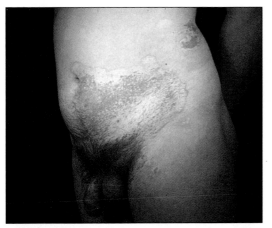

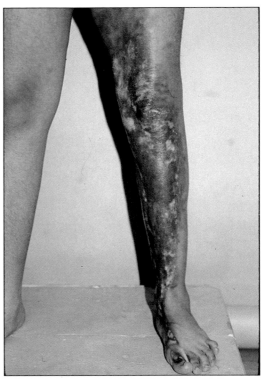

Color plate 1 (Fig. 4.1). Extensive morphea plaque in the abdomen. The margins are lilac and clearly defined.

Color plate 2 (Fig. 4.2). Linear scleroderma of the left lower leg involving the knee.

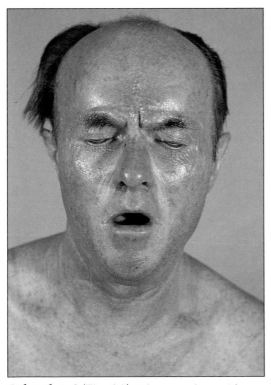

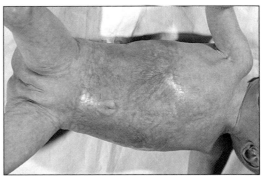

Color plate 4 (Fig. 6.2). Neonatal sclerodermiform progeria. Skin indurations involving the whole body with flexion contractures of the limbs.

Color plate 3 (Fig. 6.1). Scleromyxedema with pronounced skin indurations. The paraproteinemia was of IgG lambda type. Indurated edema and tense skin of the face.

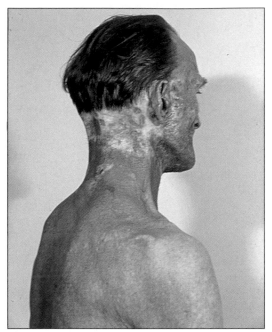

Color plate 5 (Fig. 6.3). Porphyria cutanea tarda. Sclerosis is most pronounced in the neck and face, the entire skin is irregularly hyperpigmented with atrophies and confluent indurations.

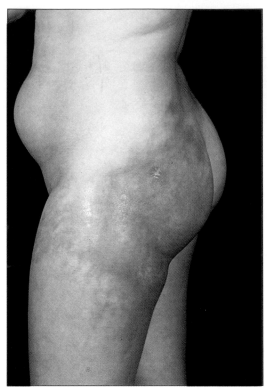

Color plate 6 (Fig. 6.6). Erythematous and indurated plaque in gluteal area after phytonadione (vitamin K) injection in a 5-year-old girl. In this case, we found extensive inflammatory changes in the fascia.

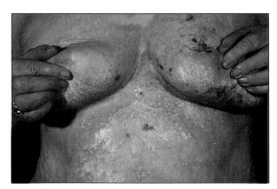

Color Plate 7 (Fig. 6.9). *A.* Widespread confluent lesions of *lichen sclerosus et atrophicus* involving almost the entire skin with numerous hemorrhagic bullae. There is similarity to localized scleroderma but the lesions are more superficial, do not involve the deep tissues and differ by a rough surface due to hyperkeratosis.

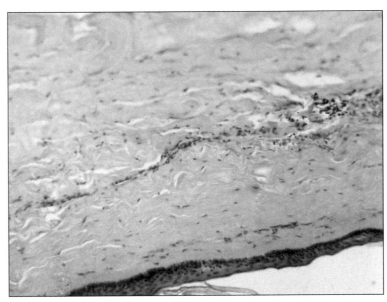

Color plate 8 (Fig. 6.9). *B.* Histology of *lichen sclerosus et atrophicus.* Characteristic hyperkeratosis with thinning of the epidermis, hydropic degeneration of basal cells and homogenization of the subepidermal zone. Slight inflammatory infiltrates beneath this zone. (H&E, magnification × 120)

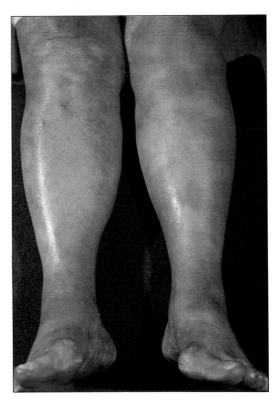

Color plate 9 (Fig. 6.10). *Sclerodermiform acrodermatitis chronica atrophicans.* Symmetrical indurations which developed in extensive erythematous lesions of the lower extremities are indistinguishable from localized scleroderma. In this patient, there was a high titer of antiborrelia antibodies and the response to penicillin was as rapid as in typical *acrodermatitis chronica atrophicans.*

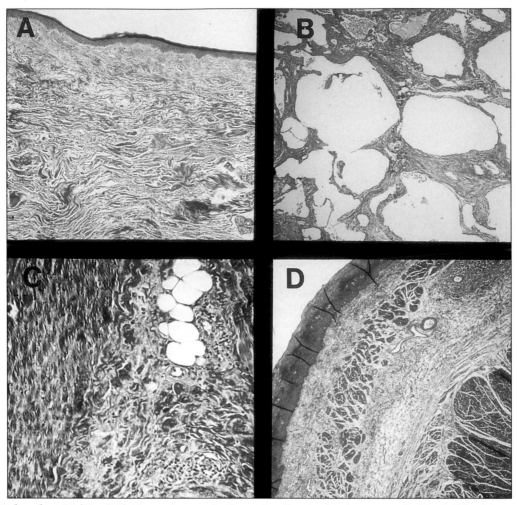

Color plate 10 (Fig. 7.1). Photomicrographs illustrating fibrosis of various organs in SSc: *A*, Skin; *B*, Lung; *C*, Heart; *D*, Esophagus. Note marked accumulation of collagen and disruption of the normal tissue architecture (Masson's trichrome stain).

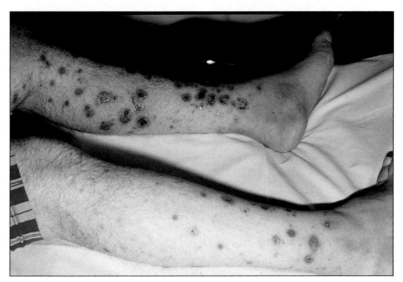

Color plate 11 (Fig. 14.1). Skin lesions caused by vasculitis in a patient with the CREST variant of progressive systemic sclerosis associated with Sjögren's syndrome.

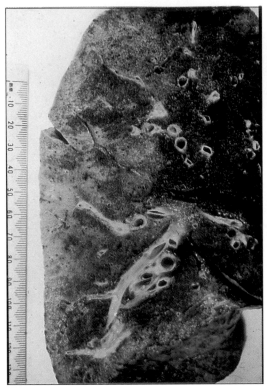

Color plate 12 (Fig. 15.1). Autopsy lung from a patient with systemic sclerosis. Pale areas of sub-pleural interstitial fibrosis are seen especially in the posterior and diaphragmatic aspects of the lower lobe. (Courtesy of Professor B. Corrin, Royal Brompton Hospital.)

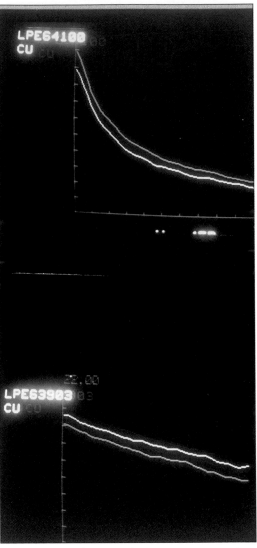

Color plate 13 (Fig. 15.7). ^{99m}Tc-DTPA scans from a patient with FASSc (*left*) and a normal individual (*right*). Note that the rate of decline of isotope from both lungs of the patient with FASSc is biexponential in pattern with a more rapid initial phase. By contrast, the rate of decline of isotope from the lung of the normal individual is monoexponential and much slower than in the patient with lung fibrosis.

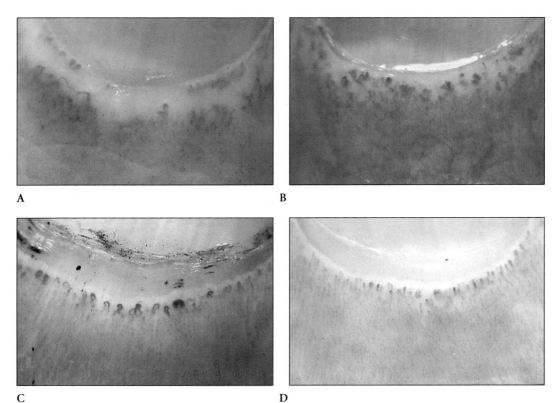

Color plate 14 (Fig. 17.3). SD-type capillary patterns seen in patients with scleroderma spectrum (SDS) disorders. *A.* "Active" pattern: extensive avascular area, destruction of capillaries with little increase in size of the remaining nailfold capillaries. *B.* "Active" pattern: extensive relatively avascular area but also exhibiting evidence of capillary neoformation—the presence of "bushy" capillaries. *C.* "Slow" pattern: enormous capillaries with little capillary loss. *D.* Numerous, moderately enlarged capillaries along the edge of the nailfold with little capillary loss—intermediate form, neither "active" nor "slow." In both 3*C* and 3*D* the capillary density along the edge of the nailfold is lower than normal, but there is not enough capillary loss to result in avascular areas.

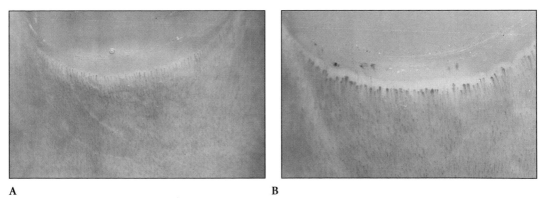

Color plate 15 (Fig. 17.5). The "white band" often observed in SSc patients' nailfolds between the endrow capillaries and the cuticle. *A.* Nailfold of a normal subject. *B.* Nailfold of a SSc patient. Note not only the slight widening of the light zone along the edge of the nailfold but also its much brighter white coloration.

I

General

A. J. BARNETT

1

History of Scleroderma

The historical sense involves a perception, not only of the pastness of the past, but also of its presence.
T S Eliot, "Tradition and the Individual Talent."

Life is a great bundle of little things.
Oliver Wendell Holmes,
"The Professor at the Breakfast Table."

So also is scleroderma.

Possible Early Cases

Scleroderma seems to be a relatively modern disease. Although not common, it is not rare and the clinical picture, particularly of the diffuse form, is so striking that it would be expected to draw the attention of physicians of past ages. Hippocrates (460–370 BC) described the case of "a certain Athenian whose skin was so indurated that it could not be pinched"(1), and Galen (130–299 AD) described an illness characterized by a "sort of obstruction of the pores with thickening, white spots, pigmentations, and absence of sweat glands"(1). Although such cases are compatible with scleroderma, it is not possible, in view of the limited descriptions, to accept them as examples of the disease we recognize today.

The first convincing case of scleroderma was described by Curzio of Naples, who wrote a monograph on the case in Italian in 1753. This case was translated into English by Watson in 1754 (2), and a description of the patient was reproduced in Rodnan and Benedet's classic paper in 1962 (2). The patient was a 17-year-old girl with "extensive tension and hardness of skin all over her body," tight eyelids, difficulty in opening her mouth, coldness of her skin, but normal sensation and no disturbance of respiratory, digestive, or renal function. The response to treatment—with warm milk, vapor baths, bleedings, and "small doses of quicksilver"—was remarkable in that, after a period of 11 months, the patient's skin had become "perfectly soft and flexible." A remission of skin sclerosis in diffuse scleroderma is fairly common, and is often attributed to the treatment given at the time; however, complete return to normality must be unique. Perhaps Curzio, like some modern physicians, looked at his result through rose-colored glasses. Other possible early cases referred to by Wolters in his review article in 1892 (2) are only slightly suggestive of the disease.

Descriptions of Scleroderma in the Nineteenth Century

Scleroderma was first established as a clinical entity and given its current name in the mid-nineteenth century with reports by Thirial (1845) (2), Forget (1847)(2), and Grisolle (1847)(2). Gintrac (1847) reviewed these cases together with five previous accounts, including that of Curzio, and called the condition "sclérodermie" (2). This name was adopted by Horteloup in his review of the subject in 1865 (2). In contrast to the apparent rarity of the condition before the 1840s, its description at this time was followed by

3

a flood of reports. Writing in Hebra's "Diseases of the Skin" in 1874, Kaposi stated that by that time more than 50 cases of "sclerema adultorum" (an alternative name) had been recorded (2). He gave two case histories of his own patients. In the first, the sclerosis affected the left arm and left leg; this would now be regarded as an example of morphea. In the second, there was diffuse sclerosis of arms, face, trunk, and legs; this would now be regarded as diffuse scleroderma. Kaposi reported on a biopsy specimen of skin from the upper arm showing accumulations of lymphocytes and a thick network of dense fibrous tissue extending into the subcutaneous tissue.

In Raynaud's thesis of 1862 on "Local Asphyxia and Symmetrical Gangrene of the Extremities" (3) it seems possible that some of the patients were suffering from scleroderma, but this cannot usually be substantiated because skin changes are not described in detail. For one 40-year-old male patient, however, it is stated that "the skin is white and hard, like parchment." Another case, described in Raynaud's "New Researches" of 1874 (4), reports a "sort of edematous puffiness which extends up to the middle part of the dorsal aspect of the hands."

Jonathan Hutchinson (1893) was much more explicit (5). He reported on a 50-year-old woman who had been subject all her life to "dead fingers," had frequent attacks of Raynaud's phenomenon (RP), had noticed the tight state of the skin of her fingers, and had several attacks of digital gangrene. He wrote: "her face is board-like and much freckled, with some stigmata" (probably telangiectasis), and that "she easily gets diarrhea" (suggestive of small bowel involvement). Hutchinson commented on the coincidence of "sclerodermia" with "Raynaud's malady" but believed that "their connection is by no means essential." He continued to publish reports on patients with hard skin, and was intrigued with the possible relationship between the apparently diverse conditions with this anomaly. In 1895, he wrote "The group of affections which have been described under the names of 'Morphea', 'Hide-bound skin', 'Sclerodermia' and 'Scleriasis Cutis' offer to

us most interesting and at the same time very difficult problems"(6). He then described illustrative cases. The first four had "modified Raynaud's phenomena" with a tendency toward production of "acroteric scleriasis." The next case, described as "aroterie morphea," had more extensive sclerosis affecting the hands and face. The next two cases had even more extensive sclerosis, the first involving the trunk and limbs (but excluding the feet, hands, and face), and the second involving all four limbs including the fingers. These latter patients did not suffer from RP. He then described five patients with patches of hard white skin, which he called "herpetiform morphea."

A description of scleroderma appears in Osler's 1894 textbook on "The Principles and Practice of Medicine"(7). He described two forms of scleroderma: "circumscribed" (equivalent to morphea) and "diffuse" (equivalent to systemic sclerosis or SSc), and wrote that patients are "apt to succumb to pulmonary complaints or to nephritis"; also, "rheumatic troubles have been noticed in some instances; in others endocarditis." In an article in 1898, in which he reported on eight cases of diffuse scleroderma, Osler gave a dramatic picture of the severe generalized form (8): "In its aggravated form, diffuse scleroderma is one of the most terrible of all human ills. Like Tithonus to wither slowly and like him to be beaten down and marred and wasted until one is literally a mummy encased in an evershrinking skin of steel is a fate not pictured in any tragedy, ancient or modern." A review of scleroderma by Lewin and Heller in 1895 included 507 case reports (2).

There was little mention of systemic involvement in the nineteenth century reports, although Auspitz (1863) (2) and Meyer (1887) (9) suggested renal involvement. Osler, in his textbook in 1894, stated that patients with scleroderma were apt to succumb to pulmonary complaints or nephritis (7). Joint problems were mentioned in case reports by Forget in 1847 (2), Dercum in 1896 (10) and 1898 (2), and Osler in 1898 (17). However, in spite of these isolated observations, the systemic nature of scleroderma was not generally recognized, and Wolters (1892) wrote: "According to all observations, scleroderma does not appear to be a disease which threatens life directly. . . . Exitus usually results from the greatest variety of disease(s) which are not directly related to the process"(2).

Subdivisions of Types of Scleroderma

SYSTEMIC SCLEROSIS AND MORPHEA

It is apparent from reading reports of cases of scleroderma from the nineteenth century that these differed greatly in the distribution of skin changes and associated symptoms. In 1817, Alibert discussed a condition called *scleremia*, which he divided into two types: a "partial" called *scleremia circumscripta* (probably linear scleroderma), and "universal" occurring primarily in children (2). In 1818, he wrote "Nothing is more bizarre, but also nothing is more interesting than the stiffened degeneration of the dermal system. It will always be for doctors a great subject of study and of meditation, such that they will add some prize to physiological researches"(2).

In 1854, Addison reported on a condition he called "true keloid," which he described in detail (2): "It has its original seat in the subcutaneous areolar tissue, and is first indicated by a white patch or opacity of the integument, of a rounded or oval shape and varying in size from that of a silver penny to that of a crown piece . . . a more or less vivid zone of redness surrounding the whole patch." This is a clear description of what would be regarded now as a patch of morphea. In 1857, Wilson described "morphea alba atrophica" (equivalent to the modern localized scleroderma en coup de sabre) and hemiatrophy of the face, and is attributed with the introduction of the term "morphea" to designate localized scleroderma (2).

It was becoming apparent that more than one condition was being referred to as scleremia or scleroderma. Duhring, in his 1881 textbook on diseases of the skin, distinguished between morphea and scleroderma with symmetrical skin stiffness (2).

Hutchinson, in 1895, devoted a separate part of his paper "On morphea and allied conditions" to *herpetiform morphea*, in which the skin lesions occurred in patches. This was in contrast to the cases described in the first part of the paper in which the skin sclerosis was symmetrical (6). He distinguished clearly between the localized form of scleroderma (his *herpetiform morphea*) and scleroderma with symmetrical skin stiffness; however, there was some confusion in terminology as he still used the term morphea as a comprehensive one to include both conditions, and was apparently unaware of the restricted use of this term introduced by Wilson and accepted by Duhring. In fact, in the early part of his paper he wrote of "Raynaud's phenomenon and acroteric morphea."

The various forms of localized scleroderma (morphea patches, scleroderma en coup de sabre, sclerodermia with hemiatrophy) are now recognized as a separate disease from the systemic form of scleroderma (or SSc), although some confusion persisted in the minds of some people up to the middle of the current century and some papers on the treatment of "scleroderma" included both conditions.

SUBDIVISIONS OF SYSTEMIC SCLEROSIS

Even after the separation of localized skin lesions, now referred to as morphea, from scleroderma with symmetrical skin stiffness, it was apparent that scleroderma with symmetrical skin involvement varied greatly in severity. Thus, Hutchinson described RP followed by sclerosis of the fingers ("modified Raynaud's phenomenon with tendency to production of acroteric sclerosis"), RP with more severe sclerosis ("Raynaud's phenomenon with tendency to morphea acroterica"), and more diffuse skin involvement ("acroteric morphea in association with general emaciation, pigmentation and papillomatosis") (6). He was, as explained previously, using the term "morphea" for general skin sclerosis rather than in its modern application of "localized sclero-derma."

In 1934, Sellei coined the term "acrosclerosis" to describe a condition characterized by RP, symmetrical stiffness of the hands and face, frequent telangiectasis, and predominance in females. He distinguished this from what he described as "true scleroderma" or *scleroderma verum* (11). According to Sellei, scleroderma verum "arises in different parts of the body and occurs in various forms—circular (scleroderma circumscriptum), ribbon-like (scleroderma en bandhes), or with irregular plaques (scleroderma diffusum)." In other words, his "true scleroderma" seemed to correspond to the various forms of morphea previously described. As outlined previously, the distinction between these conditions and scleroderma with symmetrical skin stiffness had already been made. However, the term acrosclerosis caught the imagination, and subsequent workers were concerned with the distinction between this and scleroderma with more widespread skin involvement (diffuse scleroderma).

Truelove and Whyte (1951) (12) and Ramsey (1951) (13) considered acrosclerosis and diffuse scleroderma to be distinct, whereas Leinwand et al (1954) (14) and O'Leary et al (1957) (15) considered them to be variants of the one disease. O'Leary et al found certain histological differences between the diffuse and acrosclerotic forms of the disease: the dermis was thickened in the diffuse form, thinned in the acrosclerotic form; obliterative changes in the vessels were more marked in the diffuse form; and hyperkeratosis was more marked in the acrosclerotic form. However these features were not diagnostic. In 1959, JabloÉnska et al found similar visceral changes in acrosclerotic patients and those with more diffuse skin involvement (16). However, Farmer et al, in 1961, suggested that sclerodermatous changes limited to the fingers ("sclerodactylia secondary to Raynaud's phenomenon") might be a different condition from scleroderma with more extensive skin changes,

and wrote that "systemic scleroderma" seemed to have developed in only three of 71 such patients after follow-up for 1 to 31 years (17). The extent of the skin sclerosis might influence prognosis. In 1961, Tuffanelli and Winkelmann, in their enormous series of 727 patients seen at the Mayo Clinic from 1935 through to 1958, found that in the acrosclerotic form (the great majority) the course in many patients was long and chronic, whereas in diffuse scleroderma with widespread skin involvement the course was rapid and the prognosis poor (18). It is interesting that even today there is a lack of uniformity among workers in the classification of various forms of scleroderma (SSc), and terms in use include "diffuse and limited varieties"; "Type 1, 2, and 3"; and the "CREST variant."

Description of Types of Systemic Involvement

During the first half of this century, numerous papers appeared describing involvement of particular organs or systems in scleroderma. Many of these were individual case reports, others were series of cases. These will be discussed in the following paragraphs under the headings of the various systems.

SKIN

In the nineteenth century, scleroderma was regarded mainly as a dermatological condition. The skin changes described were not confined to hardness and stiffness, but other features such as ulceration, gangrene, pigmentation, and telangiectasia were mentioned by various writers, including Raynaud and Hutchinson. Calcinosis was first described by Weber in 1878 (31) and was rediscovered in 1911 by Thiberge and Weissenbach, who described a case and included eight more cases from the literature (2). The condition was discussed in great detail in 1928 by Durham, who collected an additional 14 cases, including one of his own (1). Deposits of calcium were found not only in areas obviously involved by scleroderma but also in other regions, particularly around joints. Calcium deposits were found in tendons in one case and the buttocks in another. Chemical examinations showed the presence of calcium phosphate and carbonate, and the absence of uric acid and urates. Durham discussed various theories concerning the pathogenesis of the calcinosis, and concluded that "in view of the number of divergent opinions reviewed, it is obvious that much confirmatory work needs to be done." However, he believed that "local inflammatory changes usually are not a causative factor."

Calcinosis is now a well-recognized feature of certain cases of scleroderma and forms part of the so-called CREST (calcinosis, Raynaud's phenomenon, esophageal dysfunction, sclerodactyly, telangiectasia) syndrome. Unfortunately, there has been no progress in understanding its pathogenesis since the time of Durham.

JOINTS

Pain and swelling of joints was noted in various early reports of cases of scleroderma but was regarded as associated rheumatism. Dercum first appreciated that joint changes and other skeletal abnormalities might be part of the scleroderma process. In 1896 (in the very early days of radiology), he obtained x-ray pictures of the hands of a patient with scleroderma and observed narrowing of interphalangeal joint spaces (10). Two years later he emphasized that tendons, muscles, fascia, and joints might become involved in this disease, and that the changes in these organs might be more prominent than those in the skin, suggesting that they might be an integral part of the disease process (2). Indeed, he seems to have anticipated the concept of scleroderma as a systemic disease. Osler, in 1898, reported on "rheumatic nodules" in some of his eight patients with scleroderma and five of them experienced troubles with the joints, ranging from swelling and stiffness of the hands to frank polyarthritis (8). Joint involvement in scleroderma was reviewed by Adrian and Roderer in 1920; they concluded that the primary disturbance was in the synovial membrane (41). Joint involvement has since been recognized as a prominent feature of scleroderma and was described in various comprehensive surveys, such as that by Tuffanelli and Winkelmann in 1961 (18). They found that the onset of the disease was heralded by articular pain, swelling, and redness in 12% of patients and articular changes developed during the course of the disease in 46% of patients. Biopsy studies have been made by various workers including Rodnan (1962) who found infiltration of the synovium with lymphocytes and plasma cells in the acute stage and vascular sclerosis in the late stage (19). Tendonitis, diagnosed on the basis of presence of friction rubs, also a common feature in scleroderma, was first described by Shulman et al in 1961 (20).

BLOOD VESSELS

The association of vasospastic attacks (RP) and scleroderma was recognized early. It seems likely that some of the patients described in Raynaud's monograph in 1962 had scleroderma (3), and in a contribution to Horteloup's monograph on scleroderma in 1965, he specifically described a young man who, following a period of affection with RP, developed features of scleroderma of the face and hands (2). The temporal association of RP and scleroderma intrigued Hutchinson (1895) who listed three situations: (a) RP not associated with skin sclerosis; (b) skin sclerosis without preceding RP, which appeared subsequently; and (c) long-standing RP followed by the gradual development of sclerosis of the skin (6).

The structural basis of the vascular disturbance in scleroderma has been the subject of much study. In this respect, particular reference must be made to the work of Matsui, who in 1924 made a detailed pathological study of six patients with scleroderma and described the macroscopic and histological findings in the skin and in various internal organs (21). He found changes in blood vessels not only in the skin but also in the internal organs consisting of hypertrophy of the media and of the intima with narrowing of the lumen of small arteries, and sometimes thrombi leading to gangrene. His name will recur frequently during this chapter when referring to the discovery of pathological changes in various organs. Brown et al (1930) found that the heat elimination from the hand was low and that the "vasomotor index" (rise in skin temperature per degree rise in oral temperature during artificial pyrexia) was lower than normal (22). Lewis and Landis (1931) found that there was a greatly diminished rise in pulse volume produced by warming in subjects with sclerodactyly compared to people without this condition (23). Later (1937), Lewis used post mortem studies to demonstrate structural changes in digital arteries in the form of thickened intima, diminished lumen, and occlusions by thrombi (24). Brown and O'Leary (1925) (25) and Brown et al (1930) (22) described changes in the nailfold capillaries of patients with scleroderma studied *in vivo*: reduction in the number of loops, giant loops, and reduced flow. Capillaroscopy has recently become a popular diagnostic test for scleroderma and other connective tissue diseases.

ALIMENTARY TRACT

Although dyspeptic symptoms were mentioned in some of the nineteenth century reports, they were apparently considered to be coincidental. The first recognition of esophageal involvement in scleroderma is attributed to Ehrman (1903) who described a patient with cough and dyspnea and concluded that "the same process which was in the skin doubtlessly was also present in the pharynx and esophagus" (26). In 1916, Schmidt reported on a woman with scleroderma and dysphagia in whom an x-ray examination after swallowing bismuth paste showed a "gaping esophagus" (27). Pathological studies of the esophagus in patients with scleroderma were made by Matsui (1925) (19), who found sclerosis and hypertrophy of the muscle coat, and by Rake (1931), who found scarring of the submucosa

(28). Goetz (1945) described inflammatory changes, hypertrophy of the muscle coat, and scarcity of the ganglion cells (29). Detailed radiological studies were made by Hale and Schatzki in 1944 (30) and by Harper in 1955 (31) whose findings included aperistalsis, dilatation, stricture, and hiatus hernia.

Pathologic changes in the intestines were described in 1924 by Matsui, who reported on fibrosis of the submucosa and slight hypertrophy of the muscle coat (21), and by Kraus, who found dilatation of the stomach and duodenum (2). The first clinical recognition of bowel disease in a patient with scleroderma was made in 1931 by Rake, who reported on a patient with a long history of abdominal pain and diarrhea and an x-ray finding of dilatation of the esophagus and small and large intestines; at surgery the colon was found to be enlarged and filled with putty-like material (28). Goetz and Cole-Rous (1942) reported on a patient with scleroderma and dysphagia in whom x-ray examination showed a spastic constriction of the lower third of the esophagus, duodenal ileus, and a dilated colon (32). This patient's scleroderma problem progressed and she eventually died of bronchopneumonia following a Heller's operation for stenosis of the lower end of the esophagus. The clinical, radiologic, and pathologic findings were reported in great detail in 1945 by Goetz (29). Radiologic examination some 2 years before the patient's death showed a constricted lower end of the esophagus with dilatation above, a hypotonic stomach, dilated duodenum with slow passage of barium, dilated loops of small intestine with slow passage of barium, and saccules and stretches of narrowing and rigidity of the large bowel. These findings were broadly confirmed at necropsy. Histological changes in some organs were described. The esophagus contained an ulcer at its lower end, the muscle coat showed hypertrophy, there was infiltration with lymphocytes, and the walls of the blood vessels were thickened. The muscular coat of the colon was extremely atrophic and the blood vessels had thickened walls. The myenteric plexus was extremely prominent both in the esophagus and colon, but at the latter site there was an absence of ganglion cells.

A detailed report was made by Hale and Schatzki in 1944 on the radiological findings in 22 patients with scleroderma studied by a barium meal examination supplemented in some cases by a barium enema (30). Seven of these patients complained of dysphagia but the others had no definite symptoms. The esophagus was abnormal in 13 cases, with the main abnormalities being delayed emptying and decreased peristalsis. The small intestine was abnormal in four of 19 cases studied, with widening of the proximal loops of the bowel and marked delay in passage of the contrast material. The colon was abnormal in two of 15 patients studied, with peculiar sacculation and, in one case, rigidity and irregularity of outline in the region between the sacs.

There have since been various reports of bowel involvement in scleroderma. Abrams et al, in 1950, presented six cases illustrating involvement of the small bowel in scleroderma and demonstrated that in this instance scleroderma could be a rapidly progressive fatal disease (33). They found no correlation between the extent of the skin involvement and the severity of the bowel symptoms. Radiological features comprised dilatation and hypomotility of the bowel and segmentation of the barium contrast material. In 1953, Cullinan presented 14 cases (34) and the radiological findings in these cases were described by Harper in an addendum to Cullinan's paper. In the colon, they found regions of sacculation and "pseudo-diverticula." They were able to demonstrate that the abnormality was in the sacculation rather than in the apparently narrow intervening bowel by showing that, after a tannic acid enema, barium was retained in the saccules, whereas it was cleared from the intervening bowel. Symptoms described in bowel involvement in scleroderma have included weight loss, abdominal distension, diarrhea, and pseudoobstruction.

Scleroderma as a cause of the malabsorption syndrome was recognized in 1956 by Marshall, who reported on three patients with "collagen disease" associated with weight loss and abdominal symptoms, in two of whom scleroderma was diagnosed histologically (35). In 1957, Rosenthal demonstrated that small bowel lesions in scleroderma might produce steatorrhea (36). More recent studies have elucidated the mechanism of malabsorption in scleroderma. Salen et al, in 1966, reported on a case in which culture of the jejunal contents showed increased bacterial flora and there was improvement following correction of the bacterial overgrowth by treatment with tetracycline (37). In 1966, Kahn et al reported on four cases of scleroderma with intestinal malabsorption, proven by a D-xylose excretion test and measurement of fecal fat excretion (38); bacterial proliferation was suggested by increased urinary secretion of indican and confirmed by culture of the duodenal contents. Three of the four patients responded to treatment with the broad-spectrum antibiotics oxytetracyline and ampicillin. It was therefore demonstrated conclusively that the malabsorption in scleroderma resulted from colonization of the upper reaches of the small intestine with bacteria secondary to stasis.

LUNGS

Although several of the nineteenth century reports of patients with scleroderma contained reference to pulmonary symptoms, such as dyspnea and bronchitis, these were attributed to tightness of the skin of the chest. Hoppe-Seyler, in 1889, observed accentuation of the pulmonary second sound in a patient with scleroderma and suggested that this phenomenon was the result of interference with the pulmonary circulation (2). Von Notthafft, in 1898, made a detailed pathological examination of the lungs of a patient with this disease and found an increase in the interstitial connective tissue and thickening of the walls of arterioles (24). Further reports of these pathological changes were made in 1924 by Kraus (39) and Matsui (70).

A clear description of the radiological findings in the lungs of a patient with scleroderma was first made in 1941 by Murphy et al, who reported as follows: "Within the pulmonary fields with the exclusion of the apices and the lateral aspect of the bases there was a diffuse network-like shadow extending from the cardiac border to the periphery"(39). They proved that the shadow was caused by an abnormality of the lung by observing that the shadow disappeared after induction of a pneumothorax. Further reports of pulmonary fibrosis in patients with scleroderma were made during 1943 by Linenthal and Talkov (40) (three cases), Jackman (41) (four cases), and Lloyd and Tonkin (42) who reported on another four cases and reviewed the literature. The pathological changes in two severely affected patients were described in 1945 by Getzowa (43). Both cases exhibited hyaline fibrosis of alveolar walls accompanied by disappearance of capillaries resulting in dissolution of the partitions between alveoli producing cystic spaces, called "cystic pulmonary sclerosis." In one case, there were also areas of diffuse alveolar fibrosis without dissolution, called "compact pulmonary fibrosis."

Later studies have been directed mainly to lung function in scleroderma. Baldwin et al (1949), in a study of a series of patients with pulmonary fibrosis resulting from various causes, found that three of 14 patients who developed arterial oxygen desaturation on exercise had scleroderma (44). He believed that his findings suggested an insufficiency of alveolar respiration with minimal impairment of ventilatory function. More formal lung function studies have since been made on various series of patients with scleroderma. Some examples include the studies by Miller et al (1959, 22 patients) (45), Adhikari et al (1962, 13 patients) (46), Catherall and Rowell (1963, 31 patients) (47), and Hughes and Lee (1963, 12 patients) (48). A disturbance in lung function has been a common finding, with the most frequent abnormalities being a diffusion defect or a restrictive defect, alone or in combination. These defects may occur in the absence of symptoms or of radiological evidence of fibrosis; however, if the latter is present, the severity of the defect in pulmonary function is related to the degree of radiologic fibrosis.

HEART

Pathologic changes in hearts of patients with scleroderma were noted in several nineteenth century reports. Thus myocardial or pericardial disease is mentioned in 16 of 28 necropsies in Lewin and Heller's monograph in 1895 (2), but it is difficult to say how many of these were caused by scleroderma and how many were incidental. In 1898, Von Notthafft reported a round cell infiltration and sclerosis of cardiac muscle (2). Kraus, in 1924 (2), and Heine, in 1926 (49), observed cases of enlargement of the right side of the heart and myocardial fibrosis; Matsui (1924) reported dilatation of the right side of the heart and main pulmonary artery (21). In 1934, Brock described diffuse increase in connective tissue and hypertrophy of muscle fibers (50).

Weiss et al, in 1943, established scleroderma heart disease as a clinical entity, when they reported on a study of nine patients with scleroderma and cardiac symptoms of whom eight died (six with congestive cardiac failure) (51). Necropsy studies in two of these patients showed fibrotic changes of an unusual type in that they were not related to coronary arteries, and small numbers of myocardial fibers were preserved in the center of the lesions. Additional reports of single cases of scleroderma heart disease were made by East and Oram (1947) (52), Mathison and Palmer (1947) (53), and Hurly et al (1951) (54). In 1951, Goetz gave a detailed report with pathological findings in three cases who came to necropsy, and referred to clinical aspects of twelve other patients with scleroderma who showed features indicative of involvement of the heart (55). Symptoms included dyspnea, orthopnea, and cyanosis. ECGs were grossly abnormal showing bundle branch block or atrial fibrillation. He described four types of histological lesion: (*a*) regions with numerous capillaries, (*b*) diffuse lesions with separation of muscle fibers by young blood vessels, (*c*) frank fibrosis of the entire thickness of the myocardium, and (*d*) scattered foci of fibrosis. In 1951, Gil found cardiac symptoms in six of eight patients with severe scleroderma and cardiac enlargement in five of the eight patients (56). Barrett and O'Brien (1952) reported on the clinical features in two cases of scleroderma heart disease (57).

An extensive study of scleroderma heart disease, made in 1961 by Oram and Stokes, was based on 49 patients comprising 28 patients that were previously reported and 21 patients that were observed personally, including four necropsy studies (58). They listed the modes of presentation of cardiac involvement in scleroderma as: (*a*) heart failure with primary myocardial involvement or secondary to some other feature of the disease such as cor pulmonale, mitral incompetence, or hypertension resulting from renal involvement or treatment with adrenal steroids; (*b*) pericarditis; (*c*) cardiac pain of the nature of that in ischemic heart disease; (*d*) arrhythmias; (*e*) syncope; or (*f*) an incidental finding on clinical examination or electrocardiography. The earliest evidence of cardiac involvement was provided by ECG, which showed various abnormal features. The clinical features most suggestive of scleroderma heart disease were symptoms and signs suggestive of myocardial infarction in the absence of the chest pain characteristic of this condition. The most prominent abnormalities in their autopsy patients were either diffuse fibrosis or patches of sclerosis. Various subsequent studies have also stressed the importance of cardiac involvement in scleroderma.

KIDNEYS

The first case of acute renal failure associated with scleroderma was reported as early as 1863 by Auspitz, who described a male patient with tightness and pigmentation of the skin and who died following symptoms of rapidly progressing uremia (2). At autopsy the kidneys were small and irregular with scattered small yellow areas. Auspitz failed to recognize a relationship between the patient's kidney disease and his skin disease and, in fact, stated "there is, however, no evidence to support a causal relationship between the kidney disease and the skin disease as such." In 1887, Meyer reported on a case of scleroderma in which the kidneys showed nephritis and endarteritis (9). Osler, in his 1894 textbook, wrote that patients with scleroderma were apt to succumb to pulmonary complaints or nephritis (7). These nineteenth century writers apparently regarded renal involvement associated with scleroderma as a superadded disease.

In 1924, Matsui observed increased connective tissue around the renal tubules in patients with scleroderma, but none of his cases showed the florid vascular changes associated with scleroderma renal crisis (21). These were first described in 1938 by Masugi and Yä-Shu in a young woman dying with diffuse scleroderma in whom they found severe vessel changes not only in the skin but also in most internal organs (51). In the kidneys, there was hyperplasia of the intima of the intralobular arteries resulting in narrowing of the lumen, and fibrinoid material in the intima of these vessels and afferent arterioles, sometimes extending into the glomeruli. In 1939, Talbott et al independently described similar changes as well as cortical renal infarcts in a young woman dying from diffuse scleroderma (60).

However, acute renal failure resulting from scleroderma did not receive widespread recognition until the report by Moore and Sheehan in 1952 of three patients whose renal function was satisfactory until a few weeks before their death in acute renal failure (61). None of these patients had been severely hypertensive. At necropsy the kidneys showed similar features: normal size; irregular surface with pale and dark nodules; and, on microscopy, intimal thickening and narrow lumen of intralobular arteries, fibrinoid changes in these arteries and the afferent arterioles, and regions of ischemia and infarction. In 1956, Calvert and Owen reported on a similar case, discussed previous reports, and coined the term "true scleroderma kidney" (62). Renal disease has since been regarded as an important cause of death in scleroderma. Previously considered to be untreatable, this position has recently changed dramatically with the introduction of potent hypotensive drugs, particularly the angiotensin converting enzyme (ACE) inhibitors.

Concept of Scleroderma as a Systemic Disease

In the nineteenth century, scleroderma was regarded as a disease of the skin and, although some reports mentioned affections of other organs, these were regarded as concomitant and not part of underlying process. However, during the first half of the twentieth century numerous reports, listed previously in this chapter, describing involvement of various systems (vascular, joints, gastrointestinal, pulmonary, and renal), indicated that scleroderma was not purely a dermatological condition, but one involving numerous organs or systems. In his detailed pathological studies in six cases, Matsui (1924) found sclerotic and vascular changes not only in the skin but also in internal organs (lungs, gastrointestinal tract, and kidneys), indicating that the structural changes in scleroderma were not confined to the skin but involved the body generally (21).

The concept of scleroderma as a systemic disease was first described in detail by Goetz in 1945 (29). In a classic paper, he gave a detailed history and pathologic findings of a female patient who had presented with RP, sclerodermatous changes of acroteric distribution, and dysphagia, and whom he had followed until her death 2 years later. Goetz also referred to 12 other patients showing similar features but not examined in the same detail. He described the clinical and pathologic changes in various systems: (a) in the vasomotor system—RP, digital ulceration, decreased peripheral blood flow, and radiological evidence of absorption of the terminal phalanges; (b) in the integument–scleroderma, telangiectasia, and calcinosis; (c) in the gastrointestinal tract—dysphagia and esophageal ulceration and radiologic findings of dilatation of the esophagus, duodenum, small and large bowel, and deficient peristalsis in the affected region; (d) in the muscular system—asthenia and wasting and histological findings of atrophy and fibrosis; (e) in the heart—dyspnea, orthopnea, cyanosis, and evidence of myocardial damage and, at necropsy, extensive myocardial fibrosis of an unusual type. There were also marked pathological changes in the kidneys, liver, spleen, and lungs, and various-constitutional disturbances including loss of weight, pigmentation, loss of pubic and axillary hair, and amenorrhea suggestive of hormonal disturbance. Goetz concluded "obviously the term 'scleroderma' should be abandoned. It is quite evident today that we are dealing with a systemic disease neither solely nor primarily involving the skin. 'Scleroderma' is only the obvious and striking symptom of a generalized disease and the most serious symptoms actually arise in the viscera. . . . The term 'sclerosis' already being in use, it appears that 'progressive systemic sclerosis' would describe the condition adequately until such time as the etiology has been established." This, then, became the new name for the disease as an alternative to diffuse scleroderma, but it has recently been shortened to "systemic sclerosis," because it has become appreciated that the disease process is not always progressive. Beerman, in a review article in 1948, again emphasized the importance of visceral lesions in scleroderma, which were reported in almost every organ (63).

Subsequently, several large series of patients with scleroderma (systemic sclerosis), including both the acrosclerotic and diffuse forms, were reported with description of clinical and pathologic features and the outcome. Farmer et al (1960) reported on 271 patients (64). Many of these had evidence of visceral involvement on presentation: esophageal 64.5%, lungs 21%, heart 8.9%, kidneys 1.5%, and bowel in a few cases. Several patients died from the visceral lesions. By far the largest study ever conducted was that by Tuffanelli and Winkelmann of 722 cases published in 1961 (18). Patients were mainly of the acrosclerotic type (95%), and the ratio of female to male patients was 3:1. The age of onset covered a wide range (5–86 years) but was usually in early or middle adult life (20–60 years). RP was a common early symptom of the acrosclerotic form but not of the diffuse form. Systemic involvement of the nature described in previous reports was common. With regard to renal involvement, they stressed the frequent finding of chronic albuminuria in the absence of renal failure. Four of their patients had hepatic cirrhosis of "unknown etiology" (probably primary biliary cirrhosis). An important part of the study related to the prognosis. This was extremely variable for individual cases; however, for the group as a whole there was a survival rate of approximately 70% at 5 years and 60% at 10 years, indicating "that the prognosis of scleroderma is not as completely bleak as has been previously thought." Although no separate analysis is given for the diffuse scleroderma and the acrosclerotic form, the authors wrote that for the diffuse form "the course is rapid; the prognosis is extremely poor." Of 209 survivors responding to a follow-up letter, approximately 30% considered themselves to be improved, 45% considered their condition to be the same, and only 25% felt that their condition was worse. These findings indicated that scleroderma did not continue to progress in many patients, and justified the subsequent dropping of the word "progressive" from the proposed name of "progressive systemic sclerosis."

Attempts have been made to find prognostic indicators of the course of scleroderma. In 1960, Farmer et al considered cardiac and renal involvement, elevation of the sedimentation rate, and anemia to be poor prognostic signs (90). Winterbauer (1964) described a new syndrome of calcinosis, RP, sclerodactyly, and telangiectasia (abbreviated to "CRST syndrome") and regarded this as a relatively benign form of scleroderma (65). [The acronym CRST has later been extended to CREST as this is more euphonic and the E can be taken to indicate esophageal involvement which is also common in this syndrome.] This concept was criticized by Rowell (1965), who

found that each of these features was common in scleroderma, and that the combination of features was not uncommon and did not preclude visceral involvement (66). In the same communication Rowell suggested the omission of the word "progressive" from the term "progressive systemic sclerosis." A formal attempt to determine prognostic factors in scleroderma was made by Medsger et al in 1971, who conducted a life table analysis of 309 patients that were subdivided into various groups (67). The overall 5-year survival was 50% and the 10-year survival 40%, suggesting that they were a sicker group than those previously reported by Tuffanelli and Winkelmann. Medsger et al found that males fared worse than females, older people (>45 years) fared worse than younger people, and Blacks fared worse than Caucasians, but the most important factor was the nature and extent of visceral involvement. Best prognosis was for those with no lung, heart, or renal involvement; worst prognosis (all dead within 9 months) was in those with kidney involvement. Intermediate values were obtained for those with heart and lung involvement, with heart involvement being more unfavorable than lung involvement.

The accumulation of such a large series as that accumulated by Tuffanelli and Winkelmann indicated that scleroderma was not a rare condition as had previously been believed, and some attempts have been made to determine its incidence and prevalence. Kurland et al (1969), in an epidemiological study of connective tissue disorders in Rochester, Minnesota, during the 10-year period of 1957 through 1967, found eight cases of "diffuse systemic sclerosis," giving a prevalence of 10.5 cases per 100,000 of the total population and a yearly incidence of 1.2 cases per 100,000 (68). Masi and d'Angela (1967) studied the mortality rate from scleroderma in Baltimore (population approximately 1,000,000) during the period of 1948 through 1963 and found a mortality rate between 2 and 4 per 1,000,000 per year (69). Medsger and Masi (1971) conducted an epidemiological study of all the hospitals in Shelby County, Tennessee, during the period of 1947 through 1968 and found an annual incidence of 2.7 new patients per 1,000,000 people (70). There was a female:male ratio of 3:1 with few childhood cases and increase in incidence with age. There was no significant difference between Blacks and Caucasians and no apparent socioeconomic variables. The figures for incidence among studies have been widely divergent and point to the difficulties in conducting such a study—related to criteria for diagnosis and problems of detection, with the likelihood of many more patients in the general community than those who appear at a hospital.

The Nature of the Disease

Early workers seem to have been content to describe scleroderma without being particularly concerned about its nature. Because the most obvious manifestation being stiffness and hardness of the skin, it was regarded as a dermatological condition. However, as described previously, evidence was gradually obtained that other organs and systems were involved and that the changes in these might be more important than those in the skin; in other words scleroderma was a multi-system disease. This presented a problem of classification among diseases, which are often classified according to the organ or system involved.

CONNECTIVE TISSUE DISEASE

In 1942, Klemperer et al suggested that diffuse scleroderma, like acute disseminated lupus erythematosus, could he regarded as a "systemic disease of connective tissue" and that "connective tissue proper can be justly regarded as a system" (71). As a result, scleroderma has been classified among the connective tissue diseases.

Since the main histological abnormality is sclerosis, or apparent increase in the connective tissue, it was natural that research should be directed for any abnormality in connective tissue, particularly collagen which is its main compo-

nent. This became an almost obsessive activity in the 1960s, and references to these researches must be selective. Results were sometimes conflicting, which could be expected because scleroderma is a chronic condition and different findings might be expected at various stages (e.g., in the early active phase and a later inactive phase).

The chemical constitution of the collagen seemed to be normal. Thus, Fleischmajer (1964) compared the properties of affected skin with non-affected skin in eight patients with scleroderma and found that the water content, hydroxyproline content, amino acid concentration, and x-ray diffraction pattern was "normal" in the sclerodermatous skin, which led him to suspect that the main abnormality was primarily in the ground substance (72). Fleischmajer found support for this latter hypothesis in the finding of increased concentration of bound hexoses in two of the subjects. However, Korting el al (1964) found an increased proportion of collagen soluble in weak salt solutions in skin affected by scleroderma (73). Several workers studied the fine structure of collagen in such skin, particularly by electron microscopy, where the main finding was an increased proportion of fine fibers resembling those found in embryos and, therefore, believed to be indicative of young collagen (Fleischmajer et al, 1971) (74), (Hayes and Rodnan, 1971) (75).

The metabolism of collagen was studied by tests directed at measuring its rate of production and rate of excretion. Uitto et al (1967) found that the incorporation of ^{14}C proline to produce ^{14}C hydroxyproline was increased in skin from scleroderma patients (76). LeRoy (1971) found an increased production of soluble collagen by tissue culture preparations of fibroblasts from scleroderma patients compared with those from normal subjects (77). Tests for excretion of urinary hydroxyproline, an index of collagen breakdown, have given conflicting results with increased excretion in only a minority of cases (Uitto et al, 1967) (77).

Studies of the metabolism of glycosaminoglycans (GAGs) also gave conflicting results. Kreysel et al (1973) found evidence of increased biosynthesis of these compounds (78), and Holzmann et al (1968) found evidence of increased excretion (79). Although there were some disagreements among the findings of various workers, the evidence in general pointed to disturbance in metabolism of both collagen and GAGs with increased production of both of these substances in scleroderma.

It may seem strange, in view of the detailed studies of metabolic disturbances in the skin of patients with scleroderma, that there have been conflicting results concerning the basic finding of its thickness. Black et al (1970) found it to be thin (80), while Hayes and Rodnan (1971) found it to be thick (75). This may be related to such factors as the type and stage of the disease and the depth of the biopsy specimen. Fleischmajer et al (1971) showed that the sclerotic process in scleroderma extends deep to the dermis into the subcutaneous tissue (74).

VASCULAR DISEASE

Vascular disturbance is common in scleroderma. RP is a common symptom; several functional studies have shown impaired ability of vessels to dilate, and various symptoms, particularly local gangrene and ulcers of the skin, are the result of obliteration of vessels. Structural changes in the vessels resulting in narrowing of the lumen or occlusion have been found in pathological studies. In fact, Matsui found such changes in all organs of the body (44). In view of the widespread vascular involvement, Norton and Nardo (1970) wrote that "sufficient evidence exists to implicate the vascular system as the primary target organ in the disease," and that the fibrosis and organ damage are secondary to the vascular abnormality (81). However, this view has not gained wide acceptance.

AUTOIMMUNE DISEASE

We are left with the possibility of some more basic pathogenic process affecting both the connective tissue and blood vessels. Recently there has been mounting evidence for immunological disturbance in scleroderma. As outlined previously, scleroderma had been linked with lupus erythematosus as a connective tissue disease, and it was suggested by Rich (1946) that "hypersensitivity" (immune disturbance) might have a role in these diseases (82). Friou (1958) used the fluorescent antibody test to demonstrate the presence of autoantibodies in systemic lupus erythematosus (SLE) (83), and it was therefore natural to apply this test also to scleroderma. Early reports of positive tests were described by Bardowil et al (1958) (84), Alexander et al (1960) (85), Hall et al (1960) (86), Beck et al (1963) (87), and Rowell and Beck (1967) (88). The percentage of positives varied among reports but increased with improved techniques, particularly the use of Hep-2 cells as antigen, so that now a positivity rate of more than 90% may be expected (Tan, 1980) (89). At first, the fluorescence was described qualitatively as "homogeneous," "speckled," or "antinucleolar." More recently, patients with scleroderma have been found to have antibodies that react with two specific cellular antigens: Scl-70 or topoisomerase in certain patients with diffuse skin involvement (Douvas et al, 1979) (90); or with the anticentromere antigen in many patients with more limited skin involvement, including many with the so-called CREST syndrome (Morai et al, 1980) (91).

Because of the high prevalence of autoantibodies in scleroderma, many workers have regarded it as an "autoimmune" disease, which has been described by Mackay and Burnet (1963) "as a condition in which structural or functional damage is produced by the action of immunological competent cells or antibodies against normal components of the body" (92). Although Mackay and Burnet included a description of scleroderma in their text, they admitted that the role of autoimmunity in this disease was uncertain. They also concluded, perhaps prophetically, "If further studies confirm that an antinuclear antibody is regularly present in the sera of patients with active scleroderma, the autoimmune status of this disease would be enhanced." Although autoantibodies had been demonstrated in sera of most patients with scleroderma, they seemed to be directed against nuclei generally and not against any particular organ, and there was no evidence that they were doing damage. However, there is now increasing evidence (beyond the scope of this discussion) of widespread immunological disturbance in scleroderma involving immunocytes and cytokines, pointing to a conclusion that scleroderma is indeed an autoimmune disease.

Views on Causation

Although there has recently been continuous progress in understanding the pathogenesis (or mechanism) of the disease, there is still ignorance of its fundamental cause and study of history does not reveal any important advances.

One of the earliest theories concerning the cause of scleroderma was that it was the result of disorder of the ductless glands. This question was discussed exhaustively in 1923 by Castle, who quoted various workers who believed the condition was caused by disordered function of thyroid, pituitary, or adrenal glands and who had attempted to treat the scleroderma with gland extracts, sometimes with apparent benefit (93). He was critical of the view that scleroderma was caused by a disorder of a particular gland and wrote "In most cases the deductions are founded on a misconception; it is surely erroneous to suppose that because the extract of a gland may improve or even cure a case, the underlying cause was a deficiency of this gland."

Some workers have considered a possible infective agent, either an acid-fast bacillus (Wuerthele-Caspe et al, 1947) (94) or a virus (Norton, 1969) (95), but their findings have not been accepted by later workers. As in other diseases of obscure origin, psychological factors have been postulated as a causative factor (Mufson, 1953) (96) but their importance has not been confirmed.

In 1969, Housset et al found an increased frequency of chromosomal abnormalities in cyto-genetic studies of patients with scleroderma when compared with control subjects (97), but, as the authors recognized, it was difficult to say whether these changes were the cause or consequence of the illness. In spite of occasional reports of scleroderma affecting several members of one family, these are rare and there does not appear to be any strong genetic influence.

There have been several observations suggesting that exposure to silica may be a causative factor in the development of scleroderma in some instances. In Scotland, Bramwell (1914) found seven patients with diffuse scleroderma among 17,000 general medical cases in hospital practice and 10,000 cases in private practice (98). Five of these were stonemasons and one was a coal miner. Erasmus (1957) encountered 17 cases in a population of 40,000 miners in Witzwatersrand in South Africa over a period of 18 months, whereas he found only one case (a miner) among 25,300 hospital patients over a similar period (99). In Pittsburgh, Pennsylvania, Rodnan et al (1967) found that of 60 consecutive men with scleroderma, 26 had been coal miners or had been engaged in other occupations causing exposure to silicious dust (100). This led them to perform an epidemiological study involving 10 hospitals comparing the prevalence of scleroderma in miners and non-miners. They found a prevalence of scleroderma in 17 out of 100,000 miners compared with 6 out of 100,000 male non-miners.

There have been isolated reports of scleroderma or scleroderma-like illness occurring after exposure to certain other chemicals: vinyl chloride (Wilson, 1967) (101), industrial solvents (Owens and Medsger, 1988) (102), and silicone breast implants (Kumagi et al, 1984) (103). Many of the patients affected by the "toxic epidemic syndrome" in Spain, which has been attributed to the contamination of cooking oil, later developed scleroderma-like syndromes (104).

Obviously these cases in which a possible causative factor was found account for only a small minority of reported cases of scleroderma. A general view has developed that scleroderma is the result of an immunological disturbance, the cause of which is obscure, but that trigger factors, such as exposure to certain chemicals, may operate in some cases.

Treatments

Numerous forms of treatment for scleroderma have been tried by various workers, depending on ideas current at the time on the cause or nature of the disease. Usually benefit was claimed, but in view of the variable course of the disease and the possibility of remission, the favorable results must be considered with some skepticism. The concept of the double-blind, placebo-controlled trial with statistical analysis is a relatively recent innovation and also difficult to carry out in a chronic disease such as scleroderma.

Some of the earlier treatments used for scleroderma will be mentioned briefly. There was a widespread view among early workers that scleroderma was caused by a disorder of the ductless glands. Osler (1898) discussed his experience with treatment with thyroid gland extract in eight cases and was not favorably impressed (8). He wrote "Altogether my personal experience and the results as recorded in the literature do not favor the treatment of the disease by thyroid gland extract. It may be tried without harm."

Endocrine replacement therapy continued to be used by some workers in the early part of this century, and the various reports were discussed in Castle's review in 1923 (93). Asboe-Hansen (1962) claimed benefit from d-thyroxine (a non-calorigenic isomer of thyroid hormone) (105). On the supposition of disturbed calcium metabolism in scleroderma, treatment with the chelating agent ethylenediaminetetraacetic acid (EDTA) was introduced by Klein and Hanis in 1955 (106) and held favor over a period of about 10 years, but has since been discarded.

Following the demonstration of benefit from treatment with adrenal steroids and corticotrophin in rheumatic diseases, these were used for the treatment of scleroderma. Bayles et al (1960), in a small trial of injections of corticotrophin in four patients, reported clinical benefit (general well being, loosening of skin, less pain, increased mobility of joints) during administration of the drug but return to the previous state within a few weeks of stopping (107). Zion et al (1955), in a somewhat larger trial of 14 patients using corticotrophin or cortisone, or a combination of these hormones, found similar improvement in 13 patients, but this was graded moderate to marked in only four cases, and in no case was the benefit maintained when the treatment was temporarily discontinued (108). Doubts concerning benefit from adrenal steroids or corticotrophin and the probability of undesirable side effects have led to the gradual withdrawal of treatment with these drugs. Other anti-inflammatory drugs, including colchicine derivatives (Housset, 1967) (109) and salazopyrin (Dover, 1971) (110), have had a short run.

Several anti-fibrotic drugs have been used from time to time. Casten and Boucek (1958) reported significant improvement in skin tightness, RP, and trophic ulceration following injections of relaxin—the hormone that causes softening of the uterine cervix and pubic ligaments during pregnancy (111). The preparation used was of animal origin, and treatment by this means was ceased following a fatal anaphylactic reaction in one patient. However, the substance has since been produced by genetic engineering and there is further interest in its use. Zarafonetis (1959) claimed remarkable benefit from potassium paraaminobenzoic acid (POTABA) (112) but this was not confirmed by other workers. Harris and Sjoerdsma (1966) reported that administration of D-penicillamine produced solubilization of collagen and increased urinary excretion of its breakdown product hydroxyproline (113). Various people have since used D-penicillamine for the treatment of scleroderma with varying results. The largest trial of this drug in scleroderma was that of Steen et al (1982) (115). These workers compared the results of treatment with D-penicillamine in 73 patients with diffuse skin changes and early disease (<three years dura- tion) with those of 45 similar (diffuse skin changes and early disease less than three years duration), but not randomized, patients who did not receive the drug. They reported decreased ex- tent and degree of skin thickening, reduced rate of new visceral involvement, and increased sur- vival rate in the treated patients compared with the non-treated patients. D-penicillamine has se- rious toxic effects, and its use is now confined to patients with early disease and diffuse skin in- volvement. Dimethyl sulphoxide (DMSO) was introduced for the treatment of scleroderma by Scherbel et al in 1965 (161). This solvent experi- enced considerable popularity among some workers until recent times. It is a by-product of the paper industry, is soluble both in water and oils, passes readily through the skin, and has been claimed to have a softening effect on collagen. However, its place in therapy has not been es- tablished. Korting and Holzmann (1967) have claimed that progesterone and related substances ("gestagens") have a softening effect on collagen and have reported a beneficial effect in sclero- derma patients (117).

After reviewing all of these treatments, and others not mentioned here, it is apparent that, although benefit was claimed by their originators

Antibiotic therapy has been suggested on the supposition of a possible infective agent in scle- roderma. Ottolenghi (1961) (118) and Øhlen- schlaeger and Tissot (1967) (119) have claimed benefit from the use of a derivative of penicillin G. With the evidence of an immunologic distur- bance in many cases of scleroderma, some work- ers have tried the administration of immunosup- pressive agents, such as G-thioguanine by Demis et al (1968) (120), but the results of the treatment have not been impressive. A rather strange treat- ment introduced by Rotstein et al (1963) was with epsilon-aminocaproic acid (EACA), an anti- fibrinolytic agent, on the idea that the patho- logical changes in scleroderma are the result of the products of clot lysis (121). These workers claimed benefit in 22 of 26 patients treated!

and their early successors, most have not with- stood the test of time, and a controlled trial with objective measurements would seem the only valid means of establishing the value of a treat- ment. New treatments are still being tried and successes claimed, but history teaches us that we should suspend judgment until these treatments have been duplicated by several independent ob- servers.

In spite of the negative or doubtful results of the treatments listed in this chapter, the outlook for patients with scleroderma has recently be- come much better. This is because of the im- proved management of the effects of scleroder- ma. For example, ACE inhibitors are used to treat acute renal involvement, potent vasodilators for ischemic features, and inhibitors of acid secre- tion in the stomach for reflux esophagitis; how- ever, these developments may be too recent to be included in a chapter on history.

Conclusion

Although attempts have been made to trace re- ports of scleroderma in the writings of ancient physicians, these inferences are conjectural and the first acceptable case report is that of Curzio in Italy in 1753. Scleroderma was first recognized as a clinical entity and given its name by French workers in the mid-nineteenth century. It was then regarded as a skin disease, although some workers recognized an association with RP. Although symptoms suggestive of systemic in- volvement were mentioned in some of the early reports, these were regarded as associated prob- lems and not as part of the disease.

During the first half of the twentieth century, reports accumulated of both pathological and clinical involvement of organs other than the skin: joints, alimentary canal, lungs, heart, and kidneys. At this time, researchers recognized that scleroderma was a multi-system disease and it was given a new name "progressive systemic scle- rosis."

Discussions took place concerning the various subdivisions of scleroderma. It was recognized early that there was a "localized form" with discrete skin lesions in the absence of involvement of other systems. This was considered to be a separate condition, and was listed under the various forms of morphea. The systemic form (systemic sclerosis) also varied greatly in its manifestations and severity, and a distinction was made between the acroteric form (acrosclerosis) and the diffuse form, but most workers concluded that they were variants of the same disease.

The nature of scleroderma (systemic sclerosis) remains a mystery. It was pointed out that there was widespread involvement of connective tissue, which is an important part of all organs; therefore, scleroderma was included among the connective tissue diseases. It was also stressed that there was widespread involvement of blood vessels, and it was even suggested that this might be the primary lesion. Immunologic disturbance, particularly the presence of antinuclear antibodies, was found in various connective tissue diseases including scleroderma. Consequently, this led to the concept of scleroderma as an autoimmune disease. Although there was no direct evidence that the auto-antibodies were harmful, recent work has shown that certain auto- antibodies are specific to scleroderma. In addition, other immune disturbances, particularly involving cytokines, have been described.

No specific cause for scleroderma has been found, but there is evidence for certain trigger factors. For example, exposure to silica and certain industrial chemicals appear to act as trigger factors in some cases. Specific treatments for scleroderma have generally been ineffective. However recent advances in the management of certain effects of the disease have improved prognosis and made the condition of patients much more tolerable. Scleroderma has proven to be a complicated and intriguing problem and we await a major breakthrough, particularly concerning its cause and treatment.

References

1. Durham RA. Scleroderma and calcinosis. Arch Intern Med 1928;42:467a.
2. Rodnan GP, Benedek TG. An historical account of the study of progressive systemic sclerosis. Ann Intern Med 1962;57:305.
3. Raynaud M. On local asphyxia and symmetrieal gangrene of the extremities, 1864. London: The New Sydenham Society, 1888.
4. Raynaud M. New researches on the nature and treatment of local asphysia of the extremities, 1874. London: The New Sydenham Society, 1888.
5. Hutchinson J. Congenital defects and inherited proclivities. Arch Surg 1883;4:305.
6. Hutchinson J. On morphea and allied conditions. Arch Surg 1895;6:350.
7. Osler W. The principles and practice of medicine. New York: Appleton, 1894:993.
8. Osler W. On diffuse scleroderma; with special reference to diagnosis, and the use of thyroid gland extract. J Cutan Genito-urinary Dis 1895; 16:49.
9. Quoted from Sachner MA. Arthritis Rheum 1962;5:184.
10. Dercum FX. Scleroderma. J Nerv Ment Dis 1896; 21:431. (loc. cit.).
11. Sellei J. The diagnosis and treatment of scleroderma and some of its kindred. Br J Dermatol Syph 1934;46:523.
12. Truelove SC, Whyte HM. Acrosclerosis. Br Med J 1951;2:873.
13. Ramsey AS. Acrosclerosis. Br Med J 1951;2:877.
14. Leinwand I, Duryee AW, Richter MN. Scleroderma (based on a study of over 150 cases). Ann Intern Med 1954;41:1003.
15. O'Leary PA, Montgomery H, Ragdale WE. Dermatopathology of various types of scleroderma. Arch Dermatol 1954;75:78.
16. Jablónska S, Bubnow B, Lukasiak B. Acrosclerosis: A disease sui generis or a variety of diffuse scleroderma? Br J Dermatol 1959;71:123.
17. Farmer RG, Gifford RW Jr, Hines EA Jr. Raynaud's disease with sclerodactylia: A follow-up study of seventy-one patients. Circulation 1961; 23:13.
18. Tuffanelli DL, Winkelmann RK. Systemic scleroderma: Clinical study of 722 cases. Arch Dermatol 1961;84:359.
19. Rodnan GP. The nature of joint involvement in progressive systemic sclerosis (diffuse scleroderma): Clinical study and pathologic examination

of synovium in twenty-nine patients. Ann Intern Med 1962;56:422.

20. Shulman LE, Kurban AK, Harvey AM. Tendon friction rubs in progressive systemic sclerosis (scleroderma). Arthritis Rheum 1961;4:438.

21. Matsui S. Über die Pathologie und Pathogenese von Sclerodermia universalis. Tokyo University College of Medicine Medizinische Facultat Mitterlungen 1924;31:55.

22. Brown GE, O'Leary PA, Adson AW. Diagnostic and physiologic studies in certain forms of scleroderma. Ann Intern Med 1930;4:531.

23. Lewis T, Landis EM. Further observations on a variety of Raynaud's disease; with special reference to arteriolar defects and to scleroderma. Heart 1931;15:329.

24. Lewis T. The patholgical changes in the arteries supplying the fingers in warm-handed people and in cases of so-called Raynaud's disease. Clin Sci 1937;3:287.

25. Brown GE, O'Leary PA. Skin capillaries in scleroderma. Arch Intern Med 1925;36:73.

26. Ehrman S. Über die Beziehung der Sklerodermie zu den Autotoxischen erythem. Wien Med Wochenschr 1903;53:1097.

27. Schmidt R. Sklerodermie mit Dysphagie. Deutsch Med Wochenschr 1916;42:1023.

28. Rake G. On the pathology and pathogenesis of scleroderma. Johns Hopkins Hosp Bull 1931; 48:212.

29. Goetz RH. The pathology of progressive systemic sclerosis (generalized scleroderma) with special reference to changes in the viscera. Clin Proc (S Afr) 1945;4:337.

30. Hale CH, Schatzki R. The roentgenological appearance of the gastrointestinal tract in scleroderma. Am J Roentgenol 1944;51:409.

31. Harper RAK. The radiological manifestations of diffuse systemic sclerosis (scleroderma). Proc R Soc Med 1950;46:512.

32. Goetz RH, Cole-Rous M. Note on a case showing Raynaud's phenomenon and additional manifestations. Clin Proc (S Afr) 1942;1:244.

33. Abrams NL, Carnes WH, Eaton J. Alimentary tract in disseminated scleroderma. Arch Intern Med 1954;94:61.

34. Cullinan ER. Scleroderma (diffuse systemic sclerosis). Proc R Soc Med 1953;46:507.

35. Marshall I. Collagen disease of the small bowel. N Engl J Med 1956;255:978.

36. Rosenthal FD. Small intestinal lesions with steatorrhoea in diffuse systemic sclerosis (scleroderma). Gastroenterology 1957;32:332.

37. Salen G, Goldstein F, Wirts CW. Malabsorption in intestinal scleroderma; relation to bacterial flora and treatment with antibiotics. Ann Intern Med 1966;64:834.

38. Kahn IJ, Jeffries GH, Sleisenger MH. Malabsorption in intestinal scleroderma; correction by antibiotics. N Engl J Med 1966;274:1339.

39. Murphy JR, Krainin P, Gerson MJ. Scleroderma with pulmonary fibrosis. JAMA 1941;116:499.

40. Linenthal H, Talkov R. Pulmonary fibrosis in Raynaud's disease. N Engl J Med 1941;223:682.

41. Jackman J. Roentgen features of scleroderma and acrosclerosis. Radiology 1943;40:163.

42. Lloyd WE, Tonkin RD. Pulmonary fibrosis in generalized scleroderma: Review of the literature and report of four further cases. Thorax 1948;3: 241.

43. Getzowa S. Cystic and compact pulmonary sclerosis in progressive scleroderma. Arch Pathol 1945;40:99.

44. Baldwin E deF, Cournand A, Richards DW Jr. Pulmonary insufficiency II. A study of thirty-nine cases of pulmonary fibrosis. Medicine 1949;28:1.

45. Miller RD, Fowler WS, Helmolz FH Jr. Scleroderma of lungs. Mayo Clin Proc 1959;34:66.

46. Adhikari PK, et al. Pulmonary function in scleroderma: Its relation to changes in chest roentgenogram and in the skin of the thorax. Am Rev Respir Dis 1962;86:823.

47. Catterall M, Rowell NR. Respiratory function studies in patients with certain connective tissue diseases. Br J Dermatol Syph 1965;77:221.

48. Hughes DTD, Lee FI. Lung function in patients with systemic sclerosis. Thorax 1963;18:16.

49. Heine J. Über eine eigenartiges krankheitsbild von diffuser sklerosis der haut und innerer organe. Virchows Arch Path Anat 1926;262:351.

50. Brock WG. Dermatomyositis and diffuse scleroderma; differential diagnosis and reports of cases. Arch Dermatol Syph 1934;30:227.

51. Weiss S, Stead EA Jr, Warren JV, Bailey OT. Scleroderma heart disease; with a consideration of certain other visceral manifestations of scleroderma. Arch Intern Med 1943;71:749.

52. East T, Oram S. The heart in scleroderma. Br Heart J 1947;9:167.

53. Mathison AK, Palmer JD. Diffuse scleroderma with involvement of the heart; report of a case. Am Heart J 1947;33:366.

54. Hurly J, Coe J, Weher L. Scleroderma heart disease. Am Heart J 1951;42:758.

55. Goetz RH. The heart in generalized scleroderma; progressive systemic sclerosis. Angiology 1951;2: 555.

56. Gil JR. Clinical and visceral lesions and endocrine

disturbances in eight cases of diffuse scleroderma. Ann Intern Med 1951;34:862.

57. Barritt DW, O'Brien W. Heart disease in scleroderma. Br Heart J 1952;14:421.

58. Oram S, Stokes W. The heart in scleroderma. Br Heart J 1961;23:243.

59. Masugi M, Yä-Shu. Die diffuse sklerodermie und ihre gefassanderung. Virchows Arch Pathol Anat 1938;302:39.

60. Talbott JH, Gall EA, Consolazio WV, Coombs FS. Dermatomyositis with scleroderma, calcinosis and renal endarteritis associated with focal corticol necrosis; report of a case in which the condition simulated Addison's disease, with comment on metabolic and pathological studies. Arch Intern Med 1939;63:476.

61. Moore HC, Sheehan HL. The kidney in scleroderma. Lancet 1952;1:68.

62. Calvert RJ, Owen TK. True scleroderma kidney. Lancet 1956;2:19.

63. Beerman H. The visceral manifestations of scleroderma; a review of the recent literature. Am J Med Sci 1948;216:458.

64. Farmer RG, Gifford RW, Hines EA. Prognostic significance of Raynaud's phenomenon and other clinical characteristics of systemic scleroderma. A study of 271 cases. Circulation 1960;21:1088.

65. Winterbauer RH. Multiple telangiectasis, Raynaud's phenomenon, sclerodactyly and subcutaneous calcinosis: a syndrome mimicking hemorrhagic telangiectasia. Johns Hopkins Hosp Bull 1964;114:361.

66. Rowell NR. Systemic sclerosis. Br Med J 1968; 1:514.

67. Medsger TA Jr, Masi AT, Rodnan GP, Benedek TG. Survival with systemic sclerosis (scleroderma); a life-table analysis of clinical and demographic factors in 309 patients. Ann Intern Med 1971;75:369.

68. Kurland LT, Hauser WA, Ferguson RH, Holley KE. Epidemiologic features of diffuse connective tissue disorders in Rochester, Minnesota, 1951 through 1967 with special reference to systemic lupus erythematosis. Mayo Clin Proc 1969;44:649.

69. Masi AT, d'Angelo WA. Epidemiology of fatal systemic sclerosis (diffuse scleroderma); a fifteen year survey in Baltimore. Ann Intern Med 1967; 66:870.

70. Medsger TA, Masi AT. Epidemiology of systemic sclerosis (scleroderma). Ann Intern Med 1971;74: 714.

71. Klemperer P, Pollack AD, Baehr G. Diffuse collagen disease; acute disseminated lupus erythematosus and diffuse scleroderma. JAMA 1942; 119:331.

72. Fleischmajer R. The collagen in scleroderma. Arch Dermatol 1964;89:437.

73. Korting GW, Holzmann H, Kühn K. Biochemische bindgeweibanalysen bei progressiver sklerodermie. Klin Wochenschr 1964;42:248.

74. Fleischmajer R, Damiano V, Nedwick A. Scleroderma and the subcutaneous tissue. Science 1971; 171:1019.

75. Hayes RL, Rodnan GP. The ultrastructure of skin in progressive systemic sclerosis (scleroderma). Am J Path 1971;63:433.

76. Uitto J, Laitinen O, Hannusekela M, Mustakallio KK. The collagen in dermatomyositis, lupus erythematosus and scleroderma. Scand J Clin Lab Invest 1967;95(suppl):41.

77. LeRoy EC. Connective tissue synthesis by scleroderma skin fibroblasts in cell culture. J Exp Med 1972;135:1362.

78. Kreysel HW, Köhler H, Kleine TO. Biosynthese von glycosaminoglycanen in der haut bei der progressiven sklerodermie. Klin Wochenschr 1973; 51:214.

79. Holzmann H, Korting GW, Morsches B. Zur beeinflussung der mucopolysaccharide in serum und urin von sklerodermiekranken durch gestagen-behandlung. Arch Klin Exp Dermatol 1968; 231:156.

80. Black MM, Bottoms E, Shuster SL. Skin collagen and thickness in systemic sclerosis. Br J Dermatol 1970;83:552.

81. Norton WL, Nardo JM. Vascular disease in progressive systemic sclerosis (scleroderma). Ann Intern Med 1970;73:317.

82. Rich AR. Hypersensitivity in disease with special reference to periarteritis nodosa, rheumatic fever, disseminated lupus erythematosus and rheumatoid arthritis. Harvey Lectures 1946/7, Series 42: 106.

83. Friou GJ, Finch SC, Detre KD. Interaction of nuclei and globulin from lupus erythematosus serum demonstrated with fluorescent antibody. J Immunol 1958;80:324.

84. Bardawil WA, Toy BL, Galins N, Bayles TB. Disseminated lupus erythematosus and dermatomyositis as manifestations of sensitization to DNA protein. 1. An immunohistochemical approach. Am J Pathol 1958;34:607.

85. Alexander WRM, Brenner JM, Duthie JJR. Incidence of antinuclear factor in human sera. Ann Rheum Dis 1960;19:338.

86. Hall AP, et al. The relations between the antinuclear, rheumatoid and LE-cell factors in the systemic rheumatic diseases. N Engl J Med 1960; 263:769.

87. Beck JS, Anderson JR, Gray KJ, Rowell NR. Antinuclear and precipitating autoantibodies in progressive systemic sclerosis. Lancet 1963;2:1188.

88. Rowell NR, Beck JS. The diagnostic value of an antinuclear antibody in clinical dermatology. Arch Dermatol 1967;96:290.

89. Tan EM, et al. Diversity of antinuclear antibodies in progressive systemic sclerosis. Anticentromere antibody and its relationship to CREST syndrome. Arthritis Rheum 1980;23:617.

90. Douvas AS, Achten M, Tan EM. Identification of a nuclear factor (Scl-70) as a unique target of human antinuclear antibodies in scleroderma. J Biol Chem 1979;254:10514.

91. Morai Y, et al. Autoantibody to centromere (kinetochord) in scleroderma sera. Proc Natl Acad Sci USA 1980;77:1627.

92. Mackay IM, Burnet FM. Autoimmune diseases: Pathogenesis, chemistry and therapy. Springfield, Thomas, 1963.

93. Castle WF. The endocrine causation of scleroderma, including morphea. Br J Dermatol Syph 1923;35:255.

94. Wuerthele-Caspe V, Brodkin E, Mermod C. Etiology of scleroderma: A preliminary report. J Med Soc NJ 1947;44:256.

95. Norton WL. Endothelial inclusions in active lesions of systemic lupus erythematosus. J Lab Clin Med 1969;74:369.

96. Mufson I. An etiology of scleroderma. Ann Intern Med 1953;39:1219.

97. Housset E, Emerit I, Boulon A, de Grouchy J. Anomalies chromoscomiques dans la sclérodermie generalisée. Une étude de dix malades. C R Acad Sci (Paris) 1969;269:413.

98. Bramwell B. Diffuse scleroderma: Its occurrence in stone masons; its treatment by fibrinolysin–elevations in temperature due to fibrinolysin injections. Edinb Med J 1914;12:387.

99. Erasmus LD. Scleroderma in gold-miners on the Witzwatersrand with particular reference to pulmonary manifestations. S Afr J Lab Clin Med 1957;3:209.

100. Rodnan GP, Benedek TG, Medsger TA Jr, Cammarata RJ. The association of progressive systemic sclerosis (scleroderma) with coal miners' pneumoconiosis and other forms of silicosis. Ann Intern Med 1967;66:323.

101. Wilson RH, McCormack WE, Tatum CF, Creech JL. Occupational acro-osteolysis. Report of 31 cases. JAMA 1967;201:577.

102. Owens GR, Medsger TA. Systemic sclerosis secondary to industrial exposure. Am J Med 1988;85:114.

103. Kumagai Y, Shiokowa Y, Medsger TA Jr, Rodnan GP. Clinical spectrum of connective tissue disease after cosmetic surgery. Observation of eighteen patients and a review of the literature. Arthritis Rheum 1984;27:1.

104. Toxic Epidemic Study Group. Toxic epidemic syndrome, Spain 1981. Lancet 1982;2:697.

105. Asboe-Hansen G. Treatment of scleroderma with dextro-thyroxine. Excepta Med Int Cong 1962;55:1305.

106. Klein R, Harris SB. Treatment of scleroderma, sclerodactylia and calcinosis by chelation (EDTA). Am J Med 1955;19:798.

107. Bayles TB, Stout CF, Stillman JS, Lever W. The treatment of scleroderma with adrenotrophic hormone: Preliminary observations. Proceedings of the First Clinical ACTH Conference. Philadelphia, Blakiston, 1950.

108. Zion MM, Goldberg B, Suzman MM. Corticotrophin and cortisone in the treatment of scleroderma. Q J Med N S 1955;24:215.

109. Housset E. Interêt de certains dérivés de la colchicine dans le traitement des syndromes sclérodermiques. Ann Dermatol Syph (Paris) 1967;94:31.

110. Dover N. Salazopyrine (azulfidine) treatment in scleroderma. Isr J Med Sci 1971;7:1301.

111. Casten GC, Boucek RJ. Use of relaxin in the treatment of scleroderma. JAMA 1958;166:319.

112. Zarafonetis, CJD. Antifibrotic treatment with POTABA. Am J Med Sci 1964;248:550.

113. Harris ED Jr, Sjoerdsma A. Effect of penicillamine on human collagen and its possible application to treatment of scleroderma. Lancet 1966;2:996.

115. Steen VD, Medsger TA Jr, Rodnan GP. D-penicillamine therapy in progressive systemic sclerosis (scleroderma). A retrospective analysis. Ann Intern Med 1982;97:652.

116. Scherbel AL, McCormack LJ, Poppo MJ. Alteration of collagen in generalized scleroderma (progressive systemic sclerosis) after treatment with methyl sulphoxide. Cleve Clin Q 1965;32:47.

117. Korting GW, Holzmann H. Gestagen-Behandlung der sklerodermie. Aesthetic Med (Berlin) 1967;16:291.

118. Ottolenghi F. An antibiotic with anti-sclerodermic activity: the diethylamino-ethylester hydriodide salt of penicillin G. Dermatologica 1961;123:331.

119. Øhlenschlaeger K, Tissot J. Scleroderma treatment with the diethylamino-ethylester hydriodide salt of penicillin G. Dermatologica 1967;134:129.

120. Demis DJ, Brown CS, Crosby WH. Thioguanine in the treatment of certain autoimmune, immunologic and related diseases. Am J Med 1964;37:195.

121. Rotstein J, Gilbert M, Estrin J. Antifibrinolytic drug in treatment of progressive systemic sclerosis. JAMA 1963;184:517.

ALAN J. SILMAN
CAROL M. BLACK
KENNETH I. WELSH

2

Epidemiology, Demographics, Genetics

THIS CHAPTER REVIEWS DATA on the occurrence of scleroderma, or systemic sclerosis (SSc), as well as the genetic and environmental risk factors associated with this disease. Given that much of the epidemiology of scleroderma is related to the occurrence of Raynaud's Phenomenon (RP), we have also added a short section covering the main epidemiological aspects of this latter condition.

Introduction

Interpretation of available data on the occurrence of scleroderma is only possible in the presence of a clear definition of disease that is universally accepted and distinguishes clearly between scleroderma and mortality on the one hand and closely related but clinically distinct disorders on the other hand. Diseases like scleroderma, which are variable in their presentation and course and rely on clinical observation for diagnosis, are notoriously difficult to define in a sufficiently rigorous manner for epidemiological purposes. There is not a single diagnostic test available for scleroderma and, until 1980, there were no published criteria that could be used. It can be argued, however, that the skin involvement in the disease is sufficiently obvious and clinically distinct to obviate the need for specific criteria. There is, however, substantial variation among clinicians in their assessment of skin involvement (1).

DISEASE CRITERIA

Criteria for scleroderma were developed by a subcommittee of the American Rheumatism Association (ARA). This subcommittee surveyed 264 patients from 29 centers with "definite" scleroderma, according to the physicians, and compared the clinical findings with some 400 patients with systemic lupus erythematosus (SLE), dermatomyositis (DM), polymyositis (PM), or RP (2). All the patients studied were within 2 years of diagnosis with an average delay since first symptoms of approximately 6 years. The criteria that emerged were not surprising, given the choice of subjects (Table 2.1). These criteria were 97% sensitive, had a specificity of 98% to 99% compared to the SLE patients, and a specificity of 94% compared to the RP patients. The single criterion of proximal scleroderma was 100% specific and 91% sensitive. It is likely that a very different set of criteria would have emerged if dermatological patients had been used as the "controls." Another problem with the criteria is that proximal scleroderma is not infrequently absent from patients with the limited cutaneous form of the disease (discussed later in this chapter). Thus, the criteria are likely to be insensitive for that group, who account for up to 50% of patients in published clinical series. Consequently, in 56 consecutive new patients from New Zealand, the ARA criteria were only 69% sensitive (3,4). By contrast, the criterion of proximal scleroderma was present in all of a heavily selected population of 46 Belgian patients (5).

Table 2.1. Classification Criteria for Scleroderma[a]

I	Proximal Skin Scleroderma
	or 2 of
II	Sclerodactyly
	Digital Pitting Scars/Pulp Loss
	Bibasilar Pulmonary Fibrosis

Definitions

Skin scleroderma:	Tightness, thickening and non-pitting in duration excluding local forms of scleroderma
Sclerodactyly:	Scleroderma skin change involving the fingers or toes.
Pulp loss:	Loss of substance of digital finger pad.

[a]Source: Subcommittee 1980 (2)

CLASSIFICATION

For clinical classification purposes, scleroderma is usefully subdivided into the "limited" and the "diffuse" cutaneous forms (6). In the limited form (lcSSc), the skin involvement is limited to the extremities—distal to the elbows, knees, and above the clavicles—and the patient has a low risk of internal organ involvement. The anticentromere antibody (antikinetochore) is frequently, but not universally, present. Included within the subgroup is the CREST syndrome of calcinosis, Raynaud's, esophageal hypomotility, sclerodactyly (see Table 2.1), and telangiectasia. By contrast, the diffuse form (dcSSc) is distinguished by skin involvement proximal to the elbows, knees, and below the clavicles. These patients have an increased frequency of internal organ involvement. The Scl-70 antibody (topoisomerase-1) is frequently present, but the association is less strong than that between anticentromere and lcSSc. These clinical and serological differences are not absolute, and although they are useful for prognostic purposes, it has been considered preferable for epidemiological purposes to consider scleroderma as a single disease entity. One consequence of this "lumping" is that if there is etiological heterogeneity, which seems likely, then associations may be missed by combining disparate groups for study.

It is important, however, to distinguish localized scleroderma, which was previously known as morphea. Localized scleroderma is not widespread in its anatomical distribution, does not produce internal organ involvement, and is immunologically distinct. Therefore, it is not considered further in this review.

Occurrence

Scleroderma is a rare disease that renders population-based surveys impractical on the grounds of size and cost. As a consequence, virtually all of the descriptive epidemiology is derived from either prospective or retrospective review of patients, and often only their medical records, based on their attendance at health service institutions serving a defined denominator population. Population mortality data have also been used as a surrogate for incidence.

POPULATION MORTALITY RATES

The advantages of using mortality data are: (*a*) they are frequently readily available for national and sub-national population groups, for example by region, social class, and ethnic origin; and (*b*) in a disease like scleroderma, with a high and relatively constant case fatality rate, patterns of incidence in different groups are reflected by similar patterns in population mortality. The major drawbacks are, of course, the difficulties in standardizing diagnosis and completion of death certificates, and these are a source of both within- and between-population variation. The available mortality rate data are summarized in Table 2.2.

The overall annual average population mortality in Baltimore, Maryland, during the period of 1949 through 1963, was 1.3 and 2.2 per million, respectively, in Caucasian males and females (7). All subsequent studies have produced very similar results. Thus, in the United States as a whole during the period of 1959 through 1961, the annual rates for Caucasian males and females were 1.0 and 2.1 per million, respectively (8), and during 1969 through 1977 were 1.5 and 3.5 per million, respectively (9). Data from US male veterans for 1963 through 1968 were also similar at

Table 2.2. Mortality Rates from Scleroderma in National and Subnational Populations

Reference	Country	Period	Mortality Rate/Million Males	Mortality Rate/Million Females
Cobb (1971) (8)	USA	1959–61	1.0	2.1
Masi & D'Angelo (1967) (7)	USA (Baltimore)	1949–63	1.3	2.2
Medsger & Masi (1978) (10)	USA (male veterans)	1963–68	1.4	
Hochberg et al (1985) (9)	USA	1969–77	1.5	3.5
Silman (1990) (11)	UK	1974–85	0.9	3.8

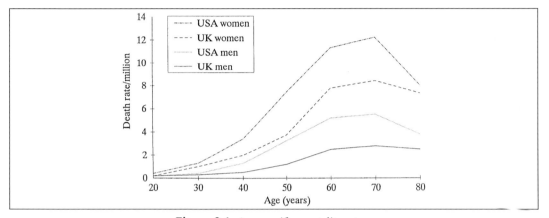

Figure 2.1. Age-specific mortality rates.

1.4 per million (10). Recent data from the United Kingdom during the period of 1974 through 1985 are also similar, with rates of 1 and 4 per million, respectively, for Caucasian males and females (11). The age-specific population mortality curves that were derived from these data for both the US and the UK are shown in Figure 2.1. These curves clearly demonstrate the rarity of the disease under the age of 25 (at least as a cause of death) and the relatively slow increase in mortality with increasing age until the seventh decade. These data also suggest that scleroderma is apparently a disease with a relatively stable occurrence (at least in mortality terms) both over time and between populations.

INCIDENCE

As stated previously, incidence data are mainly based on retrospective reviews of patients who attend clinics. There have been 10 published reports of scleroderma incidence (Table 2.3). The published crude rates vary between 2 and 10 per million total population, although the most recent data from the Pittsburgh group suggest an even higher rate (12). The rates, however, are relatively consistent among the countries for which data are available. Differences in age structure among populations will obviously influence the overall rates. The Mayo Clinic studies (13,14) have the advantage that the nature of the health care system is such that all patients within their denominator population of Olmsted County, Minnesota, are likely to be ascertained, whereas in other studies complete ascertainment has to be assumed. However, the Olmsted population is small and the confidence intervals are wide (e.g., 0–6 per million for males, 7–25 per million for females) (14). In the UK study (15), multiple methods of case ascertainment were used to compensate for under-ascertainment from hospital registers. The degree of overlap between the ascertainment methods was not sufficiently large to preclude under-ascertainment.

AGE, SEX, AND TIME TRENDS

All of the incidence studies demonstrate a female excess over males (see Table 2.3) ranging from 3:1 to 8:1. This female excess is more marked in early adult life (15,16) when the ratio is approximately 7:1; however, the excess narrows to 2:1 in the fifth and subsequent decades.

The age-specific incidence curves (Fig. 2.2), as with the mortality curves, show the rarity of the disease under the age of 25 and the peak in incidence in the fifth and sixth decades. However, compared to other autoimmune diseases, there is only a modest effect of age. Scleroderma can occur in childhood (17) but is very rare, particularly in its CREST form (18). Conversely, scleroderma is well described in the elderly (age 80+) (19) and, in contrast to childhood scleroderma, is frequently benign with the CREST form the typical pattern (20). One artifactual explanation for this apparent age effect is that it might reflect the relatively late or missed presentation of those forms of the disease associated with slow progression and good survival.

Despite the population mortality data showing little variation in rates over time, in those populations with estimates of incidence over a reasonable time period, there has been an increase in occurrence. Thus, in Shelby County, Tennessee, the rates (per million) were 0.6 during 1947 through 1952, 1.5 during 1953 through 1957, 4.1 during 1958 through 1962, and 4.5 during 1963 through 1968 (16). A similar analysis of

Table 2.3. Incidence Studies of Scleroderma

Reference	Country/Population	Period	Incidence Per Million			Female:Male
			Males	Females	Both	
Kurland et al (1969) (13)	USA/Rochester	1951–67			1.2	
Medsger & Masi (1971) (16)	USA/Tennessee (Caucasians)	1947–68	1.2	3.6	2.7	3:1
Bosmansky et al (1971) (130)	Czechoslovakia	1961–69			7	
Medsger & Masi (1978) (10)	USA/Male Army Veterans	1963–68	2.3			
Michet et al (1985) (14)	USA/Rochester	1951–79	2	16	10	8:1
Wigley & Borman (1980) (3)	New Zealand/South Island	1950–73			2.3	
Eason et al (1981) (27)	New Zealand/Auckland	1970–79			6.3	
Medsger (1985) (21)	USA/Pittsburgh	1963–72			10.0	
Steen et al (1988) (12)	USA/Pittsburgh	1973–82			19.1	
Silman et al (1988) (15)	UK/West Midlands	1980–85	1.1	6.2	3.7	5.5:1

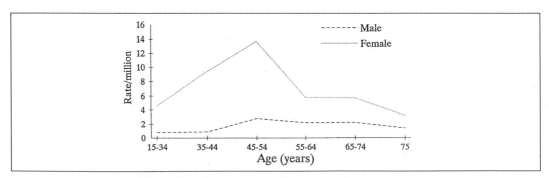

Figure 2.2. Age-specific incidence rates of scleroderma.

the period 1963 to 1985 in Allegheny County (Pittsburgh), Pennsylvania, showed the same phenomenon of an increasing trend (12,21). Whether such increases represent a true underlying increase or improved case ascertainment is unanswered. Scleroderma is not a recently recognized disease and it seems intuitively unlikely, given the long-standing high reputation of the Pittsburgh group in treating the disease, that case ascertainment and diagnostic accuracy are responsible.

PREVALENCE

Paradoxically, prevalence is a more difficult measurement of disease occurrence to derive from the available data sources. This reflects the lack of cross-sectional population-based surveys and the requirement to estimate prevalence from retrospective ascertainment of hospital series of patients alive at a particular date, i.e., "prevalence day." The difficulties inherent in such an approach are reflected by the wide variation in rates reported from different studies (Table 2.4). The Mayo Clinic data are difficult to interpret given the lack of a single male case alive at "prevalence day" (14). The data from Tennessee are derived from the results of incidence (16). The UK data were derived using multiple methods of ascertainment, including primary care and the patient self-help organization, in addition to hospital clinics (15). The only true community-based survey was from South Carolina (22). This was a multi-phase survey that began with a questionnaire survey for the symptoms of RP in 7000 residents. Samples of both the positive and negative respondents were followed up, and the authors could only derive estimates of prevalence under a series of assumptions about the occurrence of scleroderma in those patients who were not seen. Furthermore, these estimates were derived from only two cases, which yielded a minimum prevalence (subject to a wide confidence interval) of 290 per million. In addition, a further five patients were identified with what the authors termed "scleroderma spectrum disorders." These

were patients whose clinical features were insufficient to satisfy the ARA criteria but who had some features of scleroderma. The conclusion from considering the available data is that, as with most other chronic disorders, scleroderma varies in severity, and, thus, epidemiological studies based only on diagnosed cases ascertained by specialist clinics will underestimate the true occurrence of pathology in the community.

GEOGRAPHICAL DISTRIBUTION: AMONG COUNTRIES

Scleroderma has been described in a substantial number of non-Western populations including Japan (23), USSR (24), Nigeria (25), Mexico (26), and Polynesians in New Zealand (27). The disease is manifestly not confined to European Caucasians. There are, however, few epidemiological data to determine whether there are real differences among countries. The prevalence in Japan was estimated to be approximately 7 per million, which is substantially lower than that seen in Western countries (23).

The Nigerian experience, from the very limited data provided, would suggest that scleroderma in Black African populations fails to be seen, to any important extent, in the main connective tissue disease center (25). The disease is not rare, however, in African-American populations in the United States. Indeed, in the Southern US the rates in African-Americans are slightly higher than in Caucasians both in males, 1.6 and 1.2 per million, respectively, and in females, 4.3 and 3.6 per million, respectively (16). Nationally in the US, the incidence in male army veterans was substantially higher in African-Americans than in Caucasians: 7.1 versus 1.9 per million, respectively (10). The rate in Polynesian New Zealanders is similar to that seen in New Zealanders of European extraction (27). By contrast, no cases were diagnosed in Aborigines among a personal series of 179 Australian patients (28). Again, these data lack a denominator for accurate comparison.

Table 2.4. Prevalence Studies of Scleroderma

Reference	Country/Population	Source of Data	Date	Prevalence per Million		
				Males	Females	Both
Kurland et al (1969) (13)	USA/Olmsted County	Mayo Clinic	1968			105
Medsger & Masi (1971) (16)	USA/Tennessee	Multi Institutions	1942–52			4
			1953–57			7
			1958–62			21
			1963–68			28
Asboe Hansen (1985) (131)	Denmark Hospitals	Multi	1977–79			126
Michet et al (1985) (14)	USA/Olmsted County	Mayo Clinic	1980		253[a]	
Hautstein et al (1985) (97)	East Germany Institutions	Two	1980–81	20		
	East Germany/Leipzig	Two Institutions	1980–81			100
Silman et al (1985) (15)	UK/West Midlands	Multi Institutions	1986	12.8	47.9	
Maricq et al (1989) (22)	USA/South Carolina	Community Survey	1988		290[b]	30.8

[a]No male cases detected.
[b]Minimum estimate.

GEOGRAPHIC DISTRIBUTION: WITHIN COUNTRIES

There does not appear to be any urban/rural difference in occurrence (10). Studies within most countries investigated have shown some geographical variation in rates. Thus, the incidence in US male veterans was greater, after adjustment for race, in those living in the South Atlantic and East South-Central regions of the US (10). A similar geographic distribution was observed in the US national mortality analysis (9). In the UK, rates in South and West London were higher than those observed in the West Midlands, which are some 100 miles away. Further analysis at electoral ward level of those living in South/West London showed a non-random distribution with a clustering of cases in small areas. One interesting feature of that study was the apparent clustering in those areas adjacent to major international airports (11). A cluster of patients with a variety of connective tissue diseases was also described from Georgia (US), but formal analysis could not confirm a significant increase in prevalence (29). A clearer cluster was reported from Italy in a region near Rome (30). Others have reviewed the possibility of geographical clustering, which remains an interesting but unproven suggestion (31).

Genetics

The strongest genetic factor in the classic disease is gender—as mentioned previously, the majority of scleroderma patients are female. A genetic predisposition to SSc is suggested by the familial clustering of scleroderma with other autoimmune diseases, but families with more than one case of actual scleroderma are uncommon (32, 33). There are fewer than 20 reports in the English language literature of first-degree relatives of patients with SSc having SSc themselves: these reports include parent and child and siblings sharing the disease. Recently, there has been the first report in the English language literature of

scleroderma in identical twins (34). Between siblings, the difference in age of onset is typically 10 years, and the differences between affected parents and children indicate that a shared environment rather than disease development at a pre-programmed age is the major predisposing factor within families. This may also be supported by the finding of higher than expected frequency of autoantibodies in the spouses of SSc patients as well as blood relatives (35,36).

The genetic contribution to disease susceptibility will be considered under the headings of *Induced Chromosomal Damage* and *Role of Major Histocompatibility Complex in Genetic Susceptibility*, together with the relationship of each of these to autoantibody production and clinical practice (Fig. 2.3).

INDUCED CHROMOSOMAL DAMAGE

As discussed later in this chapter, chemicals and toxins are capable of inducing SSc, but it is not known if these agents act upon an already genetically susceptible background or if they themselves can induce genetic change. Bleomycin is known to be a clastogenic (chromosome-breaking) agent, but it is not known if there is a link between this function of the drug and the onset of a SSc-like disease. Much of the work relating to chromosomal abnormalities in SSc was performed several years ago. Since the original work of Housset et al in 1969 (37), which showed increased chromosomal breakage rate, deletions and acentric fragments both in patients' lymphocytes and in fibroblasts have been shown to be a consistent feature of the disease (38). Only recently have attempts been made to utilize the new DNA technology in order to re-address the question of chromosome damage in SSc. In addition to the abnormalities described above (i.e., increased breakage rate, deletions, and acentric fragments), and presumably causally related to them, there is evidence for clastogenic activity in both sera and cell extracts from SSc patients (39,40). The serum factors increase the rate of chromosomal aberrations of normal cells *in vitro*,

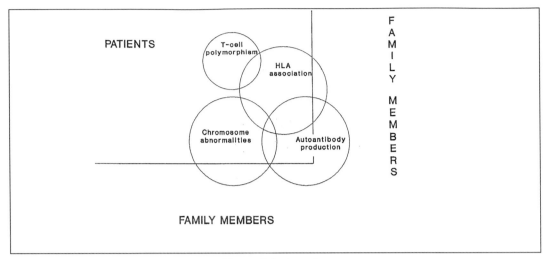

Figure 2.3. Genetics.

and activity can be abolished by the addition of superoxide dismutase, a substance involved in the protection of DNA from damage by oxygen radicals (41). Exogenous factors associated with induction of chromosomal aberrations include ionizing radiation, clastogenic viruses, and a variety of chemicals. SSc patients are not known for their photosensitivity, and there is but weak evidence as yet for a viral etiology for SSc, although the possibility should remain open. However, there is a clear association between the exposure to known clastogenic chemical agents and the development of SSc and similar fibrotic disorders. Bleomycin, one of the most studied of these agents, is a good example. It can induce a fibrotic disease that closely resembles idiopathic SSc (42). An extract of betel nuts also induces oral submucosal fibrosis (43) in a proportion of individuals who chew them. Histologically, this entity is remarkably similar to the fibrosis seen in SSc (44). The disorder has an association with DR3 (45), as does lung fibrosis in the context SSc (46).

The phenomenon of increased chromosomal breakage rate (ICBR) has also been described in the first degree relatives of SSc patients (47,48), but the clastogenic serum factor is not found in these relatives. Although SSc is not included among the classic chromosomal instability syndromes, interestingly it does share a particular clinical feature with one of them: ataxia telangiectasia (AT). Dermatological signs are always a feature of AT, and the fibroblasts of these patients show more chromosomal abnormalities than do the lymphocytes (49,50). In addition, the fibroblasts from AT patients produce elevated levels of fibronectin and procollagen, type I and II. For scleroderma, there are no data to indicate whether a specific aberration among general chromosomal abnormalities is common to all SSc patients. Microscopic karyotyping has been used to analyze these defects, but it is probable that many chromosomal abnormalities are invisible to this method of investigation. An example is the report by Lamb et al (51), who demonstrated a submicroscopic abnormality in a patient with a-thalassemia by a molecular approach using DNA probes. The implication of specific loci in certain tumors has also been achieved by detecting chromosomal deletions using DNA probes for polymorphic markers on autosomal chromosome arms. By analogy with karyotyping, the term allelotyping has been coined to refer to chromosomal analysis using DNA markers for each chromosomal arm. To give an example, in one study (52), the allelotyping of colorectal carcinoma tissue revealed that among a variable number of aberrations involving many chromosomes, allelic deletion of chr. 17p was common to all patients. This led directly to the identification of a gene and its mutant forms on 17p, which are implicated in the etiology of the disease.

In 1993, Artlett et al (53) characterized genetic alterations at the molecular level in the scleroderma genome using variable number tandem repeats (VNTR). Peripheral lymphocytes from 49 scleroderma and 45 control families and paired fibroblast cell lines from the "affected" and "unaffected" skin of 30 patients were examined for chromosomal abnormalities. There were significant rises in the level of VNTR mutations in scleroderma patients (36.7%, n = 18), their siblings (16.3%, n = 13), and offspring (21.7%, n = 15). VNTR mutations in the control group were 0.6% (n = 5). These mutations did not correlate with the presence of autoantibodies and no patient was taking a known clastogenic drug. Differences were also seen in the VNTR lengths between fibroblast and lymphocyte DNA from the same patient as measured by size alteration of one of the alleles. The reason for the genomic changes remains unknown, but the presence of a hitherto unrecognized clastogen is a possibility.

Although the cause of chromosomal abnormalities in SSc is not known, the high rate of chromosomal instability seen in first-degree relatives of patients makes it likely that this phenomenon is partially relevant to the etiology of SSc. Early work has shown that in certain patients with RP this instability could predict the subsequent development of SSc (50). More recently, an attempt has been made to localize the fragile sites relevant to scleroderma and relate them to autoantibody production (54). In this study, 1100 metaphases from 11 patients showed 171 breaks (15.5% vs. controls of 1.7%). The most common fragile site mapped to 3p15, but no relationship with disease specific antibodies was observed.

The tumor literature has interesting pieces of information that might relate to chromosomal abnormalities in SSc. One of these is the presence in some SSc patients of small numbers of dmins (double minute chromosomes) previously thought to be specific to certain murine and human tumor types (55).

ROLE OF MAJOR HISTOCOMPATIBILITY COMPLEX IN GENETIC SUSCEPTIBILITY

Serological Studies

Initial studies of the major histocompatibility complex (MHC) alleles in SSc patients using serological methods indicated an increased frequency of class I and class II alleles, although no pattern common to all ethnic groups emerged and the strength and nature of the association was also controversial. The lack of correlation might be explained by three factors:

(1) Ethnic Variability: it is known that in different ethnic groups different degrees of linkage disequilibrium occur between HLA antigens;
(2) Geographic and Environmental Variability: there appears to be a growing number of possible environmental triggers capable of inducing scleroderma;
(3) Clinical Heterogeneity: here there is the problem of uniformity in terms of diagnosis and accurate subsetting.

Table 2.5 summarizes much of the MHC data available, and Figure 2.4 depicts some of the HLA genes relevant to SSc.

Early negative MHC studies in the US (56,57) were followed by weak positive associations with the Class I MHC antigen HLA Bw35 and the class II MHC antigen DR1, particularly in dcSSc (58). In contrast, two European studies demonstrated DR1 as associated with lcSSc or the CREST syndrome (59,60). In Canada, Gladman et al (60) had shown a stronger association with DR5 in severe disease: American studies linked this gene to the overall disease and British and Australian work defined an association with limited disease.

Table 2.5. Disease Subsets, MHC Class II Antigens and Autoantibodies

Allele	First Author	Year	Size of Population	Geo	Disease Association	Autoantibody Association
DR1	Lynch (57)	1982	237	USA	dcSSc	
	Whiteside (132)	1985	125	USA	Weak dcSSc	ACA
	Alarcon (64)	1985	44	USA	SSc	
	Livingstone (65)	1987	35	USA	Weak SSc	
	Steen (133)	1988	191	USA	lcSSc	ACA
	Black (62)	1984	54	EUR	lcSSc	ACA
	Luderschmidt (59)	1987	136	EUR	CREST	ACA
	Genth (134)	1990	118	EUR	SSc	ACA
DR1 & 4	Briggs (68)	1993	115	EUR	SSc	ACA
DR2	Kondo (135)	1985		JAP	SSc	—
DRw6	Sasaki (136)	1991	families	JAP	SSc familial	ACA
DR3	Germain (63)	1981	14	USA	CREST	
	Livingstone (65)	1987	35	USA	lcSSc	
	Kallenberg (60)	1981	28	EUR	SSc	
	Ercilla (61)	1981	21	EUR	SSc	
	Black (58)	1983	21	EUR	Severe VCD	
	Black (62)	1984	54	EUR	Weak dcSSc	
	Myers (137)	1989	21	EUR	IPF	
	Luderschmidt (59)	1987	136	EUR	Male SSc	
Drw52a	Briggs (46)	1992	75	EUR	IPF	
	Langevitz (73)	1992	126	CAN	PHT	
DR5	Gladman (59a)	1981	34	CAN	Severe	
	Alarcon (64)	1985	44	USA	SSc	
	Livingstone (65)	1987	35	USA	Weak SSc	
	Steen (133)	1988	206	USA	dcSSc	Scl-70
	Harvey (44)	1983	44	EUR	VCD	
	Black (62)	1984	54	EUR	lcSSc	ACA
	Luderschmidt (59)	1987	136	EUR	SSC	ACA & Scl-70
	Genth (134)	1990	118	EUR	SSc	ACA
	Barnett (138)	1989	46	AUS	dcSSc	
DR11	Dunckley (139)	1989	41	AUS	SSc	
DRw15	Jazwinska (140)	1990	18	JAP	SSc	
DQA2	Briggs (68)	1993	115	UK	SSc	
DQ57	Reveille (70)	1992	116	USA	SSc	ACA
DQB1, DQw3	Reveille (71)	1992	161	USA	SSc	Scl-70
DQB1	Kuwana (74)	1993	62	JAP	SSc	Scl-70
DPB1	Briggs (68)	1993	115	UK	SSc	Scl-70

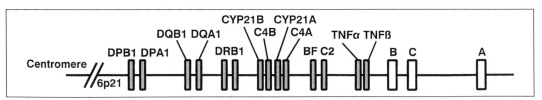

Figure 2.4. Some of the HLA genes on chromosome 6 relevant to scleroderma.

Early reports from the European mainland showed an increase in the "common" autoimmune disease associated haplotype HLA A1, B8, DR3 (61,62). In the initial studies in the UK, this was particularly associated with diffuse disease (59), an association interestingly found in vinylchloride-induced scleroderma of the severe variety (63). In contrast, three North American studies showed DR3 to be associated with limited forms of scleroderma (64–66). Both DR3 and DR5 genes are linked to DRw52, and Livingstone et al (66) suggested in 1987 that this could be the primary MHC Class II allele associated with SSc. To answer such a question a more detailed analysis of the MHC was required using modern technology.

The class III genes have been less well studied in scleroderma. C4 typing, especially the assignment of null phenotypes, is technically difficult, and family studies considered necessary for positive assignment of null alleles. This may explain the relative paucity of studies. In an early study, we reported an association between C4AQ0 and SSc which, unlike the C4AQ0 association in SLE, is not entirely dependent on the co-expression of DR3 (67). This association has not been found by other groups, although one report suggested that homozygous C4BQ0 is associated with SSc (68). Since our initial report we have confirmed our data on a larger series of UK patients by performing restriction fragment length polymorphism (RFLP) analysis on both the C4 allotypes and the C4 genes (69). In addition, the demonstration of C4 activation in SSc provides further evidence that null C4 alleles contribute to the disease process (70).

DNA

Current technology permits MHC analysis at the DNA level either by RFLP or by oligonucleotide probes, which are specific either for particular alleles or for sequences that determine specific motifs or epitopes. These techniques have substantially improved the accuracy and specificity with which the DR loci (DRB, DQA, DQB, DPA and DPB) can be identified. Many alleles defined serologically and by RFLP can be further subdivided when they are compared at the level of the genomic DNA sequence. For example, the alleles that determine DR4 can be resolved into DRB10401/0418 and those that determine DR1 into DRB10101/0104. Because of the sequence information known for most alleles, HLA associations can now be seen in terms of specific epitopes or amino-acid residues. In addition, DNA analysis permits better definition of linkage groups. The gene for DR3 is linked to that for DR52a or DR52b. Linkage of DR3 to DR52a is a property of an extended MHC haplotype common only in western European populations which, in addition, comprises HLA A1-B8 and a non-detected C4 locus (C4AQO) DQB0201 and, to a lesser extent, DPB0101.

Taking advantage of this technology, Briggs et al studied a large group of patients (n = 115) in order to redefine the association of the MHC with SSc (69). Class II alleles (DRB, DQA, DPB) were tested by a combination of RFLP analysis and oligonucleotide probing with polymerase chain reaction amplification, and C4 was tested by protein phenotyping and RFLP analysis. The analysis of multiple loci in a single study allows discrimination of primary and secondary associations and the relative contribution of the different alleles. Correlations were made between disease status, pulmonary fibrosis, and the expression of scleroderma-related antibodies.

Analysis showed that: (*a*) C4A null alleles provide the strongest correlation of the MHC with SSc (Table 2.6); (*b*) DQA2 is an additional primary susceptibility marker, and the previously reported DR3 and DR11 associations are secondary because of linkage disequilibrium (Table 2.7); (*c*) DR52a is the primary MHC marker for pulmonary fibrosis in SSc (Table 2.8); (*d*) Class II allele frequencies differ between female and male patients; and (*e*) ACA expression is associated with DR1 and DR4 (a finding compatible with Reveille's results described below), while acidic residues at position 69 in DPB are associated with expression of anti-Scl-70. When UK

Table 2.6. Association Between C4 Polymorphisms[a]

Group	All Cases		Limited Cutaneous		Diffuse Cutaneous		Controls	
Phenotype	80	(%)	43	(%)	37	(%)	307	(%)
AQO, QO	2	(2.5)	0	(0.0)	2	(5.4)	8	(2.6)
BQO, QO	3	(3.8)		(0.0)	3	(8.1)	9	(2.9)
TaqI RFLV[b]	80	(%)	39	(%)	41	(%)	70	(%)
7.0 kb	79	(98.8)	39	(100.0)	40	(97.6)	69	(98.6)
6.4 kb	29	(36.3)[c]	15	(38.5)	14	(34.1)	15	(21.4)
6.0 kb	61	(76.3)	29	(74.4)	32	(78.0)	51	(72.9)
5.4 kb	37	(46.3)	20	(51.3)	17	(41.5)	41	(58.6)

[a]The C4 phenotype was analyzed at the protein level.
[b]RFLV = restriction fragment length variant.
[c]Significantly different from controls, $p < .05$, unadjusted for multiple testing.

Table 2.7. HLA Class II Results: DRB and DQA by RFLP

Group	All Cases		Limited Cutaneous		Diffuse Cutaneous		Controls	
Allele	115	(%)	62	(%)	53	(%)	142	(%)
DR1	22	(19.1)	14	(22.6)	8	(15.1)	20	(14.1)
DR2 (15)	20	(17.4)[a]	11	(17.7)	9	(17.0)	48	(33.8)
DR3	49	(42.6)[b]	25	(40.3)	24	(45.3)	40	(28.2)
DR4	47	(40.9)	24	(38.7)	23	(43.4)	57	(40.1)
DR11	20	(17.4)[b]	10	(16.1)	10	(18.9)	11	(7.7)
DR12	2	(1.7)	1	(1.6)	1	(1.9)	1	(0.7)
DR6(w9)	8	(7.0)	5	(8.1)	3	(5.7)	13	(9.2)
DR6(w16)	1	(0.9)	0	(0.0)	1	(1.9)	1	(0.7)
DR(w18)	6	(5.2)	3	(4.8)	3	(5.7)	12	(8.5)
DR6(w19)	7	(6.1)	1	(1.6)	6	(11.3)	5	(3.5)
DR7	20	(17.4)[b]	11	(17.7)	9	(17.0)	40	(28.1)
DR8	7	(6.1)	2	(3.2)`	5	(9.4)	5	(3.5)
DR10	1	(0.9)	1	(1.6)	0	(0.0)	0	(0.0)
DR52a	43	(37.4)	22	(35.5)	21	(39.6)	13	(26.7)
DR52b	37	(32.2)	19	(32.3)	17	(32.1)	41	(28.9)
DR52c	7	(6.1)	1	(1.6)	6	(11.3)	5	(3.5)
DR53	63	(54.8)	34	(54.8)	29	(54.7)	86	(58.4)
DR3/52a	39	(33.9)[b]	20	(33.3)	19	(35.9)	33	(23.2)
DR3/52b	12	(10.4)	7	(11.3)	5	(9.4)	8	(5.6)
DQA1a	30	(26.1)	19	(30.6)	11	(20.8)	31	(21.7)
DQA1b	32	(27.8)	15	(22.6)	18	(34.0)	53	(41.3)
DQA1c	7	(6.1)	3	(4.8)	4	(7.5)	10	(7.0)
DAQ2	67	(58.3)[a]	36	(58.1)	31	(58.5)	59	(41.3)
DAQ3	63	(53.4)	34	(56.5)	29	(49.1)	86	(61.4)

Significant differences compared to controls are indicated as [a]$p < .01$, [b]$p < .05$. Results are thus unadjusted for multiple significance testing.

and US data are now compared, it is noticeable that the presence of the B8,DR3,DQ2 haplotype is less common in American patients (71,72). One of the results in Reveille's work is that the DQ antigens DQ7 and DQ5 are more common. The two data sets are consistent if one "corrects" for this haplotype. Reveille and Stephens also reported a negative overall disease association with HLA-DP (71–73).

The CYP locus controlling 21-hydroxylase production is complex, polymorphic, and an attractive candidate region for a disease with a strong gender bias. It maps close to C4 and is partially deleted on B8 haplotypes.

Table 2.8. MHC Class II Alleles Associated with Pulmonary Fibrosis (PF)

Group			DR3		Drw52a		DR3/DRw52a	
		n	n	(%)	n	(%)	n	(%)
All	PF+	42	22[b]	(52.3)	21[d]	(50.0)	19[d]	(45.2)
	PF−	33	8	(24.2)	4	(12.0)	2	(6.1)
Limited	PF+	18	11	(61.1)	11	(61.1)	10[c]	(55.6)
	PF−	19	3	(15.8)	2	(10.5)	0	—
Diffuse	PF+	24	11	(45.8)	10	(41.7)	9	(37.5)
	PF−	14	5	(35.7)	2	(14.3)	2	(14.3)
Morphea		30	8	(26.7)	13	(43.3)	8	(26.7)
CFA[a]		16	4	(25.0)	7	(43.8)	4	(25.0)
Normal		142	48	(28.2)	38	(26.7)	33	(23.2)

[a]CFA = Cryptogenic fibrosing alveolitis.
Significant differences compared to controls are indicated as [b]$p < .05$, [c]$p < .01$, [d]$p < .001$ but compared to those without pulmonary fibrosis.

THE MHC, AUTOANTIBODY PRODUCTION, AND CLINICAL RELEVANCE

As indicated in previous paragraphs, the HLA associations with scleroderma are many and varied. Thus, SSc differs from many other autoimmune rheumatological diseases, such as rheumatoid arthritis (RA), SLE, and ankylosing spondylitis (AS), in that it does not have a strong primary HLA association. SSc does have a strong and clinically useful association between the B8-DR3-DR52-DQB2 haplotype and the development of lung fibrosis (46). Pulmonary disease is now the major cause of death in SSc, and the presence of DR52a and anti-Scl-70 permits the prediction of pulmonary disease in individual patients (RR = 16.7). It is not formally known whether the association is with severe pulmonary hypertension or with lung fibrosis. The original DR3 association described by Lynch et al (59) was found to be with lung fibrosis. It has now been shown that the association was not with DR3 *per se* but with another and so far unidentified gene on the common HLA-DR3-bearing haplotype. Thus, for example, morphea patients bearing the DR3 haplotype were not susceptible to lung fibrosis. A Canadian group has now linked the same haplotype with pulmonary hypertension in SSc (74), but they did not exclude the possibility of the link being with the development of fibrosis. A combined study would probably be necessary to prove the point, because pulmonary hypertension may occur secondary to pulmonary fibrosis in some patients. The common genetic background would probably stop such a study from localizing the primary gene(s). Transracial gene mapping would therefore be of value. The Japanese, for example, have different HLA associations with SSc, suggesting that combined studies might identify a primary gene within the MHC that would link with population-dependent markers.

In the absence of a strong association, one is left with the question of why there are so many weak and partially reproducible links with so many different antigens. Some of the explanations may themselves be important. Thus, when families typed in 1984 were re-studied using DNA technology, the association with HLA-DR5 had vanished. This turned out not to be due to typing errors, as was originally thought, but to the fact that 9 of 13 individuals who had typed serologically as HLA-DR5 had died between studies, resulting in a loss of statistical association in the survivors. Also, we have observed that the incidence of HLA-DR4 in SSc in the UK can depend on how the patients are drawn from the rheumatology clinic and how the evidence for arthritis is interpreted at presentation. Subtyping of HLA-DR4 in our SSc patients shows that they have the same incidence of the rheumatoid motif as HLA-DR4 positive patients with rheumatoid arthritis.

One area where there is high but not absolute agreement among different studies is in the definition of which MHC antigen links with the presence or absence of individual autoantibodies. As both MHC and antinuclear antibody (ANA) definition became more sophisticated with the advance of new techniques, so the association between them has become tighter and tighter. However, linkage disequilibrium still makes it difficult to define the gene and sequence of interest. Antitopoisomerase-1 (Scl-70) has been associated with HLA DR2 or DR5. In 1992, Reveille et al (71) ascribed this link to HLA-DQB alleles in linkage disequilibrium with DR2 and DR5 and more specifically to alleles bearing uncharged polar amino acid residues at position 30 of outermost domain. Alternative candidates were positions 38 (alanine) and position 77 (threonine) of these same alleles. Japanese studies show an association of Scl-70 with the presence of a tyrosine at position 26 of the HLA DQB1 outermost domain (75). In English patients, the Scl-70 antibody association is with an acidic residue at position 69 in the DPβ chain (69). Another example of where the overall associations are consistent among groups but the sequence of interest is in dispute relates to ACA. Reveille et al (72) have described a 100% association between ACA and the presence of a polar amino acid, either tyrosine or glycine, at position 26 in the cleft region of the DQB1 alleles DQ5 and DQ7. Earlier results from ourselves and others had suggested an association with HLA DR1 and HLA DR4. The DQ7 association of DR4 and DQ5 association of DR1, mentioned above, explains this association. Our own data on HLA DQ-typed patients support the Reveille data with the proviso that an alternative or additional candidate for the primary association could be in HLA-DP (76). However, Fox et al (77) do not support the Reveille data. The authors state: "The presence of a polar residue at position 26 is neither necessary nor sufficient for ACA production and that since responses to ACA are directed at multiple epitopes it would be surprising if a single (or limited number of) peptide-binding sites was responsible for directing responses to such a wide variety of epitopes." A unifying hypothesis would be that each epitope of ACA induces an MHC-dependent and MHC-directed response. Hence, if the assay only measured one antibody then it would always be MHC-restricted. If the assay measures five antibodies against different epitopes, then any MHC restriction would vanish because each individual antibody would have a different MHC association. In practice, MHC association would reappear as up to five separate associations as assays for all five antibodies become distinct. We are of the school which believes that each IgG antibody against a well-defined target epitope will have an MHC-driven association. We would not expect persistent IgM antibodies to show the same association.

T CELL RECEPTORS IN SSc

Although most genetic interest in SSc has centered on the MHC, there are few family data to support the influence of a single inherited characteristic, and interest is turning toward more complex gene interactions and the action of outside agents on susceptible genetic backgrounds. Thus, IgG antibody production is governed by not only the stimulating antigen, the MHC, the immunoglobulin gene families, and the time of stimulus in relation to family expression but also the αβ T cell receptor whose influence is complex. Receptor responsiveness is influenced by the family repertoire, the timing of exposure relative to the expressed repertoire, and the cell on which the αβ T cell repertoire is expressed (e.g., CD4 or CD8).

Currently, studies on SSc T cells are limited both in scope and reproducibility, principally because the system is so complex and SSc so variable that it may take years before constant patterns emerge (92–94). Kahan et al (80) have shown that T cells (both CD4 and CD8) bearing the "memory" marker CD29 are of increased frequency in SSc patients. The CD45RA population analysis supported the hypothesis that these cells were converting from naive T cells. As the authors point out, this conversion can increase adhesion molecule expression and give the cells a greater ability to participate in adhesion-dependent reactions, a factor that may be of considerable importance in the pathogenesis of scleroderma. Kratz et al (81) suggested a role for γ/δ T cells in SSc based on their observation that 41% carry the 11.3 kb Puv II fragment of the T cell receptor γ/δ gene (compared with 21.7% of controls). Sakamoto et al (82) observed that the small proportion of T cells carrying the α/β receptors but lacking the above markers (double-negative T cells) are themselves restricted in V beta expression. Several groups have reported that γ/δ cells can be antigen-restricted and recognize MHC class I and class II antigens, and there are many papers linking such cells with the skin and gut. Gruschwitz et al (83) have described γ/δ cell enrichment in the dermis of chickens with hereditary systemic sclerosis. The position within the dermis determines the CD4:CD8 ratio observed.

In addition to the genetic factors discussed, there are other "constitutional" effects that may be important in disease susceptibility.

Non-Genetic Host Factors

ASSOCIATION WITH CANCER

There have been some interesting suggestions of specific cancer risks with scleroderma (84), although the direction of the link (cause or effect) is unclear. A cluster of breast cancer cases was reported in women with scleroderma (85), but a subsequent formal epidemiological study could not confirm an excess of breast cancer. It did suggest that in some women there was a temporal relationship between the onset of the two diseases (86). There have been similar case reports of the simultaneous co-occurrence of scleroderma with ovarian cancer (87), but the possibility that such

reports represent random events cannot be ruled out. There is also an increased rate of lung cancer in scleroderma patients (86), which seems to be independent of cigarette smoking but related to the presence of pulmonary fibrosis (88). This is perhaps not a surprising result given the association of lung cancer with pulmonary fibrosis from occupational causes.

REPRODUCTIVE AND GYNECOLOGICAL FACTORS

The female excess in incidence, particularly in young women, has generated a number of studies looking for possible reproductive and gynecological factors in disease susceptibility. The major feature of interest has been in the interrelations between scleroderma and pregnancy (89). Much interest has centered on the effect of scleroderma on pregnancy outcome. Thus, although clinical case series of women with established scleroderma have suggested an increased reproductive loss as a consequence of the disease, this risk might not be as large as originally thought (90). The studies discussed in the following paragraphs refer to the converse hypothesis; that is, prior reproductive problems might be either a marker, or indeed, casually related to the subsequent development of scleroderma. The methodological problem in attempting to address this issue even in prospective studies is that dating disease onset is very difficult. It is thus not possible to exclude the explanation that in a disease with a long latent or subclinical period, the occurrence of adverse reproductive events, occur as a consequence rather than as a cause of disease.

In general, scleroderma patients appear to have a reduced fertility prior to disease presentation, even when the disease is delayed in onset to the fifth and subsequent decades (91–93). The latter study was of interest in that two control groups were used: a patient series with RP and a general population group. The reduced fertility was only observed in comparison to a community control group, and there were no differences in

Table 2.9. Case Control Studies of Spontaneous Abortion Rates Prior to Clinical Onset of Scleroderma

Reference	Cases			Controls			Odds Ratio (95% CI) (%)
	Women (N)	Pregnancies (N)	Spontaneous Abortions (%)	Women (N)	Pregnancies (N)	Spontaneous Abortions	
Giordano (1985) (141)	86	299	16.7	86	332	9.6	1.9 (1.2–3.0)
Silman & Black (1988) (91)	115		28.7[a]	115		17.4	1.9 (1.0–3.6)
Steen et al (1989) (90)[b]	48	47	15	48[c]	77	15	0.9 (0.3–2.6)
McHugh et al (1989) (142)	28	63	33[d]	117[c]	264	15	2.8 (1.5–5.7)
Englert et al (1992) (93)	204	331	14.8	233[e]	310	18.1	0.8 (0.5–1.2)
				189[f]	221	12.7	1.2 (0.7–0.8)

[a]Percentage of women.
[b]Includes only women who had pregnancy both before and after disease onset.
[c]Controls were rheumatoid arthritis women.
[d]All pregnancy losses.
[e]Raynauds controls.
[f]Community controls

comparison to a group of Raynaud's women. This is consistent with other observations of reduced fertility in women with apparently primary Raynaud's (94,95). The authors of the latter study suggested that the vasospasm induced by Raynaud's could impair fertility. Thus, the fertility problem in women prior to the onset of scleroderma can be explained by the frequent existence of Raynaud's for some years prior to disease onset. In addition to infertility, however, women who are able to conceive and subsequently develop scleroderma also have an increased rate of reporting delayed (>1 year) conception compared to normal controls (93).

A second avenue of inquiry has been the possibility that there is an increased rate of early reproductive loss (spontaneous abortion) in women prior to the onset of their scleroderma. Those studies with available data are reviewed in Table 2.9 and the results are not consistent. Indeed, the most recent studies, and probably methodologically the most sound studies, found no increase in this loss. The study by Englert et al (93) suggested an increased rate of low birth weight babies prior to disease onset, but this might be a reflection of the vasospasm mentioned above.

Environmental Factors

Unlike many of the rheumatic diseases, there is a considerable amount of literature suggesting that environmental factors may explain the occurrence, in some individuals, of scleroderma. These exposures can broadly be subdivided into silica, organic solvents, and drugs, and are summarized in the following paragraphs. A complete review is found in Chapters 5 and 10. In addition, two specific syndromes are related to, but are not identical to, scleroderma are of interest: the (Spanish) Toxic Oil Syndrome and the L-tryptophan eosinophilia-myalgia syndrome. These "pseudoscleroderma" syndromes are also considered in detail in Chapters 5 and 10. A list of the major exposures said to be associated with scleroderma is provided in Table 2.10. A recent case report (96)

suggested that vibration, well described as a cause of RP *per se*, may also lead to scleroderma.

The epidemiological question of interest is the contribution made by "known" environmental exposures to the overall incidence of scleroderma. Thus, a number of the agents listed in Table 2.10 are derived from single case reports. In general, the female excess normally observed in scleroderma is lost when only those with a known environmental exposure are studied. Indeed, male scleroderma patients may be predominantly explained by an environmental exposure (97), particularly in mining areas. On the other hand, a recent study in the UK failed to reveal any of the reported occupational exposure in over 80% of male cases (98).

SILICA

The first suspicion that silica dust may lead to scleroderma came from reports of a series of 17 gold miners in South Africa (99). This association has also been suggested by other reports (100,101). Indeed, Scottish stone masons were probably the first occupational group to be described with scleroderma (102). The high attributable risk of silica dust exposure for scleroderma in men has become apparent. The most important epidemiological study comes from Pittsburgh, Pennsylvania (103): of 60 men diagnosed between 1955 and 1965, 26 (43%) were either coal miners or were in other occupations which exposed them to silica dust. This exposure frequency was higher than that observed in local hospital controls (19%) or in the fathers or husbands of female scleroderma patients (22%). It was estimated from those data that the prevalence of scleroderma in male coal miners is twice that in the normal female population. In a similar study from what was known as East Germany, 77% of a large series of male patients had been exposed to silica of whom 39 actually had silicosis. The relative risk of scleroderma was 25 with occupational exposure and 110 with frank radiological silicosis (97). One intriguing anecdote that is reminiscent of the asbestosis story, was of

Table 2.10. Environmental Agents Implicated in Scleroderma

A Silica dust:		coal miners gold miners stone masons scouring powder

B Organic chemicals:
  (a) Aromatic hydrocarbons:
	toluene
	benzene
	xylene
	aromatic mixes: white spirit
	                 dieselene	

(b) Aliphatic hydrocarbons: (i) Chlorinated	vinyl chloride trichlorethylene perchlorethylene	

(ii) Non-Chlroinated:
    (iii) Epoxy resins
    (iv) Biogenic amines:
    (v) Urea formaldehyde foam insulation
	naphtha-n-hexane
	
	metaphenylenediamine	

C Drugs:	bleomycin carbidopa L-5-hydroxytryptophan pentazocine cocaine appetite suppressants e.g., breast augmentation:	 diethyl proprion fenfluramine hydrochloride silicone paraffin
D Toxic oil E L-Tryptophan		

a husband and wife pair who both developed scleroderma. The husband had silica exposure and it was suggested that the wife became affected by inhaling dust from his clothes (104)! Other occupational exposures to silica may be important, such as a recent case that was described after exposure to scouring powder containing crystalline silica (105).

ORGANIC SOLVENTS

There have been several case reports of patients with scleroderma after exposure to a variety of organic solvents: both aromatics, such as toluene, benzene, and white spirit (106–108), and non-halogenated and halogenated diphatics, such as perchlorethylene (109) and trichlorethylene (110–112). Some groups of workers seem particularly at risk, such as those in the dry cleaning and similar industries. Vinyl chloride disease is a well-recognized complication of those who clean the reactors after polymerization. This disorder is characterized by osteolysis of the phalanges, dyspnea, fatigue, liver disease (including fibrosis and angiosarcoma), and hematological change in addition to RP and sclerodermatous skin change. Vinyl chloride exposure is well-recognized as a cause of scleroderma (113). The immunogenetics of susceptibility to scleroderma in this group of workers is well described (62). This clinical and genetic study of "affected" and "unaffected" workers in a UK vinyl chloride plant showed HLA DR5 to be a strong susceptibility marker and the A1 B8 DR3 haplotype to define severity. Other organic chemicals, including the so-called biogenic amines used both in epoxy resin manufacturing (114) and other processes (115), have also been implicated. Exposure to urea formaldehyde is a further possible occupational cause (116).

OTHER LIFESTYLE FACTORS

There are few data on other lifestyle factors in scleroderma. There was an excess rate of smoking prior to disease onset in one study of US males and an increased rate of moderate alcohol consumption when compared to a similarly drawn control group (10). The only other finding of note is the as yet uncorroborated suggestion that there is a higher rate of pet ownership (cats and dogs) in female scleroderma patients, particularly those owning more than one pet compared to friend controls (117).

Epidemiology of Raynaud's Phenomenon

CLASSIFICATION OF RAYNAUD'S PHENOMENON

Maurice Raynaud's (118) original definition of RP as episodic, symmetrical, acral vasospasm characterized by pallor, cyanosis, suffusion, and a sense of fullness and tautness which may be painful, has been used as a descriptive tool for ascertaining cases for epidemiological study. Difficulty in classification arises from the blurred division between a normal and an abnormal cold response, the realization that the condition is rarely present at the time of examination, and the fact that there is little agreement on the minimum number of features required for a positive diagnosis. In addition to this, there is a confusing nomenclature attributed to the condition, such as the somewhat arbitrary distinction between Raynaud's Syndrome and Raynaud's Disease, (119).

The color changes of the digits during an attack of RP are in fact the only symptom whose diagnosis can be objectively ascertained. This creates difficulties for epidemiological studies, which rely on verbal description alone to distinguish normal from abnormal color changes. To avoid such misclassification, a solution was proposed by Maricq and Weinrich (120) who combined simple questions with color charts and photographs. Initial testing of this system with 48 patients and 246 controls showed a sensitivity of 90% and a specificity of 100%.

O'Keeffe et al (121) validated these criteria in a similar study using unselected hospital employees. In practice, a simple questionnaire had a sensitivity of 100% and a specificity of 94% against the use of color charts as a "gold standard." Similar results were obtained by comparison of color charts with a clinical assessment. In comparison, the color charts proved valuable as part of the epidemiological survey, with 9% of women and 4% of men in the study being diagnosed as having the condition.

Brennan et al (122) also assessed the validity of the color charts in 1993, with a study that also tested the reliability of two other methods used in classifying RP: (*a*) a questionnaire based on criteria derived from a group of clinicians, and (*b*) a consensus opinion from clinicians. Only a moderate level of agreement existed between the methods. That study also concluded that the color chart is too insensitive for RP diagnosis, and a structured questionnaire based on perceived clinicians' opinions could not reproduce clinicians' classification in practice. However, by supplying clinicians with a standard description, a reliable classification of RP was obtained.

RAYNAUD'S PHENOMENON AND SCLERODERMA

RP is clearly a central clinical feature in the clinical presentation of scleroderma, and it is appropriate to consider the occurrence of the former in attempting to understand the epidemiology of scleroderma. The large majority of subjects with RP do not have or will not develop scleroderma, but the relationship between the two is far from clear. In hospital series of patients with RP who are clearly selected toward those with severe disease, there is a substantial proportion of individuals both with features of connective tissue disease "at baseline" as well as those who will develop such a disorder on follow-up (123,124). Given the selection factors involved, it is difficult to accurately estimate the proportion in the population with RP who will develop connective tissue disease in general, or scleroderma in particular, on prolonged follow-up. The only true population study that combined a search for both RP and scleroderma (22) suggested that there might be a spectrum from RP to complete scleroderma, which indicates that any artificial separation might be hazardous. Indeed, RP might thus be considered as a marker for the subsequent development of scleroderma, albeit a low risk one.

PRIMARY AND SECONDARY RAYNAUD'S PHENOMENON

Criteria for distinguishing primary from secondary RP have been described (125). Primary RP is digital vasospastic disease not associated with a specific known cause, and thorough clinical and laboratory evaluation has been proposed as a requirement to determine that there are no associated conditions present. Specifically, the criteria are as follows:

Episodic attacks of acral pallor or cyanosis,
Strong and symmetric pulses,
No evidence of digital pitting, ulceration, or gangrene,
Normal nailfold capillaries,
Negative antinuclear test,
Normal erythrocyte sedimentation rate (Westergren).

When Allen and Brown (126) supplemented their own ideas for RP classification, it was suggested that a minimum 2-year follow-up period was required for further evaluation. The more recent recommendations appear to indicate that this is unnecessary, as patients with conditions matching these criteria tend not to develop a secondary disease.

Secondary RP occurs in association with other disorders, such as scleroderma. The proposed features that define secondary RP are as follows:

Abnormal nailfold capillary pattern,
Positive antinuclear tests,
Digital pitting or gangrene,
Esophageal abnormalities (e.g., long transit time),
Small intestine abnormalities (e.g., atrophy on biopsy),
Colonic abnormalities (e.g., abnormal motility),
Pulmonary abnormalities (e.g., x-ray interstitial changes),
Cardiac abnormalities (e.g., by electrocardiogram),
Renal abnormalities (e.g., reduced renal blood flow).

In practice, any feature of undifferentiated connective tissue disease or of various scleroderma-like illness meets the criteria for secondary RP. In LeRoy and Medsger's series of 240 patients with primary RP, 52% satisfied the criteria. Of the remainder, 87% were positive for one or more of three features of connective tissue disease (125).

More recently, Planchon et al (127) have carried out a 6-year study of 194 subjects (aged 10 to 86 years) with RP. Using Allen and Brown's (126) criteria for classification, plus nailfold capillaroscopy and negative serological examination, they showed that there was a correlation between patient age, disease duration, and the decade of onset.

PREVALENCE OF RAYNAUD'S PHENOMENON.

Many studies of RP have been carried out over the past 60 years (Table 2.11). As shown in Table 2.11, the studies have varied widely in their case definition used reflecting some of the difficulties listed above. Some of the discrepancies may reflect true geographical variation, with the studies from western Europe showing prevalence rates in the teens compared with rates under 10% for North American populations. In this regard, it is of interest that in identically conceived studies carried out in France and the US (128) the oc-

Table 2.11. Prevalence of Raynaud's Phenomenon

Reference	Method	Country/Population	Prevalence Males n	%	Females n	%	Age Range (Years)
Lewis & Pickering (1934) (143)	Interviews with medical students and nurses.	USA	62	25.0	60	30.0	19 to 45
Fessel (1975) (144)	Questionnaires from patients in General Practice (GP).	USA USA	29,486 32,098	10.7 10.3	24,739 25,012	16.2 17.2	— —
Olsen & Nielsen (1978) (145)	Postal questionnaire plus clinical investigation.	Denmark (Copenhagen)	—	—	67	22.0	21 to 50
Heslop et al (1983) (146)	Random sample from GP; postal questionnaire plus interview.	England (Hampshire)	260	8.3	260	17.6	20 to 59
Maricq et al (1986) (147)	Random subjects given short questionnaire and interview.	US Caucasian US African-American (South Carolina)	508 169	3.0 4.5	762 313	4.5 2.5	Over 18 Over 18
Leppert et al (1987) (148)	Postal questions, interview and examination.	Sweden (Västeras)	—	—	3000	15.6	18 to 59
Silman et al (1990) (129)	Postal Questionnaires. Questionnaires while attending General Practice	England England London Merseyside Chesire	231 357 105 150 102	11.3 15.7 18.0 8.0 15.0	182 762 294 252 216	18.7 20.6 26.0 13.0 13.0	Over 14 Over 14
Weinrich et al (1990) (149)	Respondents from data survey, given interviews and then screening.	US Caucasian US African-American (South Carolina)	1780 572	2.8 2.3	2037 857	3.8 5.3	18 to 86 18 to 86
Harada et al (1991) (150)	Interviews with symptoms manual with typical photo.	Japan	1875	3.3	1998	2.5	20 to 69
O'Keefe et al (1992) (121)	Questionnaire, clincal interview and color charts.	USA (Burlington, MA)	150	4.0	600	9.0	21 to 60
Bartelink et al (1992) (151)	Questionnaires completed by patients in General Practice.	Netherlands		0.5		2.9	
Riera et al (1993) (152)	Occupational: questopmmaore, capillaroscopic examination.	Spain (Girona)	988	3.2	479	4.7	16 to 64
Maricq et al (1993) (128)	Probability sample after random phone interviews.	France (Tarentaise, Sacoie) USA (Charleston, SC)	835 1353	13.5 4.3	1165 1608	20.1 5.7	Over 18 Over 18
Inaba et al (1993) (153)	Health tests plus interviews, using symptoms manual.	Japan (Gifu)	332	3.0	731	3.4	30 to 91

currence of RP in the former was three times that of the latter.

In virtually all studies, the frequency in females was higher than that for males, with a female excess of 1.5 to 2. There are limited data on changing prevalence with age, but in one UK study (129) there was a remarkably flat age distribution in both males and females throughout adulthood. The explanation for this presumably lies in the onset of new cases occurring in early adult life, or even childhood, in a disorder which persists throughout life and is not associated with a selectively increased mortality.

Few studies have examined in detail ethnic influences, and indeed the interpretation of color differences is potentially problematic when comparing different skin colors. In studies in the US, the prevalence was not importantly different between Caucasians and African-Americans.

References

1. Brennan P, Silman AJ, Black C, Bernstein R, Coppock J, Maddison P, Sheerin T, et al. Reliability of skin involvement measures in scleroderma. Br J Rheumatol 1992;31:457–460.
2. Subcommittee for Scleroderma Criteria of the American Rheumatism Association Diagnostic and Therapeutic Criteria Committee. Preliminary criteria for the classification of systemic sclerosis (scleroderma). Arthritis Rheum 1980;23: 581–590.
3. Wigley RD, Borman B. Medical geography and the etiology of the rare connective tissue. Soc Sci Med 1980;14D:175–183.
4. Tan PLJ, Wigley RD, Borman B. Clinical criteria for systemic sclerosis. Arthritis Rheum 1981;24: 1589–1590.
5. Jannssens X, Herman L, Mielants H, Verbruggen G, Veys EM. Disease manifestations of progressive systemic sclerosis: Sensitivity and specificity. Clin Rheumatol 1987;6:532–538.
6. LeRoy EC, Black CM, Fleischmajer R, et al. Scleroderma (systemic sclerosis): Classification subsets and pathogenesis. J Rheumatol 1988;15:202–205.
7. Masi AT, D'Angleo WA. Epidemiology of fatal systemic sclerosis (diffuse scleroderma). Ann Intern Med 1967;66:870–875.
8. Cobb S. The frequency of rheumatic diseases. Cambridge, MA: Harvard University Press, 1971.
9. Hochberg MC, Lopez-Acuna D, Gittlesohn AM. Mortality from systemic sclerosis (scleroderma) in the United States, 1969–85. In: Black CM, Myers AR, eds. Systemic sclerosis (scleroderma). New York: Gower, 1985.
10. Medsger TA, Masi AT. The epidemiology of systemic sclerosis (scleroderma) among male US veterans. J Chron Dis 1978;31:73–85.
11. Silman AJ, Hicklin AJ, Black CM. Geographical clustering of scleroderma in South and West London. Br J Rheumatol 1990;29:92–96.
12. Steen V, Conte C, Santoro D, et al. Twenty year incidence survey of systemic sclerosis. Arthritis Rheum 1988;32(Suppl 14):S57.
13. Kurland LT, Hauser WA, Ferguson RH, Holley KE. Epidemiologic features of diffuse connective tissue disorders in Rochester Minnesota, 1951 through 1967, with special reference to systemic lupus erythematosus. Mayo Clin Proc 1969;44: 649–663.
14. Michet CJ, McKenna CH, Elveback LR, Kaslow RA, Kurland LT. Epidemiology of systemic lupus erythematosus and other connective tissue disease in Rochester Minnesota, 1950 through 1979. Mayo Clin Proc 1985;60:105–113.
15. Silman AJ, Jannini S, Symmons D, Bacon P. An epidemiological study of scleroderma in the West Midlands. Br J Rheumatol 1988;27:286–290.
16. Medsger TA, Masi AT. Epidemiology of systemic sclerosis (scleroderma). Ann Intern Med 1971;74: 714–721.
17. Ansell BM, Nasseh GA, Bywaters EGL. Scleroderma in childhood. Ann Rheum Dis 1976;35:189–197.
18. Burge SM, Ryan TJ, Dawber RPR. Case report: Juvenile onset systemic sclerosis. J R Soc Med 1984; 77:793–794.
19. Dalziel JA, Wilcox GK. Progressive systemic sclerosis in the elderly. Postgrad Med J 1979;55:192–193.
20. Editorial. Systemic sclerosis in old age. Br Med J 1979;2:1313–1314.
21. Medsger TA Jr. Epidemiology of progressive systemic sclerosis. In: Black CM, Myers AR, eds. Systemic sclerosis (scleroderma). New York: Gower, 1985;53–59.
22. Maricq HR, Weinrich MC, Keil JE, et al. Prevalence of scleroderma spectrum disorders in the general population of South Carolina. Arthritis Rheum 1989;32:998–1006.
23. Shinkai H. Epidemiology of progressive systemic sclerosis in Japan. In: Black CM, Myers AR, eds.

Systemic sclerosis (scleroderma). New York: Gower, 1985, 79–81.

24. Guseva NG, Folomeeva OM, Oskilko TG. Familial systemic sclerosis: A follow up study of concordant monozygotic twins. Ter Arkh 1981;53:43–47.

25. Somorin AO, Mordi VIN. Connective tissue disease in Nigeria with emphasis on scleroderma. Cent Afr J Med 1980;26:59–63.

26. de Kasep GI, Alarcon-Segovia D. Preliminary epidemiologic data on progressive systemic sclerosis. In: Black CM, Myers AR, eds. Systemic sclerosis (scleroderma). New York: Gower, 1985, 70–71.

27. Eason RJ, Tan PL, Gow PJ. Progressive systemic sclerosis in Auckland: A ten year review with emphasis on prognostic features. Aust NZ J Med 1981; 11:657–662.

28. Barnett AJ. Epidemiology of systemic sclerosis (scleroderma) in Australia. In: Black CM, Myers AR, eds. Systemic sclerosis (scleroderma). New York: Gower, 1985, 82–83.

29. Freni-Titulaer LWJ, Kelley DB, Grow AG, et al. Connective tissue disease in South Eastern Georgia: A case-control study. Am J Epidemiol 1989; 130:404–409.

30. Valesini G, Litta A, Bonavita MS, Luan FL, Purpura M, Mariani M, Balsano F. Geographical clustering of scleroderma in a rural area in the province of Rome. Clin Exp Rheum 1993;11:41–47.

31. Maricq HR. Geographical clustering of scleroderma. Br J Rheumatol 1990;29:241–244.

32. Molta CT, Khan MA, Aponte CJ, Reynolds TL, Macintyre SS. Familial occurence of systemic sclerosis, rheumatoid arthritis and other immunological disorders: Report of two kindreds with study of HLA antigens and review of the literature. Clin Exp Rheumatol 1989;7:229–236.

33. Arnett FC, Bias WB, McLean RH, Engel M, Duvic M, Goldstein R, Freni-Titulaer L, et al. Connective tissue disease in Southeast Georgia. A community based study of immunogentic markers and autoantibodies. J Rheumatol 1990;17:1029–1035.

34. Cook NJ, Silman AJ, Propert J, Cawley MID. Features of systemic sclerosis (scleroderma) in an identical twin pair. Br J Rheumatol 1993;32:926–928.

35. Pereira S, Black C, Welsh K, Ansell B, Jayson M, Maddison P, Rowell N. Autoantibodies and immunogenetics in 30 patients with systemic sclerosis and their families. J Rheumatol 1987;14:760–765.

36. Maddison PJ, Stephens C, McHugh N, Briggs D, Welsh KI, Harvey G, Whyte J, Black CM. Connec-

tive tissue disease and autoantibodies in the kindreds of 63 patients with systemic sclerosis. Medicine 1993;72;2:103–112.

37. Housset E, Emerit I, Baulon A, et al. Anomalies chromosomiques dans la sclérodermie généralisée. Études de 10 malades. Cr Hebd Seanc Acad Sci (Paris) 1969;269.

38. Emerit I, Housset E, Grouchy J de, et al. Chromosomal breakage in diffuse scleroderma. A study of 27 patients. Biomedicine 1971;16:648.

39. Wolff DJ, White-Needleman B, Wasserman SS, Schwartz S. Spontaneous and clastogen-induced chromosomal breakage in scleroderma. J Rheumatol 1991;18:6.

40. Emerit I, Levy A, Housset E. Sclerodermie généralisée et cassures chromosomiques. Mise en évidence d'un "facteur cassant" dans la serum des maladies. Ann Genet 1973;16:135.

41. Emerit I. Chromosomal instability in collagen disease. J Rheumatol 1980;39:84–90.

42. Finch WR, Buckingham RB, Rodnan GP, et al. Scleroderma induced by Bleomycin. In Current topics in rheumatology. New York: Gower, 1985.

43. Stich HF, Stich W. Chromosome damaging activity of saliva of betel and tobacco chewers. Cancer Lett 1982;15:193–202.

44. Harvey W. Submucous fibrosis. In Proceedings of the scleroderma symposium. Welwyn Garden City, New Jersey: Smith Kline and French Laboratories Ltd, 1983.

45. Canniff JP, Batchelor JR, Dodi IA, Harvey W. HLA-typing in oral submucous fibrosis. Tissue Antigens 1985;26:138–142.

46. Briggs DC, Vaughan R, Welsh KI, et al. Immunogenetic prediction of publmonary fibrosis in systemic sclerosis. Lancet 1992;338:661–662.

47. Emerit I. Chromosmal breakage in systemic sclerosis and related disorders. Dermatologica 1976; 153:145–156.

48. Rittner G, Schwanitz G, Baur MP, et al. Family studies in scleroderma (systemic sclerosis) demonstrating an HLA-linked increased chromosmal breakage rate in cultured lymphocytes. Hum Genet 1988;81:64–70.

49. Patterson MC, Smith BP, Knight PA, Anderson AK. Ataxia telangiectasia. An inherited human disease involving radiosensitivity, malignancy and defective DNA repair. In: Castellani A, ed. Research in photobiology. New York: Plenum Press, 1977;207–218.

50. Emerit I, Housset E, Feingold J. Chromosomal breakage and scleroderma. Studies in family members. J Lab Clin Med 1976;88:81.

51. Lamb J, Wilkie AOM, Harris PC, et al. Detection of breakpoints in submicroscopic chromosomal

translocation, illustrating an important mechanism for genetic disease. Lancet 1989;ii:819–826.

52. Hastie ND, Dempster M, Dunlop, et al. Telomere reduction in human colorectal carcinoma and with ageing. Nature 1990;346:866–868.

53. Artlett C, Vancheeswaran R, Black C, Welsh K. Variable number tandem repeat and fingerprint analysis of scleroderma family DNA. Am Coll Rheumatol 1993;S182:B244.

54. Tsay GT, Lan J-L, Li S-Y. Chromosome studies in systemic sclerosis with consideration of antibodies to topoisomerase I. Ann Rheum Dis 1992;51:624–626.

55. Birnbaum NS, Rodnan GP, Rabin BS, et al. Histocompatibility antigens in progressive systemic sclerosis (scleroderma). J Rheumatol 1977;4:425–428.

56. Majsky A, Kobikova M, Stava Z. HLA and systemic scleroderma. Tissue Antigens 1979;14:359–360.

57. Lynch CJ, Singh G, Whiteside TL, et al. Histocompatibility antigens in progressive systemic sclerosis (scleroderma). J Clin Immunol 1982;2:314–318.

58. Black CM, Welsh KI, Walker AE, et al. Genetic susceptibility to scleroderma-like syndrome induced by vinyl chloride. Lancet 1983;i:53–55.

59. Luderschmidt C, Scholz S, Mehlhaff E, et al. Association of progressive systemic scleroderma to several HLA-B and HLA-DR alleles. Arch Dermatol 1987;123:1188–1191.

60. Gladman DD, Keystone EC, Baron M, et al. Increased frequency of DR5 in scleroderma. Arthritis Rheum 1981;24:854–856.

61. Kallenberg CGM, Van der Voort-Beelen JM, D'Amaro J. Increased frequency of B8/DR3 and association of the haplotype with impaired cellular response. Clin Exp Immunol 1981;43:481–485.

62. Black CM, Welsh IK, Maddison PJ, et al. HLA antigens, autoantibodies and clinical subsets of scleroderma. Br J Rheumatol 1984;23:267–271.

63. Germain BF, Espinoza LR, Bergen LL, et al. Increased prevalence of DRw3 in the CREST syndrome. Arthritis Rheum 1981;24:857–859.

64. Alarcon GS, Philips RM, Wasner CK, et al. DR antigens in systemic sclerosis: Lack of clinical correlations. Tissue Antigens 1985;26:156–158.

65. Livingstone JZ, Scott TE, Wigley FM, et al. Systemic sclerosis (scleroderma): Clinical, genetic and serological subsets. J Rheumatol 1987;14:512–518.

66. Briggs DC, Welsh KI, Pereira RS, Black CM. A strong association between null alleles at the CRA locus in the major histocompatibility complex and systemic sclerosis. Arthritis Rheum 1986;29:1274–1277.

67. Rittner C. Chromosomes and complement in scleroderma. In: Proceedings of the scleroderma symposisum. Welwyn Garden City, New Jersey: Smith Kline and French Laboratories Ltd, 1983.

68. Briggs D, Stephens C, Vaughan R, Welsh K, Black C. A molecular and serologic analysis of the major histocompatibility complex and complement component C4 in systemic sclerosis. Arthritis Rheum 1993;36:943–954.

69. Senaldi G, Vergani D, McWhirter A, et al. Complement activation in progressive systemic sclerosis. Lancet 1987;i:1143–1144.

70. Reveille JD, Owerbach D, Goldstein R, Moreda R, Isern RA, Arnett FC. Association of polar amino acids at Position 26 of the HLA-DQB1 first domain with the anticentromere autoantibody response in systemic sclerosis (scleroderma). J Clin Invest 1992;89:1208–1213.

71. Reveille JD, Durban E, MacLeod-St Clair MJ, Goldstein R, Moreda R, Altman RD, Arnett FC. Association of amino acid sequences in the HLA-DQB1 first domain with the antitopoisomerase 1. Autoantibody response in scleroderma (progressive systemic sclerosis). J Clin Invest 1992;90:973–980.

72. Stephens C. HLA DP in scleroderma: No primary association. Tissue Antigens (in press).

73. Langevitz P, Buskila D, Gladman DD, Darlington GA, Farewell VT, Lee P. HLA alleles in systemic sclerosis: Association with pulmonary hypertension and outcome. Br J Rheumatol 1992;31:609–613.

74. Kuwana M, Kaburaki J, Okano Y, Inoko H, Tsuji K. The HLA-DR and DQ genes control the autoimmune response to DNA topoisomerase 1 in systemic sclerosis (Scleroderma). J Clin Invest 1993;92:1296–1301.

75. McHugh NJ, Whyte J, Artlett C, Briggs DC, Stephens CO, Olsen NJ, Gusseva NG, et al. Anticentromere antibodies (ACA) in systemic sclerosis patients and their relatives: A serological and HLA study. Clin Exp Rheumatol 1994;96:267–274.

76. Fox RI, Kang H-I. Genetics and environmental factors in systemic sclerosis. Curr Opin Rheumatol 1992;4:857–861.

77. Postlethwaite AE, Kang AH. Cellular immunity in systemic sclerosis. In: Jayson MIV, Black CM, eds. Systemic sclerosis (scleroderma). Chichester, UK: John Wiley & Sons, 1988.

78. White-Needleman B. Immunologic aspects of scleroderma. Curr Opin Rheumatol 1992;4:862–868.

79. Yurovsky VV, Sutton PA, Schulze DH, Wigley FM, Wise RA, Howard RF, White B. Expansion of selected Vδ1+ $\gamma\delta$ T cells in systemic sclerosis patients. J Immunol 1994;153:881–891.

80. Kahan A, Kahan A, Picard F, Menkes CJ, Amor B. Abnormalities of T-lymphocyte subsets in systemic sclerosis demonstrated with anti-CD45RA and anti-CD29 monoclonal antibodies. Ann Rheum Dis 1991;50:354–358.

81. Kratz LE, Boughman JA, Pincus T, Cohen DI, White-Needleman B. Association of scleroderma with a T cell antigen receptor gamma gene restriction fragment length polymorphism. Arthritis Rheum 1990;33(4):569–573.

82. Sakamoto A, Sumida T, Maeda T, Itoh M, Asai T, Takahashi H, Yoshida S, et al. T cell receptor V beta repertoire of double-negative alpha/beta T cells in patients with systemic sclerosis. Arthritis Rheum 1992;35(8):944–948.

83. Gruschwitz MS, Moormann S, Kromer G, Sgonc R, Dietrich H, Boeck G, Gershwin ME, et al. Phenotypic analysis of skin infiltrates in comparison with peripheral blood lymphocytes, spleen cells and thymocytes in early avian scleroderma. J Autoimmun 1991;4(4):577–593.

84. Duncan SC, Winkelman RK. Cancer and scleroderma. Arch Dermatol 1970;115:950–955.

85. Lee P, Alderdice C, Wilkinson S, Keystone EC, Urowitz MB. Malignancy in progressive systemic sclerosis–association with breast carcinoma. J Rheumatol 1983;10(4):665–666.

86. Roumm AD, Medsger TA. Cancer and systemic sclerosis. A epidemiological study. J Rheumatol 1985;12:1336–1340.

87. Young R, Towbin B, Isern R. Scleroderma and ovarian carcinoma. Br J Rheumatol 1990;29:314.

88. Peters-Golden M, Wise RA, Hochberg M, Stevens MB, Wigley FM. Incidence of lung cancer in systemic sclerosis. J Rheumatol 1985;12:1136–1139.

89. Silman AJ. Pregnancy and scleroderma. Am J Reprod Immunol 1992;28:238–240.

90. Steen VD, et al. Pregnancy in women with scleroderma. Arthritis Rheum 1989;32:151–157.

91. Silman AJ, Black CM. Increased incidence of spontaneous abortion infertility in women with scleroderma. Ann Rheum Dis 1988;47:441–444.

92. Ballou SP, Morley JJ, Kushner I. Pregnancy and systemic sclerosis. Arthritis Rheum 1984;27(3):295–298.

93. Englert H, McNeil D, Brennan P, Black C, Silman AJ. Reproductive function prior to disease onset in women with scleroderma. J Rheumatol 1992;19(10):1575–1579.

94. de Trafford JC, Lafferty K, Potter CE, Roberts VC, Cotton LT. An epidemiological survey of Raynaud's phenomenon. Eur J Vasc Surg 1988;2:167–170.

95. Kahl LE, Blair C, Ramsey-Goldman R, Steen VD. Pregnancy outcomes in women with primary Raynaud's phenomenon. Arthritis Rheum 1990;33:1249–1255.

96. Pelmear PL, Roos JO, Maehle WM. Occupationally induced scleroderma. J Occup Med 1992;34:20–25.

97. Haustein UF, Ziegler V. Environmentally induced systemic sclerosis-like disorders. Int J Dermatol 1985;24:147–151.

98. Silman AJ, Jones S. What is the contribution of occupational environmental factors to the occurrence of scleroderma in men? Ann Rheum Dis 1992;51:1322–1324.

99. Erasmus LD. Scleroderma in gold miners on the Witzwaterzrand with particular reference to pulmonary manifestations. S Afr J Lab Clin Med 1957;3:209–231.

100. Bernstein R, Prinsloo I, Zwi S, Andrew MJA, Dawson B, et al. Chromosomal aberrations in occupational-associated progressive systemic sclerosis. S Afr Med J 1980;58:235–237.

101. Cowie RL. Silica dust exposed mine workers with scleroderma (systemic sclerosis). Chest 1987;92:260.

102. Bramwell B. Diffuse scleroderma: Its frequency, its occurrence in stone masons, its treatment by fibrolysin-elevations of temperature due to fibrolysin injections. Edinburgh Med J 1914;12:387.

103. Rodnan GP, Benedek TG, Medsger TA, Cammaratta RJ. The association of progressive systemic sclerosis (scleroderma) with coal miners pneumoconiosis and other forms of silicosis. Ann Intern Med 1967;66:323–334.

104. Christy WC, Rodnan GP. Conjugal progressive systemic sclerosis (scleroderma): Report of the disease in husband and wife. Arthritis Rheum 1984;27:1180–1182.

105. Mehlhorn VJ, Gerloach CH, Ziegler V. Occupational progressive systemic sclerosis through scouring powder. Dermatosen 1990;38:180–185.

106. Walder BK. Solvents and scleroderma. Lancet 1965;2:436–437.

107. Walder BK. Do solvents cause scleroderma? Int Soc Trop Dermatol 1983;22:157–158.

108. Czirjak L, Katalin D, Schlammadinger J, Suranyi P, Tamasi L, Szegedi GY. Progressive systemic sclerosis occurring in patients exposed to chemicals. Int J Dermatol 1987;26:374.

109. Sparrow GP. A connective tissue disorder similar to vinyl chloride disease in a patient exposed to perchlorethylene. Clin Dermatol 1977;2:17–22.

110. Reinl W. Sclerodermic durch trichlorethylen (trans). Bull Hygiene 1957;32:678.

111. Saihan EM, Burton JL, Heaton KW. A new syndrome with pigmentation, scleroderma, gynaecomastia, Raynauds and peripheral neuropathy. Br J Dermatol 1978;99:437.

112. Lockey JE, Kelley CR, Cannon GW, et al. Progressive systemic sclerosis associated with exposure to trichloroethylene. J Occup Med 1987;29:493.

113. Veltman C, Lange CE, Juhe S, Stein G, Bachner V. Clinical manifestations and course of vinyl chloride disease. Ann NY Acad Sci 1975;246:6–17.

114. Yamakage A, Ishikawa H, Saito Y, et al. Occupational scleroderma-like disorders occurring in men engaged in the polymerization of epoxy resins. Dermatologica 1980;161:33–44.

115. Owens GR, Medsger TA. Systemic scleroderma secondary to occupational exposure. Am J Med 1988;85:114–116.

116. Rush PJ, Chaiton A. Scleroderma, renal failure and death associated with exposure to urea formaldehyde foam insulation. J Rheumatol 1986;13: 2:475.

117. Silman AJ, Jones S. Pet ownership: A possible risk factor for scleroderma. Br J Rheumatol 1990;29: 494.

118. Raynaud M. De l'asphyxic locale et de la gangrene symetrique des extremities. Paris, Rignoux, 1862. See selected monographs for translation, 1888.

119. Wigley FM. Raynaud's phenomenon. Curr Opin Rheumatol 1993;5:773–784.

120. Maricq HR, Weinrich MC. Diagnosis of Raynaud's phenomenon assisted by color charts. J Rheumatol 1988;15:454–459.

121. O'Keeffe ST, Tsapatsaris P, Beetham WP. Color chart assisted diagnosis of Raynaud's phenomenon in an unselected hospital employee population. J Rheumatol 1992;19:1415–1417.

122. Brennan P, Silman A, Black C, Bernstein R, Coppock J, Maddospm P, Sheeran T, et al. Validity and reliability of three methods used in the diagnosis of Raynaud's Phenomenon. Br Soc Rheumatol 1993;32:357–361.

123. Kallenberg CGM, Wouda AA, Hauw T. Systemic involvement in immunologic findings in patients presenting with Raynaud's phenomenon. Am J Med 1980;69:675–680.

124. Kallenberg CGM, Wouda AA, Hoet MH, van Venrooij WJ. Development of connective tissue disease in patients presenting with Raynaud's phenomenon: A six year follow up with emphasis on the predictive value. Ann Rheum Dis 1988;46:634–641.

125. LeRoy EC, Medsger TA. Raynaud's phenomenon: A proposal for classification. Clin Exp Rheumatol 1992;10:485–488.

126. Allen EV, Brown GE. Raynaud's disease: A critical review of minimal requisites for diagnosis. Am J Med Sci 1932;183:187–200.

127. Planchon B, Pistorius M-A, Beurrier P, De Faucal P. Primary Raynaud's phenomenon. Age of onset and pathogenesis in a prospective study of 424 patients. Angiology J Vasc Dis 1994;45:677–686.

128. Maricq HR, Carpentier PH, Weinrich MC, Keil JE, Franco A, Drouet P, Poncot OCM, et al. Geographic variation in the prevalence of Raynaud's phenomenon: Charleston, SC, USA, vs Tarentaise, Savoie, France. J Rheumatol 1993;20:70–76.

129. Silman AJ, Holligan S, Brennan P, Maddison P. Prevalence of symptoms of Raynaud's phenomenon in general practice. Br Med J 1990;301:590–592.

130. Bosmanski K, Zitnan D, Urbanek T, Svec U. Incidence of diffuse disorders of the connective tissue with special reference to systemic lupus erythematosus in a selected district in the years 1961–1969. Fysiatr Reumatol Vestn 1971;49:267–272.

131. Asboe-Hansen G. Epidemiology of systemic sclerosis in Denmark. In: Black CM, Myers AR, eds. Systemic sclerosis (scleroderma). New York: Gower, 1985.

132. Whiteside TL, Medsger Jr TA, Rodnan GP. Studies of the HLA antigens in systemic sclerosis. In: Black CM, Myers AR, eds. Systemic sclerosis (scleroderma). New York: Gower, 1985.

133. Steen VD, Powell DL, Medsger Jr TA. Clinical correlations and prognosis based on serum autoantibodies in patients with systemic sclerosis. Arthritis Rheum 1988;31:196–203.

134. Genth E, Mierau R, Genetsky P, et al. Immunogenetics associations of scleroderma-related antinuclear antibodies. Arthritis Rheum 1990;33: 657–665.

135. Kondo H, Yoshii M, Kashiwazaki S, et al. Histocompatibility antigens in progressive systemic sclerosis. In: Black DM, Myers AR, eds. Systemic sclerosis (scleroderma). New York: Gower, 1985.

136. Sasaki T, Denpo K, Ono H, Nakajima J. HLA in systemic scleroderma (PSS) and familial scleroderma. J Dermatol 1991;18:18–24.

137. Myers AR, Briggs DC, Black CM, et al. Class II major histocompatibility complex antigens and pulmonary fibrosis in systemic sclerosis. Arthritis Rheum 1989;32(Suppl):S77.

138. Barnett AJ, Tait BD, Barnett MA, Toh BH. T-lymphocyte subset abnormalities and HLA antigens in scleroderma (systemic sclerosis). Clin Exp Immunol 1989;76:24–29.

139. Dunckley H, Jazwinska EC, Gatenby PA, Serjeatson SW. DNA DR-typing shows HL-DRw11

RFLPs are increased in frequency in both progressive systemic sclerosis and CREST variants of scleroderma. Tissue Antigens 1989;33:418–420.

140. Jazwinska EC, Olive C, Dunckley H, et al. HLA-DRw15 is increased in frequency in Japanese scleroderma patients. Dis Markers 1990;8:323-3-26.

141. Giordano M, Valentini G, Luroli S, Giordano A. Pregnancy and systemic sclerosis (letter). Arthritis Rheum 1985b;28:237–238.

142. McHugh NJ, Reilly PA, McHugh LA. Pregnancy outcome and autoantibodies in connective tissue disease. J Rhematol 1989;16:43–46.

143. Lewis T, Pickering GW. Observations upon maladies in which the blood supply to digits ceases intermittently or permanently, and upon bilateral gangrene of digits: observations relevant to so-called "Raynaud's phenomenon." Clin Sci 1933;1:327.

144. Fessel WJ. Rheumatology for clinicians. New York: Stratton, 1975:214.

145. Olsen N, Nielson SL. Prevalence of primary Raynaud's phenomenon in young females. Scand J Clin Lab Invest 1978;38:761–764.

146. Heslop J, Coggon D, Acheson ED. The prevalence of intermittent digital ischemia (Raynaud's phenomenon) in a general practice. J R Coll Gen Pract 1983;33:85–89.

147. Maricq HR, Weinrich MC, Keil JE, LeRoy EC. Prevalence of Raynaud phenomenon in the general population. A preliminary study by questionnaire. J Chronic Dis 1986;39:423–427.

148. Leppert J, Aberg H, Ringqvist I, Sorensson S. Raynaud's phenomenon in a female population: Prevalence and association with other conditions. Angiology 1987;38:871–877.

149. Weinrich MC, Maricq HR, Keil JE, McGregor AR, Diat F. Prevalence of Raynaud's phenomenon in the adult population of South Carolina. J Clin Epidemiol 1990;43:1343–1349.

150. Harada N, Ueda A, Takegata S. Prevalence of Raynaud's phenomenon in Japanese males and females. J Clin Epidemiol 1991;44:649–655.

151. Bartelink ML, Wollersheim H, van de Lisdounk E, Spuijt R, van Weel C. Prevalence of Raynaud's phenomenon. Neth J Med 1992;41:149–152.

152. Riera G, Vilardell M, Vaque J, Fonollosa V, Bermejo B. Prevalence of Raynaud's phenomenon in a healthy Spanish population. J Rheumatol 1993;20:66–69.

153. Inaba R, Maeda M, Fujita S, Kashiki N, et al. Prevalence of Raynaud's phenomenon and specific clinical signs related to progressive systemic sclerosis in the general population of Japan. Int J Dermatol 1993;32:652–655.

THOMAS A. MEDSGER, JR.
VIRGINIA D. STEEN

3

Classification, Prognosis

Classification

PURPOSES OF DISEASE CLASSIFICATION

Disease classification criteria are used to establish, with reasonable certainty, that a group of patients has a particular disorder and to compare those patients directly with other case series in the medical literature (1). Systemic sclerosis (SSc) is a particularly challenging problem for classification, because it includes a very broad spectrum of disease.

CLASSIFICATION CRITERIA

Preliminary criteria for SSc were developed during the Scleroderma Criteria Cooperative Study (SCCS), which was a multicenter prospective study of 264 scleroderma patients and more than 400 comparison patients. These criteria were published in 1980 (2) (Table 3.1). Comparison groups included systemic lupus erythematosus (SLE), polymyositis-dermatomyositis (PM-DM), and Raynaud's disease. All patients were evaluated within 2 years of first diagnosis, and the diagnosis was confirmed 2 years after entry. Only 12 patients (1.5%) were excluded because of a subsequent change in diagnosis.

The major criterion for definite SSc was skin thickening proximal to the metacarpophalangeal joints. Minor criteria were also proposed (see Table 3.1). These criteria had a 97% sensitivity and 98% specificity. They clearly point out that skin thickening is distinctive for SSc, occurring

rarely in comparison patients with SLE or polymyositis. An important limitation of these criteria is that they do not perform as well in patients with SSc and limited cutaneous involvement (CREST syndrome). In retrospect, most of the patients entered by SCCS center physicians had diffuse cutaneous involvement. Thus, the final criteria serve best to differentiate diffuse but not limited disease from the comparison conditions. In one series, 24 (15%) of 164 consecutive scleroderma patients, all with "complete" CREST syndrome, failed to satisfy the 1980 criteria (3). Among 1500 University of Pittsburgh patients evaluated between 1972 and 1993, excluding those with scleroderma in overlap, 68 (5%) have not satisfied SCCS criteria even after a mean follow-up of 2 years. An important goal for future revisions of these classification criteria should be the inclusion of patients who have limited or no skin thickening (systemic sclerosis *sine* scleroderma).

The converse is the issue of how often patients with SSc satisfy published classification or diagnostic criteria for other connective tissue diseases such as SLE or PM-DM. This question has not been formally addressed in any literature reports. Using the University of Pittsburgh computer data base, we found that 87 of 1499 (6%) definite SSc patients, excluding those diagnosed with overlap syndromes, satisfied the 1982 revised American College of Rheumatology (ACR) classification criteria for SLE (4). This relatively high proportion is in part attributable to the high frequency of serositis (39%), joint findings (66%),

Table 3.1. Numbers of Patients Who Satisfied Either Major or Minor Criteria for Systemic Sclerosis Grouped According to the Committee's Diagnostic Categories

	Systemic Sclerosis		Comparison Patients		
	Definite N = 264	Probable N = 35	SLE N = 172	PM/DM N = 120	Raynaud's N = 121
Major criterion					
Proximal scleroderma	239	18	1	0	0
Minor criteria[a]	(25)	(17)	(171)	(120)	(121)
Sclerodactyly	19	8	1	4	11
Digital pitting scars	15	7	15	8	18
Bibasilar pulmonary fibrosis	8	1	11	22	3
Two or more minor criteria	17	4	0	3	6
Proposed criteria satisfied	256	22	1	3	6
(percent)	(97%)	(63%)	(1%)	(3%)	(5%)

[a]Applies to the number of patients who did not satisfy the major criterion, as shown in parentheses.

and positive antinuclear antibodies (ANAs) (89%) in the SSc patients. Twenty-three (1.3%) of these SSc patients satisfied the Bohan and Peter diagnostic criteria for definite PM-DM (5). Almost all patients who satisfy two or more of these three criteria sets would be considered to have SSc "in overlap."

CLASSIFICATION BASED ON CLINICAL AND LABORATORY FEATURES

The most widely accepted subsets of SSc, based on clinical and laboratory features, are diffuse cutaneous (dcSSC) and limited (or absent) cutaneous disease (lcSSc). A patient with skin thickening proximal to the elbow and knee (i.e., affecting the upper arms, thighs, and/or trunk) is considered to have diffuse disease. However, this subset distinction also depends on other important findings, which have been summarized in an editorial co-authored by several well-recognized experts (6) (Table 3.2). A rapid pace of skin thickening (reaching the forearm within several months) occurs in diffuse involvement but not in limited cutaneous involvement. The latter group most typically still has sclerodactyly after 5 to 10 years. These guidelines are not mutually exclusive, leaving some patients difficult to classify with confidence.

Several attempts have been made to create a classification with three (7) or even four (8) clinical subsets. The proposed "intermediate" categories are not convincing, because the patients included have no distinctive clinical, laboratory, or serologic features.

CLASSIFICATION BASED ON SERUM AUTOANTIBODIES

Two major serum autoantibodies in SSc patients have been recognized since 1980: anticentromere and anti-topoisomerase I antibodies. Anti-topoisomerase I is specific to SSc; two-thirds of patients with this autoantibody have diffuse skin involvement and pulmonary interstitial fibrosis (9). Antibody reactivity to epitope region (ER) 4 on the topoisomerase I molecule greatly increases the risk of diffuse cutaneous disease, pulmonary fibrosis, and reduced survival (10). Anticentromere antibody is present primarily in patients with limited cutaneous SSc (lcSSc). These patients have a low frequency of heart, lung, and renal disease, although the serious complication of pulmonary arterial hypertension (without fibrosis) occurs in up to 20% of this subgroup (11). Anti-U1 ribonucleoprotein (RNP) antibody classically has been associated with SSc in overlap with lupus and/or polymyositis—so-

Table 3.2. Subsets of Systemic Sclerosis (SSc)

Diffuse Cutaneous SSc (DSSc)[a]

Onset of Raynaud's within 1 year of skin changes
   (puffy or hidebound)
Truncal and acral skin involvement
Presence of tendon friction rubs
Early and significant incidence of interstitial lung disease,
   oliguric renal failure, diffuse gastrointestinal disease, and
   myocardial invcolvement
Absence of anticentromere antibodies (ACA)
Nailfold capillary dilatation and capillary destruction[b]
Antitopoisomerase antibodies (30% of patients)

Limited Cutaneous SSc (LSSc)

Raynaud's for years (occasionally decades)
Skin involvement limited to hands, face, feet and forearms
   (acral) or absent
A significant late incidence of pulmonary hypertension,
   with or without interstitial lung disease, trigeminal
   neuralgia, skin calcifications, telangiectasia
A high incidence of ACA (70–80%)
Dilated nailfold capillary loops, usually without capillary
   dropout[b]

[a]Experienced observers note some patients with dSSc who do not develop organ insufficiency and suggest the term chronic dSSc for these patients.
[b]Nailfold capillary dilation and destruction may also be seen in patients with dermatomyositis, overlap syndromes, and undifferentiated connective tissue disease. These syndromes may be considered as part of the spectrum of scleroderma-associated disorders.

called "mixed connective tissue disease" (MCTD) (12). Features not usually found in SSc but linked to U1RNP are rheumatoid-like inflammatory polyarthritis, leukopenia, and trigeminal neuropathy (13).

SSc patients' sera have been shown to contain other ANAs, most often with nucleolar staining patterns on immunofluorescence testing. Well-characterized nucleolar antigens to which these antibodies are directed include Th RNP, fibrillarin (U3RNP), and PM-Scl. Anti-Th RNP antibody is relatively specific to lcSSc, but its usefulness as a marker for more serious visceral complications is unclear (14). Anti-fibrillarin antibody has a high frequency among African-Americans with SSc and is associated with skeletal muscle disease and pulmonary arterial hypertension (15). Anti-PM-Scl antibody identifies a subset of patients with a high prevalence of skeletal myositis (16). Antibodies to the RNA poly-

merase complex enzymes (RNA polymerase I, II, and III) have nucleolar and/or speckled nuclear staining and are specific for SSc. Compared with antitopoisomerase I, the anti-RNA polymerase antibodies identify a higher proportion of individuals with diffuse cutaneous disease, increased skin thickness, and renal involvement, and a lower proportion with lung and skeletal muscle disease (17,18). In our experience, the seven autoantibodies described in this section identify nearly 90% of all SSc patients (Fig. 3.1).

Future classification schemes must include all of the clinically distinctive and pathophysiologically meaningful subsets of SSc patients currently recognized. In addition to the obvious cutaneous features, other clinical and immunologic data should be considered in such analyses. It is hoped that classification research will lead to more accurate patient subgrouping, which will in turn facilitate the conduct of both laboratory investigations and therapeutic intervention trials (1,19).

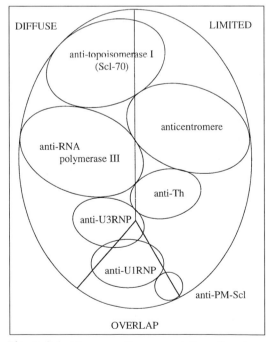

Figure 3.1. Diagrammatic representation of serologic subsets in systemic sclerosis.

Prognosis

PROBLEMS IN DETERMINING OUTCOME

Estimating outcome in SSc is particularly difficult for several reasons (20,21). First, SSc is a disorder of remarkable clinical heterogeneity. Today, most patients should be correctly classified as having diffuse or limited cutaneous involvement (see previous discussion under *Classification*), but additional variants not yet described are likely to exist. Although most rheumatologists understand the differences between disease subsets, other primary care physicians are not so aware of these important distinctions. Unfortunately, many earlier treatment studies (22–25) included combinations of patients with various subtypes and stages of disease without stratification. Thus, it is often very difficult or impossible to interpret the results of these trials. The differences in natural history of disease in these patient subsets have major implications for prognosis, patient and family education, anticipating future complications, and monitoring and treating patients.

The second reason for the difficulty in estimating the outcome of SSc is a lack of standardized terminology for organ system involvement. Scleroderma lung disease is defined by some investigators as pleural thickening on chest roentgenogram, reduced vital capacity, reduced diffusing capacity for carbon monoxide (DLCO), or bibasilar rales on physical examination, while other authors require dyspnea on exertion and pulmonary fibrosis on chest roentgenogram. Different definitions may make the results of two studies difficult to compare. In the circumstance where heavy emphasis is placed on patients' symptoms, such as the frequency and severity of Raynaud's phenomenon (RP), more objective methods of measurement are needed. The psychological status of the patient and a prominent placebo effect in therapy trials must be considered. Most importantly, we need to be precise in defining all outcome measurements and prognostic terms.

A third problem is that there are no standardized, widely accepted methods to measure "disease stage" or "disease activity." If generally accepted definitions of stage and activity could be developed, clinical research studies and therapeutic trials would be comparable and prognostic information would be more meaningful. Basic research to identify pathogenic mechanisms of scleroderma also would benefit from such precise definitions. An attempt to develop an SSc severity index has been initiated recently (26).

Fourth, studies in SSc must be of adequate size and duration to answer important outcome questions. Cross-sectional reports are inferior to those of longitudinal design. The latter typically require 2 years of observation for clinical endpoints and 4 years for survival outcome. Multicenter efforts are often necessary to locate adequate numbers of patients with the desired variants and stages of disease.

NATURAL HISTORY OF DISEASE

The natural history of SSc is best understood by reviewing the two major variants and their early and late stages (Fig. 3.2). For this purpose, we have arbitrarily defined early (<3 years) and late (6+ years) for diffuse cutaneous SSc and early (<5 years) and late (10+ years) for limited cutaneous SSc, both measured from the time of the first symptom attributable to SSc (see Tables 3.3 and 3.4).

Early Diffuse Cutaneous Disease

Patients with early diffuse scleroderma are sometimes difficult to diagnose. They often have fatigue, arthralgias, carpal tunnel syndrome, puffy fingers, swollen feet and legs, and a positive serum ANA test prior to developing RP or skin thickening (see Table 3.2). Helpful clues at this point, when the diagnosis is not clear, include capillary dropout on nailfold microscopy (27), the presence of palpable tendon friction rubs, and serum anti-topoisomerase I antibody (9). After this prodromal phase, there is most often a rapid progression of the disease. Sclerodactyly

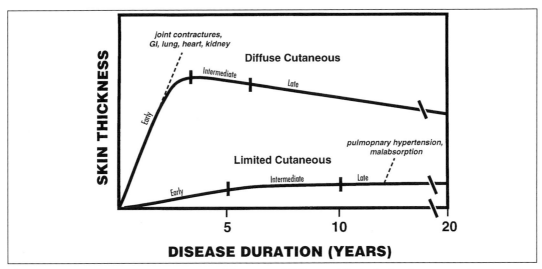

Figure 3.2. Diagrammatic representation of the stages of diffuse and limited scleroderma over time, including the typical relationships between skin thickness and selected organ system involvements.

begins first, but within 6 to 12 months skin thickening progresses proximally on the arms and legs, sometimes but not always affecting the trunk. Arthralgias, alone or with true synovitis in a rheumatoid distribution, are common in early diffuse scleroderma. Tendon friction rubs (resulting from fibrous tenosynovitis), which may be painful or asymptomatic, are most commonly palpated in the palms, wrists, and ankles. The combination of accelerated skin thickening, tendon, and joint involvement often leads to severe contractures with marked decrease in function within the first 12 months after disease onset. RP may result in fingertip ulcerations, while ulcers found over the dorsal surface of the proximal interphalangeal joints are more likely caused by a combination of flexion contractures, skin stretching and thinning, trauma, and circulatory insufficiency. Muscle involvement, either inflammatory or non-inflammatory, can cause proximal muscle atrophy and weakness.

Visceral changes are frequent in early diffuse scleroderma. Figure 3.3 graphically displays the onset of visceral disease in relation to time after disease onset. Gastrointestinal involvement, particularly esophageal dysmotility, is present in 50% of patients at the time of initial evaluation

and occurs in some individuals with no complaints of dysphagia or heartburn. More severe small intestinal hypomotility may develop later but is uncommon. Pulmonary interstitial changes are also frequent in early diffuse disease (approximately 50%). In some patients, a mononuclear cell inflammatory component has been identified by bronchoalveolar lavage (28,29). A rapid decline in forced vital capacity suggests severe and progressive interstitial lung disease. Subclinical evidence of heart disease (from electrocardiogram, echocardiogram, or thallium perfusion scan) is more common than symptomatic heart disease (30). The latter occurs in less than 10% of patients with diffuse skin thickening. The most dramatic complication of early diffuse cutaneous disease is renal involvement with malignant arterial hypertension, so-called "scleroderma renal crisis." Eighty percent of patients with renal crisis develop this condition during the first 4 years of the illness (31).

Late Diffuse Cutaneous Disease

We consider the change from early to late diffuse disease to occur when skin thickening has passed its peak extent and severity and has begun to regress. Worsening of skin thickening in the late

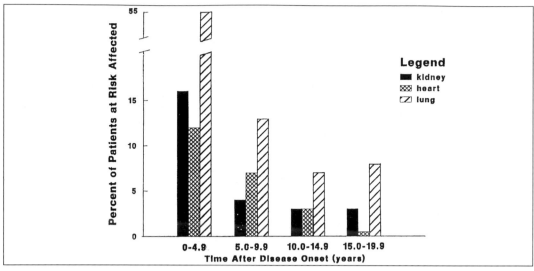

Figure 3.3. Timing of internal organ involvement during course of disease in 560 patients with diffuse sclero-derma.

stage of diffuse scleroderma is uncommon. Cutaneous improvement almost always begins in areas that have been affected last, i.e., anterior chest, abdomen, and upper arms. Once diminished proximal skin thickening is obvious (32), arthralgias and tendon rubs also decrease, allowing patients to be more functional. Unfortunately, hand and digital contractures that occurred early in the disease most often cannot be reversed (Table 3.3). However, systemic features, such as fatigue, frequently subside and renewed energy and sense of well-being return.

After several years, telangiectasias and calcinosis may appear and be indistinguishable from such findings in patients with limited scleroderma. Considering these late findings and the regression of cutaneous changes, which is often dramatic leaving only residual sclerodactyly, late stage diffuse disease can be misdiagnosed as limited disease. The presence of severe hand contractures and one of the serum autoantibodies characteristic of diffuse disease suggest that such patients initially had the diffuse cutaneous variant.

Although the fibrotic process in internal organs evident earlier in the disease may continue to progress slowly, it is unusual for there to be new visceral involvement after peak skin thickening. In late stages, complications result from fibrotic and atrophic changes rather than inflammatory events. The gastrointestinal problems include a flaccid, atonic esophagus or esophageal stricture and small intestinal hypomotility, which may result in malabsorption. If pulmonary fibrosis is present, it is typically benign, producing no symptoms or only mild dyspnea on exertion. In this stage, pulmonary function deterioration, if it occurs, is slow, although smokers may experience more accelerated functional loss (33,34). In some cases, pulmonary insufficiency not evident in early disease supervenes, resulting in respiratory failure. Secondary pulmonary hypertension with cor pulmonale and death caused by bacterial pneumonia, hypoxia, or arrhythmia are common in this circumstance.

Heart disease is the least predictable of the visceral involvements during late stage diffuse scleroderma. Thallium perfusion scan defects, decreased left ventricular function, conduction disturbances, electrocardiographic abnormalities, or echocardiographic evidence of pericardial effusion can be seen in patients with either early or late disease (35–37). The abnormalities found during early disease may persist asymptomatically without progression or evolve to serious left ventricular dysfunction, life-threatening arrhythmia, or, rarely, pericardial tamponade. Both ventricular ectopy and supraventricular tachycardia are associated with increased mortality (38).

As noted in previous paragraphs, only a few episodes of renal crisis occur in late diffuse cutaneous disease. Some investigators believe that mild hypertension, proteinuria, or azotemia developing at any time during the course of scleroderma represent evidence of "scleroderma kidney" (39,40). Our experience suggests that only a small proportion of diffuse disease patients (<4%) have unexplained azotemia or proteinuria, and that these patients do not subsequently develop end-stage renal disease (41).

Early Limited Cutaneous Disease

Detailed information on early limited cutaneous involvement is relatively unavailable because people with this condition often do not seek medical attention. Patients with limited scleroderma most often have RP, with or without digital tip ulcerations, for years (often 1 or more decades) before other clinical manifestations of SSc appear (Table 3.4). Next, they typically experience mild digital puffiness or heartburn, which may be the reason for seeking medical attention. Excessive fatigue and severe arthralgias are unusual, and true synovitis and tendon friction rubs are rare. Calcinosis and telangiectasias, which are considered classic markers of this variant (often termed CREST syndrome), often require years or even decades to develop and thus cannot be relied on to assist in classification during this early stage. The presence of skin thickening restricted to distal extremities (fingers, hands, distal forearms) for several years and the presence of serum anticentromere antibody are strong clues to classification as the limited cutaneous variant. Gastrointestinal symptoms and objective findings are frequent and indistinguishable from those encountered in diffuse disease. Pulmonary interstitial fibrosis is also similar in type to that seen in diffuse disease but is far less common, perhaps because of an apparent "protective" effect of anticentromere antibody (42). Myocardial and renal scleroderma are rare in the limited cutaneous subtype (see Fig. 3.3).

Late Limited Cutaneous Disease

In late stage limited cutaneous involvement, skin changes remain stable. The most remarkable finding is an increase in the number of mat-like

Table 3.3. Clinical Characterisitics of University of Pittsburgh Patients with Diffuse Cutaneous Scleroderma with Early Disease (Less than 3 Years of Symptoms) and Late Disease (More than 6 Years of Symptoms)

	Early (<3 years) (n = 425)	Late (6+ years) (n = 319)	Significance
Symptom duration (years)	2.2	12.0	$P < .001$
Fatigue	83%	71%	$P < .01$
Arthralgias	52%	49%	
Puffy fingers	58%	35%	$P < .0001$
Tendon friction rubs	67%	27%	$P < .0001$
Carpal tunnel	27%	10%	$P < .01$
Joint contractures	88%	93%	
Muscle weakness	39%	50%	$P < .01$
Raynaud's phenomenon	89%	94%	
Digital ulcers	22%	47%	$P < .0001$
Total skin thickness score	40	28	$P < .001$
Calcinosis	10%	53%	$P < .0001$
Telangiectasias	51%	82%	$P < .0001$

Table 3.4. Clinical Characterisitics of Patients with Limited Cutaneous Scleroderma with Early Disease (Less than 5 Years of Symptoms) and Late Disease (More than 10 Years of Symptoms)

	Early (<5 years) (n = 175)	Late (10+ years) (n = 417)	Significance
Symptom duration (years)	3.7	22.0	$P < .001$
Fatigue	69%	74%	
Arthralgias	32%	40%	
Puffy fingers	69%	63%	
Tendon friction rubs	5%	8%	
Carpal tunnel syndrome	19%	16%	
Joint contractures	47%	60%	$P < .01$
Muscle weakness	23%	44%	$P < .0001$
Raynaud's phenomenon	91%	98%	$P < .01$
Digital ulcers	24%	43%	$P < .0001$
Total skin thickness score	6	9	
Calcinosis	28%	59%	$P < .001$
Telangiectasias	75%	93%	$P < .001$

telangiectasias (more than 90% of patients), especially on the fingers, lips, and face, and the appearance of subcutaneous calcinosis affecting the fingers, forearms (elbows), and knees (more than 50% of patients) (see Table 3.4). Digital tip ischemia may lead to ulcerations or gangrene with secondary bacterial infection. The occurrence of inflammatory ulcerative calcinosis or digital ischemic ulcers with secondary bacterial infection at these sites may result in significant disability.

In this late stage, esophageal reflux and stricture are frequently severe. Although far less common, small bowel malabsorption with recurrent episodes of pseudo-obstruction may progress and become life-threatening. Pulmonary interstitial fibrosis may be present and progressive, but clinically meaningful myocardial and/or renal involvement are rare in this type and stage of disease.

The most serious problem in late limited scleroderma is the development of pulmonary arterial hypertension, which is uniformly fatal. This complication typically occurs many years after the onset of RP, most often in patients who have had few other scleroderma problems (43). Rapid progression of dyspnea over the course of several months is the most frequent initial symptom.

Once hypoxemia and/or secondary right heart failure develop, the mean survival is less than 2 years. If a scleroderma patient has MCTD clinical features with serum anti-U1RNP antibody, pulmonary arterial vasculitis may be detected (44). However, in typical uncomplicated scleroderma, there is non-inflammatory subintimal proliferation of small and medium-sized pulmonary arteries without significant interstitial fibrosis (45). Another problem that can occur in late limited disease is vasculitis affecting the skin (palpable purpura) and peripheral nervous system (sensory neuropathy or mononeuritis multiplex). This complication has been observed to be associated with Sjögren's syndrome (46).

MORTALITY AND SURVIVAL

For the total United States population, age-adjusted mortality for scleroderma has increased significantly, from 2.68 per million in 1969 to 3.08 per million in 1977, with rates for women being twice those for men (47). Similar results have been reported in England and Wales during 1968–1985, where the crude female to male ratio was more than 4:1 (48). It is most likely that increased physician awareness and more accurate coding of death certificates account for such trends, but other factors may contribute, including a true increase in disease incidence in these populations. African-American females have more severe SSc; mortality studies in the United States have shown a two- to three-fold increased average annual age-adjusted mortality in African-American females compared with Caucasian females (47,49). In one of these reports, mortality rates peaked earlier among African-Americans (age range 45–64) than among Caucasians (age range 55–74) (47).

Survival in SSc is variable, but a number of factors identified at the time of first evaluation have been confirmed to be adverse prognostic features by most investigators who have studied patients during the past 50 years (50). A comprehensive summary of the results of studies including more than 2,000 patients has been published, and ten of these reports are summarized in Table 3-5 (21,51–59). Although criteria for inclusion of patients and starting times varied somewhat, cumulative survival rates using the life-table method for populations including all ages and both males and females were typically 60% to 70% at 5 years and 40% to 50% at 10 years after first physician diagnosis or after enrolling at a medical center. Patients older than 40 to 50 years at diagnosis had significantly reduced survival in most reports, men had worse survival than women in three publications, and in two series African-Americans had reduced survival, especially during the first 6 to 12 months. There was nearly uniform agreement that skin thickening affecting the trunk carried a poor prognosis, primarily because of its high correlation with serious visceral disease (60). Involvement of the kidney, heart, and lung at entry or during the course of the illness were also significantly associated with poor survival. For patients in whom these three internal organs were not affected at entry, other factors predicting death included elevated erythrocyte sedimentation rate, anemia, proteinuria, hypoproteinemia, heavy alcohol use (Caucasians only), and heavy cigarette use (first year only).

It is important to separate patients into diffuse and limited cutaneous disease categories for purposes of survival analysis. This has been done by several investigators (8,61,62) with the expected result of better survival in patients with limited skin involvement. Interestingly, within these subgroups the presence of serum anticentromere or antitopoisomerase I antibody did not influence survival (62).

The most striking success in therapeutic intervention for SSc in recent decades has been for "renal crisis." In the 1970s, with the advent of more potent antihypertensive agents, dialysis, and renal transplantation, some patients survived this complication, which previously had been uniformly fatal (63). After 1980, angiotensin converting enzyme (ACE) inhibitors became widely available and resulted in a dramatic increase in survival of renal crisis patients (64). The 1-year cumulative survival rate has improved from 20% before the widespread availability of ACE inhibitors to 68% after the routine use of these drugs (65).

In our experience, the overall 10-year cumulative survival from first physician diagnosis during 1980–1989 was 62%: 56% in diffuse cutaneous involvement and 69% in limited cutaneous involvement. It is likely that studies performed during the 1990s will demonstrate even better outcome. Earlier diagnosis, inclusion of mild cases, better overall medical care, and such life-saving interventions as the use of ACE inhibitors in "renal crisis" should account for improved prognosis.

The causes of death in SSc according to disease subset and stage have changed over the past 20 years (Table 3.6). In our referral series, scleroderma-related kidney, heart, and lung involvement are the leading causes of death in early diffuse disease, while pulmonary arterial hypertension and non-sclerodermatous causes are most prevalent in the late limited cutaneous involvement variant. Today, pulmonary interstitial fibrosis has replaced "scleroderma renal crisis" as the single most frequent cause of death.

Table 3.5. Selected Survival Studies in Systemic Sclerosis[a]

Reference	Number of Patients	Cumulative Survival (Life-Table Method)		Early Factors or Organ Involvements Significantly Associated with Poor Survival		
		5 yr	10 yr	Demographic	Clinical	Laboratory
Farmer (1960) (51)	236		51[b]	Age > 40	Heart Kidney Trunk skin	ESR > 50 mm/h (Westergren) Anemia
Tuffanelli (1962) (52)	727	70+	59		Trunk skin	
Bennett (1971) (53)	67	73	40	Age > 40	Lung Trunk skin	BUN > 40 mg/dl ECG abnormal
Medsger (1971) (54)	309	60	35	Age > 45 Males African-Americans	Lung Heart Kidney	
Medsger (1973) (55)	358	44		Age > 50 African-Americans Heavy alcohol and cigarette use	Lung Heart Kidney	ESR > 32 mm/h Anemia Proterinuria
Barnett (1978) (56)	113	70	55	Age > 40 Males	Heart Kidney Trunk skin	
Eason (1981) (57)	47	60	42	Lung Heart Kidney Non-CRST		
Wynn (1985) (58)	64	69	51	Age > 50	S3 gallop Corticosteroid use Trunk skin	
Giordano (1986) (8)	90	72	32			
Altman (1991) (59)	264	63	42	Age > 64	Kidney Heart Lung Intestine	Anemia Serum protein ≤ 6 g/dl

[a]Modified from reference 21 and reprinted by permission of the publisher
[b]Percentage of patients alive (years of follow-up)

Table 3.6. Causes of Death in Patients in the University of Pittsburgh Scleroderma Data Base Decreased during 1970–1989

Causes of Death	1970–1979[a] (n = 125)	1980–1989[a] (n = 339)
Scleroderma	83 (66%)	176 (52%)
Kidney	34 (27%)	41 (12%)
Heart	12 (10%)	29 (9%)
Lung:Fibrosis	5 (4%)	30 (9%)
Lung: Pulmonary Hypertension	15 (12%)	40 (12%)
GI Tract	15 (12%)	24 (7%)
Other	2 (2%)	12 (4%)
Non-Scleroderma	36 (29%)	149 (44%)
Unknown	6 (5%)	14 (4%)

[a]Based on 463 patients evaluated during 1970–1979 and 1166 patients evaluated during 1980–1989.

MORBIDITY

Important outcomes in addition to survival are morbidity and disability from visceral disease as well as from cutaneous, joint, and tendon involvement. Functional assessments have documented marked deficits in the ability to perform activities of daily living (66,67). Using the Health Assessment Questionnaire (HAQ), we found a mean disability index of 1.02 for patients with diffuse cutaneous involvement and 0.67 for those with the limited cutaneous variant (68). Comparable figures are 0.82 for rheumatoid arthritis patients and 0.67 for persons with SLE (69,70). The HAQ disability index scores correlate well with the extent of skin thickening, loss of fist closure, proximal muscle weakness, and tendon friction rubs but not with the presence of digital ulcers. Involvement of the skin, tendons, joints, and vasculature result in the hands being uniformly and often severely affected, but an adequate outcome instrument to measure hand dysfunction in SSc has not been developed to date.

Patient lifestyle, psychosocial, and iatrogenic factors may also play important roles in scleroderma outcomes. Cigarette smoking is recognized to have an adverse influence on RP and pulmonary interstitial fibrosis (34). Predictors of poor psychosocial adjustment to illness in SSc patients include lower formal educational level, more functional disability, illness-related uncertainty, and reduced levels of "hardiness" and satisfaction with social support (71). Nonsteroidal anti-inflammatory drugs, prescribed to ameliorate joint and tendon discomfort, may cause gastritis and exacerbate reflux esophagitis. Calcium channel blocking agents, commonly used in the management of RP, also reduce lower esophageal sphincter pressure, thus potentially aggravating reflux esophagitis and exacerbating small intestinal hypomotility. Corticosteroids are sometimes used to treat the inflammatory phase of early diffuse scleroderma, but it is precisely in these patients that steroids may be implicated in the precipitation of "renal crisis" (72), particularly of the normotensive variety (73). Agents intended to induce remission of early diffuse disease may themselves have serious adverse effects. For example, D-penicillamine, one of the more popular drugs prescribed today, cannot be tolerated by approximately 20% of scleroderma patients (74). Several rare adverse effects of this drug, such as aplastic anemia, pemphigus, nephrotic syndrome, and myasthenia gravis, may be debilitating but are rarely either persistent or fatal. Immunosuppressive drugs, particularly alkylating agents, have been implicated in the subsequent development of malignancy (75,76), as is the case in other rheumatic diseases (77).

The direct costs of physician visits, medications, laboratory tests, physical and occupational therapy, hospitalizations, and indirect costs of illness (work time lost, help from others) for the scleroderma patient are high. Although no formal studies have been published, we suspect that costs for diffuse scleroderma are considerably greater than those for rheumatoid arthritis during the first 5 years of disease.

References

1. Fries JF, Hochberg M, Medsger TA Jr, Hunder GG, Bombardier C, et al. Criteria for rheumatic disease: Different types and different functions. Arthritis Rheum 1994;37:454–462.

2. Masi AT, Rodnan GP, Medsger TA Jr, Altman R, D'Angelo W, Fries J, LeRoy EC, et al. Preliminary criteria for the classification of systemic sclerosis (scleroderma). Arthritis Rheum 1980;23:581–590.
3. Vayssairat M, Baudot N, Abuaf N, Johanet C. Long-term follow-up study of 184 patients with definite systemic sclerosis: Classification considerations. Clin Rheumatol 1992;11:356–363.
4. Tan EM, Cohen AS, Fries JF, Masi AT, McShane DJ, Rothfield NF, Schaller JG, et al. The 1982 revised criteria for the classification of systemic lupus erythematosus. Arthritis Rheum 1982;25:1271–1277.
5. Bohan A, Peter JB, Bowman RL, Pearson CM. A computer-assisted analysis of 153 patients with polymyositis and dermatomyositis. Medicine (Baltimore) 1977;56:255–286.
6. LeRoy EC, Black C, Fleischmajer R, Jabłónska S, Krieg T, Medsger TA Jr, Rowell N, et al. Scleroderma (systemic sclerosis): Classification, subsets and pathogenesis. J Rheumatol 1988;15:202–205.
7. Masi AT. Classification of systemic sclerosis (scleroderma): Relationship of cutaneous subgroups in early disease to outcome and serologic reactivity. J Rheumatol 1988;15:894–898.
8. Giordano M, Valenti G, Migliaresi S, Picillo U, Vatti M. Different antibody patterns and different prognoses in patients with scleroderma with various extent of skin sclerosis. J Rheumatol 1986;13:911–916.
9. Steen VD, Powell DL, Medsger TA Jr. Clinical correlations and prognosis based on serum autoantibodies in patients with systemic sclerosis. Arthritis Rheum 1988;31:196–203.
10. Kuwana M, Kaburaki J, Mimori T, et al. Autoantigenic epitopes on DNA topoisomerase I: Clinical and immunogenetic associations in systemic sclerosis. Arthritis Rheum 1993;36:1406–1413.
11. Tan EM, Rodnan GP, Garcia I, et al. Diversity of antinuclear antibodies in progressive systemic sclerosis (scleroderma): Anticentromere antibody and its relationship to CREST syndrome. Arthritis Rheum 1980;23:617–625.
12. Sharp GC, et al. Mixed connective tissue disease: An apparently distinct rheumatic disease syndrome associated with a specific antibody to an extractable nuclear antigen (ENA). Am J Med 1972;52:148–159.
13. Farrell DA, Medsger TA Jr. Trigeminal neuropathy in progressive systemic sclerosis. Am J Med 1982;73:57–62.
14. Okano Y, Medsger TA Jr. Autoantibody to Th ribonucleoprotein (nucleolar 7–2 RNA protein particle) in patients with systemic sclerosis (scleroderma). Arthritis Rheum 1990;33:1822–1828.
15. Okano Y, Steen VD, Medsger TA Jr. Autoantibody to U3 nucleolar ribonucleoprotein (fibrillarin) in patients with systemic sclerosis. Arthritis Rheum 1992;35:95–100.
16. Oddis CV, Okano Y, Rudert WA, et al. Serum autoantibody to the nucleolar antigen PM-Scl: Clinical and immunogenetic associations. Arthritis Rheum 1992;35:1211–1217.
17. Okano Y, Steen VD, Medsger TA Jr. Antibody reactive with RNA polymerase III in systemic sclerosis. Ann Intern Med 1993;119:1005–1013.
18. Kuwana M, Kaburaki J, Mimori T, et al. Autoantibody reactive with three classes of RNA polymerases in sera from patients with systemic sclerosis. J Clin Invest 1993;91:1399–1404.
19. Masi AT. Clinical-epidemiological perspective of systemic sclerosis (scleroderma). In: Jayson MIV, Black CM, eds. Systemic sclerosis (scleroderma). Chichester, UK: John Wiley & Sons, Ltd, 1988; 7–31.
20. Medsger TA Jr. Treatment of systemic sclerosis. Rheum Dis Clin North Am 1989;15:513–531.
21. Steen VD, Medsger TA Jr. Systemic sclerosis. In: Bellamy N, ed. Prognosis in the rheumatic diseases. London: Kluwer Academic Publishers, 1991;213–232.
22. Steigerwald JC. Progressive systemic sclerosis: Management. III. Immunosuppressive agents. Clin Rheum Dis 1979;5:289–294.
23. Alarcon-Segovia D. Progressive systemic sclerosis: Management. IV. Colchicine. Clin Rheum Dis 1979;5:294–302.
24. Jayson MIV, Lovell C, Black CM, et al. Penicillamine therapy in systemic sclerosis. Proc R Soc Med 1977;70(suppl 3):82–88.
25. Furst DE, Clements PH, Hillis S, et al. Immunosuppression with chlorambucil vs. placebo for scleroderma: Results of a 3-year parallel, randomized, double-blind study. Arthritis Rheum 1989;32:584–593.
26. Medsger TA Jr, Silman AJ, Steen VD, et al. Development of a severity index for systemic sclerosis. Arthritis Rheum 1994;37(9):S260.
27. Maricq HR, Spencer-Green G, LeRoy EC. Skin capillary abnormalities as indicators of organ involvement in scleroderma (systemic sclerosis). Am J Med 1976;61:862–870.
28. Owens GR, Paradis IL, Gryzan S, et al. The role of inflammation in the lung disease of systemic sclerosis: Comparison with idiopathic pulmonary fibrosis. J Lab Clin Med 1986;107:253–262.
29. Silver RM, Metcalf JF, Stanley JH, et al. Interstitial lung disease in scleroderma: Analysis by bronchoalveolar lavage. Arthritis Rheum 1984;27:1254–1261.
30. Follansbee W. The cardiovascular manifestations of systemic sclerosis (scleroderma). Curr Probl Cardiol 1986;11:242–298.

31. Steen VD, Medsger TA Jr, Osial TA Jr, et al. Factors predicting development of renal involvement in progressive systemic sclerosis. Am J Med 1984;76: 779–786.

32. Black C, Dieppe PK, Huskisson T, et al. Regressive systemic sclerosis. Ann Rheum Dis 1986;45:384–388.

33. Schneider PD, Wise RA, Hochberg MC, et al. Serial pulmonary function in systemic sclerosis. Am J Med 1982;73:385–394.

34. Steen VD, Owens GR, Fino GJ, et al. Pulmonary involvement in systemic sclerosis (scleroderma). Arthritis Rheum 1985;28:759–767.

35. Follansbee WP, Curtiss EI, Rahko PS, et al. The electrocardiogram in systemic sclerosis (scleroderm): A study of 102 consecutive cases with functional correlations and a review of the literature. Am J Med 1985;79:183–192.

36. Smith JW, Clements PJ, Levisman J, et al. Echocardographic features of progressive systemic sclerosis (PSS): Correlation with hemodynamic and post-mortem studies. Am J Med 1979;66:28–33.

37. Follansbee WP, Curtiss EI, Medsger TA Jr, et al. Physiologic abnormalities of cardiac function in progressive systemic sclerosis with diffuse scleroderma. N Engl J Med 1984;310:142–148.

38. Kostis JB, Seibold JR, Turkevich D, et al. The prognostic importance of cardiac arrhythmias in systemic sclerosis. Am J Med 1988;84:1007–1015.

39. Cannon PJ, Hassar M, Case DB, et al. The relationship of hypertension and renal failure in scleroderma (progressive systemic sclerosis) to structural and functional abnormalities of the renal cortical circulation. Medicine 1974;53:1–46.

40. LeRoy EC, Fleischman RM. The management of renal scleroderma: Experience with dialysis, nephrectomy and transplantation. Am J Med 1978; 64:974–978.

41. Steen VD, Syed A, Johnson JP, Conte CG, Medsger TA Jr. Renal disease in systemic sclerosis. Arthritis Rheum 1993;36(9):S131.

42. Steen VD, Medsger TA Jr, Rodnan GP, et al. Clinical associations of anticentromere antibody (ACA) in patients with progressive systemic sclerosis. Arthritis Rheum 1984;27:125–131.

43. Stupi AM, Steen VD, Medsger TA Jr, et al. Pulmonary hypertension (PHT) in the CREST syndrome variant of progressive systemic sclerosis (PSS). Arthritis Rheum 1986;29:515–524.

44. Singsen BH, et al. A histologic evaluation of mixed connective tissue disease in childhood. Am J Med 1980;68:710–717.

45. Salerni R, Rodnan GP, Leon DF, et al. Pulmonary hypertension in the CREST syndrome variant of progressive systemic sclerosis (scleroderma). Ann Intern Med 1977;86:394–399.

46. Oddis CV, Eisenbeis CH Jr, Reidbord HE, et al. Vasculitis in systemic sclerosis: A subset of patients with the CREST variant, Sjögren's syndrome and neurologic complications. J Rhematol 1987;14: 942–948.

47. Hochberg MC, Lopez-Acuna D, Gittelsohn AM. Mortality from systemic sclerosis (scleroderma) in the United States, 1969–1977. In: Black CM, Myers AR, eds. Systemic sclerosis (scleroderma). New York: Gower, 1985;61–69.

48. Silman AJ. Mortality from scleroderma in England and Wales, 1968–1985. Ann Rheum Dis 1991;50: 95–96.

49. Masi AT, D'Angelo WA. Epidemiology of fatal systemic sclerosis (diffuse scleroderma): A 15-year survey in Baltimore. Ann Intern Med 1967;66:870–883.

50. Silman AJ. Scleroderma and survival. Ann Rheum Dis 1991;50:267–269.

51. Farmer RG, Gifford RW Jr, Hines EA Jr. Prognostic significance of Raynaud's phenomenon and other clinical characteristics of systemic sclerosis. Circulation 1960;21:1088–1095.

52. Tuffanelli DL, Winkelman RK. Diffuse systemic scleroderma: A comparison with acrosclerosis. Ann Intern Med 1962;57:198–203.

53. Bennett R, Bluestone R, Holt PJL, Bywaters EGL. Survival in scleroderma. Ann Rheum Dis 1971;30:581–588.

54. Medsger TA Jr, Masi AT, Rodnan GP, Benedek TG, Robinson H. Survival with systemic sclerosis (scleroderma): A life-table analysis of clinical and demographic factors in 309 patients. Ann Intern Med 1971;75:369–376.

55. Medsger TA Jr, Masi AT. Survival with scleroderma II: A life-table analysis of clinical and demographic factors in 358 male U.S. veteran patients. J Chronic Dis 1973;26:647–660.

56. Barnett AJ, Miller MH, Littlejohn GO. A survival study of patients with scleroderma diagnosed over 30 years (1953–1983): The value of a simple cutaneous classification in the early stages of the disease. J Rheumatol 1978;15:276–283.

57. Eason RJ, Tan PJ, Gow PJ. Progressive systemic sclerosis in Auckland: A ten year review with emphasis on prognostic features. Aust NZ J Med 1981;11:657.

58. Wynn J, Fineberg N, Metzer L, et al. Prediction of survival in progressive systemic sclerosis by multivariate analysis of clinical features. Am Heart J 1985;110:123–127.

59. Altman RD, Medsger TA Jr, Bloch DA, et al. Predictors of survival in systemic sclerosis (scleroderma). Arthritis Rheum 1991;34:403–413.

60. Medsger TA Jr, Masi AT. Epidemiology of systemic sclerosis (scleroderma). Ann Intern Med 1971;74: 714–721.

61. Barnett AJ, Miller MH, Littlejohn GO. A survival study of patients with scleroderma diagnosed over 30 years (1953–1983): The value of a simple cutaneous classification in the early stages of the disease. J Rheumatol 1988;15:276–283.

62. Ferri C, Berini L, Cecchetti R, Latorraca A, Marotta G, Pasero G, Neri R, Bombardieri S. Cutaneous and serologic subsets of systemic sclerosis. J Rheumatol 1991;18:1826–1832.

63. Traub YM, Shapiro AP, Rodnan GP, Medsger TA Jr, McDonald RH Jr, Steen VD, Osial TA, et al. Hypertension and renal failure (scleroderma renal crisis) in progressive systemic sclerosis: Report of a 25-year experience with 68 cases. Medicine 1983;62:335–352.

64. D'Angelo WA. Long-term survival of scleroderma renal crisis and malignant hypertension with captopril. In: Black CM, Myers AR, eds. Systemic sclerosis. New York: Gower, 1985;437–445.

65. Steen VD, Costatino JP, Shapiro AP, Medsger TA Jr. Outcome of renal crisis in systemic sclerosis: Relation to availability of angiotensin converting enzyme (ACE) inhibitors. Ann Intern Med 1990;113:352–357.

66. Coppock JS, Bacon PA. Outcome, assessment and activity. In: Jayson MIV, Black CM, eds. Systemic sclerosis (scleroderma). Chichester, UK: John Wiley & Sons, Ltd, 1988;279–288.

67. Coppock JS, England SE, Harris P, et al. Clinical measurement of the hand in scleroderma: Its relationship to hand function. Br J Rheumatol 1985;24:96.

68. Poole J, Steen VD. The use of the Health Assessment Questionnaire (HAQ) to determine physical disability in systemic sclerosis. Arthritis Care Res 1991;4:27–31.

69. Fries JF, Spitz PW, Young DY. The dimensions of health outcomes: The health assessment, disability and pain scales. J Rheumatol 1982;9:789–793.

70. Hochberg MC, Sutton JD. Physical disability and psychosocial dysfunction in systemic lupus erythematosus. J Rheumatol 1988;15:959–964.

71. Moser DK, Clements PJ, Brecht ML, et al. Predictors of psychosocial adjustment in systmic sclerosis: The influence of formal education level, functional ability, hardiness, uncertainty and social support. Arthritis Rheum 1992;36:1398–1405.

72. Steen V, Conte C, Medsger TA Jr. Case control study of corticosteriod use prior to scleroderma renal crisis. Arthritis Rheum 1994;37(9):S360.

73. Helfrich DJ, Banner B, Steen VD, et al. Renal failure in normotensive patients with systemic sclerosis. Arthritis Rheum 1989;32:1128–1134.

74. Steen VD, Blair C, Medsger TA Jr. The toxicity of D-penicillamine in systemic sclerosis. Ann Intern Med 1986;104:699–705

75. Roumm AD, Medsger TA Jr. Cancer in systemic sclerosis: An epidemiologic study. Arthritis Rheum 1985;28:344–360.

76. Medsger TA Jr. Editorial. Systemic sclerosis and malignancy—Are they related? J Rheumatol 1985;12:1041–1043.

77. Baker GL, Kahl LE, Zee BC, et al. Malignancy following treatment of rheumatoid arthritis with cyclophosphamide: A long-term case-control follow-up study. Am J Med 1987;83:1–9.

JOAN GUITART
GIUSEPPE MICALI
LAWRENCE M. SOLOMON

4

Localized Scleroderma

LOCALIZED SCLERODERMA (LS), first described by Addison in 1854 (1), is a distinct form of dermal induration confined to an asymmetrical area of the skin. Although some clinicopathological findings are similar, LS bears minimal relation to systemic sclerosis (SSc). Besides the limited skin involvement, LS differs from SSc by the absence of Raynaud's phenomenon (RP) or significant systemic involvement (2).

Although rare, LS is more common than SSc. Dermatologists tend to care for affected patients, because the lesions are often confined to the skin. Nevertheless, the extent and depth of involvement can cause significant disabilities often requiring the expert care of a multi-specialty team.

Various forms of LS have been proposed based on clinical differences, which may be real or simply a matter of convenience. The classification used by most dermatologists and rheumatologists divides the cases of LS into two groups: morphea and linear scleroderma (3,4) (Fig. 4.1). Morphea can be a single plaque (limited form), several plaques, or extensive and confluent (generalized form). The clinical presentation will determine the use of other descriptive terms such as guttate, subcutaneous, pansclerotic, or nodular types. An early study of 235 patients from the Mayo clinic showed that 54% of the cases were morphea (35% limited form, 19% generalized form) and 46% of the cases were linear scleroderma (5). The impression prevails among dermatologists that the plaque form of morphea is most prevalent.

Epidemiology

LS is rare. An epidemiological study done in the West Midlands region of England reported morphea at a rate of 2 per 1,000,000 among males and 4.7 per 1,000,000 among females (6). Females are more often affected than males by a ratio of 3:1 or 4:1. In addition, Caucasians are more commonly affected than Orientals or Blacks (4).

Although LS can occur at any age, the peak incidence is between 20 and 40 years of age (7). Generalized morphea tends to appear in the elderly, while localized plaques and linear lesions appear at younger ages (8).

Clinical Presentation

Although the lesions appear spontaneously in most cases, injury of various types may precede LS.

A prodrome of joint pains, not necessarily close to the skin involvement, occurs in up to 13% of the patients (2). Arthralgias tend to subside when the skin lesions become more noticeable.

Early manifestations are difficult to diagnose. An ill-defined plaque of edema with occasional erythema and pain precedes the typical skin lesions (2). After some weeks or months, one or more plaques with distinct features may appear (7). The plaques range from 1 to 15 cm in greatest dimension and, in contrast with PSS, are

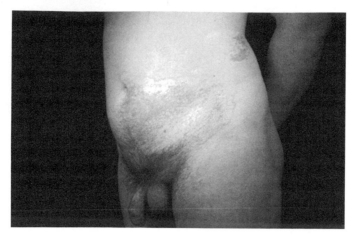

Figure 4.1. Extensive morphea plaque in the abdomen. The margins are lilac and clearly defined.

sharply defined and asymmetrical (7). The center is smooth and white-tan with various shades of pigmentation. The surface appears shiny and atrophic (Fig. 4.2). Hair and sweat are diminished or absent in advanced lesions. A lilac ring at the margin of the plaque implies active inflammation and probable progression of the disease, and a high vascular flow at the lilac ring has been identify by Laser-Doppler (9). According to Serup, perilesional hyperpigmentation (55% of patients) is seen more often than the classic lilac ring (14% of patients) (8). Perilesional hyperpigmentation probably correlates with the natural course of the lesion and may imply resolution of a prior inflamed area. It is not unusual to find new lesions while the old ones are resolving (7).

LS plaques tend to be thicker than the skin that is affected by generalized scleroderma (Fig. 4.3). In morphea, the skin is thickened by 13% to 310% in comparison to normal skin (10). The same study by Serup (8) reported that the increase of thickness was greater in the normally thinner skin of the extremities than the torso (10). The measurement of skin thickness has been done by semiquantitative clinical assessment, weighing skin biopsy specimen, ultrasound techniques, and, recently, a durometer reported by Falanga (11) to be effective and reliable. Progression of LS is also accompanied by a decrease

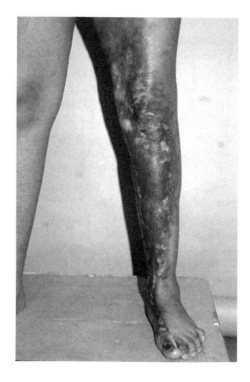

Figure 4.2. Linear scleroderma of the left lower leg involving the knee.

in extensibility, which correlates with the thickness of the lesion (12). Hypesthesia is often present when the plaques are thick (7). Eccrine gland function in LS plaques is defective with or without prior pilocarpine stimulation (13).

The trunk is the most common location of morphea, while linear scleroderma often involves the limbs (4). Axillae, perineum, and periareolar are unusual locations for both, and occurrence in the face is rare except for "en coup de sabre" (2,4,7). Calcinosis and even bone formation have been described in old plaques (14, 15,16).

Rarely, hemorrhagic bullae and ulceration may occur (16,17,18). The bullae may be caused by lymphatic blockage, friction, trauma, or even as a complication of treatment (16,19). In addition, a nodular or keloidal variant with exuberant collagen production has been described (20).

Although approximately 15% of LS patients complain of abdominal pain and migraine, internal organ involvement with the fibrotic process is rare (5). An autopsy study of 27 patients with LS showed no evidence of systemic involvement by the fibrotic process (21).

The life expectancy of children with LS appears to be normal (4), and RP has been reported in LS, but is apparently rare (8).

The esophageal symptoms in LS are mostly mild. Marked esophageal dysfunction and acid exposure in the distal esophagus are only seen in SSc (22). Esophageal dysfunctions with decreased peristaltic contractions of the upper third of the esophagus were reported in two of 14 patients with morphea (23). The significance of this finding is questionable because the lower esophagus is primarily involved in generalized scleroderma.

A patient with severe cardiomyopathy and LS has been reported (24). The patient's cardiac failure and skin lesions reverted during a course of prednisone therapy.

The inflammatory and sclerotic process in morphea in young patients lasts for approximately 3 to 5 years, and then the lesions may soften and blend with the surrounding skin, often

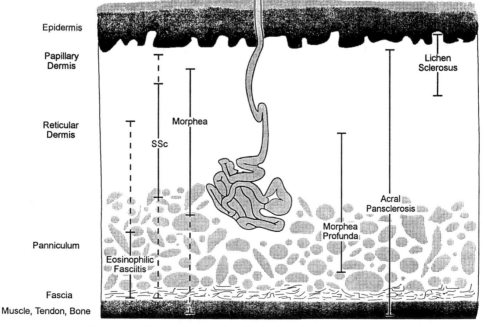

Figure 4.3. Depth of involvement in localized scleroderma and related conditions.

leaving residual pigmentary changes (7). This resolution is more likely to occur in plaque-type LS than in linear lesions on the lower limbs.

Despite the benign evolution of some patients, few patients resolve completely (4). Some residual lesions were found in 63 of 88 (72%) children with morphea (25).

Progression of LS into SSc has been described, and that occurrence may have been a coincidence (26); this type of disease progression must be extremely rare. Nailfold capillary abnormalities similar to those seen in SSc are not seen in LS; therefore, the presence of nailfold capillary abnormalities should alert the physician about the possible development of SSc (27). Mizutani reported on a patient with SSc and coexistent morphea. Outbreaks of new morphea lesions in this patient did not alter the course of SSc (28).

LINEAR SCLERODERMA

Linear scleroderma occurs as an indurated patch with pigmentary changes most commonly seen in the lower limbs (see Fig. 4.2), although the arms and the frontoparietal area can also be involved (4). The most common presentation is a single patch, but bilateral asymmetrical patches as well as coexistence with morphea has been reported (2).

Linear scleroderma is most frequently, but not exclusively, seen in childhood (5). The direction of the plaques is transverse in the trunk and longitudinal in the extremities. The distribution does not follow specific dermatomes (8). The fibrotic bands often infiltrate the soft tissues causing atrophy and sclerosis of the underlying fat, fascia, and muscle. When the plaques cross a joint, the fibrotic process may involve the articular capsule and tendons causing contractions in a significant number of patients (29,30). If the process involves the epiphyseal growth plate, disturbances of bone growth with limb asymmetry can occur. A study showed 20% of patients with lower limb involvement had significant length discrepancy of up to 7 cm. One patient with severe contracture even required amputation of

the affected leg (29). A circumferential sclerotic ring is a very rare presentation that can lead to atrophy of the entire limb (2). *Spina bifida* is frequently associated with linear scleroderma of the legs and buttocks (5).

Linear scleroderma can affect part of the face and scalp with a sharp border at the midline. The term "en coup de sabre" is used for this presentation, because the French imagined it to have some resemblance to the results of a blow with a sabre (Fig. 4.4). Disturbances of bone growth can cause significant facial deformities (2). Unlike other forms of LS, "en coup de sabre" can last for decades, sometimes extending its coverage over the years. Scarring alopecia often appears if there is frontoparietal involvement. The hair may regrow after remission of the scalp lesion.

The distribution of "en coup de sabre," like other cases of linear scleroderma, does not follow

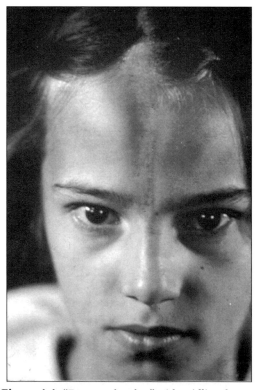

Figure 4.4. "En coup de sabre" with midline depression.

any anatomic structure. Johnston speculated that the distribution may reflect an abnormal migration of neuroectodermal cells during embryogenesis (31). This theory is supported by the frequent development of seizures, hemiparesis, and headaches during the evolution of "en coup de sabre" (4). Imaging studies of the brain have shown vascular and cerebral changes even when the patients are asymptomatic (4,32). Alterations of the sympathetic nervous system have also been found (33).

Several eye findings have been described with "en coup de sabre," probably reflecting extension of the same pathological process into internal ocular structures (34). Central corneal thickness correlates with the duration of disease (35), and heterochromia iridis and uveitis have also been described (32,36).

Cases of LS involving the perioral skin may extend into the oral cavity. Hemiatrophy of the tongue, loss of periodontal support, early loss of the primary teeth with eruption of the permanent teeth, and lack of alveolar growth have been described (37).

Parry-Romberg syndrome is closely related to linear morphea and is characterized by hemifacial atrophy with sclerodermoid features (2). Progressive hemifacial atrophy associated with other lesions of LS has been reported (38). Ocular, oral, and neural changes as well as a patch of alopecia reflect the close link with "en coup de sabre" (39).

DISABLING ACRAL PANSCLEROTIC MORPHEA OF CHILDHOOD

This variant of LS presents with deep sclerotic plaques involving the extensor aspect of the extremities, yet sparing the fingertips and toes (40). The process often extends to the fascia, muscle, and even bone. The lesions begin to appear before puberty and are accompanied by arthralgias, joint stiffness, and contractions (41). Pansclerotic morphea has a relentless progression with poor response to therapy (25). Some patients have abnormal pulmonary function tests, elec-

tromyograms, and esophageal manometry (40). How this alleged variant differs significantly from SSc progressive systemic sclerosis is not clear.

MORPHEA PROFUNDA

This subcutaneous variant of morphea has a significant inflammatory component, but because of the depth of the lesion the margins are ill-defined. Some authors have suggested that morphea profunda may be a chronic form of eosinophilic fasciitis. Arthralgias and myalgias are frequently present. Flexion contractures of the joints and carpal tunnel syndrome may also occur (41). A deep biopsy will show inflammation of the entire panniculus with dermal fibrosis confined largely to the deep dermis (42). The infiltrate includes eosinophils in a significant number of cases (43). Pulmonary and esophageal sclerosis with eosinophilia are often found (44).

GUTTATE MORPHEA

The lesions of guttate morphea are smaller and more numerous than localized morphea plaques, although both types often coexist (45). The shoulders and chest are frequently involved. The epidermis is thin and atrophic, resembling *lichen sclerosus et atrophicus*. The latter is less extensive and has distinct pathological features (Fig. 4.3 and Differential Diagnosis section later in this chapter).

ATROPHODERMA OF PASINI AND PIERINI

This controversial entity is probably an atrophic disease or distinct form of morphea with characteristic clinical features. The patches are similar to morphea, but they are depressed with a slate-gray color and without the lilac ring (46). The back is commonly involved. Coexistence with classic morphea has been described (47,48). The pathology is similar to morphea with a propensity for epidermal atrophy and dermal thinning.

The pathological changes are often so minimal that the biopsy needs to be compared side-by-side with a specimen from nearby non-affected skin (49).

Differential Diagnosis

Many cutaneous diseases can have sclerodermoid changes simulating LS. Sarcoidosis and sclerosing basal cell carcinoma often appear as facial annular lesions with an atrophic center and red or hyperpigmented rim, simulating morphea (50). Only a histopathologic examination of the tissue can lead to a certain diagnosis.

Lichen sclerosus consists of thin and atrophic plaques that resemble the guttate form of LS. Clinically, *lichen sclerosus* differs from morphea by the presence of keratotic plugs at the surface. Hydropic degeneration of the basal cells with edema and homogenization of the papillary dermal collagen are also unique findings of *lichen sclerosus* (45). The coexistence of LS and *lichen sclerosus et atrophicus* in the same patient and even within the same lesion has been observed (51,52).

Lipodystrophy and lupus panniculitis can mimic morphea profunda with similar depressed sclerotic plaques (41). Morpheaform lesions have also been observed in phenylketonuria, graft versus host disease, *porphyria cutanea tarda*, and Borrelia infection (2,8). Exposure to certain chemicals such as vinyl chloride, perchlorethylene (e.g., in coal and gold mining), and contaminated L-tryptophan, and toxic oil syndrome can also produce sclerotic lesions, although a presentation resembling SSc is more common (8).

Melorheostosis is a rare disease that presents with endosteal densities of the long bones, limb pain, and skin lesions resembling linear scleroderma (53).

Eosinophilic fasciitis may also develop sclerotic plaques resembling morphea (3). Increased collagen production and type I procollagen mRNA levels in fibroblasts cultured from eosinophilic fasciitis lesions have been reported (54). Other clinical and laboratory findings are similar and suggest a close relationship between SSc and LS. Distinguishing features include a rapid course, frequent onset after intense physical exercise, high eosinophilia, and good response to systemic steroids. RP and systemic involvement are rare (41). Eosinophilic fascitis is commonly associated with lymphoproliferative and myeloproliferative disorders (55). Joint contractures can develop rapidly and the retraction of the subcutaneous tissue can create cutaneous grooves delineating muscle groups and veins (56). Multiple morphea lesions have been repeatedly noted in eosinophilic fascitis patients (57).

Laboratory Abnormalities

Although many blood tests may be abnormal in LS patients, most patients with limited disease have no significant blood changes and there is no specific test to identify affected patients.

Eosinophilia is more common in LS (31% of patients) than in SSc (7% of patients) (56). Linear scleroderma, generalized morphea, morphea profunda, and acral pansclerotic morphea are particularly prone to eosinophilia. The level of eosinophilia correlates with the extent of skin involvement and is, in general, associated with active inflammatory disease and high erythrocyte sedimentation rate (56). A significant number of LS patients have hypergammaglobulinemia (4). According to Falanga a high level of IgG in linear scleroderma patients correlates positively with the development of joint contractures (58).

Rheumatoid factor is positive in 25% to 40% of the patients, and the titer also correlates with the severity of the disease (4). Complement levels are normal with the exception of one report of hereditary deficiency of C2 in a patient with linear scleroderma (59). A weak association was found in morphea patients with HLA DR2, A3 and B7 antigens (60).

Antinuclear antibodies (ANA) are detected in 23% to 67% of LS patients (4,61). The percentage is significantly higher when a monolayer of Hep-2 cells is used as a substrate (62). The highest frequency of ANA was found to be positive among children with linear scleroderma (63). Patients with extensive generalized morphea and deep soft tissue involvement also frequently have a positive ANA, but the titer does not correlate with disease activity (63). The most frequently found specific ANA in LS is anti-ss-DNA found in approximately 40% of the patients (64). A positive ss-DNA pattern may indicate a prolonged course with extensive cutaneous involvement (62). IgM is the most common isotope for anti-ss-DNA in LS, although a significant number of patients with linear scleroderma have IgA and some generalized morphea patients have IgG (64). A unique immunofluorescence pattern has been identified by chromosome spreads which, although not identical, resembles the anti-centromere antibody pattern (65). This anti-centromere-like pattern differs from other patterns by not being paired or uniform, and also by staining at the periphery of the chromosomes and not the chromosomes themselves (63). The specificity of the antibody for most of the LS patients is not clearly defined, but differs from Scl-70, dsDNA, and histones (65). An increased incidence of organ-specific antibodies with associated autoimmune disorders has been detected in patients with LS and their relatives (66). A high titer of anti-fibronectin antibodies has also been reported in one patient (67). Autoantibodies in LS could be an epiphenomenon associated with tissue damage. The inconsistency of a positive ANA, which often appears late in the clinical course, or changes the antigenic specificity, questions its significance.

Pathology

The histopathological findings of LS are not easily distinguishable from SSc. A skin biopsy should be deep enough to include the subcutaneous adipose tissue, which is often involved in LS (68). The epidermis is for the most part unremarkable in LS, but when the papillary dermis is altered by the sclerotic process, epidermal atrophy with loss of rete pegs or even acanthosis may be seen. A case of perforating morphea with transepidermal elimination of elastolytic material has been reported (69).

Edema and homogeneous degeneration of collagen fibers have been described as an early feature; however, this is difficult to distinguish from normal.

A deep, primarily perivascular, and to a lesser extent interstitial, inflammatory cellular infiltrate is the main finding in early stages. This infiltrate is composed of lymphocytes with some macrophages, mast cells, eosinophils, and plasma cells, and extends from the deep dermis to the subcutaneous fat (3). The extent, depth, and density of the infiltrate is variable and correlates with the clinical findings (Figs. 4.5 and 4.6, see also Fig. 4.3). While most of the cases involve the upper panniculus, morphea profunda extends deeper to involve the entire panniculus. Even the fascia, skeletal muscle, tendons, and periosteum can be involved in the pansclerotic form. The inflamed soft tissue is eventually replaced by the fibrotic process. Conversely, the infiltrate may involve the upper reticular and papillary dermis with hyalinization of the collagen resembling *lichen sclerosus*. Combined features of morphea and *lichen sclerosus* are not rare (51,52,70).

With time, the dermis becomes thickened by broad, closely packed collagen bundles, which may appear homogeneous and deeply eosinophilic. The three-dimensional orientation of the collagen fibers is lost and replaced by new collagen fibers oriented parallel to the epidermis (16). Interstitial hyaluronic acid is decreased in the center but increased at the periphery of the lesion (71).

The subcutaneous and periappendageal fat is progressively lost and replaced by collagen with focal mucoid and hyalin changes. Dystrophic calcinosis and even ossification can occasionally be seen (14,15,72).

Cutaneous appendages (e.g., hair follicle and sweat glands) are entrapped by the fibrous stroma

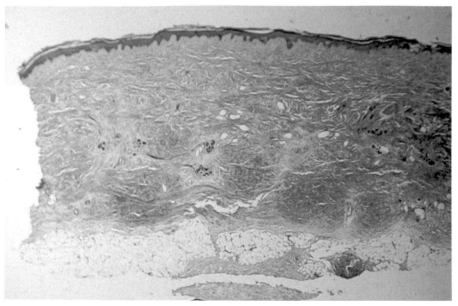

Figure 4.5. Low power view of morphea biopsy with dense collagen bands in the lower dermis.

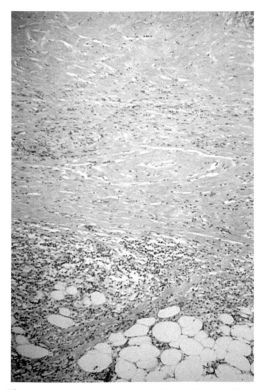

Figure 4.6. The lower dermis shows dense collagen bundles with a mononuclear cell infiltrate.

with loss of the periappendageal fat pad (Fig. 4.7). The skin appendages often became atrophic or even disappear.

Eventually, as the lesion resolves, the inflammatory infiltrate disappears and the thickened dermis becomes thinner. Blood vessels show gradually intimal thickening with eventual obliteration of the lumen and replacement by fibrosis (68).

Under electron microscopic examination, collagen fibers undergo myxedematous changes in the early stages. This process is similar to the changes seen in SSc (8).

Elastic fibers, on the contrary, are not significantly altered. Mast cells are found in the early myxedematous stage but not in fibrotic areas.

The increased number of fibroblasts and myofibroblasts originates from activated pericytes of small nerves and vessels. Activated pericytes are also responsible for the thickening of the basal lamina of blood vessels (3). Myofibroblasts display features of the fibroblast, such as abundant rough endoplasmic reticulum, and features of smooth muscle cells, such as α-smooth muscle actin filaments and contractile properties (73). Myofibroblasts are found in granulation tissue and other conditions requiring active collagen production (73). Vacuolization and degeneration of endothelial cells are found in dermal blood vessels but not in skeletal muscle capillaries. Even normal skin of patients with morphea may show endothelial cell changes by electron microscopy without associated fibrosis (8).

Etiology

Genetic, environmental, and immune factors seem to play a role in the development of LS, although the precise cause is still unknown. Genetic factors may have predisposed some individuals to rare reported cases of familial LS (74,75). A weak HLA linkage has been detected in some patients. HLA B7/DR2 may predispose some individuals to a rather mild form of morphea (60). Although congenital morphea has never been described (8), an abnormal migration and proliferation of ectodermal cells during embryogenesis may be the cause of "en coup de sabre" (31). Injury of various types has been implicated. Local trauma preceded LS lesions in up to 23% of the patients reported in one study (2). Prior immobilization of the affected limb has also been reported as a possible cause (7). Other reported forms of preceding injury include radiotherapy, BCG vaccination, and measles (7,76, 77). Neurological injury is often seen in LS patients, in particular among patients with linear scleroderma (5). Transverse myelitis, *spina bifida*, spinal surgery, or even trauma to peripheral nerves has been reported (3,78). A case of linear scleroderma in the mandibular branch of the trigeminal nerve was reported following a mandibular nerve block (79).

LS has also been reported following measles and varicella (7,80). Late lesions of *Borrelia burgdorferi* infection include morphea and *acrodermatitis chronica atrophicans*, which may resemble linear scleroderma (2). Other late cutaneous findings in Lyme disease are anetoderma, atrophoderma,

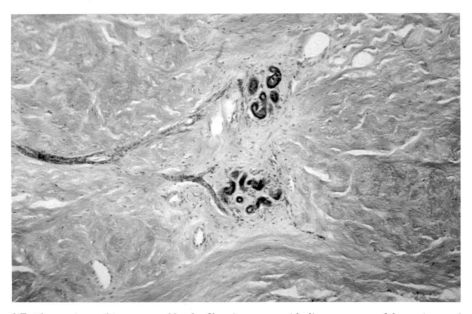

Figure 4.7. The eccrine coil is entrapped by the fibrotic process with disappearance of the periappendageal fat pad.

lichen sclerosus et atrophicus, eosinophilic fascitis, and progressive hemifacial atrophy, all of which are similar to LS (81,82). Whether single lesions of LS can be induced by the spirochete is controversial. Spirochetes have been visualized in morphea lesions, and borrelia antibodies have been detected in some affected patients (83). A positive association from areas where *B. burgdorferi* seroconversion is prevalent in the general population supports the infectious origin of some cases of a morphea-like eruption (84). The resolution of morphea lesions after penicillin treatment further lends support to an infectious origin of some cases. Peripheral nerve involvement with dysesthesias within the plaque has been noted in borrelia-induced lesions (85).

Both LS and systemic scleroderma have been reported after silicone gel prosthetic implants, especially after trauma with rupture of the capsule (86). Silicone related LS lesions can appear distant from the implant site (87).

Morphea-like patches were reported in a patient with rheumatoid arthritis during a course of D-penicillamine treatment (88). Similar cases have been reported following treatment with valproate sodium, phytonadione injections, bleomycin injections, and even immunotherapy with irradiated melanoma cells (89,90,91).

The possible autoimmune origin of LS is suggested by the frequent finding of autoantibodies in LS patients and also by the morpheaform lesions seen in chronic graft-versus-host disease (92). An increased incidence of autoimmune disorders has been noted in LS patients, but does not alter the evolution and, therefore, the prognosis of LS (2,66). Lesions of subacute cutaneous lupus erythematosus have been noted to precede morphea plaques (93).

Pathogenesis

Several hypotheses exist regarding the pathogenesis of LS. Most of the ideas are based on research done with PSS, which, despite similar pathological findings, is not the same disease. The initial pathologic event may be endothelial cell swelling and vacuolization, probably inflicted by increased proteolytic enzymes or oxygen-free radicals (94). The resulting tissue hypoxia and inflammation may activate fibroblasts, thereby inducing fibrosis as a repair process. Mast cells may also be implicated in the initial vascular insult (95). Biochemical studies have shown that the development of morphea is similar to the natural process of growth, regeneration, and repair (8). Platelet aggregation with release of platelet-derived growth factor (PDGF) and transforming growth factor-β (TGFβ) may modulate fibroblast function, although the possible action of platelets does not suffice to explain scleroderma.

Linear scleroderma may be initiated by neurological injury. Neuropeptides, such as bradykinin and substance P, may stimulate Interleukin 1 production with subsequent fibroblast and pericyte activation (78). Ablation of the cervical sympathetic ganglion in experimental animals superficially reproduced the changes of Parry-Romberg's disease, supporting the theory of neural injury for this variant of LS (33).

An abnormal migration of ectodermal cells during embryogenesis has been suggested as the initial step in "en coup de sabre." The hyperresponsive fibroblasts at the site of future lesions are activated by an unknown stimulus later in life (2).

The inflammatory event leading to LS may be triggered by an autoimmune process. Clumping between different chromosome groups was detected in metaphase lymphocytes from scleroderma patients (96). Damaged nuclear material may focally become a strong antigenic stimulus attracting mononuclear cells, which could secrete cytokines and stimulate fibroblasts.

TGFβ, which may stimulate type I collagen production, is increased in lesional skin (97). TGFβ also down-regulates lymphocyte proliferation and is often increased in other inflammatory dermatosis without a fibrotic component (98). Therefore, TGFβ may regulate the inflammatory infiltrate, but is less likely to regulate the fibrotic process. Hatamochi demonstrated an increase in type I collagen mRNA in early-passage fibroblasts derived from inflammatory LS lesions, but not from late sclerotic LS lesions. These data lend credence to the notion that the inflammatory cells are directly involved in the fibroblast stimulation and collagen production (99). Decreases in thickness of late LS lesions reflects hypofunction and inhibition of fibroblasts (8).

In summary, multiple signaling pathways are probably involved in the activation of fibroblasts and increased collagen production in LS. Neurological injury, autoimmunity, and abnormal cell migration during embryogenesis may partially or totally induce LS lesions.

Treatment

There is no standard treatment for LS (2). The majority of the treatment trials reported include few cases and lack adequate controls. Evaluation of treatment modalities is further complicated by the natural tendency of the disease for improvement over variable time periods (4).

If the lesions are limited and asymptomatic, treatment is not necessary and resolution may occur spontaneously (7). Emollients and low concentration, weak topical steroids may be required to relieve a sense of dryness and pruritus (2). It is also claimed that etretinate has induced skin "softening" in an uncontrolled study (100). Sunscreens may help improve residual hyperpigmentation (2).

A moderate dose of systemic steroids may help control inflammation during the early stages and may possibly prevent further extension. Intralesional injection of triamcinolone acetonide (5–10 mg/ml) at the margins, and even at the center of the lesions, may also halt the fibrotic process. Injections are repeated every 3 to 4 weeks unless atrophy occurs (7).

Active exercise and orthopedic devices are important to prevent joint contractures, especially in linear scleroderma. Physical and occupational therapy may be needed to treat disabilities of advanced LS lesions. Surgical release of tendons and articular capsular contractions is performed occasionally, but only when the lesions are quiescent (4). Plastic surgical repair and fat autotransplantation may help some patients with "en coup de sabre" and Parry-Romberg syndrome (101).

The use of drugs with potentially significant side effects should be limited, because most patients have limited purely cutaneous involvement. Falanga studied the treatment of severe and extensive LS with D-penicillamine (102). The dose used was 2–5 mg/kg over 15 to 53 months, with improvement beginning in 3 to 6 months. Seven (64%) of 11 patients demonstrated decreased active inflammation, skin softening, decreased contractures, and growth improvement of the affected limb. (102). One patient exhibited nephrotic syndrome, but did not develop renal insufficiency. D-penicillamine used in combination with prednisone (102) and pyridoxine (103) were also reported to show good results. Limited studies and reports using various experimental drugs have shown variable results, which are difficult to interpret.

Some degree of improvement has been attributed to phenytoin (104), potassium p-aminobenzoate (105), vitamin E (106), salazopyrine (107), and cyclophenyl (108), among others. Immunosuppressive drugs have given variable results (109). Penicillin was successfully used in Europe for Borrelia-induced morphea lesions (110). Penetrating lesions of LS, such as pansclerotic morphea, respond very poorly to any treatment modality (40). A decreased level of type I and type III procollagen mRNA in cultured LS fibroblasts that were exposed to interferon-α and interferon-γ suggests that this might be a promising drug for testing in LS (110).

References

1. Fox TC. Note on the history of scleroderma in England. Br J Dermatol 1892;4:101.
2. Falanga V. Localized scleroderma. Med Clin North Am 1989;73(5):1143–1156.
3. Schachter RK. Localized scleroderma. Curr Opin Rheum 1990;2:947–955.

4. Krafchik BR. Localized cutaneous scleroderma. Semin Dermatol 1992;1:65–72.
5. Christianson HB, Dorsey CS, O'Leary PA, et al. Localized scleroderma: A clinical study of 235 cases. Arch Dermatol 1956;74:629–639.
6. Silman A, Jannini S, Symmons D, et al. An epidemiological study of scleroderma in the West Midlands. Br J Rheumatol 1988;27:286-290.
7. Rowell NR, Goodfield MJD. Localized morphea. In: Champion RH, Burton JL, Ebling FJG, eds. Rook, Wilkinson, Ebling textbook of dermatology, 5th ed. Oxford: Blackwell Scientific Publication, 1992.
8. Serup J. Clinical appearance of skin lesions and disturbances of pigmentation in localized scleroderma. Acta Derm Venereol (Stock) 1984;64:485-492.
9. Serup J, Kristensen JK. Blood flow of morphea plaques as measured by laser-Doppler flowmetry. Arch Dermatol Res 1984;276:322–325.
10. Serup J. Decrease skin thickness of pigmented spots appearing in localized scleroderma (morphea). Measurement of skin thickness by 15 Mhz pulsed ultrasound. Arch Dermatol Res 1984;276: 135–137.
11. Falanga V, Bucalo B. Use of a durometer to assess skin hardness. J Am Acad Dermatol 1993;29: 47–51.
12. Kalis B, De Rigal J, Leonard F, et al. *In vivo* study of scleroderma by non-invasive techniques. Br J Dermatol 1990;122:785–791.
13. Serup J. Localized scleroderma (morphea): Study of eccrine gland function and skin microtopography. J Dermatol (Tokyo) 1984;11:269–276.
14. Monroe AB, Burgdorf WH, Sheward S. Plate like cutaneous osteoma. J Am Acad Dermatol 1987; 16(2):481–484.
15. Hazel PG, Askari A. Localized scleroderma with cutaneous calcinosis. A distinctive variant. Arch Dermatol 1979;115(7):871–872.
16. Taylor RM. Sclerosing disorders. In: Farmer ER, Hood AF, eds. Pathology of the skin. Connecticut: Appleton and Lange, l990. Norwalk, CT.
17. Tosti A, Melino M, Bardazzi F. Hemorrhagic bullous lesions in morphea. Cutis 1989;44(2):118–119.
18. Kobayasi T, Willeberg A, Serup J, et al. Generalized morphea with blisters. Acta Derm Venereol (Stockh) 1990;70(5):454–456.
19. Joly P, Lampert A, Thomine E, et al. Development of pseudobullous morphea and scleroderma-like illness during therapy with L-hydroxytryptophan and carbidopa. J Am Acad Dermatol 1991;25(2): 332–333.
20. Jablonska S, Rodnan GP. Localized forms of scleroderma. Clin Rheum Dis 1979;5:215–220.
21. Piper WN, Helwig EB. Progressive systemic sclerosis. Arch Dermatol 1955;72:535–546.
22. Zaninotto G, Peserico A, Costantini M, et al. Esophageal motility and lower esophageal sphincter competence in progressive systemic sclerosis and localized scleroderma. Scand J Gastroenterol 1989; 24(1):95–102.
23. Weihrauch TR, Korting GW. Manometric assessment of esophageal involvement in PSS, morphea and Raynaud's disease. Br J Dermatol 1982;107: 325–332.
24. Moore EC, Cohen F, Farooki Z, et al. Focal scleroderma and severe cardiomyopathy. Patient report and brief review. Am J Dis Child 1991; 145:229–231.
25. Torok E, Ablonezy E. Morphea in children. Clin Exp Dermatol 1986;11:607–612.
26. Rossi P, Fossaluzza V, Gonano L. J Rheumatol 1985;12(3):629–630.
27. Maricq HR. Capillary abnormalities, Raynaud phenomenon and systemic sclerosis in patients with localized scleroderma. Arch Dermatol 1992; 128(5):630–632.
28. Mizutani H, Tanaka H, Okada H, et al. Palindromic morphea: Multiple recurrences of morphea in a patient with systemic sclerosis. J Dermatol (Tokyo) 1992;19(5):298–301.
29. Kornreich HK, King KK, Bernstein BH, et al. Scleroderma in childhood. Arthritis Rheum 1977; 20:343–350.
30. Larregue M, Ziegler JE, Lauret P, et al. Sclerodermie en bande chez l'enfant (a propos de 27 cas). Ann Dermatol Venereol 1986;113:207–224.
31. Johnston MC. The neural crest in abnormalities of the face and brain. In: Bergsma D, Paul NW, eds. Morphogenesis and malformations of the face and brain. New York: Alan R Liss, 1975.
32. Luer W, Jockel D, Henze T, et al. Progressive inflammatory lesions of the brain parenchyma in localized scleroderma of the head. J Neurol 1990;237(6):379–381.
33. Resende LA, Dal Pai V, Alves A. Experimental study of progressive hemifacial hemiatrophy: Effects of cervical sympathectomy in animals. Rev Neurol (Paris) 1991;147:609–611.
34. Segal P, Jablonska S, Mrzyglod S. Ocular changes in linear scleroderma. Am J Opthalmol 1961;51: 807–813.
35. Serup J, Serup L. Increase central corneal thickness in localized scleroderma (morphea). Metab Pediatr Syst Opthalmol 1985;8:11–14.
36. Stone RA, Scheie HG. Periorbital scleroderma as

sociated with heterochromia iridis. Am J Opthalmol 1980;90:858–860.

37. Seou WK, Young W. Localized scleroderma in childhood: Review of the literature and case report. Pediatr Dent 19829(3):240–244.

38. Tan E, Kurkcuoglu N, Atalag M, et al. Progressive hemifacial atrophy with localized scleroderma. Eur Neurol 1989;29(1):15–17.

39. Auvinet C, Glacet-Bernard A, Coscas G, et al. Parry-Romberg progressive facial hemiatrophy and localized scleroderma. Nosologic and pathogenic problems. J Fr Ophtalmol 1989;12(3):169–173.

40. Diaz-Perez JL, Connolly SM, Winkelmann RK. Disabling pansclerotic morphea of children. Arch Dermatol 1980;116:169–173.

41. Doyle JA, Connolly SM, Winkelmann RK. Cutaneous and subcutaneous inflammatory sclerosis syndromes. Arch Dermatol 1982;118:886–890.

42. Su WP, Person JR. Morphea profunda: A new concept and a histopathologic study of 23 cases. Am J Dermatopathol 1981;3(3):251–260.

43. Peters MS, Su Wp. Eosinophils in lupus panniculitis and morphea profunda. J Cutan Pathol 1991;18(3):189–192.

44. Person JR, Su WPD. Subcutaneous morphea: A clinical study of 16 cases. Br J Dermatol 1979;100: 371–380.

45. Lever WF, Schaumburg-Lever G. Histopathology of the skin, 7th ed. Philadelphia: JB Lippincott, 1990.

46. Canizares O, Sachs PM, Jaimovich L, et al. Idiopathic atrophoderma of Pasini and Pierini. Arch Dermatol 1958;77:42–60.

47. Kee CE, Brothers WS, New W. Idiopathic atrophoderma of Pasini and Pierini with coexistent morphea. Arch Dermatol 1960;82:154–157.

48. Murphy PK, Hymes SR, Fenske NA. Concomitant unilateral idiopathic atrophoderma of Pasini and Pierini and morphea. Int J Dermatol 1990;29: 281–283.

49. Mehregan AH, Hashimoto K. Changes of collagen and ground substance. In: Pinkus H, Mehregan AH. A guide to dermatohistopathology. Norwalk, CT: Appleton and Lange, 1991.

50. Hess SP, Agudelo CA, White WL, et al. Ichthyosiform and morpheaform sarcoidosis. Clin Exp Rheumatol 1990;8(2):171–175.

51. Uitto J, Santa Cruz DJ, Bauer AB, et al. Morphea and lichen sclerosus et atrophicus. J Am Acad Dermatol 1980;3:271–279.

52. Shono S, Imura M, Ota M, et al. Lichen sclerosus et atrophicus, morphea, and coexistence of both diseases. Arch Dermatol 1991;127:1352–1356.

53. Soffa DJ, Sire DJ, Dodson JH. Melorheostosis with linear sclerodermatous skin changes. Radiology 1975;114:577–578.

54. Kahari VM, Heino J, Niskanen L, et al. Eosinophilic fascitis. Increased collagen production and type I procollagen mRNA levels in fibroblasts cultured from involved skin. Arch Dermatol 1990; 126:613–617.

55. Lakhanpal S, Ginsburg WW, Michet CJ, et al. Eosinophilic fasciitis: Clinical spectrum and therapeutic responses in 52 cases. Semin Arthritis Rheum 1988;17(4):221–231.

56. Falanga V, Medsger TA. Frequency levels and significance of blood eosinophilia in systemic sclerosis, localized scleroderma and eosinophilic fasciitis. J Am Acad Dermatol 1987;17:648.

57. Hulshof MM, Boom MW, Dijkmans BA. Multiple plaques of morphea developing in a patient with eosinophilic fasciitis. Arch Dermatol 1992;128: 1128–1129.

58. Falanga V, Medsger TA, Reichlin M, et al. Linear scleroderma. Clinical spectrum, prognosis and laboratory abnormalities. Ann Intern Med 1986; 104:849.

59. Hulsmans RFHJ, Asghar SS, Siddiqui AH, et al. Hereditary deficience of C2 in association with linear scleroderma en coup de sabre. Arch Dermatol 1986;122:76–79.

60. Kuhnl P, Sibrowski W, Broehm BO, et al. Association of HLA antigens with PSS and morphea. Tissue Antigens 1989;34:207–209.

61. Scharffetter K, Kind P, Wollny-Protzel D, et al. Scleroderma. Z Hautkr 1990;65(3):245–246.

62. Falanga V, Medsger TA, Reichlin M. Antinuclear and anti-single-stranded DNA antibodies in morphea and generalized morphea. Arch Dermatol 1987;123(3):350–353.

63. Jablonska S, Blaszczyk M, Chozelski T,P et al. Clinical relevance of immunologic findings in scleroderma. Clin Dermatol 1992;10(4):407–419.

64. Ruffatti A, Peserico A, Rondinone R, et al. Prevalence and characteristics of anti-single-stranded DNA antibodies in localized scleroderma. Arch Dermatol 1991;127:1180–1183.

65. Kikuchi K, Tekahara K, Ishibashi Y. Antinuclear antibodies in localized scleroderma: Unique staining in chromosome spreads. J Am Acad Dermatol 1989;21(6):1301–1303.

66. Harrington CI, Dunsmore IR. An investigation into the incidence of autoimmune disorders in patients with localized scleroderma. Br J Dermatol 1989;120:645–648.

67. Stefanato CM, Gorkiewicz PA, Jarzebek-Chlorzelska M, et al. Morphea with high titer of

fibronectin antibodies. Int J Dermatol 1992;31: 190–192.

68. Fleischmajer R, Nedwich A. Generalized morphea. Histology of the dermis and subcutaneous tissue. Arch Dermatol 1972;106:509–514.

69. Barr RJ, Siegel JM, Graham JH. Elastosis perforans serpiginosa associated with morphea. J Am Acad Dermatol 1980;3:19–22.

70. Tremaine R, Adam JE, Orizaga M. Morphea coexisting with lichen sclerosus et atrophicus. Int J Dermatol 1990;29(7):486–489.

71. Moller R, Serup J, Amitzboll T. Glycosaminoglycans in localized scleroderma. Connect Tissue Res 1985;13:227–236.

72. Nagy E, Nagy-Vezekenyi K, Dobransky I. Osteosis and calcinosis in scleroderma circumscripta linearis. Z Hautkr 1990;65(2):190–192.

73. Sappino AP, Masouye I, Saurat JH, et al. Smooth muscle differentiation in scleroderma fibroblastic cells. Am J Pathol 1990;137(3):585–591.

74. Taj M, Ahmad A. Familial localized scleroderma (morphea). Arch Dermatol 1977;113:1132–1133.

75. Wadud MA, Bose BK, Al-Nasir T. Familial localized scleroderma from Bangladesh: Two case reports. Bangladesh Med Res Counc Bull 1989; 15(1):15–19.

76. Colver GB, Rodger A, Mortimer PS, et al. Post-irradiation morphea. Br J Dermatol 1989;120: 831–835.

77. Trattner A, Figer A, David M, et al. Circumscribed scleroderma induced by postlumpectomy radiation therapy. Cancer 1991;68:2131–2133.

78. Littman BH. Linear scleroderma: A response to neurologic injury? Report and literature review. J Rheumatol 1989;16:1135–1140.

79. Kingery LB. Scleroderma following nerve injury, report of a case. Arch Dermatol Syph 1922;5: 579–583.

80. Spirer Z, Ilie B, Pick IA, et al. Localized scleroderma following varicella in a 3-year-old girl with IgA deficiency. Acta Paediatr Scand 1979;68: 783–785.

81. Ross SA, Sanchez JL, Taboas JO. Spiroquetal forms in the dermal lesions of morphea and lichen sclerous et atrophicus. Am J Dermatopathol 1990;12(4):357–362.

82. Malane MS, Grant-Kels JM, Feder HM, et al. Diagnosis of Lyme disease based on dermatologic manifestations. Ann Intern Med 1991;114(6): 490–498.

83. Aberer E, Stanek G, Ertl M, et al. Evidence of spiroquetal origin of circumscribed scleroderma (morphea). Acta Derm Venereol (Stockh) 1987; 67:225–231.

84. Lecerf V, Bagot M, Revuz L, et al. Borrelia burgdorferi and localized scleroderma. Arch Dermatol 1989;125:297–300.

85. Aberer E, Kollegger H, Kristoferitsch W, et al. Neuroborreliosis in morphea and lichen sclerous et atrophicus. J Am Acad Dermatol 1988;19: 820–825.

86. Press RI, et al. Antinuclear antibodies in women with silicone breast implants. Lancet 1992;340: 1304.

87. Sahn EE, Garen PD, Silver RM, et al. Scleroderma following augmentation mammoplasty. Report of a case and review of the literature. Arch Dermatol 1990;126(9):1198–1202.

88. Bernstein RM, Hall MA, Gostelow BE. Morphea-like reaction to D-penicillamine therapy. Ann Rheum Dis 1981;40(1):42–44.

89. Goihman-Yahr M, Leal G, Essenfeld-Yahr E. Generalized morphea: A side effect of valproate sodium? Arch Dermatol 1980;116(6):621.

90. Pujol RM, Puig L, Moreno A, et al. Pseudoscleroderma secondary to phytonadione (vitamin K) injections. Cutis 1989;43:365–368.

91. Lacour JP, Caldani C, Thyss A, et al. Vitiligo-like depigmentation and morphea after specific intralymphatic immunotherapy for malignant melanoma. Dermatology 1992;184:283–285.

92. Van Vlotten WA, Scheffer E, Dooren LJ. Localized scleroderma like lesions after bone marrow transplantation in man. A chronic graft-versus-host reaction. Br J Dermatol 1977;96:337–341.

93. Rao BK, Coldiron B, Freeman RG, et al. Subacute cutaneous lupus erythematosus lesions progressing to morphea. J Am Acad Dermatol 1990;23: 1019–1022.

94. Murrell DF. A radical proposal for the pathogenesis of scleroderma. J Am Acad Dermatol 1993; 28:78–85.

95. Claman HN. Mast cells and fibrosis: The relevance to scleroderma. Rheum Dis Clin North Am 1990;16:141–151.

96. Sherer GK, Jackson BB, LeRoy EC. Chromosome breakage and sister chromatid exchange frequencies in scleroderma. Arthritis Rheum 1981;24: 1409–1413.

97. LeRoy EC, Smith EA, Kahaleh MB, et al. A strategy for determining the pathogenesis of systemic sclerosis. Arthritis Rheum 1989;32:817–825.

98. Kerhl JH, Wakefield LM, Roberts AB, et al. Production of TGF-beta by human T lymphocytes and its potential role in the regulation of T cell growth. J Exp Med 1986;63:1037–1050.

99. Hatamochi A, Ono M, Arakawa M, et al. Analysis of collagen gene expression by cultured fibrob-

lasts in morphea. Br J Dermatol 1992;126: 216–221.

100. Neuhofer J, Fritsch P,. Treatment of localized scleroderma and lichen sclerosus with etretinate. Acta Derm Venereol (Stochk) 1984;64:171–174.

101. Milan MF, Bennett JE. Scleroderma en coup de sabre. Ann Plast Surg 1983;10:364–367.

102. Falanga V, Medsger TA Jr. D-penicillamine in the treatment of localized scleroderma. Arch Dermatol 1990;126:609–612.

103. Moynahan EJ. Morphea (localized cutaneous scleroderma) treated with low dosage penicillamine (4 cases including en coup de sabre). Proc R Soc Med 1973;66:1083–1085.

104. Nelder KH. Treatment of localized scleroderma with phenytoin. Cutis 1978;22:569–572.

105. Guillon M, Priestley GC, Heyworth R. Effects of paraminobenzoate on skin fibroblasts from lichen sclerosus et atrophicus and morphea (abstr). Br J Dermatol 1987;119:454.

106. Humbert PG, Dupond JL, Rocheford A, et al. Localized scleroderma response to 1,25-dihydrovitamin D3. Clin Exp Dermatol 1990;15:396–398.

107. Czarnecki DB, Taft EH. Generalized morphea successfully treated with salazopyrine. Acta Derm Venereol (Stochk) 1982;62:81–82.

108. Pachor ML, Nicolis F, Lunardi C, et al. Morphea: Treatment of two cases with cyclophen. Clin Exp Rheumatol 1987;5(3):293–294.

109. Worle B, Hein R, Krieg T, et al. Cyclosporin in localized and systemic scleroderma—A clinical study. Dermatologica 1990;181(3):215–220.

110. Kahari VM, Heino J, Vuorio T, et al. Interferon-alpha and interferon-gamma reduce excessive collagen synthesis and procollagen mRNA levels of scleroderma fibroblasts in culture. Biochim Biophys Acta 1988;18:45–50.

5

Scleroderma and Pseudoscleroderma: Environmental Exposure

SCLERODERMA, or scleroderma-like conditions, have been reported to be associated with a variety of chemical and environmental exposures ever since the early part of the twentieth century, when Bramwell noted the occurrence of scleroderma in five stonemasons exposed to silica (1). In more recent years, other chemicals and environmental exposures have been implicated (2,3), and the list of chemicals and drugs reported to be associated with scleroderma, or scleroderma-like conditions, continues to grow (Table 5.1).

Cases of scleroderma related to environmental exposures often are marked by cutaneous lesions that resemble idiopathic scleroderma clinically and histologically, yet they may differ from idiopathic scleroderma in the distribution of the cutaneous lesions, by the presence or absence of typical visceral changes of systemic sclerosis (SSc), or by the presence of unique clinical features not generally associated with scleroderma. For these reasons, the term *pseudoscleroderma* has been applied to some of these diverse conditions. Within the pseudoscleroderma group, certain conditions bear a striking resemblance to one another, suggesting a possible common etiology or pathogenesis. This is best illustrated by the similar nature of the toxic oil syndrome (TOS) and the eosinophilia-myalgia syndrome (EMS) (Table 5.2).

The female preponderance seen in idiopathic scleroderma is often not seen when certain occupational exposures are implicated as a cause of the disease. It has even been suggested that environmental exposure may be the major cause of scleroderma among males (4). Depending upon the study, as many as 56% to 77% of male scleroderma patients have been reported to have an occupational exposure risk (5,6). A survey of scleroderma patients in the UK found no occupational risk, but the total number of cases and controls was small (7).

Although some differences may exist between the toxic pseudosclerodermas and idiopathic scleroderma, many similarities exist. In each, an altered immune response is believed to result in the activation of fibroblasts and the synthesis of excessive amounts of connective tissue. Studies of the epidemiology, the immunogenetic susceptibility, and the pathogenesis of the pseudosclerodermas may yield information that not only may prevent future occurrences of environmentally- or occupationally-related pseudoscleroderma, but also may provide insight into the etiology and pathogenesis of idiopathic scleroderma.

Silica, Silicosis, and Silicone

Exposure to elemental silicon (Si) has been associated with a variety of connective tissue diseases, most notably scleroderma. This association was first made in Scottish workers exposed to silica dust (silicon dioxide, SiO_2). Bramwell reported the occurrence of scleroderma in nine of 27,000 patients in his general medical practice, five of whom were stonemasons (1). Typical features of scleroderma were described, including Raynaud's

Table 5.1. Chemicals and Toxins Implicated in Scleroderma and Pseudoscleroderma

Silica and Silicone exposure
Adulterated rapeseed oil (Toxic Oil Syndrome)
Contaminated L-tryptophan (Eosinophilia-Myalgia Syndrome)
Other biogenic amines: 5-hyroxytryptophan, appetite suppressants, bromocriptine
Vinyl chloride monomer (Vinyl Chloride Disease)
Epoxy resin vapor
Organic solvents: Trichloroethylene, trichloroethane, perchlorethylene, toluene, benzene, xylene, methylene chloride, meta-phenylenediamine
Bleomycin
Pentazocine

Table 5.2. Clinical manifestations of acute DFE, TOS and EMS[*]

Clinical Features	DFE	TOS	EMS
Gender	F = M	F > M	F >> M
Age, mean (yrs.)	45	47	49
Precipitant (% cases)	exercise (30%)	adulterated rapeseed oil (~100%)	contaminated L-tryptophan (98%)
Occurrence	sporadic	epidemic	epidemic
Peak onset	N/A	1981	1989
Fever	+/−	+ + + +	+ +
Myalgia	+	+ + + +	+ + + +
Alopecia	+/−	+ + + +	+ +
Rash	+/−	+ + +	+ + +
Scleroderma-like lesions	+ + + +	+ +	+ +
Arthralgia/arthritis	+ +	+ + + +	+ + +
Dyspnea/infiltrate	+/−	+ + + +	+ + +
Peripheral neuropathy	+/−	+ +	+ +
Cardiac disease	+/−	+	+
Pulmonary hypertension	+/−	+	+/−
Hepatic disease	+/−	+	+/−
Thromboemboli	+/−	+	+/−

[*] Abbreviations: DFE, diffuse fasciitis with eosinophilia; TOS, toxic oil syndrome; EMS, eosinophilia-myalgia syndrome; N/A, not applicable
+ + + + ≥ 75% cases   + + + ≥ 50-75% cases   + + ≥ 25-50% cases   + ≥ 25% cases
+/− ≤ 5% or absent

phenomenon (RP), digital ulcers, swollen and hidebound skin over the hands, telangiectasias, and arthralgia.

The association of scleroderma and silica exposure received little attention until Erasmus reported the occurrence of scleroderma among 17 South African goldminers exposed to high concentrations of silica (8). Later, the association of scleroderma with silica exposure and silicosis was confirmed in American and German coalminers (4,9). German investigators estimated the likelihood of developing scleroderma to be 25-fold higher in persons exposed to silica and 110-fold higher in persons with silicosis (4). Although a later study of 79 South African goldminers with scleroderma failed to confirm the association between scleroderma and silicosis (radiographically defined), it did find a significantly higher cumulative lifetime silica exposure in scleroderma cases compared to controls (10). Despite differences in methods and controls, reports spanning many years and from many geographic locales support an association between silica exposure and diffuse cutaneous scleroderma. The illness is typical of systemic sclerosis and in some cases there may be a fulminant pulmonary component of the disease. Antibodies to topoisomerase I (anti-Scl-70) are detectable in as many as 50% of silica-associated scleroderma cases (5,6,11). Anticentromere antibodies have also been reported (6).

The relationship between silicone and connective tissue disease (CTD), especially scleroderma, has generated much controversy and is the subject of great debate and considerable litigation. Silicone (dimethylpolysiloxane) has been used extensively in medicine and surgery (e.g., silastic or silicone gel). The longterm safety of silicone gel-filled breast implants has been questioned, but only recently has the US Food and Drug Administration required the manufacturers of breast implants to provide proof of safety of such prostheses. The medical and the general communities await the outcome of such studies to define the actual risk of scleroderma and other CTD for those exposed to silicone. Until then, opinions and decisions will be based on data derived from previously cited studies of silica exposure (silica is present in silicone gel-filled breast implants), anecdotal reports linking silicone to scleroderma and other CTD, and circumstantial evidence demonstrating Si at sites of CTD in patients with silicone gel-filled breast implants (see following paragraphs).

The term *human adjuvant disease* was coined in 1984 by Japanese investigators who reported the occurrence of CTD in two patients who received injections of paraffin and silicone for augmentation mammoplasty (12). In the 1950s and 1960s, direct injection of paraffin, silicone, or processed petroleum jelly was performed to augment breast size. Later, implantable silastic envelopes containing silicone gel or saline were employed. There have been numerous case reports or small series reporting CTD in women following such cosmetic surgery, with a latency period averaging 10 years. Of 85 cases reviewed by Hochberg in 1992, 50 patients had a definite

CTD (25 scleroderma, 13 rheumatoid arthritis (RA), eight systemic lupus erythematosus (SLE), four mixed connective tissue disease (MCTD)), and the remainder had a poorly defined syndrome often referred to as human adjuvant disease (13). The validity of the association of augmentation mammoplasty with scleroderma remains uncertain, but the unexpected preponderance of scleroderma among silicone exposed subjects with CTD is suggestive of a possible etiologic role. An initial survey failed to reveal any significant increase in the incidence of CTD, but the follow-up was relatively brief and the sample size was small and inadequate to detect an increased risk for a condition as rare as scleroderma (14). A larger multicenter case-control study noted a frequency of 0.66% for augmentation mammoplasty before diagnosis of scleroderma, which does not differ from the expected frequency of 0.65% to 1% (15). The final results of this and other ongoing case-control studies should help determine the validity of the association of scleroderma with augmentation mammoplasty.

Cases of scleroderma associated with silicone exposure resemble those of idiopathic scleroderma, with skin fibrosis in a limited (acrosclerosis) or diffuse (truncal) cutaneous distribution (16–23) or, occasionally, as morphea without systemic involvement (24,25). RP, digital ulceration, arthralgia or arthritis, and visceral involvement have been reported. At least two cases of scleroderma renal crisis have been reported (26,27), with reversal following silicone implant removal in one (26). Esophageal dysmotility similar to that observed in scleroderma, but without skin changes, RP, or antinuclear antibodies (ANAs), has been reported in a few selected children breast-fed by mothers with silicone breast implants (28). Overall, the clinical response to removal of silicone implants has been variable; some patients have shown dramatic improvement in skin and visceral organ involvement, whereas others have had progressive, sometimes fatal, disease (23,29).

Positive ANAs occur in a variable percentage of patients, depending in part on the substrate or method employed. Western blot is more sensitive than indirect immunofluorescence tests, but even with the former the frequency of recognized ANAs may be lower than in idiopathic scleroderma (30). Generally, the more well defined the CTD the higher the likelihood of finding a positive ANA. Scleroderma-specific autoantibodies, such as antitopoisomerase-I, anticentromere, and anti-RNA polymerase I, have been detected in scleroderma patients with prior silicone exposure (30,31).

Elemental Si is present in the fibrous capsule as well as in lymph nodes and tissues involved by CTD in subjects with silicone gel-filled breast implants (21,29). Using electron probe microanalysis, Si was detected in skin involved by scleroderma but not in clinically uninvolved skin (29). In a second patient with interstitial lung disease and features of scleroderma and SLE, silicon was present in alveolar macrophages (29). Similar findings were noted in the capsule surrounding the breast implants, among foamy macrophages containing vacuoles with small residual fragments of refractile, nonpolarizeable material containing silicon (Fig. 5.1) (21,29). Similar histologic and electron microscopic features have been described in axillary lymph nodes (21). Taken together, these studies demonstrate that silicone or silicon may escape from breast implants (even without frank rupture) and may migrate beyond the capsule to regional lymph nodes and distant sites where an inflammatory and fibrotic process may ensue. The actual role of silicon in this process remains to be determined, but experimental evidence indicates that Si might trigger persistent inflammatory and fibrotic reactions (21). Subcutaneous injection of silicone in animals is followed by a local inflammatory response with accumulation of vacuolated macrophages that ingest silica, followed by chronic inflammation and the development of fibrosis (33). Furthermore, silicone may be converted *in vivo* to silica, which has been shown experimentally to exert profound effects on the immune system (33,34).

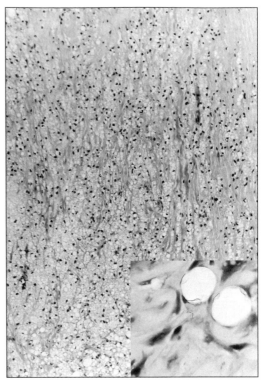

Figure 5.1. Fibrous capsule of breast implant containing numerous foamy macrophages. (*Inset*) Many vacuoles contain small residual fragments of refractile, nonpolarizable material near the rim of the vacuole (*arrow*) (hematoxylin-eosin, original magnifications x80 and x400). (Reproduced with permission from Silver RM, Sahn EE, Allen JA, et al. Demonstration of silicon in sites of connective tissue disesase in patients with silicone–gel breast implants. Arch Dermatol 1993;129:63–68.)

Toxic Oil Syndrome

In May 1981, a new food-borne disease that came to be known as the toxic oil syndrome (TOS) occurred in epidemic proportions in Spain (35). Approximately 20,000 individuals were affected, with more than 800 deaths to date. The majority of those surviving continue to display symptoms and signs to a varying degree. Epidemiological studies of TOS showed a strong association with the ingestion of adulterated rapeseed oil (36). Rapeseed oil denatured with aniline was sold door-to-door or in weekly open-air markets, supposedly as pure olive oil in 5-liter plastic containers (37). Virtually all studies support the conclusion that adulterated rapeseed oil was the vehicle of the TOS agent. The precise agent was never identified, but case-associated oils were contaminated with fatty acid anilides and aniline. A dose-response relationship existed between the level of aniline and anilide contamination and the risk of a family member developing TOS (38).

The vast majority of toxicity studies of case-associated oils in experimental animals were negative (39). One possible etiologic agent, 3-aminophenyl-1,2-propanediol, was present in some case-associated oils and was present after simulated refining procedures with oils containing aniline. In only one toxicological study did 3-aminophenyl-1,2-propanediol produce tissue toxicity when administered to mice (40). Of interest is the identification of a similarly structured compound, 3-(phenylamino)alanine (PAA), in batches of L-tryptophan implicated in the EMS epidemic (41), described below.

TOS affected children and adults, with a female:male ratio of 1.5:1. The clinical course was divided into three phases: an acute phase (months 1–2), an intermediate phase (months 2–4), and a chronic phase (month 4 onward).

The acute phase was marked by a nonproductive cough, chest tightness, and dyspnea. Other symptoms consisted of fever, malaise, headache, edema, myalgia, arthralgia, pruritus, and rash. Eosinophilia was observed in more than 85% of patients during the acute phase. Serum levels of IgE, triglycerides, and hepatic transaminases often were elevated. Chest radiography revealed generalized alveolar-interstitial infiltrates and pleural effusions. The clinical picture was consistent with non-cardiogenic pulmonary edema, and secondary respiratory failure was a frequent cause of death during the acute phase.

The majority of patients evolved to an intermediate phase 2 to 4 months after onset. Edema of the skin and subcutaneous tissue, a prominent feature of this phase, often progressed to fibrosis with contracture formation. Other cutaneous manifestations included alopecia and hyperpigmented papules. Severe myalgia and muscle cramps occurred. In some patients, a sensory neuropathy developed. Thromboembolic complications also occurred, and in some patients were fatal.

The chronic phase was marked by the occurrence of peripheral neuropathy (37%), hepatomegaly (32%), scleroderma-like skin changes (22%), and pulmonary hypertension (10%)(42). Skin changes more closely resembled those of eosinophilic fasciitis and EMS (see below) than idiopathic scleroderma. The eosinophilia resolved, and later the fibrosis of the skin and subcutis evolved to an atrophic stage. Death attributable to pulmonary hypertension continues to be reported during the chronic phase.

The distinctive lesion of TOS is a non-necrotizing vasculitis affecting mainly the intima (an "endovasculitis") and involving vessels of every type and size in nearly every organ (43). Damage extends from the intima into the media and adventitia without fibrinoid necrosis, and consists of a mixed inflammatory infiltrate (lymphocytes, histiocytes, and eosinophils). Subintimal fibrosis ensued, and thromboembolic complications were related to the endovasculitis.

Skin lesions in the acute phase were marked by edema of the papillary dermis with superficial and deep perivascular inflammatory infiltrates. In the intermediate phase, scleroderma-like lesions were characterized by fibrosis and vascular changes in the deep dermis and panniculus. Mucin deposits were present in papular lesions. Eventually, dermal sclerosis occurred with loss of hair follicles and sebaceous glands.

Empiric treatment consisted of antibiotics, corticosteroids, d-penicillamine, immunosuppressive agents, plasmapheresis, vasodilators, and anti-oxidants. No convincing effect was noted for any such therapy. Corticosteroid therapy may have ameliorated the acute pulmonary edema and eosinophilia but did not appear to prevent chronic disease. Pulmonary hypertension and neuromuscular disease remain difficult chronic problems with no effective treatment.

Eosinophilia-Myalgia Syndrome

A seemingly new illness was first described in the United States in late 1989, when physicians in New Mexico reported the occurrence of generalized myalgia and eosinophilia in three women, each of whom had a prior history of ingesting the amino acid, L-tryptophan (44). The illness was linked to the ingestion of L-tryptophan and reached epidemic proportions in late 1989. It quickly subsided when L-tryptophan-containing products were recalled. This illness, now known as the eosinophilia-myalgia syndrome (EMS), frequently was complicated by the occurrence of scleroderma-like hardening of the skin and subcutaneous tissues. EMS shares many features with eosinophilic fasciitis (45,46), as well as with the toxic oil syndrome (TOS)(35,47)(Table 5.2).

During the 1980s, L-tryptophan was used for a number of conditions, such as depression, insomnia, obesity, and premenstrual syndrome, based on its metabolic role as a precursor for the synthesis of the neurotransmitter serotonin (5-hydroxytryptamine). In addition to its role in the synthesis of serotonin, L-tryptophan is also metabolized via kynurenine to nicotinamide dinucleotide (NAD) and nicotinic acid, or niacin. In fact, the vast majority of ingested L-tryptophan is metabolized via the kynurenine pathway, and only a fraction is metabolized to serotonin (Fig. 5.2).

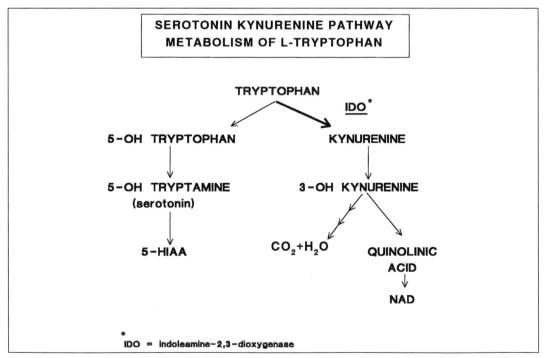

Figure 5-2. Serotonin and kynurenine pathways of metabolism of L-tryptophan. During the active phase of the eosinophilia-myalgia syndrome, the toxic oil syndrome, and eosinophilic fasciitis, kynurenine and quinolinic acid levels are elevated, probably as a result of induction of the enzyme indoleamine-2,3-dioxygenase (IDO).

Alteration in L-tryptophan metabolism has been described in a number of inflammatory and rheumatic conditions, including scleroderma and eosinophilic fasciitis (48). Of interest was the observation in 1981 by Sternberg et al of altered metabolism of L-tryptophan in a patient with a scleroderma-like illness associated with the ingestion of 5-hydroxytryptophan (49). Several similar cases have been described (50,51), all closely resembling cases of EMS. Although elevated levels of kynurenine were initially attributed to a possible inborn error of metabolism, subsequent studies suggest that in these conditions it was due to the induction of indoleamine-2,3-dioxygenase (IDO), with shunting of L-tryptophan via the kynurenine pathway (Fig. 5.2).

During the active, eosinophilic phase of the illness, untreated EMS patients had low plasma levels of L-tryptophan and high plasma levels of kynurenine and its breakdown product, quinolinic acid (52). Plasma neopterin, a marker of interferon-γ, was elevated and correlated with quinolinic acid (53). When given a loading dose of L-tryptophan, such patients demonstrated enhanced kynurenine and quinolinic acid synthesis (54). Corticosteroid-treated EMS patients metabolized L-tryptophan in a manner similar to age- and sex-matched healthy controls. Thus, the handling of L-tryptophan in EMS and related conditions is the result of cytokine induction of IDO and not related to an inborn error of metabolism. Identical findings have been reported in patients with TOS (53).

Federal and state health agencies in the United States acted swiftly to define EMS and to investigate its etiology (55). The Centers for Disease Control (CDC) established the following case definition for surveillance purposes: (*a*) eosinophil count $> 1 \times 10^9$/L, (*b*) generalized myalgia of sufficient severity to limit activity, and (*c*) exclusion of neoplasm or infection to account for the syndrome (56). As of August 1, 1992, the CDC reported 1,511 cases of EMS and 38 deaths from neurologic, cardiac, and pulmonary complications. In view of the passive surveillance system in the United States and the rigid case definition, it is estimated that only one-half of those patients meeting the surveillance case definition were reported, and that there may be another 3,000 individuals who consumed L-tryptophan and are now exhibiting symptoms consistent with EMS but do not meet the full surveillance criteria.

Several case-control studies showed a very strong association of EMS with the ingestion of L-tryptophan (57–59). A study from Minnesota found that 29 of 30 (97%) EMS patients and 21 of 35 controls (60%) had consumed L-tryptophan manufactured by a single manufacturer (odds ratio 19.3, p<.001) (57). A trace-back study in Oregon yielded similar results (58). A study of 418 L-tryptophan users from a single psychiatry practice showed that the risk of developing EMS was related to increasing the dose of L-tryptophan, as well as increased age of the user (60). These and other studies suggested that contamination during the manufacture of L-tryptophan was responsible for the epidemic, and that the attack rate might have been influenced by cofactors such as age.

The manufacturing process employed by the implicated company involved a bacterial fermentation process with subsequent filtration and purification. Late in 1988, a genetically modified strain of *Bacillus amyloliquefaciens* that yielded increased amounts of L-tryptophan was introduced. At about the same time, the filtration process was modified to reduce the amount of activated carbon and to bypass a reverse osmosis membrane filter. In a case-control study, significant associations between lots used by case patients and changes in the manufacturing process were confirmed (57). Initial high-performance liquid chromatography of the company's L-tryptophan demonstrated several peaks, one (peak E) strongly associated with the syndrome (57).

The structure of peak E was confirmed as 1,1'-ethylidenebis(L-tryptophan)(EBT)(61). A recent case-control study of over 500 patients attending a single medical clinic revealed an attack rate of 2.2%, and a significant association between EMS and ingestion of L-tryptophan containing a high concentration of EBT (70 µg/g)(adjusted odds ratio = 35.9, 95% CI 1.9–675.3, p = .02)(62). UV-5, a second trace contaminant of L-tryptophan, was subsequently identified as 3-(phenylamino)alanine (PAA), and it, too, has been linked epidemiologically to the EMS epidemic (41). Its structure is similar to a putative etiologic agent of TOS, 3-aminophenyl-1,2-propanediol (41). Other trace contaminants present in implicated batches of L-tryptophan (peaks AAA, C, FF, OO and 200) have also been associated with the EMS epidemic (63). Peak 200 has been identified as 2[3-indolymethyl]-L-tryptophan; structures of the other peaks are unknown at this time.

These elegant epidemiologic studies showing an association between contaminants and the EMS epidemic cannot address the issue of causation. The latter can only be determined by animal studies in which purified chemical constituents of implicated batches of L-tryptophan are administered alone or in combination to animals presumed to be susceptible to the disease. Several such studies have been reported and others are now underway. Implicated L-tryptophan and synthesized EBT have been shown to induce inflammation and fibrosis of the fascia and perimysium of female Lewis rats (64,65). Recently, a second model has been proposed employing C57/BL6 mice, in which daily intraperitoneal administration of EBT yields significant inflammation and fibrosis of the dermis, fascia, and perimysium, consistent with those changes observed in subjects with EMS (66). Mast cells, also seen in EMS lesions, have been observed in each of these proposed models. In neither model has tissue or blood eosinophilia been observed.

EMS is a multisystem disease that, in its acute phase, often has a flu-like onset with fever, rash, arthralgia, and dyspnea, as well as the characteristic myalgia and eosinophilia. Nearly one-third of all patients required hospitalization. The majority of patients were Caucasian females, a reflection of the ingestion patterns of L-tryptophan rather than race or gender susceptibility. The median daily dose of L-tryptophan ingested was 1.5 g.

Myalgia was nearly universal and often was diffuse and debilitating (67,68). Serum levels of creatine kinase were usually normal, but aldolase levels were often elevated. Severe muscle cramps occurred, and for many patients this has been a persistent and debilitating feature of the chronic phase of EMS, similar to TOS. The pathogenesis of the myalgia and cramps is not known. Ischemia and neuropathic changes may underlie their pathogenesis, but myonecrosis was not seen. An acquired metabolic abnormality is also possible, given the recent observation of abnormal P-31 magnetic resonance spectroscopy of skeletal muscle (69).

Eosinophilia is one criterion for the case definition of EMS and was present in most but probably not all patients. Overall, the median percentage of eosinophils was 39% and the median eosinophil count was more than 5×10^9/L (70). Serum and urine levels of two eosinophil granule products, major basic protein and eosinophil-derived neurotoxin, were elevated in some patients, signifying eosinophil activation and degranulation (71). Similarly, tissue levels of eosinophil granule proteins also appeared to have been accentuated (71). Interleukin-5, a cytokine that stimulates eosinophil production and enhances eosinophil survival, was detectable in the serum of some EMS patients (72). Eosinophilia resolved promptly after the administration of glucocorticoids.

Skin rash or induration was present in the majority of patients with EMS (52,67,68). Erythematous macules, sometimes pruritic, were often present on the trunk and extremities during the acute phase. Papular eruptions (papular mucinosis) occurred in some patients (73). Subcutaneous edema, sometimes massive, occurred in many patients, affecting the upper and lower extremities. Edema often evolved to a tense, woody induration with a *peau d'orange* quality similar to that seen in patients with eosinophilic fasciitis and TOS. Unlike scleroderma, the face and the acral portions of the body were usually spared by the indurative process. Also, EMS patients generally did not have RP, nor did they have abnormal nailfold capillaries (52). Alopecia affecting the scalp and the body was sometimes present in the early phase of EMS.

Many EMS patients had dyspnea and cough during the early phase of the illness (74–77), but respiratory complaints were less frequent and severe than in TOS, where noncardiogenic pulmonary edema was severe and sometimes fatal. Nevertheless, one carefully conducted study found a high incidence of pulmonary symptoms in EMS patients (77). The study found frequent abnormalities in diffusing capacity and maximal static respiratory pressures, suggesting the presence of parenchymal lung involvement and respiratory muscle weakness. Linear opacities with or without pleural effusions were frequently seen on chest radiographs and usually resolved with corticosteroid therapy. Interstitial pneumonitis with eosinophilia and perivascular inflammation was evident on lung biopsy. Bronchoalveolar lavage (BAL) fluid also contained eosinophils (78). In some patients, pulmonary vascular disease was present and sometimes fatal. Unlike TOS, few cases of late-onset pulmonary hypertension have been reported during the first four years of follow-up of EMS patients.

Peripheral neuropathy occurred in many EMS patients (68,79–82). Diffuse and localized paresthesia or hyperesthesia were frequent. An ascending polyneuropathy occurred rarely, but two-thirds of the known deaths from EMS were related to complications secondary to progressive polyneuropathy and myopathy, such as respiratory failure, pneumonia, and sepsis (83). Central nervous system involvement also has been described (84–86). A few patients were reported to have had acute encephalopathy. Magnetic resonance imaging revealed multiple white-matter lesions in some cases, and one autopsy showed a perivascular lymphocytic infiltrate and meningitis (87). In several cases, central nervous system signs and symptoms appeared long after the eosinophilia had resolved.

A major concern is the possible occurrence of neurocognitive dysfunction. Although a thorough, controlled study has yet to be performed,

a number of investigators have reported the presence of neurocognitive dysfunction such as memory impairment, difficulty concentrating, difficulty remembering words or names of persons, etc., in as many as 60% of EMS patients (88,89). Neither the actual prevalence nor the pathogenesis of this aspect of EMS is known at this time. Potential neurotoxic mediators in EMS include eosinophil-derived neurotoxin and the kynurenine metabolite, quinolinic acid. Significant elevations of quinolinic acid were detected not only in the plasma (52), but also in the cerebrospinal fluid of EMS patients (54,80).

Cardiac involvement was implicated in the death of some EMS patients but, overall, cardiac disease was not a major feature of the illness. Pathologic lesions in the coronary arteries, neural structures, and conducting system in three patients provided a basis for significant cardiac electrical instability and sudden death (90). Similar lesions were observed in cardiac tissue of patients with TOS (91). One case of severe restrictive cardiomyopathy in conjunction with deposition of eosinophil major basic protein along the fibrotic endocardial-myocardial interface has been reported (92).

Full-thickness biopsies of skin lesions show an inflammatory and fibrosing process affecting the dermis and subcutaneous tissue including the fascia and extending to the perimysium (Fig. 5.3). A perivascular mononuclear cell infiltrate is seen, with or without eosinophils. Endothelial cells appear swollen, but true vasculitis is rare. Similar lesions were seen in patients with TOS, although results of full-thickness biopsies were seldom reported. Inflammation and fibrosis affecting the subcutaneous fat, septa, and fascia are also seen in eosinophilic fasciitis, but dermal changes appear to be more prominent in EMS (93,94).

Reactive mesenchymal cells sharing features of histiocytes and fibroblasts are present in the deep fascia (95). Expression of mRNA for types I and VI collagen, as well as transforming growth factor-β_1 (TGF-β), is increased in affected fascia (96,97), supporting a role for cytokine-driven fi-

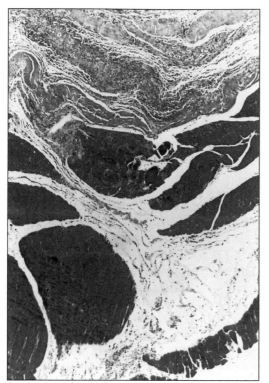

Figure 5.3. Fascia and muscle from a patient with the eosinophilia-myalgia syndrome (hematoxylin-eosin, magnification x 50). The fascia is thickened and contains an inflammatory cell infiltrate composed of lymphocytes, macrophages and plasma cells. The inflammatory cell infiltrate extends into the connective tissue of the underlying skeletal muscle, but is not associated with muscle cell degeneration. (Reproduced with permission from Silver RM, Heyes MP, Maize JC, et al. Scleroderma, fasciitis, and eosinophilia associated with the ingestion of tryptophan. N Eng J Med 1990;322: 874–881.)

brosis. In addition to the increased expression of TGF-β, there is evidence of increased production of other cytokines, including interferon-γ (53), IL-4 (98), and IL-5 (72). The nature of the dermal lymphocytic infiltrate has not been well characterized. Fascial and muscle specimens contain predominantly T lymphocytes (most are CD8+) and macrophages; B lymphocytes and eosinophils are present but make up only a fraction of the cellular infiltrate (99).

Optimal treatment of EMS, as well as its natural history, remain to be determined. As was the case in TOS, for many patients EMS has become a chronic disease, with more than 50% of patients reporting myalgia, muscle cramps, fatigue, paresthesias, and scleroderma-like skin changes at follow-up 18 to 24 months after disease onset (100). In one population-based cohort, the course during the initial 4 to 6 months was severe, followed by a gradual decrease in myalgia, pulmonary complications, skin rash, and edema (101). Despite the early improvement, most patients remained symptomatic 12 months after onset of disease (102). Myalgia and fatigue persisted in the majority of cases, and only 26% reported that they were able to perform all normal daily activities. Cognitive difficulties appear to have developed later in the course of the disease, and significant improvement in such symptoms has not been observed (100).

Treatment has generally been empiric and uncontrolled. Eosinophilia, edema, and pneumonitis usually resolved promptly after the initiation of glucocorticoid therapy, but disease duration does not appear to have been affected, and symptoms often returned after withdrawal of glucocorticoids. A variety of other agents including nonsteroidal anti-inflammatory drugs, cyclophosphamide, azathioprine, cyclosporin A, methotrexate, plasmapheresis, d-penicillamine, antimalarials, and octreotide have been employed, but none have shown consistent beneficial effects (103).

Vinyl Chloride Disease

Exposure to vinyl chloride ($CH_2=CHCl$) has been associated with a scleroderma-like illness referred to as occupational acro-osteolysis (3). Large-scale production of polyvinyl chloride (PVC) began in the 1930s in the US and Germany (104). During the mid-1950s, health hazards of chronic occupational exposure to vinyl chloride monomer (VCM) began to be reported. Workers at plants producing VCM presented with symptoms of RP ("toxic angioneurosis") (105,106). Findings included vasospasm of the digital arteries, swollen fingers, induration of the skin on the volar surface of the forearms, paresthesias, CNS symptoms such as headache, decreased memory and insomnia, mild hemolysis, and a destructive lesion of the distal phalanges in the hands (acro-osteolysis). Microvascular abnormalities on wide-field capillary microscopy resembling those seen in idiopathic scleroderma were noted in many subjects with vinyl chloride disease (107).

Less than 3% of exposed workers developed acro-osteolysis (108). Long-term reactor cleaning was most frequently associated with RP and acro-osteolysis (108). Susceptibility to vinyl chloride disease was reported to be associated with the presence of HLA-DR5, and progressive disease was linked to the presence of the A1, B8, DR3 haplotype in UK workers (109,110). The ANA was generally negative, and neither anticentromere nor anti-topoisomerase I antibodies were detected (109).

Skin changes suggestive of scleroderma included thickening of the skin over the fingers, hands and forearms, sometimes accompanied by puffiness or coarsening of the face. Raised nodules or ivory-colored plaques of indurated skin were seen over the hands and forearms (111). Biopsy showed dermal sclerosis without epidermal atrophy (112). Unlike idiopathic scleroderma, digital pitting scars, esophageal dysmotility, renal disease, and cardiac disease were generally absent. Pulmonary disease was noted in some cases (109), but a relationship to vinyl chloride exposure is uncertain (104). Noncirrhotic portal hypertension and hepatic angiosarcoma occurred as late sequelae in some cases.

Skin lesions regressed after cessation of exposure to vinyl chloride. Serious cases of vinyl chloride disease can be avoided by controlling exposure to VCM and screening exposed employees for RP and radiographic signs of early acro-osteolysis.

Organic Solvents

Since the initial report in 1957 of scleroderma occurring in a woman with a 2-year history of exposure to trichloroethylene (113), more than 50 such cases have appeared in the literature (2,114–123). A high percentage of Hungarian (28%) and UK (30%) scleroderma patients have been reported to have a history of solvent exposure (7,121). Although a case-control study did not confirm an increased risk, the number of subjects was small (7). Recently, two cases of eosinophilic fasciitis were reported in association with trichlorethylene exposure (124).

Organic solvents reported to be associated with scleroderma include trichloroethylene, trichloroethane, benzene, xylene, methylene chloride, toluene, perchlorethylene, and meta-phenylenediamine. The organic solvent implicated most often is trichloroethylene ($CHCl=CCl_2$). It and perchlorethylene ($CCl_2=CCl_2$) are similar in structure to vinyl chloride.

Scleroderma in subjects with solvent exposure generally is indistinguishable from cases of idiopathic scleroderma. Duration and intensity of exposure prior to onset of disease vary. Most cases are characterized by diffuse cutaneous involvement and are accompanied by RP and visceral organ disease. The nailfold capillaries are abnormal and the ANA is positive. The disease usually does not subside with an end to solvent exposure, and fatal cases have been reported.

Amines

Workers engaged in the polymerization of epoxy resins have been reported to develop a scleroderma-like condition. In 1980, Japanese investigators first described this illness in six of 233 workers with a history of brief exposure to vapor of epoxy resins (125). The patients had erythema and edema, which evolved to generalized dermal sclerosis and alopecia. Skin changes were accompanied by weakness and muscle atrophy. RP was not present, nor were ANA's detected. Skin biopsies revealed deposits of melanin in the epidermis and increased collagen deposition in the dermis, as well as panniculitis, which evolved to fibrosis of the subcutaneous adipose tissue. Thickening of the fascia and a low-grade inflammation of the perimysium was seen. The authors concluded that the histologic picture was more consistent with morphea than with scleroderma. Skin and muscle abnormalities improved gradually with removal from exposure to the resin plus protease and corticosteroid therapy.

Nine chemicals were present in the epoxy resin vapor. Intraperitoneal injection of one compound, bis(4-amino-3-methyl-cyclohexyl)methane, produced skin sclerosis in a murine model (125). Three additional compounds also produced skin changes in some animals, but bis(4-amino-3-methyl-cyclohexyl)methane was suspected to be the etiologic agent. It had been added to the polymerization process as a new type of plasticizer at the time of the occurrence of the illness.

Further outbreaks of scleroderma or morphea related to epoxy resin exposure have not been reported, but other amines have been linked to the development of scleroderma-like conditions. EMS is the most recent example (see previous paragraphs). The similar illness associated with 5-hydroxytryptophan has also been discussed. Other amines associated with morphea or scleroderma-like conditions include bromocriptine (126,127), various appetite suppressants (128, 129), and 5-hydroxytryptamine (serotonin) in patients with the carcinoid syndrome (130,131). Fibrosis is a complication of other amines, such as methysergide (132), and pulmonary hypertension has been reported to occur in association with certain appetite suppressants, such as aminorex and fenfluramine (133,134).

Bleomycin

RP and scleroderma occur in some cancer patients treated with bleomycin (135–137). Bleo-mycins are a group of related glycopeptide antibiotics isolated from *Streptomyces verticillus* that differ from one another in the terminal amine. Cutaneous lesions in cases associated with bleomycin are indistinguishable from idiopathic scleroderma, and lesional fibroblasts synthesize increased quantities of glycosoaminoglycan and collagen (136). Rats injected with bleomycin develop weight loss, alopecia, hyperpigmentation, and skin tightness (138). Histologic findings are consistent with those of idiopathic scleroderma. Features of systemic sclerosis may not be present, and the ANA is variably positive (137). Partial resolution occurs after cessation of bleomycin and may be hastened by the addition of corticosteroids (137).

The mechanism whereby bleomycin induces scleroderma is unknown, but vascular injury may be the primary process. The earliest pathologic lesion in experimental animal models of bleomycin-induced pulmonary fibrosis is endothelial cell injury (139). It is of interest that vascular abnormalities, such as RP, occur frequently (22 of 60 cases) in men treated with bleomycin and vinblastine for testicular carcinoma (140). Even low-dose bleomycin injected locally may be followed by the development of RP (141). Thus, vascular injury may be the primary insult whereby bleomycin induces scleroderma.

Pentazocine

Cutaneous sclerosis complicating intramuscular injections of the analgesic pentazocine is readily distinguishable from idiopathic scleroderma. Brawny induration and deep penetrating ulcers around the sites of injection are characteristic. Such changes may be accompanied by a fibrous myopathy, joint contractures, neuropathy, and soft tissue calcification (142,143). The skin of the face and fingers is spared, and patients do not have visceral organ involvement. Histologic findings include dermal fibrosis extending to the panniculus with varying degrees of inflammation, small vessel thrombosis, intimal proliferation, and lymphohistiocytic perivascular inflammation (144).

Conclusion

A variety of environmental exposures have been linked to scleroderma and scleroderma-like conditions. It is likely that other chemicals or toxins will be found to be associated with the onset of such conditions. Although some of the environmentally linked conditions differ clinically from idiopathic scleroderma, they all share the propensity to produce inflammation and fibrosis of the skin and subcutaneous tissue. Only a fraction of those exposed to such chemicals or environmental agents will develop a sclerodermatous condition. The host's immunogenetic background, as well as other potential co-factors, probably are important determinants of susceptibility to these conditions. It is hoped that knowledge gained from the study of these endemic and epidemic cases of scleroderma-like disorders will not only help to prevent future occurrences but may also lead to improved understanding of the pathogenesis of idiopathic scleroderma. Only then will rational forms of therapy be developed.

References

1. Bramwell B. Diffuse sclerdermia: Its frequency; its occurrence in stone-masons; its treatment by fibrolysin—elevations of temperature due to fibrolysin injections. Edinburgh Med J 1914;12: 387–401.
2. Owens GR, Medsger TA. Systemic sclerosis secondary to occupational exposure. Am J Med 1988;85:114–116.
3. Straniero NR, Furst DE. Environmentally-induced systemic sclerosis-like illness. Baillieres Clin Rheumatol 1989;3:63–79.
4. Haustein UF, Ziegler V. Environmentally induced systemic sclerosis-like disorders. Int J Dermatol 1985;24:147–151.
5. Gabay C, Kahn M-F. Les sclerodermies masculines: Role de l'exposition professionnelle. Schweiz Med Wochenschr 1992;122:1746–1752.
6. Haustein U-F, Ziegler V, Herrmann K, et al. Silica-induced scleroderma. J Am Acad Dermatol 1990;22:444–448.
7. Silman AJ, Jones S. What is the contribution of occupational environmental factors to the occurrence of scleroderma in men? Ann Rheum Dis 1992;51:1322–1324.
8. Erasmus LD. Scleroderma in gold-miners on the Witwatersrand with particular reference to pulmonary manifestations. S Afr J Lab Clin Med 1957;3:209–231.
9. Rodnan GP, Benedek TG, Medsger Jr TA, et al. The association of progressive systemic sclerosis (scleroderma) with coal miners' pneumoconiosis and other forms of silicosis. Ann Intern Med 1967;66:323–334.
10. Sluis-Cremer GK, Hessel P, Nizdo EH, et al. Silica, silicosis, and progressive systemic sclerosis. Br J Indust Med 1985;42:838–843.
11. McHugh NJ, Whyte J, Harvey G, et al. Anti-topoisomerase-1 antibodies are found in the majority of males with silica-associated systemic sclerosis and all inhibit topoisomerase-1 function. Arthritis Rheum 1992;35:S67.
12. Miyoshi K, Miyaoka T, Kobayashi Y, et al. Hypergamma-globulinemia by prolonged adjuvanticity in man: Disorders developed after augmentation mammoplasty. Ijishimpo 1964;2122:9–14.
13. Hochberg MC. Cosmetic surgical procedures and connective tissue disease: The Cleopatra syndrome revisited. Ann Intern Med 1993;118: 981–983.
14. Weisman MH, Vecchione TF, Albert D, et al. Connective-tissue disease following breast augmentation: A preliminary test of the human adjuvant disease hypothesis. Plast Reconstr Surg 1988;82: 626–630.
15. Wigley FM, Miller R, Hochberg MC, et al. Augmentation mammoplasty in patients with systemic sclerosis: Data from the Baltimore scleroderma research center and Pittsburgh scleroderma data bank. Arthritis Rheum 1992;35: S46.
16. Kumagai Y, Abe C, Shiokawa Y. Scleroderma after cosmetic surgery. Four cases of human adjuvant disease. Arthritis Rheum 1979;22:532–537.
17. Kondo H, Kumagai Y, and Shiokawa Y. Scleroderma following cosmetic surgery ("adjuvant disease"): A review of nine cases reported in Japan. In: Black C, Myers AR, eds. Current topics in rheumatology—systemic sclerosis (scleroderma). New York: Gower, 1985;135–137.
18. Endo LP, Edwards NL, Longley S, et al. Silicone and rheumatic diseases. Semin Arthritis Rheum 1987;17:112–118.

19. Brozena SJ, Fenske NA, Cruse CW, et al. Human adjuvant disease following augmentation mammoplasty. Arch Dermatol 1988;124:1383–1386.

20. Spiera, H. Scleroderma after silicone augmentation mammoplasty. JAMA 1988;260:236–238.

21. Varga J, Schumacher R, Jimenez SA. Systemic sclerosis after augmentation mammoplasty with silicone implants. Ann Intern Med 1989;111:377–383.

22. Marik PE, Kark AL, Zambakides A. Scleroderma after silicone augmentation mammoplasty. A report of 2 cases. Sr Afr Med J 1990;77:212–213.

23. Spiera H, Kerr LD. Scleroderma following silicone implantation: A cumulative experience of 11 cases. J Rheumatol 1993;20:958–961.

24. Sahn EE, Garen PD, Silver RM, et al. Scleroderma following augmentation mammoplasty. Report of a case and review of the literature. Arch Dermatol 1990;126:1198–1202.

25. Lazar AP, Lazar P. Localized morphea after silicone gel breast implantation: More evidence for a cause and effect relationship. Arch Dermatol 1991;127:263.

26. Gutierrez V, Espinoza LR. Progressive systemic sclerosis complicated by severe hypertension: Reversal after silicone implant removal. Am J Med 1990;89:390–392.

27. Hitoshi S, Ito Y, Takehara K, et al. A case of malignant hypertension and scleroderma after cosmetic surgery. Jpn J Med 1991;30:97–100.

28. Levine JJ, Ilowite NT. Scleroderma-like esophageal disease in children breast-fed by mothers with silicone breast implants. JAMA 1994;271:213–216.

29. Silver RM, Sahn EE, Allen JA, et al. Demonstration of silicon in sites of connective tissue disease in patients with silicone-gel breast implants. Arch Dermatol 1993;129:63–68.

30. Bridges AJ, Conley C, Wang G, et al. A clinical and immunologic evaluation of women with silicone breast implants and symptoms of rheumatic disease. Ann Intern Med 1993;118:929–936.

31. Press RI, Peebles CL, Kumagai Y, et al. Antinuclear autoantibodies in women with silicone breast implants. Lancet 1992;340:1304–1307.

32. Ballantyne DL, Rees TD, Seidman I. Silicone fluid: Response to massive subcutaneous injections of dimethylpolysulfaxone fluid in animals. Plast Reconstr Surg 1965;36:629–631.

33. Allison AC, Harrington JS, Birbeck M. An examination of the cytotoxic effects of silica on macrophages. J Exp Med 1966;124:141–154.

34. Mancino D, Vuotto ML, Minucci M. Effects of crystalline silica on antibody production to T-dependent and T-independent antigens on BALB/c mice. Int Arch Allergy Appl Immunol 1984;73:10–13.

35. Toxic Epidemic Syndrome Study Group. Toxic epidemic syndrome, Spain, 1981. Lancet 1982;II:697–702.

36. Tabuenca JM. Toxic-allergic syndrome caused by ingestion of rapeseed oil denatured with aniline. Lancet 1981;II:567–568.

37. Kilbourne EM, Posada de la Paz M, Abaitua Borda I. In: Toxic oil syndrome. Current knowledge and future perspectives. WHO Regional Publications, European Series 1992;42:5–26.

38. Kilbourne EM, Bernert JT Jr, Posada de la Paz M, et al. Chemical correlates of pathogenicity of oils related to the toxic oil syndrome in Spain. Am J Epidemiol 1988;127:1210–1227.

39. Aldridge WN. In: Toxic oil syndrome. Current knowledge and future perspectives. WHO Regional Publications, European Series 1992;42:67–98.

40. Pagani R, Portoles MT, Gavilanes FG, et al. The microviscosity of liver plasma membranes of rats fed with oleoylanilide. Biochem J 1984;218:125–129.

41. Mayeno AN, Belongia EA, Lin F, et al. 3-(Phenylamino)alanine, a novel aniline-derived amino acid associated with the eosinophilia-myalgia syndrome: A link to the toxic oil syndrome? Mayo Clin Proc 1992;67:1134–1139.

42. Abaitua Borda I, Posada de la Paz M. In: Toxic oil syndrome. Current knowledge and future perspectives. WHO Regional Publications, European Series 1992;42:27–38.

43. Martinez-Tello FJ, Tellez I. In: Toxic oil syndrome. Current knowledge and future perspectives. WHO Regional Publications, European Series 1992;42:39–66.

44. Hertzman PA, Blevins WL, Mayer J, et al. Association of the eosinophilia-myalgia syndrome with the ingestion of L-tryptophan. N Engl J Med 1990;322:869–873.

45. Shulman LE. Diffuse fasciitis with eosinophilia: A new syndrome? Trans Assoc Am Physicians 1975;88:70–86.

46. Varga J, Griffin R, Newman JH, Jimenez, SA. Eosinophilic fasciitis is clinically distinguishable from the eosinophilia-myalgia syndrome and is not associated with L-tryptophan use. J Rheumatol 1991;18:259–263.

47. Philen RM, Posada M. Toxic oil syndrome and eosinophilia-myalgia syndrome: May 8–10, 1991, World Health Organization meeting report. Semin Arthritis Rheum 1993;23:104–124.

48. Houpt JB, Ogryzlo MA, Hunt M. Tryptophan metabolism in man (with special reference to rheumatoid arthritis and scleroderma). Semin Arthritis Rheum 1973;2:333–353.
49. Sternberg EM, van Woert MH, Young SN, et al. Development of a scleroderma-like illness during therapy with L-5-hydroxy-tryptophan and carbidopa. N Engl J Med 1980;303:782–787.
50. Auffranc JC, Berbis P, Fabre JF, et al. Syndrome sclerodermiforme et poikilodermique observe au cours d'un traitement par carbidopa et 5-hydroxy-tryptophanne. Ann Dermatol Venereol 1985;112:691–692.
51. Joly P, Lampert A, Thomine E, et al. Development of pseudobullous morphea and scleroderma-like illness during therapy with L-5-hydroxytryptophan and carbidopa. J Am Acad Dermatol 1991;25:332–333.
52. Silver RM, Heyes MP, Maize JC, et al. Scleroderma, fasciitis, and eosinophilia associated with the ingestion of tryptophan. N Engl J Med 1990;322:874–881.
53. Silver RM, Sutherland SE, Carreira P, et al. Alterations in tryptophan metabolism in the toxic oil syndrome and in the eosinophilia-myalgia syndrome. J Rheumatol 1992;19:69–73.
54. Silver RM, McKinley K, Smith EA, et al. Tryptophan metabolism via the kynurenine pathway in patients with the eosinophilia myalgia syndrome. Arthritis Rheum 1992;35:1097–1105.
55. Eosinophilia-myalgia syndrome and L-tryptophan-containing products—New Mexico, Minnesota, Oregon, and New York, 1989. MMWR 1989;38:785–788.
56. Eosinophilia-myalgia syndrome—New Mexico. JAMA 1989;262:3116.
57. Belongia EA, Hedberg CW, Gleich GJ, et al. An investigation of the cause of the eosinophilia-myalgia syndrome associated with tryptophan use. N Engl J Med 1990;323:357–365.
58. Slutsker L, Hoesly FC, Miller L, et al. Eosinophilia-myalgia syndrome associated with exposure to tryptophan from a single manufacturer. JAMA 1990;264:213–217.
59. Eidson M, Philen RM, Sewell CM, et al. L-tryptophan and eosinophilia-myalgia syndrome in New Mexico. Lancet 1990;335:645–648.
60. Kamb ML, Murphy JJ, Jones JL, et al. Eosinophilia-myalgia syndrome in L-tryptophan-exposed patients. JAMA 1992;267:77–82.
61. Mayeno AN, Lin F, Foote CS, et al. Characterization of "Peak E," a novel amino acid associated with eosinophilia-myalgia syndrome. Science 1990;250:1707–1708.
62. Henning KJ, Jean-Baptiste E, Singh T, et al. Eosinophilia-myalgia syndrome in patients ingesting a single source of L-tryptophan. J Rheumatol 1993;20:273–278.
63. Hill RH Jr, Caudill SP, Philen RM, et al. Contaminants in L-tryptophan associated with eosinophilia myalgia syndrome. Arch Environ Contam Toxicol 1993;25:134–142.
64. Crofford LJ, Rader JI, Dalakas MC, et al. L-tryptophan implicated in human eosinophilia-myalgia syndrome causes fasciitis and perimyositis in the Lewis rat. J Clin Invest 1990;86:1757–1763.
65. Love LA, Rader JI, Crofford LJ, et al. Pathological and immunological effects of ingesting L-tryptophan and 1,1'-ethylidenebis(L-tryptophan) in Lewis rats. J Clin Invest 1993;91:804–811.
66. Silver RM, Ludwicka A, Hampton M, et al. A murine model of the eosinophilia-myalgia syndrome induced by 1,1'-ethylidenebis(L-tryptophan). J Clin Invest (In press).
67. Clauw DJ, Nashel DJ, Katz P. Tryptophan-associated eosinophilic connective-tissue disease. A new clinical entity? JAMA 1990;263:1502–1506.
68. Kaufman LD, Seidman RJ, Gruber BL. L-Tryptophan-associated eosinophilic perimyositis, neuritis, and fasciitis. A clinicopathologic and laboratory study of 25 patients. Medicine 1990;69:187–199.
69. Clauw DJ, Hewes B, Nelson M, et al. P-31 magnetic resonance spectroscopy of skeletal muscle in the eosinophilia myalgia syndrome. J Rheumatol 1994;21:654–657.
70. Hertzman P, Falk H, Kilbourne EM, et al. The eosinophilia-myalgia syndrome: The Los Alamos conference. J Rheumatol 1991;18:867–873.
71. Martin RW, Duffy J, Engel AG, et al. The clinical spectrum of the eosinophilia-myalgia syndrome associated with L-tryptophan ingestion. Clinical features in 20 patients and aspects of pathophysiology. Ann Intern Med 1990;113:124–134.
72. Owen WF Jr, Petersen J, Sheff DM, et al. Hypodense eosinophils and interleukin 5 activity in the blood of patients with the eosinophilia-myalgia syndrome. Proc Natl Acad Sci USA 1990;87:8647–8651.
73. Kaufman L, Seidman R, Phillips M, et al. Cutaneous manifestations of the L-tryptophan-associated eosinophilia-myalgia syndrome: A spectrum of sclerodermatous skin disease. J Am Acad Dermatol 1990;23:1063–1069.
74. Tazelaar HD, Myers JL, Drage CW, et al. Pulmonary disease associated with L-tryptophan-induced eosinophilic myalgia syndrome. Clinical

and pathologic features. Chest 1990;97:1032–1036.

75. Strumpf IJ, Drucker RD, Anders KH, et al. Acute eosinophilic pulmonary disease associated with the ingestion of L-tryptophan-containing products. Chest 1991;99:8–13.

76. Banner A, Borochovitz D. Acute respiratory failure caused by pulmonary vasculitis after L-tryptophan ingestion. Am Rev Respir Dis 1991;143:661–664.

77. Read CA, Clauw D, Weir C, et al. Dyspnea and pulmonary function in the L-tryptophan-associated eosinophilia-myalgia syndrome. Chest 1992;101:1282–1286.

78. Campagna AC, Blanc PD, Criswell LA, et al. Pulmonary manifestations of the eosinophilia-myalgia syndrome associated with tryptophan ingestion. Chest 1992;101:1274–1281.

79. Smith BE, Dyck PJ. Peripheral neuropathy in the eosinophilia-myalgia syndrome associated with L-tryptophan ingestion. Neurology 1990;40:1035–1040.

80. Heiman-Patterson TD, Bird, SJ, Parry GJ, et al. Peripheral neuropathy associated with eosinophilia-myalgia syndrome. Ann Neurol 1990;28:522–528.

81. Donofrio PD, Stanton C, Miller VS, et al. Demyelinating polyneuropathy in eosinophilia-myalgia syndrome. Muscle Nerve 1992;15:796–805.

82. Tolander LM, Bamford CR, Yoshino MT, et al. Neurologic complications of the tryptophan-associated eosinophilia myalgia syndrome. Arch Neurol 1991;48:436–438.

83. Swygert LA, Back EE, Auerbach SB, et al. Eosinophilia-myalgia syndrome: Mortality data from the US national surveillance system. J Rheumatol 1993;20:1711–1717.

84. Adair JC, Rose JW, Digre KB, et al. Acute encephalopathy associated with the eosinophilia-myalgia syndrome. Neurology 1992;42:461–462.

85. Greenfield BM, Mayer JW, Sibbitt RR. The eosinophilia myalgia syndrome and the brain. Ann Intern Med 1991;115:159–160.

86. Lynn J, Rammohan KW, Bornstein RA, et al. Central nervous system involvement in the eosinophilia-myalgia syndrome. Arch Neurol 1992;49:1082–1085.

87. Pixley JS, Eaton JM, Zweig RM. Central nervous system inflammation in the eosinophilia-myalgia syndrome. Br J Rheumatol 1992;32:174.

88. Anonymous. Eosinophilia-myalgia syndrome: Follow-up survey of patients—New York, 1990-1991. MMWR 1991;40:401–403.

89. Krupp LB, Masur DM, Kaufman LD. Neurocog-

nitive dysfunction in the eosinophilia-myalgia syndrome. Neurology 1993;43:931–936.

90. James TN, Kamb ML, Sandberg GA, et al. Postmortem studies of the heart in three fatal cases of the eosinophilia-myalgia syndrome. Ann Intern Med 1991;115:102–110.

91. James TN, Gomez-Sanchez MA, Martinez-Tello FJ, et al. Cardiac abnormalities in the toxic oil syndrome, with comparative observations on the eosinophilia-myalgia syndrome. J Am Coll Cardiol 1991;18:1367–1379.

92. Berger PB, Duffy J, Reeder GS, et al. Restrictive cardiomyopathy associated with the eosinophilia-myalgia syndrome. Mayo Clin Proc 1994;69:162–165.

93. Feldman SR, Silver RM, Maize JC. A histopathologic comparison of Shulman's syndrome (diffuse fasciitis with eosinophilia) and the fasciitis associated with the eosinophilia-myalgia syndrome. J Am Acad Dermatol 1992;26:95–100.

94. Umbert I, Winkelmann RK, Wegener L. Comparison of the pathology of fascia in eosinophilic myalgia syndrome patients and idiopathic eosinophilic fasciitis. Dermatology 1993;186:18–22.

95. Lin JD, Phelps RG, Gordon ML, et al. Pathologic manifestations of the eosinophilia myalgia syndrome: Analysis of 11 cases. Hum Pathol 1992;23:429–437.

96. Varga J, Peltonen J, Uitto JM, et al. Development of diffuse fasciitis with eosinophilia during L-tryptophan treatment: Demonstration of elevated type I collagen gene expression in affected tissues. A clinicopathologic study of four patients. Ann Intern Med 1990;112:344–351.

97. Peltonen J, Varga J, Sollberg S, et al. Elevated expression of the genes for transforming growth factor-1 and type VI collagen in diffuse fasciitis associated with the eosinophilia-myalgia syndrome. J Invest Dermatol 1991;96:20–25.

98. Kaufman LD, Gruber BL, Needleman BW. Interleukin-4 levels in the eosinophilia-myalgia syndrome. Am J Med 1991;91:664–665.

99. Emslie-Smith AM, Engel AG, Duffy J, et al. Eosinophilia myalgia syndrome: I. Immunocytochemical evidence for a T cell-mediated immune effector resopnse. Ann Neurol 1991;29:524–528.

100. Hertzman P, Clauw D, Kaufman L, et al. Eosinophilia-myalgia syndrome (EMS): Status of 205 patients and results of treatment two years after onset. Ann Int Med, in press.

101. Culpepper RC, Williams RG, Mease PJ, et al. Natural history of the eosinophilia-myalgia syndrome. Ann Intern Med 1991;115:437–442.

102. Hedberg K, Urbach D, Slutsker L, et al. Eosinophilia-myalgia syndrome. Natural history in a

population-based cohort. Arch Intern Med 1992; 152:1889–1892.

103. Kaufman LD, Seidman RJ. L-tryptophan-associated eosinophilia-myalgia syndrome: Perspective of a new illness. Rheum Dis Clin North Am 1991;17:427–441.

104. Lelbach WK, Marsteller HJ. Vinyl chloride-associated disease. In: Advances in internal medicine and pediatrics. New York: Springer Verlag, 1981.

105. Smirnova NA. Clinics of chronic intoxication by olefins and vinyl chloride. Dissertation Gor'kii (Russian text), 1959.

106. Kubota J. Occupational diseases in synthetic resin and fibre industries. (Japanese text). J Sci Labour 1957;33:1–22.

107. Maricq HR, Johnson MN, Whetstone CL, et al. Capillary abnormalities in polyvinyl chloride production workers. Examination by *in vivo* microscopy. JAMA 1976;236:1368–1371.

108. Wilson RH, McCormick WE, Tatum CF, et al. Occupational acro-osteolysis. Report of 31 cases. JAMA 1967;201:577–581.

109. Black CM, Walker AE, Catoggio LJ, et al. Genetic susceptibility to scleroderma-like syndrome induced by vinyl chloride. Lancet 1983;I:53–55.

110. Black C, Pereira S, McWhirter A, et al. Genetic susceptibility to scleroderma-like syndrome in symptomatic and asymptomatic workers exposed to vinyl chloride. J Rheumatol 1986;13: 1059–1062.

111. Veltman G, Lange CE, Juhe S, et al. Clinical manifestations and course of vinyl chloride disease. Ann NY Acad Sci 1975;246:6–17.

112. Jayson MIV, Bailey AJ, Black C, et al. Collagen studies in acro-osteolysis. Proc R Soc Med 1976;69:295–297.

113. Reinl W. Scleroderma caused by trichloroethylene? Bull Hygiene 1957;32:678–679.

114. Brasington RD, Thorpe-Swenson AJ. Systemic sclerosis associated with cutaneous exposure to solvent: Case report and review of the literature. Arthritis Rheum 1991;34:631–633.

115. Walder B. Solvents and scleroderma (letter). Lancet 1965;II:436–437.

116. Sparrow GP. A connective tissue disorder similar to vinyl chloride disease in a patient exposed to perchlorethylene. Clin Exp Dermatol 1977;2:17–22.

117. Saihan EM, Burton JL, Heaton KW. A new syndrome with pigmentation, scleroderma, gynecomastia, Raynaud's phenomenon, and peripheral neuropathy. Br J Dermatol 1978;99:437–440.

118. Lockey JE, Kelly CR, Cannon GW, et al. Progressive systemic sclerosis associated with exposure to trichloroethylene. J Occup Med 1987;29:493–496.

119. Flindt-Hansen H, Isager H. Scleroderma after occupational exposure to trichloroethylene and trichloroethane. Acta Derm Venereol (Stockh) 1987;67:263–264.

120. Yamakage A, Ishikawa H. Generalized morphea-like scleroderma occurring in people exposed to organic solvents. Dermatologica 1982;165:186–193.

121. Czirjak L, Bokk A, Csontos G, et al. Clinical findings in 61 patients with progressive systemic sclerosis. Acta Derm Venereol (Stockh) 1989;69: 533–536.

122. Bottomley WW, Sheehan-Dare RA, Hughes P, et al. A sclerodermatous syndrome with unusual features following prolonged occupational exposure to organic solvents. Br J Dermatol 1993; 128:203–206.

123. Yanez S, Moran M, Unamuno P, et al. Silica and trichloroethylene-induced progressive systemic sclerosis. Dermatology 1992;184:98–102.

124. Waller PA, Clauw D, Cupps T, et al. Fasciitis (not scleroderma) following prolonged exposure to an organic solvent (trichlorethylene): A report of two cases. J Rheumatol 1994;21:1567–1570.

125. Yamakage A, Ishikawa H, Saito Y, et al. Occupational scleroderma-like disorder occurring in men engaged in the polymerization of epoxy resins. Dermatologica 1980;161:33–44.

126. Dupont E, Olivarius B, Strong MJ. Bromocriptine-induced collagenosis-like symptomatology in Parkinson's disease (letter). Lancet 1982;I: 850–851.

127. Leshin B, Piette WW, Caplan RM. Morphea after bromocriptine therapy. Int J Dermatol 1989;28: 177–179.

128. Tomlinson IW, Jayson MIV. Systemic sclerosis after therapy with appetite suppressants. J Rheumatol 1984;11:254.

129. Aeschlimann A, de Truchis P, Kahn MF. Scleroderma after therapy with appetite suppressants. Report of four cases. Scand J Rheumatol 1990; 19:87–90.

130. Zarafonetis CJD, Lorber SH, Hanson SM. Association of functioning carcinoid syndrome and scleroderma. I. Case report. Am J Med Sci 1958; 236:1–14.

131. Fries JF, Lindgren JA, Bull JM. Scleroderma-like lesions and the carcinoid syndrome. Arch Intern Med 1973;131:550–553.

132. Graham JR, Suby HI, LeCompte PR, et al. Fibrotic disorders associated with methysergide therapy for headaches. N Engl J Med 1966;274:359–368.

133. Follath F, Burkart F, Schweizer W. Drug-induced pulmonary hypertension? Br Med J 1971;1: 265–266.

134. Douglas JG, Munro JF, Kitchin AH, et al. Pulmonary hypertension and fenfluramine. Br Med J 1981;283:881–883.

135. Cohen IS, Mosher MB, O'Keefe EJ, et al. Cutaneous toxicity of bleomycin therapy. Arch Dermatol 1973;107:553–555.

136. Finch WR, Rodnan GP, Buckingham RB, et al. Bleomycin-induced scleroderma. J Rheumatol 1980;7:651–659.

137. Kerr LD, Spiera H. Scleroderma in association with the use of bleomycin. A report of 3 cases. J Rheumatol 1992;19:294–296.

138. Mountz JD, Downs Minor MB, Turner R, et al. Bleomycin-induced cutaneous toxicity in the rat: Analysis of histopathology and ultrastructure compared with progressive systemic sclerosis. Br J Dermatol 1983;108:679–686.

139. Fasske E, Morgenroth K. Experimental bleomycin lung in mice. A contribution to the pathogenesis of pulmonary fibrosis. Lung 1983;161:133–146.

140. Vogelzang NJ, Bosl GJ, Johnson K, et al. Raynaud's phenomenon: A common toxicity after combination chemotherapy for testicular cancer. Ann Intern Med 1981;95:288–292.

141. Smith EA, Harper FE, LeRoy EC. Raynaud's phenomenon of a single digit following local intradermal bleomycin sulfate injection. Arthritis Rheum 1985;28:459–461.

142. Hertzman A, Toone E, Resnik CS. Pentazocine induced myocutaneous sclerosis. J Rheumatol 1986;13:210–214.

143. Furner BB. Parenteral pentazocine: Cutaneous complications revisited. J Am Acad Dermatol 1990;22:694–695.

144. Palestine RF, Millns JL, Spigel GT, et al. Skin manifestations of pentazocine abuse. J Am Acad Dermatol 1980;2:47–55.

STEFANIA JABŁÓNSKA
MARIA BLASZCZYK

6

Differential Diagnosis of Scleroderma-Like Disorders

THIS CHAPTER is devoted to pseudosclerodermatous conditions that, although widely different, may imitate the induration and atrophy found both in systemic and localized, exclusively cutaneous scleroderma. Pseudosclerodermatous conditions are a frequent cause of diagnostic errors because their differentiation from scleroderma can present considerable difficulty and, especially, because they fall within the scope of many specialties. Sclerodermatous changes have developed in such disparate conditions as endocrine disorders (e.g., diabetes and hypothyroidism) and malignancies (e.g., myeloma) and have been associated with environmental exposure. In those cases, the differential diagnosis between atypical scleroderma and pseudoscleroderma might be extremely difficult and the classification quite arbitrary.

This chapter does not approach the overlap syndromes, such as scleromyositis, mixed connective tissue disease, or polymyositis with sclerodermiform manifestations, because they present a separate, highly heterogeneous group of rheumatic diseases with distinctive etiology and pathogenesis. Also, Shulman's eosinophilic fasciitis, regarded previously as a scleroderma-like disease, falls within the spectrum of deep localized scleroderma and is described in Chapter 4.

Scleredema

There are two main forms of scleredema, one with an acute onset and benign course and

another with an insidious onset and extremely chronic course, often associated with diabetes (1,2).

The classical scleredema of Buschke (3), presenting as rapidly developing and progressively indurated edema on the neck, shoulder girdle, proximal parts of the upper extremities, and face, is a self-limited disease. The induration regresses within 12 to 18 months, leaving no sequelae for this form of scleredema. The edematous skin is immobile, cannot be pinched, and the facies is mask-like. Contrary to SSc, the hands are not involved. This type of scleredema, usually occurring after febrile illnesses and respiratory infections, appears to be of infectious origin and, presumably owing to the wide use of antibiotics, is currently very rare.

The cases of more widespread sclerotic cutaneous changes of long duration are frequently associated with severe insulin-resistant and/or complicated diabetes (1,4).

Scleredema is usually a relatively mild disorder, although it may be accompanied by visceral changes in the pericardium, myocardium, and/or esophagus (4,5).

PATHOLOGY/PATHOPHYSIOLOGY

Pathological examination reveals large increases in ground substance and swollen collagen fibers separated by clear spaces. The clear spaces contain mainly hyaluronic acid, since metachromasia disappears after pretreatment with hyaluronidase (2,6,7). Further, the presence of hyaluronidase was confirmed by biochemical studies.

Excessive collagen biosynthesis with a predominance of large fibers and alteration in glycosaminoglycans (GAGs) is also characteristic of diabetic thick skin (8), being more excessive in diabetic scleredema. The main difference from scleroderma is a lack of small collagen fibers in scleredema.

Insulin appears to play an important role in this disease, as shown in diabetic rats where GAG amounts are increased by insulin (9). In fact, insulin is probably responsible for mucopolysaccharide accumulation in diabetic scleredema, especially because these cases are usually associated with hyperinsulinemia.

DIFFERENTIAL DIAGNOSIS

Widespread scleredema should be differentiated from generalized morphea, scleredema associated with gammopathy or myeloma, scleromyxedema, scleromyositis, and diffuse edematous SSc (systemic sclerosis of the Hardy type).

TREATMENT

In the classic scleredema of Buschke, broad-spectrum antibiotics are effective, inducing rapid resolution. Diabetic scleredema tends to persist for years, and does not respond to antidiabetic treatment. Generally, there is also poor response to D-penicillamine and methotrexate (personal experience).

Scleredema Associated with Paraproteinemia or Myeloma

Scleredema associated with gammopathy or multiple myeloma has all the clinical and histological features of diabetic scleredema or generalized scleredema of other etiologies. The onset can be either rapid or insidious. Induration progressively involves the upper parts of the trunk and arms, causing limitation of movements and contractures in the shoulder girdle. We have observed two cases in which an IgG lambda gammopathy preceded the symptoms of multiple myeloma by several years.

PATHOLOGY/PATHOPHYSIOLOGY

Histological examination reveals dermal fibrosis and variable amounts of mucin deposits, but paraproteins are frequently not detectable in the skin (10).

One study demonstrated that serum from patients stimulated collagen production in normal skin fibroblast or autologous cell cultures (11). Circulating paraproteins may also enhance the synthesis of extracellular matrix macromolecules by dermal fibroblasts, leading to the accumulation of collagen and proteoglycans in the skin. Longer term fibroblast cultures suggested that, in these cases, the phenotypically increased procollagen production is a stable feature (12).

TREATMENT

The relation of scleroderma-like cutaneous and muscle lesions to multiple myeloma or paraproteinemia is suggested by the improvement or regression of skin changes when melphalan is used to treat the paraproteinemia (10).

Scleromyxedema

Scleromyxedema (of Gottron) is synonymous with "lichen myxedematosus" or "papular mucinosis" (13). Scleromyxedema is a scleroderma-like condition characterized by aggregated lichenoid papules that form confluent plaques, causing extensive thickening and hardening of the skin with accentuation of the skin folds.

The thickened and pendulous skin gives the impression of being too ample. The eruption involves the upper extremities, neck, upper trunk, and face, becoming progressively generalized. Because of mucin deposition, the face becomes immobile and mask-like with leonine features; the contracture of the fingers produces a scleroderma-like grip (Figs. 6.1*a* and 6.1*b*).

The main clinical difference between scleroderma and scleromyxedema is that in true scleroderma the sclerotic and atrophic skin is bound closely to underlying tissue and appears to be too tight, in contrast to the folded and pendulous skin found in scleromyxedema.

Although the disease is limited to the skin in a proportion of the patients, in long-lasting generalized cases there is a high prevalence of cardiovascular disease, neurological abnormalities, myopathy, and arthritis (14,15). Scleromyxedema with systemic involvement may imitate systemic scleroderma because sclerodactyly, Raynaud's phenomenon, esophageal immobility, and

inflammatory myopathy are frequently present. EMG findings are consistent with primary myogenic involvement, and the muscle enzymes may be moderately elevated, although the histochemical and electron microscopic studies fail to reveal mucin deposits in muscle biopsies (16).

The course of scleromyxedema is generally protracted; however, we have seen several cardiovascular complications leading to death. The patients must be consistently followed and screened for the possible development of overt myeloma or systemic manifestations.

PATHOLOGY/PHYSIOLOGY

Interestingly, scleromyxedema is associated with a gammopathy. The paraprotein is a basic IgG serum globulin with light chains mainly of the lambda type (17–19). The paraprotein is characterized by small size and absence of the antigenic portion of the Fab fragment (20). Its role in the pathogenesis of scleromyxedema is not clear because, in a proportion of patients, clinical manifestations of the disease are present for a long time before paraproteinemia is discovered.

It has been shown that serum from patients, but not isolated paraprotein, stimulates proliferation of normal fibroblasts *in vitro* (21). Another

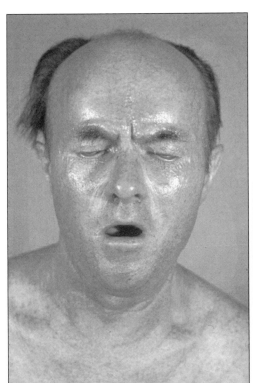

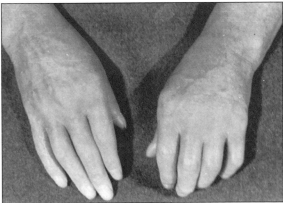

A B

Figure 6.1. Scleromyxedema with pronounced skin indurations. The paraproteinemia was of IgG lambda type. (*a*) Indurated edema and tense skin of the face. (*b*) Sclerosis of the hands with some contracture of the fingers, but with no acroosteolysis and no Raynaud's phenomenon.

group found that the serum stimulated fibroblast production of hyaluronic acid and prostaglandin E, but did not result in fibroblast proliferation (22). Thus, the mucopolysaccharide deposits in the skin could be stimulated by paraprotein, while some other mechanisms appear to be responsible for fibroblast proliferation (22).

Histology reveals fibroblast and collagen proliferation throughout the dermis, with accumulation of acid mucopolysaccharides mainly in the upper dermis between the collagen fibers, which are separated by the polysaccharides. The mucinous substance is composed mainly of hyaluronic acid and can be removed by hyaluronidase.

DIFFERENTIAL DIAGNOSIS

Scleromyxedema in its early stage should be differentiated from scleredema, and in its later stage from systemic scleroderma. While clinical differentiation may be difficult, the histology is highly characteristic.

In contrast to scleredema associated with gammopathy where the paraprotein deposits in the skin do not evoke fibroblast proliferation, scleromyxedema presents an altered fibroblast/ acid mucopolysaccharide balance. Thus, although both these pseudosclerodermatous disorders are associated with paraprotein, its role is not clear and the mechanism of skin induration appears to differ substantially.

TREATMENT

Although the causal relation between cutaneous changes and abortive myeloma or gammopathy is not clear, the beneficial effects of cytostatic therapy, especially a dramatic response to melphalan (23) which has been reported with almost total regression of cutaneous involvement, favors such a relationship.

The first reported beneficial effects of retinoids (24) were not confirmed and two of our patients treated with retinoids showed no improvement.

Scleroderma-Like Lesions in Endocrine Disorders

SCLERODERMA-LIKE LESIONS IN HYPOTHYROIDISM

Abnormalities of the thyroid are not an infrequent finding in systemic scleroderma (25). We have observed cases of scleroderma, or scleroderma-like changes with coexistent hypothyroidism, in which treatment with thyroid extract produced marked improvement or almost complete regression of cutaneous and muscle changes.

SCLERODERMA-LIKE CHANGES AND JOINT CONTRACTURES IN THE HANDS OF INSULIN-DEPENDENT JUVENILE DIABETICS

Contractures of the finger joints occur in approximately 30% of juvenile insulin-dependent diabetics and are accompanied by sclerodactyly and tight skin, especially over the dorsa of the hands in a proportion of patients. Patients with these abnormalities had diabetes for 5, 6, or more, years. Some authors stated that limited joint mobility identified a population at risk for the early development of microvascular complications (26). Others did not find differences in the incidence of retinopathy or neuropathy when comparing patients with or without hand changes (27).

PATHOLOGY/PATHOPHYSIOLOGY

Scleroderma-like skin changes appear to be related to the metabolic derangements, because insulin pump treatment was found to reduce skin thickness and collagen synthesis. They are not related to immunological abnormalities and are not accompanied by Raynaud's phenomenon. Capillaroscopy discloses narrowed, tortuous capillaries with no giant loops.

TREATMENT

Insulin pump treatment of juvenile diabetics may diminish the skin thickness concurrently with a fall in the levels of glycosylated hemoglobin (28).

Werner's Syndrome

This rare hereditary syndrome is a connective tissue disorder characterized by premature senility, various endocrine disturbances, and accelerated atherosclerosis. The disease is genetically transmitted as an autosomal-recessive characteristics, is not infrequent in siblings, and abortive forms are noted in preceding generations (29).

The patients are of short stature with disproportionately thin distal limbs, compared with moderately developed trunk, bird-like face with a beak-shaped nose, and deformities of the feet, mainly due to osteoporosis. Characteristic signs of premature aging are: graying and loss of hair, early atherosclerosis, bilateral juvenile-type cataracts, predisposition to diabetes, hypogonadism, and a high-pitched, hoarse voice. The cutaneous lesions consist of atrophy and tightening of the skin, especially in the distal extremities, because of the depletion of subcutaneous fat and wasting of the muscles of the legs, hands, and feet. Trophic ulcers of the lower legs and deformed feet are significant features of the syndrome. The thinning of the nose and lips, designated as mask-like, are also of pseudo-scleroderma type.

PATHOLOGY/PATHOPHYSIOLOGY

Cultured fibroblasts from these patients grow slowly, replicate less than controls, and behave similarly to the fibroblasts from very elderly persons (30–32). The fibroblasts produce increased amounts of collagen type I and type III, as demonstrated by increased collagen mRNA, which suggests an alteration in the control of collagen synthesis at the transcriptional level (33). Collagenase-sensitive protein production in patients' fibroblasts was found to be approximately 60% higher than in normal fibroblasts, while constitutive levels of collagenase were six-fold greater than in controls (34).

DIFFERENTIAL DIAGNOSIS

The diagnosis of Werner's syndrome is usually not difficult because of its distinct clinical characteristics. However, as pronounced scleroderma-like changes occur, Werner's syndrome is not infrequently misdiagnosed as scleroderma. In scleroderma, the induration is more conspicuous on the hands, with concomitant Raynaud's phenomenon and contractures of the fingers; in Werner's syndrome, the hands and feet are thinned, with trophic ulcerations in the areas of deformities, and vascular manifestations and visceral involvement are absent. The course of Werner's syndrome is variable and the outcome depends upon the progression of atherosclerosis. About 10% of the patients develop mesenchymal tumors (35). We have observed some abortive cases, in which the symptoms became manifest either before puberty or developed later.

TREATMENT

No therapy is available at this time.

Progeria

Progeria, or Hutchinson-Gilford syndrome, is a rare disorder characterized by markedly accelerated aging and a much shorter life span (mean 10–15 years of age) than in Werner's syndrome. In fact, Werner's syndrome is often referred to as progeria of adults (36).

The onset of progeria is usually in the first year of life. Characteristic features are severe dwarfism, disproportionately small face with mandibular hypoplasia, thin beaked nose, prominent cranium with sparse hair and prominent veins, characteristic senile appearance, stooped posture, small external genitalia, and disproportionately thin limbs.

The cutaneous lesions are mainly atrophic, but the skin of the extremities may be sclerotic with almost absent subcutaneous fat. The important clinical symptom is progressive osteolysis of terminal phalanges and clavicles.

Extensive atherosclerosis is a most prominent feature, and death results from cardiovascular causes (37).

The disease seems to be transmitted as a sporadic autosomal dominant mutation, although autosomal recessive transmission has also been reported (37).

PATHOLOGY/PATHOPHYSIOLOGY

Histopathology reveals thickened, compact collagen bundles with hyalinization of the lower dermis, collagen proliferation in the subcutaneous tissue, and decreased dermal appendages. The elastic fibers are unaffected or are increased (36).

Fibroblast cultures disclose a significant reduction of fibroblast life span because of premature senescence (38). There is a six- to nine-fold increased production of tropoelastin, both at the mRNA and protein levels (39), whereas collagen synthesis is similar to control fibroblasts, with no difference in collagen types (40). It has been proposed that increased elastin gene expression in fibroblasts from progeria patients could serve as a biochemical marker of the disorder (39).

DIFFERENTIAL DIAGNOSIS

Progeria is very easily recognized because the patients are strikingly similar. Werner's syndrome differs from progeria in that the former starts later (between 15 and 30 years of age) than progeria, and premature aging (graying of hair, cataracts, and atherosclerosis) and death occur much later in Werner's syndrome, usually in the fifth decade of life.

Another premature aging syndrome in children, congenital poikiloderma of Rothmund-Thomson, has onset in the first months of life. This syndrome differs from progeria because it has striking poikilodermatous skin changes, early cataracts, and premature hair graying, while scleroderma-like induration is usually absent.

Systemic scleroderma differs from progeria because it starts later and has both vasomotor manifestations (osteolysis of phalanges in progeria is not associated with Raynaud's phenomenon) and visceral involvement.

TREATMENT

The course of the disease is progressive, the outcome is invariably fatal, and the therapy is exclusively symptomatic.

Sclerodermiform Neonatal Progeria

Although the symptoms of progeria usually appear some months after birth, there are reports of unusual neonatal progeria or progeroid syndromes that have all the characteristics of progeria but display much more pronounced scleroderma-like cutaneous changes (Fig. 6.2), run a more severe course, and have a lethal outcome in the first year of life (41–43). Some of these cases were reported as infantile scleredema (44).

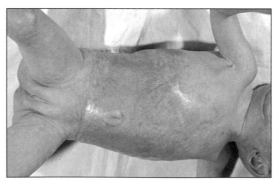

Figure 6.2. Neonatal sclerodermiform progeria. Skin indurations involving the whole body with flexion contractures of the limbs.

Restrictive Dermopathy

Restrictive dermopathy is an autosomal recessive disorder of premature born babies with a lethal outcome in the first hours, weeks, or rarely, several months of life (45–50). There are reports on parental consanguinity or multiple affected siblings.

All the children are remarkably similar, showing dysmorphic facial changes with micrognathia and microstomia, a small open mouth, a beak-like nose, low set ears, and widely spaced sutes. The hair is sparse or absent, and some children have thick rigid facial skin and develop an ectropion. The skin is taut and stretched with peeling of the superficial layers in some areas, and all infants show flexion contractures of the extremities including the hands. Restricted respiratory movements appear to be the cause of death.

PATHOLOGY/PATHOPHYSIOLOGY

One group of investigators found that the skin revealed signs of arrested morphogenesis with a hyperplastic, hyper- and parakcratotic epidermis and an aberrant pattern of keratins (46). The collagen tissue is arranged parallel to the skin surface, the dermis is thin, and subcutaneous fat is rather abundant. The dermal adnexa are arrested in their development and differentiation (46). Other investigators reported the presence of adnexal structures but an absence of elastic fibers (believed to be responsible for the tightness of the fetal skin) (48). A primary defect was suggested to be an alteration in the mechanisms regulating the morphogenesis of both the epidermis and the dermis and/or the dermal/epidermal interactions (46). Alternatively, a primary disorder of fibroblasts could lead to a decrease in skin collagen turnover; this would explain the apparent arrest in growth and differentiation of the skin (51).

Sclerodermiform Chronic Graft-Versus-Host Disease (GVHD)

Late cutaneous changes in graft-versus-host disease (GVHD) of the sclerodermatous type (52), preceded by a maculopapular and lichen planus-like eruption, may occur on the face, trunk, in the hands, and become generalized (53). Joint contractures are present in about 60% of patients surviving over 1 year; in a proportion of the patients, Sjögren's syndrome is also found. Anti-smooth muscle, antimitochondrial and antinuclear antibodies can be detected but are usually found in extensive chronic GVHD with multiple organ involvement (54).

PATHOLOGY/PATHOPHYSIOLOGY

The histology reveals features of both scleroderma and GVHD, i.e., vacuolization of basal cells, lymphocytic infiltrations, and fibrosis of the dermis and subcutis. Immunohistologic and ultrastructural study discloses, in addition to alterations at the dermal-epidermal junction, deposits of type III procollagen in the incipient sclerosis and of type I procollagen in the older lesions. Collagen fibers in the sclerotic dermis are of irregular diameter and are in close contact with mast cells, activated fibroblasts, macrophages, and lymphocytes (55).

TREATMENT

GVHD with sclerodermiform features is currently very rare, probably because of the introduction of cyclosporin A, which successfully prevents most severe complications in allograft patients. Single cases of cutaneous GVHD in spite of cylosporin A showed only acral erythema and moderate edema with no sclerosis; histologically, the GVHD was mild, although not entirely inhibited (56).

We have seen one patient, contaminated at Chernobyl, who had generalized morphea-like cutaneous changes with contractures. Skin sclerosis in this case could not be clinically distinguished from idiopathic generalized morphea. Thus, sclerodermiform GVHD provides additional evidence of the role of cell-mediated immunity in the pathogenesis of scleroderma.

Scleroderma-Like Changes of Porphyria Cutanea Tarda

Cutaneous induration is most often of the morphea type, but may simulate generalized morphea or systemic scleroderma (3,57). The changes are not accompanied by visceral involvement and are usually limited to the skin. The most affected parts of the body are the chest, the V-shaped area of the neck, the face, and hands, although the entire skin (both sun-exposed and non-sun-exposed) can present irregular confluent indurations mingled with atrophy and hyper- and depigmentation, giving the skin a mottled appearance (Fig. 6.3).

The resemblance to morphea may be so close that coexistence of porphyria cutanea tarda (PCT) and morphea has been assumed, especially since the histologic and electron microscopic examination usually reveal dermal sclerosis very similar to that of scleroderma (58,59). Cases with advanced sclerosis of the face, hands, and forearms with sclerodactyly and contractures of the fingers may be indistinguishable from SSc (3,57, 60). There is no consensus whether the cutaneous induration of PCT simulating morphea or SSc is a pseudosclerodermatous change or a chance coexistence of the two separate conditions, as reported for lupus erythematosus (61).

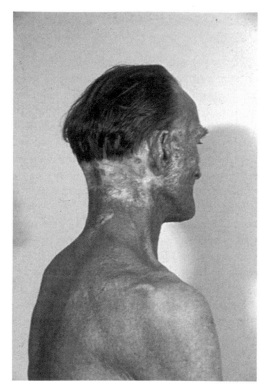

Figure 6.3. Porphyria cutanea tarda. Sclerosis is most pronounced in the neck and face, the entire skin is irregularly hyperpigmented with atrophies and confluent indurations.

PATHOLOGY/PATHOPHYSIOLOGY

Immunohistochemical and electron microscopic studies show vascular changes with reduplication of the basal lamina and a characteristic pattern of immunoglobulin deposition (62). The most probable pathogenesis appears to be related to a phototoxic insult that stimulates fibroblasts to produce sclerosis, as was shown for uro-

porphyrin I in an *in vitro* study (63). Mast cell numbers were found to be significantly increased in the scleroderma-like lesions of PCT, and it was suggested that the histamine released upon degranulation may stimulate collagen production (64), as was shown for keloid tissue.

TREATMENT

The most important finding in support of distinct pathogenesis for the sclerotic changes in scleroderma and PCT is the resolution or improvement of induration after successful therapy of PCT. The degree of improvement was proportional to the reduction of the urinary excretion of porphyrins (3,60,65).

Scleroderma-Like Lesions in Phenylketonuria

SSc-like lesions are rare in children with phenylketonuria (PKU) in whom the characteristic cutaneous abnormality is eczematous dermatitis and inadequately pigmented skin and hair.

Scleroderma-like induration usually appears in the first year of life, occupying initially the thighs and buttocks and accompanied by contractures of the legs; it later spreads over the trunk and proximal parts of the extremities (Fig. 6.4). The face and hands are usually lesion-free (66–71). In older children, the lesions resemble plaque or guttate morphea, symmetrical generalized morphea (66), or atrophoderma Pasini-Pierini (69).

PATHOLOGY/PATHOPHYSIOLOGY

The early changes mainly involve the subcutis and are symmetrical and poorly demarcated. In older, untreated children, especially with generalized skin involvement, the lesions resemble scleroderma closely, so that clinical and histological differentiation may not be possible.

The relationship of scleroderma-like lesions with PKU is quite evident, because the cutaneous changes disappear upon rapid institution of a low phenylalenine (PHA) diet at an early age, as noticed by us and others (66,67,69,71). This diet does not improve either the PKU or cutaneous lesions, nor does it prevent mental retardation, if started after the age of 2 to 3 years.

Our study on the pathomechanism of scleroderma-like changes in PKU disclosed deranged tryptophan (TRY) metabolism, mainly in the tryptamine pathway, resulting in a high tryptamine/indoleacetic acid ratio, which is also a characteristic finding in scleroderma (66,70). The increase of tryptamine/indoleacetic acid ratio paralleled the clinical condition and the phenylalanine serum level and was reversible upon early institution of PHA low diet.

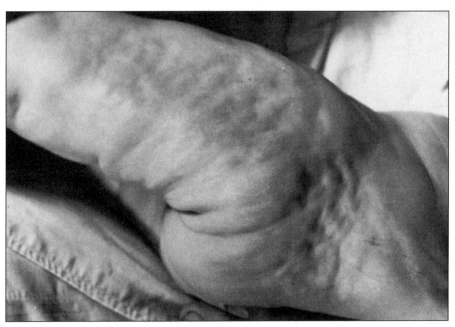

Figure 6.4. A child of 1 year and 2 months with phenylketonuria. Widespread indurations, more pronounced on the thighs and buttocks with contractures of the extremities.

THERAPY

We have observed seven cases that were followed for more than 10 years, two of which were followed for more than 20 years. We observed complete resolution of subcutaneous indurations if the PHA low diet was introduced directly after recognition of the disease and strictly maintained. In patients in whom diet was periodically not observed, scattered foci of plaque morphea appeared, which regressed under the regular PHA low diet.

Congenital Fascial Dystrophy

This rare scleroderma-like, genetically determined disorder is also known as the "stiff skin syndrome" (72). Stony hard indurations of the skin and deeper tissue were found to be more pronounced in the buttocks, thighs and legs, with limitation of joint mobility and contractures in the lower limbs (Fig. 6.5) (73–75). The disease is usually noticed in the first year of life, is not progressive, and is not accompanied by visceral involvement.

Figure 6.5. Stiff skin syndrome. Congenital fascial dystrophy. Skin indurations and stony hard deeper tissues, especially in the lower extremities, where contractures are most pronounced. Characteristic tip-top posture and small thorax with well developed muscles of the shoulder girdle.

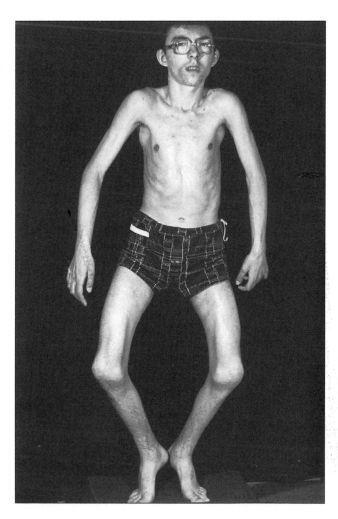

PATHOLOGY/PATHOPHYSIOLOGY

The most significant finding is a four- to six-fold increase in fascial thickness with no inflammatory infiltrates. Electron microscopy reveals amianthoid-like collagen fibers 6 to 10 times wider than normal fibers, with inadequately aggregated collagen fibrils. Fibroblast cultures showed excessive production of collagen I and III (73). We postulated a possible generalized fascial involvement, because there was an evident relationship between the extent of the indurations and thickness of the fascia in different body areas, with the most extensive changes involving the fascia lata and gluteal fascias.

The disease appears to be caused by an altered macromolecular organization of collagen fibers. It differs from scleroderma by its congenital character, onset in the first year of life, nonprogressive character, absence of visceral involvement, lack of inflammatory changes, and lack of immunological abnormalities. However, the patients are usually misdiagnosed as having scleroderma. Except for functional impairment of the lungs caused by pressure of the thickened thoracic fascia, the general condition of the patients is satisfactory, and in spite of limited joint mobility, there is no muscle involvement.

TREATMENT

The recognition of this noninflammatory involvement of the fascias is important in order to avoid unnecessary aggressive therapy.

Scleroderma-Like Changes Induced by Bleomycin

Bleomycin, an antineoplastic drug effective against carcinoma and some lymphomas, may induce cutaneous and pulmonary fibrosis. The sclerosis of the skin and gangrene of the digits may mimic systemic scleroderma (76) with contracture of the fingers. In our patients, there was also an extensive acroosteolysis with loss of the distal phalanges. Bleomycin induces fibrosis of the lung, usually affecting the lower lobes; this is a serious, sometimes fatal, complication.

The histology of the skin has all the features of scleroderma with collagen proliferation and homogenization and blood vessel damage (76).

Scleroderma-Like Plaques After Vitamin K Injection

In some predisposed individuals, oil soluble vitamin K (phytonadione) may induce erythematous and sclerodermiform plaques, appearing several weeks after injection, usually in the gluteal area (Fig. 6.6) (77). The time of appearance

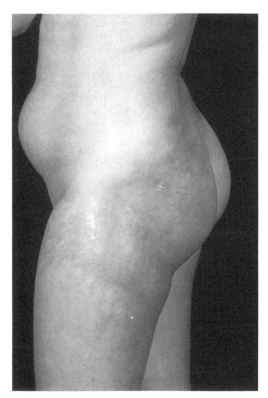

Figure 6.6. Erythematous and indurated plaque in gluteal area after phytonadione (vitamin K) injection in a 5-year-old girl. In this case, we found extensive inflammatory changes in the fascia.

after injections and positive skin tests are suggestive of delayed type hypersensitivity (78).

The changes are deep, involving the subcutis and fascia where an inflammatory reaction with numerous eosinophils may simulate eosinophilic fasciitis (79).

Progressive Facial Hemiatrophy

Progressive facial hemiatrophy, also referred to as "Parry-Romberg syndrome," is regarded as a variety of localized scleroderma (80) or as a related, but distinct, heritable skin malformation (3). Differentiation between atrophy secondary to deep involutionary scleroderma and idiopathic facial hemiatrophy is very difficult or even impossible (Fig. 6.7).

Facial hemiatrophy usually begins in the first 2 decades of life, sometimes in early childhood, and asymmetry of the face is more distinct the younger the age at the onset of the disease. The onset late in childhood does not support the presumption that facial hemiatrophy is a developmental anomaly (81).

In the idiopathic variety, atrophy is primary and affects mainly the subcutis, muscles, and bones, causing more or less pronounced asymmetry of the face. The skin itself is atrophic or uninvolved.

More than 25 years of follow-up of children whose scleroderma was localized unilaterally to the face, revealed the gradual development of confluent hemiatrophy corresponding to Parry-Romberg type, although there were cases in which preceding induration was never noticed. It

Figure 6.7. Facial hemiatrophy. Irregular atrophies involving skin, subcutaneous tissue, muscle, and bones. In this 26-year-old woman indurations appeared at the age of 6, evolving progressively into deep atrophies.

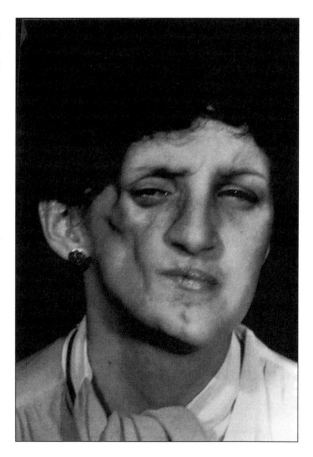

is to be presumed that such cases correspond to primary atrophic scleroderma, because linear facial scleroderma at early childhood is associated with impaired growth of the face and skull (82), which is analogous to that of affected limbs. There are no reliable histologic criteria to differentiate facial hemiatrophy from involutionary morphea. The not infrequent coexistence of facial hemiatrophy with localized scleroderma in other areas favors their close pathogenic relationship and supports the suggestion that facial hemiatrophy could be a variant of scleroderma.

Occasionally, hemiatrophy also affects the trunk on the same side or the entire half of the body (hemiatrophia progressive totalis) (83). This, however, could be an involutionary primary atrophic scleroderma distributed segmentally on the same side of the body. Both linear scleroderma of the face and facial hemiatrophy may be precipitated by the trauma (84).

PATHOLOGY/PATHOPHYSIOLOGY

Both facial hemiatrophy and involutionary scleroderma are connected with the nervous system, mainly the higher autonomic centers. The distribution of the lesions along the branches of the trigeminal nerve and, not infrequently, associated trigeminal neuralgia (84) might be a sequel of the compression of the nerve.

Some patients with facial hemiatrophy with or without coexistent morphea have elevated titers of antibody to *Borrelia burgdorferi* (85,86), and this also favors their close pathogenetic relationship.

Thus, the available data and prolonged follow-up of the patients suggest that the majority of the cases of facial hemiatrophy could be a variant of deep subcutaneous scleroderma.

Fibroblastic Rheumatism

This is a newly recognized syndrome characterized by polyarthralgia with no joint destruction and the appearance of cutaneous nodules local-

ized mainly on the dorsal aspects of the hands and forearms, preferentially in para-articular regions. The skin of the hands and forearms is indurated, with marked sclerodactyly and finger contractures (Fig. 6.8). Arthralgia also affects other joints, causing limitation of motion, especially of the elbows and shoulders (87,88).

PATHOLOGY/PATHOPHYSIOLOGY

Histologic and immunohistochemical studies reveal proliferation of fibroblasts with features of myofibroblasts and an increase in fibronectin and tenascin deposits. Electron microscopy shows fibroblasts expressing the morphological features of myofibroblasts, as in fascial fibromatosis or digital fibromatosis of childhood. In fibroblast cultures, there is reduction in collagen and non-collagen protein synthesis (88).

In the case we have followed, the nodules

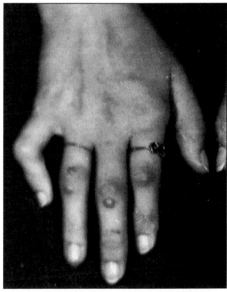

Figure 6.8. Fibroblastic rheumatism. Nodules on the dorsa of the fingers, mainly in para-articular regions, with swelling and contracture of some finger joints. In this patient, single nodules were also located on the legs. The skin nodules regressed spontaneously after several months, and joint stiffness was markedly reduced.

disappeared within several months, reappeared after some time at the knuckles, and again regressed. The histology was characteristic of fibroblastic rheumatism. This new scleroderma-like disease appears to be more common than currently recognized.

DIFFERENTIAL DIAGNOSIS

The disease should be differentiated from nodular scleroderma, which differs from fibroblastic rheumatism by a different location of nodules, a different histology (proliferation of fibroblasts, thick collagen bundles), and rheumatoid nodules (which differ clinically and histologically, by positive serology and different radiological findings). Reticulohistiocytosis is differentiated from fibroblastic rheumatism by the preference of bone destruction, its histology, and the course of the disease.

TREATMENT

The nodules of fibroblastic rheumatism may regress spontaneously or under corticosteriod therapy (88).

Localized Lipoatrophies

Local lipoatrophy is a primary, circumscribed atrophy of the subcutaneous tissues, not preceded by induration, with no muscle or bone involvement, and with virtually intact skin. The disorder may be compared to Romberg's facial hemiatrophy, differing from it with regard to the localization of the lesions, absence of bone atrophy, and absence of extensive deformities.

The lipoatrophies may appear as single or multiple foci, may be symmetrical (lipoatrophy of the ankles), or systemic (partial lipodystrophy). Except for partial lipodystrophy, they are not accompanied by any systemic disorders or muscle weakness.

GOWER'S LOCAL PANATROPHY

This type of panatrophy may appear in any location and presents mainly with atrophy of subcutaneous tissue, while the skin is somewhat thinned but otherwise intact. Slight muscle atrophy may be secondary to inflammatory vascular changes in the subcutis. Muscular strength is preserved and electromyography and muscle biopsy usually do not reveal abnormalities (3).

Differentiation from involutionary scleroderma is difficult because morphea and linear scleroderma may, on involution, leave atrophic subcutaneous tissue and muscles, closely resembling the lesions of local panatrophy. There are also no histological criteria to differentiate panatrophy from involutionary deep scleroderma.

The nature of the disorder is unknown. We have seen cases after trauma, e.g., lipoatrophy of the cheek after tooth extraction and lipoatrophy on the buttocks after injection of antibiotics several months or years earlier. Thus, the occurrence of cases presenting from onset as deep subcutaneous atrophy indicates that panatrophy could be a separate entity. It is, however, conceivable that it is a primary atrophic subcutaneous scleroderma.

ANNULAR AND SEMICIRCULAR LIPOATROPHY

In this condition, the loss of subcutaneous tissue has an annular or semicircular arrangement, usually on the thighs, although we have seen similar lesions on the arms, knees, and ankles. Atrophy involves exclusively the subcutaneous tissue while the overlying skin is intact and muscles and bone are uninvolved (89).

PATHOLOGY/PATHOPHYSIOLOGY

Histology reveals replacement of fat lobules by hyalinized connective tissue. In very early lesions, inflammatory infiltrates with neovascularization is present (89), sometimes with features of late stage panniculitis.

TREATMENT

The disease causes no symptoms and appears to be induced by light repeated trauma or pressure in women with abnormally vulnerable fatty tissue (90). Spontaneous resolution occurs within several months after pressure or trauma has been carefully avoided.

LIPOATROPHY OF THE ANKLES

This lipoatrophy may be unilateral or symmetrical, is slowly progressive, sometimes annular (91) or linear, and often manifests in a "stocking" pattern (92).

We have observed this variety of lipoatrophy most often in children or young women. There were no muscle and bone changes or other abnormalities. The general condition of the patients was invariably good. The atrophy persisted unchanged, or increased somewhat.

PATHOLOGY/PATHOPHYSIOLOGY

One patient has been seen by us at a very early stage. She presented with flat inflammatory nodules preceding the atrophy. Histological examination revealed a picture resembling panniculitis with extensive infiltrates composed of lymphocytes, histiocytes, macrophages, and fibroblasts, pronounced vascular changes, and abundant foam cells. Thus, the localized atrophy could represent the end stage of panniculitis (93).

TREATMENT

Treatment with antibiotics caused regression of the nodules, leaving atrophy, which was slowly progressive.

PARTIAL LIPODYSTROPHY WITH GLOMERULONEPHRITIS AND COMPLEMENT ABNORMALITIES

This disorder is characterized by loss of subcutaneous fat, particularly in the cheeks and, to a lesser extent, in the upper extremities and shoulders,

although it may appear in other locations. The disease is not progressive and the muscles and bones are not involved. The most important findings are accompanying abnormalities of complement (hypocomplementemia) (94), and glomerulonephritis (95).

LIPODYSTROPHIA CENTRIFUGALIS ABDOMINALIS INFANTILIS

This name was proposed for a lipoatrophy (i.e., loss of subcutaneous fat) localized to the lower abdomen and in the inguinal area, with slight scaling and redness over the depressed areas. The disease has been reported only in Japanese children, and appears to be a peculiar form of circumscribed lipoatrophy with no other accompanying abnormalities (96).

Lichen Sclerosus et Atrophicus

There is no consensus whether *lichen sclerosus et atrophicus* (LSA) is a distinct entity or a guttate variety of morphea, because LSA and scleroderma frequently appear simultaneously in the same patient (97) and both appear to represent different manifestations of one basic disease. According to Winkelmann (98), LSA could be considered a subepidermal morphea.

PATHOLOGY/PATHOPHYSIOLOGY

Typical cases of LSA differ from morphea by the porcelain white, variably indurated or atrophic papules, many with follicular plugs, distinctly outlined in confluent lesions (Fig. 6.9a), and by frequent localization in the genital area. Histology differs from morphea because LSA demonstrates vacuolar alteration at the dermal-epidermal junction, a characteristic homogeneous zone under thinned and hyperkeratotic epidermis, and subpapillary mononuclear infiltrates (Fig. 6.9b). The main feature distinguishing this histologic picture from morphea is an absence of sclerosis and inflammatory infiltrates in the

Figure 6.9. (*a*) Widespread confluent lesions of *lichen sclerosus et atrophicus* involving almost the entire skin with numerous hemorrhagic bullae. There is similarity to localized scleroderma but the lesions are more superficial, do not involve the deep tissues and differ by a rough surface due to hyperkeratosis. (*b*) Histology of *lichen sclerosus et atrophicus*. Characteristic hyperkeratosis with thinning of the epidermis, hydropic degeneration of basal cells and homogenization of the subepidermal zone. Slight inflammatory infiltrates beneath this zone. (H&E, magnification × 120)

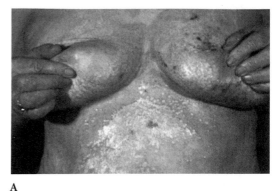

A

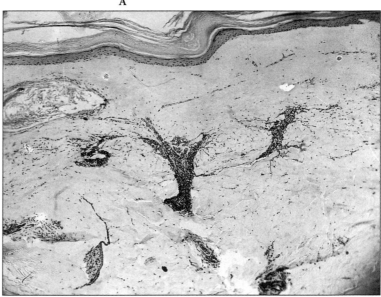

B

reticular dermis and an absence of vascular changes. The elastic fibers are absent from the subepidermal homogeneous zone, which may be the result of their destruction by an elastase-type protease isolated from human vulvar fibroblasts and found to be overproduced in LSA (99).

We and others (100) have seen clinical and histological features of both LSA and scleroderma even in the same lesion. A close relationship between LSA and scleroderma is also evidenced by cutaneous sclerosis developing as a late complication of GVHD (101,102), and which has simultaneous features of LSA and localized scleroderma, both clinically and histologically. Lichen planus-like lesions in the early stages of GVHD are also suggestive of a possible common origin for lichen planus and LSA, postulated in older literature (103). We and others have observed occurrence of all three disorders in the same patients (104). In both scleroderma and LSA, there is a higher incidence of autoimmune-related disease, especially vitiligo and alopecia areata, and a higher incidence of various autoantibodies (105).

A decreased serum level of dihydrotestosterone and free testosterone found in vulvar LSA would explain the clearing of childhood LSA at puberty (106).

Sclerodermiform Variety of *Acrodermatitis Chronica Atrophicans*

Acrodermatitis chronica atrophicans (ACA) was a disease prevalent mainly in central and eastern Europe, especially in certain forested regions where it appeared to be associated with the occurrence of the tick *Ixodes*, while in the United States only single cases were reported (107,108). Cases of ACA, a possible late manifestation of *Borrelia* infection, are currently also rare in Europe, presumably owing to the widespread use of antibiotics. *Borrelia burgdorferi* (107,108), an etiologic agent of Lyme disease, is associated with erythema chronicum migrans (ECM) and lymphadenosis benigna cutis (LBC), and possibly also some cases of ACA, morphea, LSA, progressive facial hemiatrophy, and atrophoderma Pasini-Pierini (APP) (107).

ACA starts with diffuse, poorly demarcated, violaceous or red-violaceous infiltrates on the distal parts of one extremity, and may involve all extremities. The changes spread proximally, in the lower extremities not beyond the groin and buttocks and in the upper extremities not beyond the elbows. Not infrequently, fibrous streaks are present extending from the wrist to the elbow along the ulna (ulnar streaks). The skin becomes gradually thinned and wrinkled, resembling crumpled cigarette paper, and has a mottled appearance owing to uneven pigmentations and visible veins (3).

Induration closely resembling scleroderma may develop within the violaceous infiltrates and atrophy (Fig. 6.10). Sclerodermatous changes appear more frequently on the lower extremities and fibrous streaks on the forearms (3,109). Indurated lesions resemble scleroderma so closely that they are often regarded as the coexistence of the two diseases (109). The main difference from morphea is the indistinct outlines of the erythe-matous diffuse infiltrations of ACA and the often symmetrical distribution on extremities. Morphea is more sharply outlined, surrounded by a lilac ring in the active stage, frequently also involves the deeper tissues, with possible deformities as an outcome. Gottzon (109) collected 54 cases of sclerodermatous changes among 431 cases of ACA and believed this represented the coexistence of the two diseases. There are numerous reports in the older literature of scleroderma-like lesions in ACA; other well-documented observations of coexistent ACA on the extremities and morphea on the trunk also exist

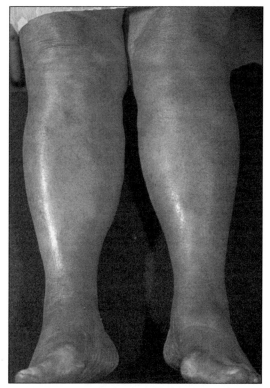

Figure 6.10. Sclerodermiform acrodermatitis chronica atrophicans. Symmetrical indurations which developed in extensive erythematous lesions of the lower extremities are indistinguishable from localized scleroderma. In this patient, there was a high titer of antiborrelia antibodies and the response to penicillin was as rapid as in typical acrodermatitis chronica atrophicans.

(3), and we have observed several cases of this type.

PATHOLOGY/PATHOPHYSIOLOGY

The histology of ACA reveals atrophy of collagen and elastic tissue in the early stages with lichenoid infiltrates in the superficial dermis (108). In the late stages, the differentiation from morphea is very difficult, because in pseudosclerodermatous ACA the connective tissue may be homogenized and compact, obscuring differences from scleroderma. Thus, also histological differentiation between sclerodermiform ACA and morphea frequently is very difficult or impossible. However, the therapeutic response distinguishes between the two diseases. In addition, a direct correlation between the occurrence of some cases of morphea with *B. burgdorferi* infection, and the simultaneous occurrence of some cases of morphea and acrodermatitis atrophicans favors a close relationship between this pseudoscleroderma and morphea (110). It is worth noting that the presence of *B. burgdorferi* was shown by serology and tissue studies in morphea (106,108), although other investigators did not confirm these findings (111,112). The reason for this discrepancy could be the geographical distribution of *B. burgdorferi* infection whose association with morphea was stronger in endemic areas and/or different strains of *B. burgdorferi*.

TREATMENT

Treatment with penicillin or other antibiotics causes rapid regression of the inflammatory and erythematous lesions of ACA and progressive but full regression of some sclerodermatous plaques. Morphea plaques in other locations may persist, although the lilac ring decreases, and improvement is noticeable after several months or years. We have observed a woman with four types of *Borrelia*-induced lesions: ECM in the forearms, ACA on the lower extremities, morphea on the back with large lilac rings, and plaques of APP elsewhere on the trunk. All four types of lesions were confirmed by histology, and anti-*Borrelia* antibodies were present in high titer. The lesions of ECM and ACA regressed rapidly under penicillin therapy, while morphea disappeared within about 2 years.

Atrophoderma Pasini-Pierini

Atrophoderma Pasini-Pierini (APP), described as idiopathic progressive atrophoderma (113), is a benign cutaneous atrophy regarded as a nosologic entity in the broad spectrum of primary atrophies (113), or as primary atrophic superficial morphea without clinical evidence of sclerosis and with no involvement of subcutaneous tissues (114).

The relationship of APP to morphea is favored both by coexistence of morphea or sclerotic foci in the central part of atrophies, and by a striking similarity of the atrophy left after regression of the morphea plaques (114,115).

PATHOLOGY/PATHOPHYSIOLOGY

The histology is similar to abortive morphea. If new morphea lesions develop simultaneously with regression of other morphea plaques, the latter are abortive and manifest as APP. However, the differences in the course and outcome of morphea and APP justify preservation of a distinct name, especially because no aggressive therapy or no therapy at all is required.

Conclusions

The described scleroderma-like conditions differ widely in clinical presentations and pathogenesis. Some closely resemble systemic or localized scleroderma (morphea). However, even in the presence of symmetrical sclerodactyly and symmetrical sclerosis elsewhere, e.g., in scleredema, scleromyxedema, or some cases of progeria, the pseudosclerodermas usually differ from SSc by the absence of Raynaud's phenomenon, visceral involvement, and specific serological markers: antitopoisomerase or anticentromere antibodies.

We believe that rheumatologists, dermatologists, pediatricians, and generalists should be aware of the divergent sclerodermiform skin indurations and atrophies; their recognition will be helpful in distinguishing true scleroderma from a scleroderma-like disease. It could also help to indicate their underlying causes.

References

1. Fleischmajer R, Faludi G, Kral S. Scleredema and diabetes mellitus. Arch Dermatol 1970;101:21.
2. Cohn BA, Wheeler CE Jr, Briggaman RA. Scleredema adultorum of Buschke and diabetes mellitus. Arch Dermatol 1970;101:27.
3. Jabłónska S. Scleroderma and pseudoscleroderma. Polish medical publishers, Warszawa 1975.
4. Wenencie PY, Powell FC, Su WPD, Perry HO. Scleredema: A review of thirty-three cases. J Am Acad Dermatol 1984;11:128.
5. Carrington PR, Sanusi JA, Winder PR, et al. Scleredema adultorum. Int J Dermatol 1984;23:514.
6. Braun-Falco O. Neues zur Histopathologie des Scleredema adultorum (Buschke). Dermatol Wochenschr 1952;125;409.
7. Fleischmajer R, Perlish JS. Glycosaminoglycans in scleroderma and scleredema. J Invest Dermatol 1972;58:129.
8. Hanna W, Frieseu D, Bombardier C, et al. Pathologic features of diabetic thick skin. J Am Acad Dermatol 1987;16:546.
9. Kofoed JA. Skin acidic glycosaminoglycans in alloxan diabetic rats. Diabetes 1970;19:732.
10. Jabłónska S, Stachow A. Scleroderma-like lesions in multiple myeloma. Dermatologica 1972;144:257.
11. Ohta A, Uitto J, Oikarinen AI, et al. Paraproteinemia in patients with scleredema. J Am Acad Dermatol 1987;16:96.
12. Oikarinen A, Ala-Kokko L, Palatsi R, et al. Scleredema and paraproteinemia. Arch Dermatol 1987;123:226.
13. Mongomery H, Underwood LJ. Lichen myxedematosus (differentiation from cutaneous myxedemas or mucoid states). J Invest Dermatol 1953;20:213.
14. McAdam LP, Pearson CM, Pitts WH, et al. Papular mucinosis with myopathy, arthritis, and eosinophilia. A histopathologic study. Arthritis Rheum 1977;20:989.
15. Fudman EJ, Galbus J, Ike RW. Scleromyxedema with systemic involvement mimics rheumatic diseases. Arthritis Rheum 1986;29:913.
16. Verity MA, Toop J, Mc Adam LP, Pearson CM. Scleromyxedema myopathy: Histochemical and electron microscopic observations. Am J Clin Pathol 1978;69:446.
17. Osserman EF, Takatsuki K. Role of an abnormal, myeloma-type, serum gamma globulin in the pathogenesis of the skin lesions of papular mucinosis (lichen myxedematosus), abstracted. J Clin Invest 1963;42:962.
18. Lawrence DA, Tye MJ, Liss M. Immunochemical analysis of the basic immunoglobulin in papular mucinosis. Immunochemistry 1972;9:41.
19. Lai A, Fat RFM, Suurmond D, et al. Scleromyxedema (lichen myxedematosus) associated with a paraprotein IgG1 of type kappa. Br J Dermatol 1973;88:107.
20. Kitamura W, Matsuoka Y, Sakamoto K, Miyagawa S. Immunochemical analysis of the monoclonal paraprotein in scleromyxedema. J Invest Dermatol 1978;70:305.
21. Harper RA, Rispler J. Lichen myxedematous serum stimulates human skin fibroblast proliferation. Science 1978;199:454.
22. Yaron M, Yaron I, Yust I, Brenner S. Lichen myxedematosus (scleromyxedema) serum stimulates hyaluronic acid and prostaglandin E production by human fibroblasts. J Rheumatol 1985;12:171.
23. Feldman P, Shapiro L, Pick AJ, Slatkin MH. Scleromyxedema: A dramatic response to melphalan. Arch Dermatol 1969;99:51.
24. Milam CP, Cohen LE, Fenske NA, Ling NS. Scleromyxedema: Therapeutic response to isotretinoin in three patients. J Am Acad Dermatol 1988;19:469.
25. Maurier-Clavreul MC, Rousset H, Claudy A. Sclérodermie et pathologie thyroidienne. Ann Dermatol Venereol 1989;116:701.
26. Rosenbloom AL, Silverstein JH, Dennis MD, Lezotte C, et al. Limited joint mobility in childhood diabetes mellitus indicates increased risk for microvascular disease. N Engl J Med 1981;305:191.
27. Garza-Elizondo MA, Diaz-Jouanen E, Franco-Casique V, et al. Joint contractures and scleroderma-like skin changes in the hands of insulin-dependent juvenile diabetics. J Rheum 1983;10:797.
28. Lieberman LS, Rosenbloom AL, Riley WJ, et al. Reduced skin thickness with pump administration of insulin. N Engl J Med 1980;303:940.
29. Epstein CJ, Martin GM, Schults AL, et al. Werner's syndrome. A review of its symptomatology,

natural history, pathologic features, genetics and relationship to the natural aging process. Medicine 1966;45:177.

30. Goldstein S, Singal DP. Alteration of fibroblast gene products *in vitro* from a subject with Werner's syndrome. Nature 1974;251:719.

31. Goldstein S. Studies on age-related disease in cultured skin fibroblasts. J Invest Dermatol 1979; 73:19.

32. Salk D. Werner's syndrome: A review of recent research with an analysis of connective tissue metabolism, growth control of cultured cells, and chromosomal aberrations. Hum Genet 1982; 62:1.

33. Arakawa M, Hatamochi A, Takeda K, Ueki H. Increased collagen synthesis accompanying elevated mRNA in cultured Werner's syndrome fibroblasts. J Invest Dermatol 1990;94:187.

34. Bauer EA, Uitto J, Tan EML, Holbrook KA. Werner's syndrome. Evidence for preferential regional expression of a generalized mesenchymal cell defect. Arch Dermatol 1988;124:90.

35. Usui M, Ishii S, Yamawaki S, Hirayama T. The occurrence of soft tissue sarcomas in three siblings with Werner's syndrome. Cancer 1984;54:2580.

36. Brown WT, Zebrower M, Kieras FJ. Progeria, a model disease for the study of accelerated aging. Basic Life Sci 1985;35:375.

37. DeBusk FL. The Hutchinson-Gilford progeria syndrome. J Pediatr 1972;90:697.

38. Goldstein S. Lifespan of cultured cells in progeria. Lancet 1969;1:424.

39. Sephal GC, Sturrock A, Giro MG, Davidson JM. Increased elastin production by progeria skin fibroblast is controlled by the steady-state levels of elastin mRNA. J Invest Dermatol 1988;90:643.

40. Rautenstrauch T, Snigula F, Krieg T, et al. Progeria: A cell culture study and clinical report of familial incidence. Eur J Pediatr 1977;124:101.

41. Moynahan EJ. Progeria (Hasting Gilford) presenting as scleroderma in early infancy. Proc R Soc Med 1962;55:233.

42. Devos EA, Leroy JG, Frijns JP, Van Den Berghe H. The Wiedemann-Rautenstrauch or neonatal progeroid syndrome. Report of a patient with consanguinous parents. Eur J Pediatr 1981;136: 245.

43. Labielle B, Dupuy P, Frey-Follezou, et al. Progeria de Hutchinson-Gilford néonatale avec atteinte cutanée sclérodermiforme. Ann Dermatol Venereol 1987;114:233.

44. Heilborn B, Saxe N. Scleredema in an infant. Arch Dermatol 1986;122:1417.

45. Witt DR, Hayden MR, Holbrook KA, et al. Restrictive dermatopathy: A newly recognized auto-

somal recessive skin dysplasia. Am J Med Genet 1986;24:631.

46. Holbrook KA, Beverly AD, Witt DR, et al. Arrested epidermal morphogenesis in three newborn infants with a fatal genetic disorder (restrictive dermopathy). J Invest Dermatol 1987;88:330.

47. Mok A, Curley R, Tolmie IL, et al. Restrictive dermopathy: A report of the case. J Med Genet 1990; 27:315.

48. Van Hoestenferghe M, Leguis E, Vandevoorde W. Restrictive dermopathy with distinct morphological abnormalities. Am J Med Genet 1990;36:297.

49. Happle R, Schuurmaus Stekhoveu J, Hamel BCJ, et al. Restrictive dermopathy in two brothers. Arch Dermatol 1992;128:232.

50. Welsh KM, Smoller BR, Holbrook KA, Johnston K. Restrictive dermopathy. Report of two affected siblings and review of the literature. Arch Dermatol 1992;128:228.

51. Paige DG, Lahe BD, Balley AJ, et al. Restrictive dermopathy: A disorder of fibroblasts. Br J Dermatol 1992;127:630.

52. Siimes MA, Johansson E, Rapola J. Scleroderma-like graft-versus-host disease as late consequence of bone marrow grafting. Lancet 1977;ii:831.

53. Saurat JH. Cutaneous manifestations of graft-versus-host disease in man. Int J Dermatol 1981; 20:249.

54. Sullivan KM, Shulman HM, Storb R. Chronic graft-versus-host disease in fifty-two patients. Adverse natural course and successful treatment with combination immunosuppression. Blood 1981;57:267.

55. Janin-Mercier A, Devergie A, Van Cauwenberge D, et al. Immunohistologic and ultrastructural study of the sclerotic skin in chronic graft-versus-host disease in man. Am J Pathol 1984;115:296.

56. Rustom KA, Pierard-Franchimont C, Pierard GE. Présentation anatomo-clinique de la maladie du greffon contre l'hôte traitée par cyclosporine A. Dermatologica 1985;171:65.

57. Grossman ME, Bickers DR, Poh-Fitzpatrick MG, et al. Porphyria cutanea tarda: Clinical features and laboratory findings in 40 patients. Am J Med 1979;67:277.

58. Parra CA, de Parra NP. Diameter of the collagen fibrils in the sclerodermatous skin of porphyria cutanea tarda. Br J Dermatol 1979;100:573.

59. Wolff K, Hönigsmann H, Rallschmeier W, et al. Microscopic and fine structural aspects of porphyrias. Acta Derm Venereol (Stockh) 1982;100 (Suppl):17.

60. Jabłónska S, Szczepanski A. Lésions sclérodermiformes dans la porphyrie cutanée. Ann Dermatol Syph 1963;90:241.

61. Doyle JA, Friedman SI. Porphyria and scleroderma: A clinical and laboratory review of 12 patients. Australas J Dermatol 1983;24:109.
62. Tuffanelli DL, Epstein JH, Epstein WL. Cutaneous porphyria. In: Beutner EH, Chorzelski TP, Bean SF, Jordon RE, eds. Immunopathology of the skin: Labeled antibody studies. Stroudsburg, PA: Dowden, Hutchinson & Ross, 1973:170.
63. Varigos G, Schlitz JR, Bickers DR. Uroporphyrin I stimulation of collagen biosynthesis in human skin fibroblasts. A unique dark effect of porphyrin. J Clin Invest 1982;69:129.
64. Torinuki W, Kudoh K, Tagami H. Increased mast cell numbers in the sclerotic skin of porphyria cutanea tarda. Dermatologica 1989;178:75.
65. Friedman SJ, Doyle JA. Sclerodermoid changes of porphyria cutanea tarda: Possible relationship to urinary uroporphyrin levels. J Am Acad Dermatol 1985;13:70.
66. Jabłónska S, Stachow A, Suffczýnska M. Skin and muscle indurations in phenylketonuria. Arch Dermatol 1967;95:443.
67. Kornreich HK, Shaw KNF. Phenylketonuria and scleroderma. J Pediatr 1968;73:571.
68. Battin J, Chavoix P, Alberty J, Henunstre JP. Phenylcétonurie avec infiltration de type sclérodermique. Pédiatrie 1970;25:777.
69. Lasser AE, Schultz BC, Beaff D, et al. Phenylketonuria and scleroderma. Arch Dermatol 1978;114:1215.
70. Jabłónska S, Stachow A, Kencka D. Phenylketonuria with sclerodermatous lesions. In: Black CM, Myers AR, eds. Systemic sclerosis (scleroderma). New York: Gower Medical, 1985:125.
71. Nova MP, Kaufman M, Halperin A. Scleroderma-like skin indurations in a child with phenylketonuria: A clinicopathologic correlation and review of the literature. J Am Acad Dermatol 1992;26:329.
72. Esterly NS, McKusick VA. Stiff skin syndrome. Pediatrics 1971;47:360.
73. Jabłónska S, Groniowski J, Krieg T, et al. Congenital fascial dystrophy: A noninflammatory disease of fascia—the stiff skin syndrome. Pediatr Dermatol 1984;2:87.
74. Jabłónska S, Schubert H, Kikuchi I. Congenital fascial dystrophy: Stiff skin syndrome—a human counterpart of the tight-skin mouse. J Am Acad Dermatol 1989;25:943.
75. Kikuchi I, Inoue S, Hamada K, Ando H. Stiff skin syndrome. Pediatr Dermatol 1985;3:48.
76. Cohen IS, Mosher MB, O'Keefe EJ. Cutaneous toxicity of bleomycin therapy. Arch Dermatol 1973;107:553.
77. Texier L, Gendre P, Gauthier O, et al. Hypodermites sclérodermiformes lombofassiéres induites par des injections medicamenteuses intramusculaires associées à la vitamin K_1. Ann Dermatol Syph (Paris) 1972;99:363.
78. Sanders MN, Windelmann RK. Cutaneous reactions to vitamin K. J Am Acad Dermatol 1988;19:699.
79. Janin-Mercier A, Mosser C, Souteyrand P, Bourges M. Subcutaneous sclerosis with fasciitis and eosinophilia after phytonadione injections. Arch Dermatol 1985;121:1421.
80. Wartenberg R. Progressive facial hemiatrophy. Arch Neurol Psychiatr 1945;54:75.
81. Lewkonia RM, Lowry RB. Progressive hemifacial atrophy (Parry-Romberg syndrome). Report with review of genetics and nosology. Am J Med Genet 1983;14:385.
82. Sanborg F, Hanson V, Kornreigh H, et al. Arthritis, myositis, and growth defects of bone in children with localized scleroderma. Arthritis Rheum 1980;23:741.
83. Braun-Falco O, Marghescu S. Über eine systematisierte neaviforme Atrophodermie. Arch Klin Exp Dermatol 1965;221:548.
84. Faim O, Guillevin L, Giroux C, et al. Neuropathie sensitive du nerf trijumeau et sclérodermie. Rev Neurol (Paris) 1989;145:236.
85. Aberer E, Klade H, Stanek G, Gebhart W. *Borrelia burgdorferi* and different types of morphea. Dermatologica 1991;182:145.
86. Abele DC, Anders KH. The many faces and phases of borreliosis II. J Am Acad Dermatol 1990;23:401.
87. Chaauat Y, Aron-Brunetiere R, Faures B. Une nouvelle entité: Le rheumatisme fibroblastique. À propos d'une observation. Rev Rheum 1980;47:345.
88. Lacour IPH, Maquart FX, Bellon G, et al. Fibroblastic rheumatism: Clinical, histological, immunohistological, ultrastructural, and biochemical study of a case. Br J Dermatol 1993;128:194.
89. Rongioletti F, Rebora A. Annular and semicircular lipoatrophies. J Am Acad Dermatol 1989;20:443.
90. Bruinsma W. Lipoatrophia annularis—an abnormal vulnerability of the fatty tissue. Dermatologica 1967;134:107.
91. Shelley WG, Izumi AK. Annular atrophy of the ankles. Arch Dermatol 1970;102:326.
92. Jabłónska S, Szczepanski A, Gorkiewicz A. Lipoatrophy of the ankles and its relation of other lipoatrophies. Acta Derm Venereol (Stockh) 1975;55:135.
93. Peters MS, Winkelmann RK. The histopathology of localized lipoatrophy. Br J Dermatol 1986;114:27.

94. Sissons JGP, West RJ, Fallows J. The complement abnormalities of lipodystrophy. N Engl J Med 1976;294:461.

95. Bouadjar B, Kaci A, Ysmail-Dahlouk M. Lipidystrophie partielle, glomerulonéphrite et hypocomplémentémie. Ann Dermatol Venereol 1991; 118:826.

96. Miroguchi M, Nanko S. Lipodystrophia centrifugalis abdominalis infantilis in dizygotic twins. J Dermatol 1982;9:139.

97. Patterson JAK, Ackerman AB. Lichen sclerosus et Trophicus is not related to morphea. A clinical and histologic study of 24 patients in whom both conditions were reputed to be present simultaneously. Am J Dermatopathol 1984;6:323.

98. Winkelmann RK. Classification and pathogenesis of scleroderma. Mayo Clin Proc 1971;46:83.

99. Godeau G, Frances C, Hornebeck W, et al. Isolation and partial characterization of an elastase-type protease in human vulvar fibroblast: Involvement in vulvar elastic tissue destruction of patients with lichen sclerosus et atrophicus. J Invest Dermatol 1982;78:270.

100. Uitto J, Santa Cruz DJ, Bauer EA, Eisen AZ. Morphea and lichen sclerosus et atrophicus. J Am Acad Dermatol 1980;2:271.

101. Shulman HM, Sale GE, Lerner KG, et al. Chronic cutaneous graft-versus-host disease in man. Am J Pathol 1978;91:545.

102. Shulman HM, Sullivan KM, Weiden PL, et al. Chronic graft-versus-host syndrome in man: A clinico-pathologic study of 20-long term Seattle patients. Am J Med 1980;69:204.

103. Grzybowski M. Über den sogenannten Lichen sclerosus. Arch Dermatol (Berlin) 1937;175: 222.

104. Connolly MG, Winkelman RK. Coexistence of lichen sclerosus, morphea, and lichen planus. Report of four cases and review of the literature. J Am Acad Dermatol 1985;12:844.

105. Meyrick Thomas RH, Ridley CM, Black MM. The association of lichen sclerosus et atrophicus and autoimmune related disease in males. Br J Dermatol 1983;109:661.

106. Friedrich EG, Kalra PS. Serum levels of sex hormones in vulvar lichen sclerosus and the effects of topical testosterone. N Engl J Med 1984;310:488.

107. Abele DC, Anders KH. The many faces and phases of borreliosis I. Lyme disease. J Am Acad Dermatol 1990;23:167.

108. Aberer E, Klade H, Hobisch G. A clinical, histological and immunohistochemical comparison of acrodermatitis chronica atrophicans and morphea. Am J Dermatopathol 1991;13:334.

109. Gottron HA. Gleichzeitiges Vorhandensein von Akrodermatitis chronica atrophicans und circumscripter Sklerodermie. Z Haut Geschlechtskr 1938;57:7.

110. Aberer E, Stanek G, Ertl M, Neumann R. Evidence for spirochetal origin of circumscribed scleroderma (morphea). Acta Derm Venereol (Stockh) 1987;67:225.

111. Hoesly JM, Mertz LE, Winkelmann RK. Localized scleroderma (morphea) and antibody to *Borrelia burgdorferi*. J Am Acad Dermatol 1987;17:455.

112. Raguin G, Boisnic S, Souteyrand P, et al. No evidence for a spirochaetal origin of localized scleroderma. Br J Dermatol 1992;127:218.

113. Canizares O. Idiopathic atrophoderma of Pasini and Pierini. Arch Dermatol 1959;79:614.

114. Jabłónska S, Szczepanski A. Atrophoderma Pasini-Pierini: Is it an entity? Dermatologica 1962; 125:226.

115. Kencka D, Błaszczyk M, Jabłónska S. Atrophoderma Pasini-Pierini is a primary atrophic abortive morphea? Dermatology 1995;190:203.

II

Pathogenesis

JOHN VARGA
SERGIO A. JIMENEZ

7

Pathogenesis of Scleroderma: Cellular Aspects

PROGRESSIVE FIBROSIS OF THE SKIN and numerous internal organs is the pathologic hallmark of systemic sclerosis (SSc, scleroderma). The fibrotic process results in disruption of the normal architecture of the affected organs, and ultimately leads to their dysfunction and failure. The extent and rate of progression of fibrosis are major factors in determining the outcome of the disease. A large number of studies have established that skin fibroblasts in SSc display a biosynthetically activated phenotype, which persists through a finite number of serial passages *in vitro*, producing increased amounts of collagen and other components of the extracellular matrix. Whereas the initial event or trigger responsible for fibroblast activation in SSc is not known, it is likely that the profound alterations in fibroblast phenotype are crucial elements in the pathogenesis of SSc. Indeed, it is the persistent activation of the genes encoding multiple extracellular matrix proteins in SSc fibroblasts which distinguishes controlled repair, such as normal wound healing, from uncontrolled connective tissue accumulation, which results in pathological fibrosis.

Inflammatory cell-derived soluble mediators can influence fibroblast growth, differentiation, and chemotaxis, as well as connective tissue macromolecule synthesis. Compelling evidence indicates that selected cytokines and growth factors are involved in the pathogenesis of the fibrotic process in SSc. It remains unclear, however, whether aberrant production or extracellular activation of these mediators, altered fibroblast responsiveness to the mediators, disrupted interaction between fibroblasts and the surrounding extracellular matrix, or impaired down-regulation of fibrogenic stimuli is responsible for uncontrolled connective tissue accumulation in SSc. Current evidence suggests that several of these mechanisms may be involved.

Excessive collagen deposition in affected tissues, as illustrated in Figure 7.1, is a central event in the pathogenesis of SSc, and is responsible for most of the clinical manifestations of this incurable disease. Pharmacological manipulation of the multiple steps involved in the complex pathway leading to exaggerated fibrogenesis offers an approach to treatment. Therefore, an understanding of the intrinsic mechanisms responsible for the normal regulation of fibroblast function, and the modulation of this process by extracellular signals may provide clues to the understanding of the molecular alterations in connective tissue cells that occur in SSc. This, in turn, may lead to the rational design of novel therapeutic interventions. In this chapter, we review current knowledge regarding fibroblast function in SSc and highlight the role that specific cellular mediators may play in the development of fibrosis.

The Connective Tissue and Fibroblasts in SSc

The extracellular matrix, a remarkably complex structure composed of a large number of distinct molecules, is not simply an inert structural scaf-

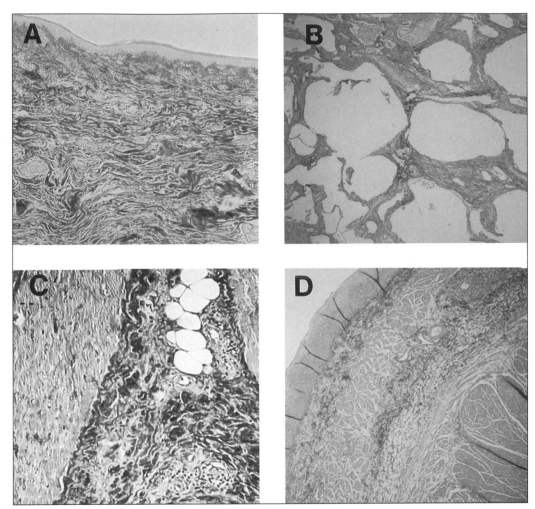

Figure 7.1. Photomicrographs illustrating fibrosis of various organs in SSc: *A*, Skin; *B*,Lung; *C*, Heart; *D*, Esophagus. Note marked accumulation of collagen and disruption of the normal tissue architecture. (Masson's trichrome stain).

fold for endothelial cells and fibroblasts, as was believed for a long time. Rather, it is an active participant in the regulation of various aspects of cell behavior, such as migration, shape, proliferation, differentiation, and biosynthesis of connective tissue macromolecules. Indeed, the extracellular matrix has been shown to play an important role in wound healing, tumor progression, and the development of fibrosis (1).

Histologic examination of affected SSc skin demonstrates that the loose dermal and subder-mal connective tissue is replaced by a dense extracellular matrix (see Fig. 7.1). Histopathologic and biochemical methods have been used to study the extracellular matrix composition of skin in SSc (2–4). While the concentration of collagen in the dermis is normal, the total amount of collagen under a constant surface area of affected skin is increased due to the increased thickness of the dermis. The marked accumulation of collagen in SSc tissues does not appear to be accompanied by abnormalities in the phenotype of the collagens (Table 7.1). Immunohistochemical studies have demonstrated markedly increased fibronectin deposition in the lower dermis in affected skin (5,6), and electronmicroscopy has revealed the accumulation of fine immature microfibrils intertwined with larger collagen fibers in a random pattern in the reticular dermis (7). These thin fibrils, which were recently identified as being composed of fibrillin, appear to cause marked disorganization of the matrix (8). Although patients with early SSc exhibit increased amounts of type III collagen deposits in the lower dermis, type I collagen production dominates in later stages of the disease. This results in a normal relative proportion of type I:type III collagens (1:4) in skin (9) and lungs (10) of patients with established SSc. Surprisingly, when total RNA was extracted from affected skin in nine patients with relatively early SSc, a greater than three-fold elevation in steady-state mRNA levels was noted for type I, but not type III collagen, when compared to healthy control skin (11). The apparent inconsistency between type I:type III collagen ratio in affected tissues determined by biochemical/immunohistochemical methods vs. quantitative mRNA analysis remains unexplained (11).

Morphologically, SSc fibroblasts display the appearance of highly active cells, with enlargement and distention of the rough endoplasmic reticulum, abundant cytoplasm, and several membrane-bound vesicles containing amorphous material presumably representing newly synthesized proteins bound for export to the extracellular space (13). In a 1974 landmark study, LeRoy demonstrated that *in vitro* skin fibroblasts from patients with SSc produce increased amounts of type I collagen compared to fibroblasts from age- and sex-matched healthy individuals (14). Subsequent studies have confirmed that the production of several connective tissue components (types I, III, VI, and VII collagens, fibronectin, decorin, and glycosaminoglycans) is up-regulated in SSc fibroblasts in culture (Fig. 7.2). The increased biosynthesis of these macromolecules is accompanied by an elevation of the steady-state levels of mRNA transcripts which is largely the result of increased transcription of the corresponding genes (15–20). Excessive collagen synthesis by SSc fibroblasts *in vitro* is not associated with alterations in the relative proportions of collagen types, indicating a coordinate up-regulation of several different genes. The persistence of the biosynthetically activated phenotype in SSc fibroblasts for several passages *in vitro* in the absence of potential extracellular activating signals suggests that fundamental alterations in the regulatory pathways controlling connective tissue gene expression have occurred in these cells. In addition to the persistent up-regulation of genes encoding multiple connective tissue proteins, SSc dermal fibroblasts also display enhanced expression of proto-oncogenes, which are known to participate in cell proliferation and activation (21,22), and of the adhesion molecules intercellular adhesion molecule-1 (ICAM-1), a ligand

Table 7.1. Biochemical Features of Connective Tissue in SSc Skin

Abnormal	Normal
Increased tissue collagen content	Collagen phenotype
Increased extractibility of tissue collagen	Collagenolytic activity[a]
Increased microfibrils (fibrillin)	
Increased activity of post-translational enzymes	
Increased glycosaminoglycan content	
Increased fibronectin content	
Increased biosynthesis of several connective tissue components	
Elevated collagen and fibronectin mRNA levels (I, III, VI, VII)	

[a]A recent study suggests impaired collagenase production by SSc fibroblasts *in vitro*.

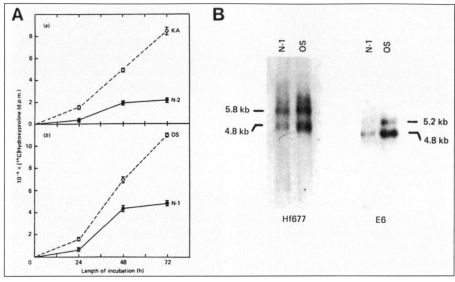

Figure 7.2. Increased collagen gene expression by SSc fibroblasts *in vitro*. A, Kinetics of collagen production by cultures of fibroblasts obtained from patients with SSc (KA, OS) and from age- and sex-matched healthy individuals (N-1 and N-2). B, Northern hybridization analysis of normal and SSc fibroblast mRNA. Total RNA was hybridized to cDNAs for human type I collagen (Hf677) and type III collagen (E6). (Reproduced with permission from Jimenez S, Feldman G, Bashey R, et al. Coordinate increase in the expression of type I and type III collagen genes in fibroblasts. Biochem J 1986;237:837.)

for T-lymphocyte receptors, and β1 integrin, a cell receptor for various extracellular matrix components (23–26). The results from studies of connective tissue metabolism by SSc fibroblasts in monolayer cultures were confirmed by observations from *in situ* hybridizations of SSc skin employing collagen cDNAs (27–29). These studies demonstrated elevated collagen mRNA transcripts in subpopulations of fibroblasts, especially in cells within the reticular dermis and in perivascular locations (Fig. 7.3). In contrast to SSc, fibroblasts in normal skin show very low level of collagen gene expression.

Whereas monolayer cultures have been utilized extensively to study the biosynthetic characteristics of normal and SSc fibroblasts, it is recognized that cell behavior in this system may differ markedly from the *in vivo* situation. In particular, fibroblasts in monolayer cultures are not surrounded by extracellular matrix. Normal fibroblasts propagated *in vitro* in a three-dimensional collagen lattice, a situation which mimics

more closely the physiologic environment than monolayer cultures, cause contraction of the surrounding gel, and drastically reduce the rate of collagen production and the levels of type I collagen mRNA (30,31). The low level of collagen synthesis under these conditions, which resembles that of fibroblasts in the normal resting dermis, results from a combination of transcriptional and post-transcriptional regulatory events (32). Integrins of the β1 family on the surface of fibroblasts appear to be involved in mediating these effects. However, the mechanisms by which signals from the surrounding extracellular matrix are transmitted to fibroblasts and alter the expression of a specific set of genes have not been investigated in detail. In striking contrast to normal fibroblasts, SSc fibroblasts cultured in three-dimensional lattices fail to down-regulate collagen synthesis while maintaining their ability to contract the gel (33). The apparent failure of SSc fibroblasts to down-regulate collagen biosynthesis when cultured in three-dimensional matrices

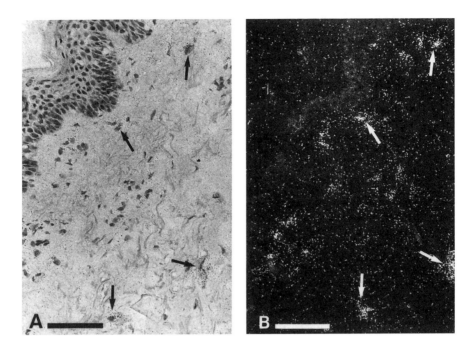

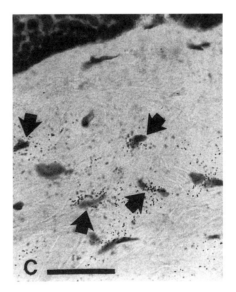

Figure 7.3. *In situ* hybridization of a skin biopsy sample from a patient with SSc with type I collagen cDNA. Note the presence of autoradiographic grains representing radiolabeled cDNA/mRNA hybrids on scattered fibroblasts (arrows). *A*, bright field; *B*, dark field; *C* higher magnification reveals the cytoplasmic localization of signals. Bar=100 μμμm in *A* and *B*, 50 μmμm in *C*. (Reproduced with permission from Peltonen J, Kähäri L, Jaakkola S, et al. Evaluation of transforming growth factor-β1 and type procollagen gene expression in fibrotic skin diseases by *in situ* hybridization. J Invest Dermatol 1989;94:365.)

may reflect alterations in fibroblast-matrix receptor function, and may be important in the development of fibrosis. The study of the modulation of collagen synthesis in fibroblasts propagated in three-dimensional matrices promises to be a fruitful area for further investigation.

Collagen

The collagens constitute a superfamily of related but genetically distinct proteins (34). At least 17 distinct human collagens, coded for by at least 25 separate genes localized on different chromosomes have been reported to date. Type I collagen is a heterotrimer widely distributed in all connective tissues, and accounts for greater than 50% of the dry weight of the skin. Type III collagen, a homotrimer, has similar tissue distribution to type I collagen, but is a relatively minor component in the skin (representing < 20% of all collagens), whereas it is abundant in major blood vessels and fetal tissues. Collagen types IV and VII are normally found only at the dermal-epidermal junction, although in SSc, an abnormal accumulation of type VII collagen throughout the dermis has been recently demonstrated (35). Type V collagen is a minor component of the skin, whereas type VI collagen is present in substantial amounts, and is a major gene product of cultured skin fibroblasts (36). Currently, the function of collagen types V and VI in the skin is unknown.

The biosynthesis of collagen is a complex process which can be regulated at several levels (37). Following secretion into the extracellular space, the amino- and carboxy-terminal propeptides of newly synthesized procollagen are enzymatically cleaved off, with subsequent spontaneous self-assembly of the cleaved molecules into collagen fibers. To attain optimal tensile strength, secreted collagen fibers must be stabilized by the formation of intermolecular cross-links. Recent evidence suggests that type III collagen and the small proteoglycan, decorin, modulate type I collagen fiber size during em-

bryonic development and in pathological conditions of fibrosis (3,8). Both amino- and carboxy-terminal propeptides of the human $\alpha 1$ chain of type I collagen, as well as chemically synthesized oligopeptide homologues of the carboxy-terminal propeptide, can selectively inhibit fibroblast collagen synthesis *in vitro* (38). It has been suggested that inhibition by procollagen propeptides may have a physiologic role in feedback modulation of collagen production. One report suggests that the down-regulation of collagen synthesis by amino-terminal propeptides *in vitro* may be impaired in SSc fibroblasts (39).

STRUCTURE AND REGULATION OF THE TYPE I COLLAGEN GENES

Type I collagen is the major interstitial fiber-forming collagen in the skin. The gene for the $\alpha 1$ chain of human type I procollagen (designated COL1A1) is 18 kb long (40). This complex gene contains 51 exons and intervening sequences (introns) of varying sizes. The pattern of exon structure and size is conserved among different collagen types, suggesting a common evolutionary origin. The COL1A1 gene contains multiple polyadenylation signals at the 3′ end, resulting in mRNA transcripts of two sizes which differ in the lengths of their untranslated 3′ regions. The functional significance of the multiple mRNA species is unknown.

During physiologic processes of tissue remodeling, the expression of collagen genes is tightly controlled, primarily by the modulation of transcriptional activity. Transcriptional modulation of eukaryotic genes is typically accomplished by the interaction between conserved cis-acting elements of the gene located in the first intron and in the 5′ flanking region, and DNA-binding nuclear proteins (trans-acting factors) which specifically recognize these cis elements. Binding of the trans-acting factors to their cognate cis elements in the gene increases (or decreases) RNA polymerase II activity, altering the rate of transcription. A complex array of positive and negative regulatory elements has been characterized in the genes coding for the two chains of type I collagen (34). Binding sites for the transcription factors NF-1 and Sp-1 have been identified in the promoter and first intron of these genes, and implicated as being potentially important in regulating their constitutive expression (41,42). Additional cis-acting elements with either stimulatory or inhibitory function have been identified in the proximal promoter regions of the type I collagen genes (43,44). The multiplicity of regulatory sequences within the collagen promoters suggests that the relative amount/activity of specific trans-acting factors ultimately determines the transcriptional activity of collagen genes in a given cell.

It should be noted that in addition to the interaction between cis-acting enhancer elements and their cognate trans-acting DNA binding proteins, other mechanisms may also be important in the regulation of collagen gene expression. For instance, it has been shown that the macromolecular organization of chromatin affects the transcriptional activity of genes in eukaryotic cells. The chromatin structure of the COL1A1 gene in normal human fibroblasts has been partially characterized by determining the distribution of DNAse hypersensitive sites (indicative of transcriptionally active regions of the DNA). However, there are no comparative data concerning the distribution of DNAse I hypersensitive sites in COL1A1 in SSc fibroblasts (45). An additional mechanism that may be important in modulating collagen gene expression is DNA methylation (46). In most eukaryotic cell lines examined, an inverse correlation exists between the degree of DNA methylation and the transcriptional activity of the gene in that cell type (47). *In vivo* demethylation of cytosine nucleotides in the collagen promoter region could cause increased transcriptional activity of the gene and excessive production of collagen, thereby contributing to the development of fibrosis. However, to date, the methylation status of collagen genes in SSc fibroblasts has not been studied.

Immune Activation and the Involvement of Cytokines in the Pathogenesis of Fibrosis in SSc

Alterations in humoral and cellular immune regulation have long been recognized in SSc. Prominent among the immunological alterations is the development of autoantibodies directed against a broad spectrum of antigens in the serum of most SSc patients. While the detection of specific autoantibodies is helpful in the diagnosis and classification of patients with SSc, it remains unsettled whether humoral autoimmunity is involved in the pathogenesis of clinical manifestations of the disease. Although the pathological hallmark of SSc skin is a thickened, homogenous dermis with densely packed collagen fibers and a paucity of cells, careful histological examination of tissues from patients with disease of relatively short duration (< 2 years) demonstrates mononuclear inflammatory cells near blood vessels, nerves, and dermal appendages (48–50). Although extensive inflammatory cell infiltration may be seen in specimens without significant fibrosis, the degree of cutaneous inflammation generally shows a positive correlation with the extent and progression of skin fibrosis (50). By analogy to wound healing, a form of controlled repair, the "inflammatory phase" in SSc appears to precede the reparative (fibrotic) phase.

Various immune cells have been implicated in the pathogenesis of SSc. T helper lymphocytes, monocyte/macrophages, mast cells, and basophils have all been shown to be increased or activated in the circulation or tissues of patients with SSc (50–52). T lymphocytes predominate in the cutaneous infiltrates in early SSc, whereas B-lymphocytes are uncommon. A majority of infiltrating T cells express Class II major histocompatibility markers, indicating that they are activated (50,51). Further analysis has shown a reduced suppressor T cell population within the infiltrates (53,54). In lesional skin of patients with early SSc, CD3+/CD4+ lymphocytes predominate, whereas in late stages, CD4+ lymphocytes are most common (6,54). These cells display α/β T cell receptors, while γ/δ positive T cells are uncommon (26). An association between tissue infiltration with activated immune cells and abnormal fibrogenesis is prominent not only in SSc, but also in other fibrotic conditions and animal models of fibrosis, such as bacterial cell wall-induced hepatic granulomas and an avian model of SSc (55,56).

The participation of mononuclear leukocytes in the pathogenesis of SSc is supported by evidence of their activation in peripheral blood. For instance, circulating mononuclear cells from patients with SSc show enhanced expression of c-*ras*, c-*myc* and c-*myb* proto-oncogenes (57,58). Furthermore, an activated subpopulation of peripheral blood mononuclear cells displays increased adhesiveness to vascular endothelium *in vitro* compared to normal mononuclear cells (59). *In situ*, the expression of the VLA-1 and β1 integrins is elevated in infiltrating lymphocytes in the affected dermis, particularly in cells that are in close proximity to collagen fibers (Fig. 7.4) (25). The increased expression of adhesion molecules on immune cells in SSc indicates prior activation of these cells. The adhesion molecules may be crucial for the binding of inflammatory cell to endothelial cells, and for their passage through the vascular wall and localization within the lesional tissue. The finding of elevated cytokine production in SSc further supports the concept that immunocompetent cells play a role in the pathogenesis of the disease. Mitogen-stimulated peripheral blood lymphocytes from SSc patients secrete more TNFα, IL-1, and IL-2 than do normal lymphocytes (60,61), and the levels of several cytokines, including IL-2, IL-4, IL-6, and IL-8, as well as soluble IL-2 receptors, are increased in SSc sera (61–64). Furthermore, circulating levels of adenosine deaminase, a marker for T cell activation, are elevated in patients with SSc (65).

SSc fibroblasts *in vitro* display increased adhesion to resting and activated normal T cells and to interstitial collagens, and retract collagen lattices *in vitro* more rapidly than do normal fibroblasts (66,67). Each of these observations could be explained by increased expression of cell-cell and cell-matrix adhesion molecules, such as β1 integrins and ICAM-1 on the surface of SSc fibroblasts (24,25,68,69). These molecules play a major role in the "homing" of pathogenetic lymphocytes to skin and their adhesion to tissue fibroblasts (70).

In situ hybridization techniques have proved to be powerful tools for the detailed examination of the temporal and spatial distribution of activated inflammatory cells and fibroblasts in SSc skin. These studies have shown that dermal fibroblasts displaying elevated levels of collagen mRNA transcripts, indicative of on-going collagen synthesis, are frequently localized in perivascular areas, generally in the vicinity of activated inflammatory cells (27–29,71). Similarly, enhanced expression of ICAM-1 is seen on fibroblasts that are close to infiltrating inflammatory cells (26). Immune cells are a rich source of cytokines, which exert paracrine, juxtacrine, or autocrine effects that result in the regulation of crucial cellular processes. Cytokines are highly pleiotropic polypeptides causing a variety of responses in different target cells, and triggering the synthesis of additional cytokines, which, in turn, may accentuate or abrogate the response. The close association of infiltrating immune cells and biosynthetically activated fibroblasts in SSc tissues suggests that direct immune cell-fibroblast interactions, or immune cell-derived informational molecules may be responsible for fibroblast activation in SSc.

Modulation of Connective Tissue Accumulation by Cytokines

In 1976, Johnson and Ziff demonstrated that supernates from mitogen-stimulated normal human mononuclear cells enhanced the proliferation and collagen synthesis by embryonic fibroblasts *in vitro* (72). These pioneering studies have stimulated an entire field of investigation focusing on the regulation of fibroblast function by cytokines. During the 1980s, it became appar-

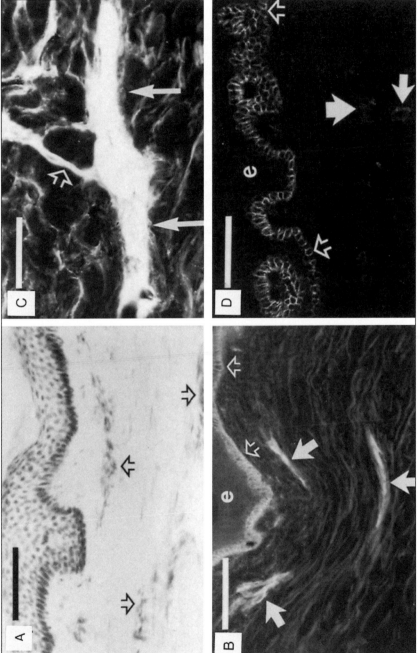

Figure 7.4. Immunodetection of β1 integrin epitopes in SSc skin. *A*, photomicrograph of SSc skin. Note the presence of inflammatory cell infiltrates (arrows). *B*, SSc skin showing intense staining with monoclonal antibody for β1 integrin associated with inflammatory cells (solid arrow). *C*, higher magnification of *B*, showing staining of inflammatory cells with β1 integrin antibody (solid arrow). β1 integrin epitopes are also seen between collagen bundles (open arrow). *D*, Immunostaining of normal skin with monoclonal antibody to β1 integrin. Staining of keratinocytes (open arrow) and occasional endothelial cells (solid arrow) is seen. (Bars= 300 μmμm, except *D*1 where bar= 75 μmμm) e= epidermis. (Reproduced with permission from Sollberg S, Peltonen J, Uitto J, et al. Elevated expression of β1 and β2 integrins, endothelial adhesion molecule 1 and leukocyte adhesion molecule 1 in the skin of patients with systemic sclerosis of recent onset. Arthritis Rheum 1992;35:290.)

ent that soluble products released from inflammatory cells can profoundly alter fibroblast behavior. It was shown that lymphocytes and monocytes elaborate factors that can stimulate or inhibit fibroblast collagen synthesis, proliferation, and chemotaxis (73–76). In the *in vivo* milieu, fibroblasts are potential targets for several cytokines that may exert additive or antagonistic effects on collagen synthesis and accumulation. Thus, the balance between stimulatory and inhibitory signals that modulate fibroblast proliferation, chemotaxis, collagen synthesis, and the production of matrix- degrading proteinases, may determine whether controlled repair (as in normal wound healing), or uncontrolled pathological fibrosis will ensue in response to injury (as in SSc). This balance is normally maintained by a remarkably complex interplay of extracellular signals acting on fibroblasts.

The identification and characterization of specific cytokines, and the cloning of the corresponding genes, has provided investigators with ready access to pure or recombinant forms of these molecules. This, in turn, has allowed the examination of specific effects of cytokines on fibroblast function. A majority of these studies have been carried out *in vitro* employing monolayer cultures of fibroblasts. Only a few studies have examined the response of fibroblasts propagated in three-dimensional collagen lattices to extracellular signals.

The Effect of Specific Cytokines on Collagen Metabolism

A growing number of cytokines and growth factors have been found to modulate collagen biosynthesis by fibroblasts (Table 7.2). The physiologic role and potential pathologic significance of some of these interactions has been demonstrated, whereas others remain to be established.

INTERFERONS (IFNS)

The interferons (IFNs) comprise three antigenically distinct types (α, β, and γ), which are se-

Table 7.2. Modulation of Fibroblast Collagen Biosynthesis by Cellular Mediators

Stimulation:	Inhibition:
TGFβ	Interferons (α, γ)
IL-1[a]	TNFα
Il-4	FGFs (Acidic and basic)
IL-6	EGF
Leukotriene B4	Prostaglandins (E1 and E2)
	IL-8
	IL-10

[a]IL-1 can up- or down-regulate collagen synthesis *in vitro*.

creted by mononuclear cells, fibroblasts and activated T-lymphocytes, and natural killer cells, respectively. Originally characterized by their ability to induce an anti-viral state, IFNs have since been shown to display anti-proliferative, immunomodulatory, and tumoricidal effects (77), and to induce the expression of the major histocompatibility antigens of classes I, II, and III on a variety of cell types. These cellular responses are initiated by binding of IFN to specific cell surface receptors, followed by changes in the expression of several cellular genes. A variety of secondary intracellular messengers have been implicated in these effects.

The most potent inhibitor of collagen production by human mesenchymal cells is the T cell-derived IFNγ (78–80). The inhibition is selective and is associated with a corresponding decrease in types I, II, and III procollagen mRNA levels (80–83). IFNγ also abrogates the stimulatory effects of transforming growth factor-β (TGFβ) on collagen production (84,85). The molecular mechanisms involved in down-regulation of type I collagen gene expression by IFNγ appear to be complex. Both transcriptional and post-transcriptional mechanisms, such as a decrease in mRNA stability, have been invoked to account for these effects (86,87).

These *in vitro* observations suggest that IFNs may play a role in physiologic modulation of collagen accumulation. However, the involvement of IFNs in wound healing or other states of controlled repair has not been firmly established to date. Furthermore, there is no evidence that biosynthetically activated fibroblasts in SSc or related fibrotic conditions have lost their responsiveness to the inhibition by IFNs, since both IFNγ and -α reduced the excessive collagen synthesis and elevated collagen mRNA levels in SSc skin fibroblasts cultivated in monolayers (Fig. 7.5), or in three-dimensional collagen lattice cultures (88–90). This inhibition persisted for at least 18 cell doublings *in vitro* following exposure to IFN (91). IFNγ also inhibited collagen production and type I procollagen mRNA levels in lung fibroblasts from patients with pulmonary fibrosis (92). *In vitro*, the production of IFNγ by mononuclear cells from SSc patients is markedly reduced compared to normal mononuclear cells (61,93). Furthermore, in contrast to other cytokines, serum levels of IFNγ are undetectable in many SSc patients (93). Therefore, abnormal production of IFNγ may play a role in the development of fibrosis in SSc. The IFNs display potent anti-fibrotic effects *in vivo* as well as *in vitro*. For instance, in a murine model of tissue repair and fibrosis the thickness and collagen content of the fibrous capsule surrounding a subcutaneously implanted osmotic pump filled with IFNγ was

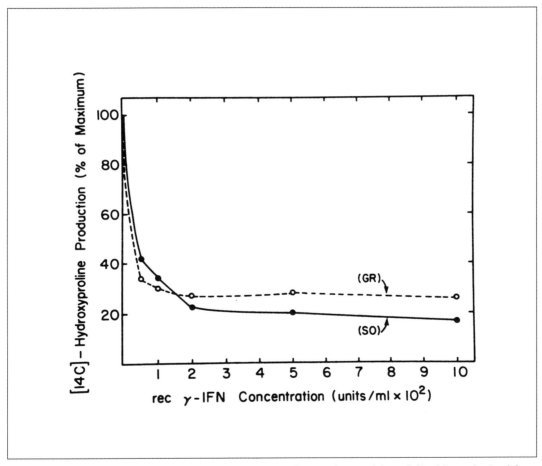

Figure 7.5. Inhibition of collagen synthesis by IFNγ. Confluent cultures of dermal fibroblasts obtained from SSc patients were treated with increasing concentrations of IFNγ. Collagen production was determined by measurement of radiolabeled hydroxyproline. (Reproduced with permission from Rosenbloom J, Feldman G, Freundlich B, et al. Inhibition of excessive scleroderma fibroblast collagen synthesis by recombinant gamma interferon. Arthritis Rheum 1986;29:851.)

markedly reduced compared to that surrounding a pump excreting saline (94). IFNγ ameliorated bleomycin- and schistosomiasis-induced lung and liver fibrosis, respectively, in mice (95,96). The potent effects of the IFNs on collagen synthesis prompted the evaluation of IFNs as potential therapeutic agents in cutaneous fibrosis (97–99). Injection of IFNα into keloids, a localized form of cutaneous fibrosis, resulted in persistent normalization of the activated phenotype of lesional fibroblasts (97). Treatment of SSc patients with IFNγ or IFNα for 4 to 6 months in open, uncontrolled studies resulted in moderate improvement in skin fibrosis, as assessed by skin score measurements (98,99). IFNα administration resulted in inhibition of type I collagen synthesis in fibroblasts derived from the "uninvolved" skin cultured *ex vivo*, whereas no inhibition was observed in fibroblasts from the "involved" skin (98). In contrast, fibroblasts from the involved skin of some, but not all, SSc patients treated with IFNγ showed markedly reduced collagen synthesis and decreased type I collagen mRNA levels compared to fibroblasts derived from pre-treatment biopsies of the same areas (Varga J, Jimenez SA, unpublished observations). These changes in collagen gene expression persisted for several passages *in vitro*. In light of their ability to cause potent, selective, and persistent down-regulation of collagen gene expression in normal and fibrotic fibroblasts, and to prevent the development of fibrosis in animal models, the IFNs hold promise as potential therapeutic agents in SSc.

TUMOR NECROSIS FACTORS (TNF)

The TNF "family" consists of the structurally and functionally related peptides TNFα (cachectin), a monocyte/macrophage product, and TNFβ (lymphotoxin), a lymphocyte product. TNFα and TNFβ bind to the same cell surface receptors and display similar biological activities (100). Originally believed to be tumoricidal cytokines, the TNFs are now recognized as major inflammatory mediators. TNFα stimulates collagenase and stromelysin synthesis (101), and is implicated in the progressive matrix degradation characteristic of rheumatoid arthritis and other forms of destructive synovitis. TNFα also exerts potent effects on the biosynthesis of collagen and other connective tissue components. Because of its effects on metalloproteinases, as well as on connective tissue production, angiogenesis, and fibroblast proliferation, TNFα appears to play an important role in tissue remodeling.

The effects of TNFα on collagen biosynthesis occur by both direct and indirect mechanisms. In human dermal and lung fibroblasts, TNFα inhibits the synthesis of types I and III collagen and abrogates the stimulation of collagen gene expression induced by TGFβ (85,102–105). The inhibition involves transcriptional modulation and is cycloheximide-sensitive, indicating that *de novo* protein synthesis is required. TNFα also down-regulates the expression of other extracellular matrix genes, including elastin and fibronectin (106). These effects may be mediated in part through endogenously produced prostaglandin E (PGE) and interleukin-1 (IL-1), because TNFα causes increased PGE release and IL-1 mRNA accumulation in fibroblasts (105). In preadipocytes, TNFα decreased, whereas in fully differentiated adipocytes it increased type I collagen mRNA levels, indicating that the effects of TNFα on collagen production *in vitro* may depend on the target cell type and state of differentiation (107). In contrast to its negative effects on connective tissue synthesis, TNFα stimulates fibroblast proliferation, and has been implicated in the development of pulmonary fibrosis in bleomycin-treated mice (108). Therefore, the net effect of TNFα on connective tissue accumulation may be determined by the degree of endogenous PGE and IL-1 synthesis by target cells, as well as by the extent of fibroblast proliferation in affected tissues.

INTERLEUKIN-1 (IL-1)

The IL-1 family of proteins consists of three structurally related polypeptides. IL-1α and β are the products of distinct genes, but display substantial amino acid sequence homology, share multiple biological activities, and bind to the same receptors. IL-1 receptor antagonists inhibit the activities of both IL-1s by blocking their binding to cell surface receptors (109). The IL-1s are produced mainly by activated monocyte/ macrophages, lymphocytes, neutrophils, and endothelial cells. In the skin, IL-1 expression can also be demonstrated in fibroblasts and keratinocytes. IL-1β has potent effects on connective tissue accumulation. *In vitro*, IL-1β stimulates the production of collagenase and related matrix-degrading metalloproteinases. In contrast, it inhibits collagen synthesis in adult dermal and lung fibroblasts, hepatic Ito cells, and osteoblastic cells (104,110–112). Other studies, however, showed that IL-1 stimulates collagen gene expression in fibroblasts and synovial cells (113–115). Therefore, the experimental conditions, as well as the type of target cell, may determine the cellular response to IL-1 *in vitro*.

Most of the evidence suggests that the inhibitory effects of IL-1 on collagen production are transcriptionally mediated; however, in some studies with dermal fibroblasts or Ito cells, IL-1 did not alter the steady-state mRNA levels or the transcriptional activity of the type I collagen genes (104,112,115). Fibroblasts, like most cells, express surface receptors for IL-1, and in SSc fibroblasts, increased expression of IL-1β receptors has been demonstrated (116). The signal transduction pathways activated by IL-1 that result in modulation of collagen gene expression involve protein kinase C as well as endogenous prostaglandins, because IL-1 is a potent inducer of PGE_2 production by fibroblasts (112,117). Blocking IL-1-induced PGE synthesis with indomethacin abolished the inhibitory effects of IL-1 on collagen production in synovial cells, but not in lung fibroblasts *in vitro* (105,113). In view of the contradictory results obtained from studies of modulation of extracellular matrix production by IL-1 *in vitro*, the net *in vivo* effects of this cytokine on connective tissue accumulation are difficult to predict, and may depend on the

relative concentrations of other cytokines in the milieu of the target organs. Interestingly, the administration of an IL-1 receptor antagonist prevented the development of pulmonary fibrosis in mice induced by bleomycin or silica, suggesting that in these models of fibrosis IL-1 plays a profibrotic role (118). Indeed, SSc fibroblasts in contrast to normal fibroblasts have been shown to constitutively express high levels of IL-1 mRNA (119).

OTHER INTERLEUKINS

IL-4 is secreted primarily by TH_2 lymphocytes and mast cells (120). This cytokine stimulates the expression of HLA class II molecules on a variety of cell types, promotes growth of IL-2 dependent T-lymphocytes, and inhibits IL-1 and TNFα secretion. Receptors for IL-4 have been identified on human dermal and synovial fibroblasts, as well as on B and T cells, macrophages, and mast cells. *In vitro*, IL-4 stimulates fibroblast proliferation and chemotaxis (121), and at high concentrations, it stimulates type I and type III collagen synthesis and transcription (122,123). Therefore, IL-4 may be viewed as a fibrogenic cytokine. A role for IL-4 in the pathogenesis of SSc is suggested by the observation that serum levels of IL-4 are elevated in some patients with SSc (65).

IL-6 is a pleiotropic cytokine secreted by T_{H2} lymphocytes and other inflammatory cells. TFGβ, platelet-derived growth factor (PDGF), IL-1, IL-4, and TNFα can induce IL-6 production in endothelial and smooth muscle cells, keratinocytes, and fibroblasts (124). IL-6 activates T and B lymphocytes, and inhibits TNF secretion. Increased expression of IL-6 in epithelial cells of SSc patients was demonstrated by *in situ* hybridization (125). In comparison to dermal fibroblasts from healthy individuals, SSc-derived fibroblasts constitutively produced 6- to 30-fold higher levels of IL-6 *in vitro* (126). IL-6 stimulated the production of collagen, glycosaminoglycans, and tissue inhibitor of metalloproteinases (TIMP) by normal dermal fibroblasts, although it had no effect on collagen synthesis by rheumatoid synovial cells *in vitro* (127–129). The constitutive secretion of the profibrotic IL-6 by SSc fibroblasts may be involved in an autocrine loop in the development of fibrosis.

IL-8 is a potent neutrophil and monocyte chemoattractant, and angiogenic factor (130, 131). IL-8 production in a variety of cell types, including endothelial cells and fibroblasts, is induced at a transcriptional level by IL-1 and TNFα. IL-8 belongs to a superfamily of proinflammatory mediators known as "chemokines." Although members of this cytokine family display homology to the connective tissue activating peptide (132), IL-8 inhibits the expression of types I and III collagen genes in human fibroblasts *in vitro* (133). In addition to their well-recognized role in inflammation, involvement of chemokines in normal and pathologic tissue repair is suggested by the *in situ* demonstration of their corresponding mRNA transcripts in granulation tissue in the late stages of wound healing (134) and the observation that alveolar macrophages from SSc patients with lung fibrosis produce increased amounts of IL-8 (135). IL-8 is detectable in the serum of 20% of SSc patients, and anti-IL-8 autoantibody titers are significantly elevated compared to healthy controls (66). Because inflammatory mediators induce IL-8 production by fibroblasts which express specific IL-8 receptors, it has been suggested that an autocrine collagen synthesis-inhibitory loop involving IL-8 may exist. This inhibitory mechanism may be interrupted by anti-IL-8 autoantibodies in SSc and may contribute to the fibrotic process.

IL-10 is secreted by T_{H2} cells and B cells, as well as by monocytes and macrophages (136). In contrast to the previously listed interleukins, IL-10 is a potent anti-inflammatory mediator, which suppresses proliferation and cytokine synthesis by the Th1 subset of T cells *in vitro*. The inhibitory effects of IL-10 on the production of IFNγ and TNFα suggest that this cytokine may indirectly stimulate connective tissue accumulation. Recent data indicate that, in contrast to the other T_{H2}-derived interleukins (IL-4 and IL-6), IL-10 directly inhibits type I collagen gene expression in fibroblasts (137). To date, the expression of IL-10 in fibrotic diseases has not been studied.

TRANSFORMING GROWTH FACTOR-B (TGFB)

The TGFβs are cytokines with remarkably pleiotropic *in vitro* and *in vivo* activity, originally identified by their ability to cause transformation of fibroblasts *in vitro* (138). The TGFβs comprise a family of five distinct gene products having substantial sequence homology. The prototype of the family, TGFβ1 is a homodimer of 25 kD, which is highly conserved among mammals. At least one isoform of TGFβ is secreted from most cells in an inactive precursor form. Latent TGFβ undergoes extracellular activation by poorly understood mechanisms, and binds to specific receptors present on virtually all cell types. The TGFβs influence a variety of important physiologic processes by regulating the expression of two broad categories of genes: (*a*) those involved in cellular growth and differentiation, and (*b*) those involved in modulating the accumulation of the extracellular matrix. TGFβ is a potent fibrogenic growth factor that plays a critical role in the maintenance of connective tissue by modulating the synthesis, deposition, and turnover of extracellular matrix (Table 7.3) (139).

During embryogenesis, TGFβ is associated with tissues of mesenchymal origin (connective tissue, bone, cartilage), and is especially abundant in areas undergoing morphogenesis (140). *In vitro*, TGFβ stimulates the synthesis of several extracellular matrix components (Fig. 7.6), and up-regulates the cellular expression of matrix receptors involved in recognition and adhesion (141–148). Furthermore, it inhibits the production of matrix-degrading metalloproteinases and stimulates the expression of their inhibitors (149). *In vivo*, TGFβ produces fibrosis and angiogenesis when injected subcutaneously into newborn mice (141), and accelerates incisional wound healing (150).

Table 7.3. Regulation of Genes Involved in Extracellular Matrix Synthesis, Deposition, and Turnover by TGFβ

Stimulation	Cell Type	Inhibition	Cell Type
Extracellular Matrix Components		*Proteases*	
Collagen α1(I)	Fibroblast	Collagenase I	Fibroblast
Collagen α2(I)	Fibroblast	Stromelysin	Fibroblast
Collagen α1(III)	Fibroblast	Gelatinase	Fibroblast
Collagen α2(V)	Fibroblast	Plasminogen Activator	Adenocarcenoma
Collagen α1(II)	Chondrocyte	Plasminogen	Fibroblast
Fibronectin	Fibroblast		
Osteonectin (SPARC)	Osteosarcoma	*Cytokines*	
Proteoglycans	Chondrocyte	IFNγ	Mononuclear
Thrombospondin	Fibroblast		cells
Laminin	Fibroblast		
Decorin[a]	Fibroblast		
Tenascin	Colon Carcinoma		
Adhesion/Recognition Molecules			
Integrins	Various		
LFA-1	Monocytic cells		
Cytokines			
TGFβ (autoinduction)	Various		
PDGF-B (c-sis)	Various		
PDGF-A	Endothelial		
Receptors			
EGF	Breast Carcinoma		
PDGF-B	Fibroblast		
Protease Inhibitors			
TIMP	Fibroblast		
Plasminogen Activator Inhibitor-1	Various		

[a]Decorin has been shown to be stimulated or inhibited by TGFβ.

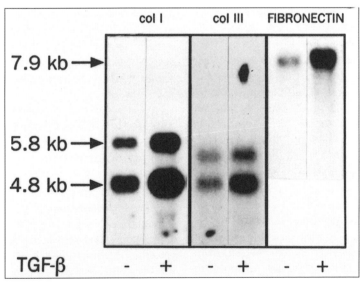

Figure 7.6. Regulation of types I and III procollagen and fibronectin mRNA levels by TGFβ. Confluent cultures of normal skin fibroblasts were treated with TGFβ, and total RNA was analyzed by Northern hybridization analysis. *Lane* 1, control; *Lane* 2, TGFβ-treated.

The intracellular pathways mediating the diverse effects of the TGFβs on fibroblasts are not completely understood. Of the three cellular TGFβ receptors that have been identified, only the types I and II are signalling receptors (151). Since the type II receptor is a serine/threonine protein kinase (152), and TGFβ activates protein kinase C (153), protein phosphorylation may be involved in the cellular responses to TGFβ. However, the intracellular targets of TGFβ receptor kinase activity have not been identified. Early-immediate genes, activated rapidly in response to TGFβ, may function as secondary messengers, and appear to be necessary for the autoinduction of TGFβ1 gene expression (154,155).

The half-life of TGFβ is short; however, by inducing its own synthesis as well as the synthesis of other cytokines, cytokine receptors, and oncogenes, the short-term cellular response to TGFβ may be amplified and transformed into persistent effects. The increase in collagen synthesis is among the best characterized responses to TGFβ. In TGFβ-treated fibroblasts, elevated collagen mRNA levels result primarily from transcriptional up-regulation, although under certain conditions stabilization of mRNA may also contribute to the increased transcript levels (146,156). In the murine COL2A1 gene, a segment approximately 300 bp upstream from the transcription start site is reported to be necessary and sufficient for its transcriptional stimulation by TGFβ (157). This region of the gene includes a potential binding site for the transcription factor nuclear factor-1 (NF-1). A 3 bp substitution mutation in this site which abolished NF-1 binding resulted in loss of inducibility of COL1A2 expression by TGFβ, indicating a functional requirement for NF-1 binding in TGFβ responsiveness. In contrast to the murine gene, induction of rat COL1A1 promoter activity by TGFβ was reported to be mediated via a short segment localized approximately 1600 bp upstream from the transcription start site, and did not appear to involve NF-1 binding (158,159). In the human COL1A2 gene, a putative TGFβ-responsive element containing a potential Sp1 binding site has

been localized at −378/−108 bp (160). In the human COL1A1 gene, a TGFβ response element is located between −340 and −84 bp upstream from the transcription initiation site and contains several potential Sp1 binding sites (161).

In addition to its effects on fibroblast chemotaxis, adhesion to the matrix and synthesis of collagen and other extracellular matrix components, TGFβ regulates certain fibroblast functions indirectly. For instance, TGFβ induces endogenous production of PDGF and IL-6 by fibroblasts (162,163). It also modulates target cell responses to basic fibroblast growth factor (βFGF), IL-6, and other cytokines by regulating the expression of specific cellular surface receptors (164,165). The indirect effects of TGFβ may be involved in the complex paracrine/autocrine networks which amplify and perpetuate fibrogenetic responses *in vivo*.

Although SSc and normal fibroblasts appear to have comparable TGFβ receptor numbers and binding affinities (166), the response of SSc fibroblasts to TGFβ *in vitro* differs from that of normal fibroblasts. For instance, TGFβ markedly increases glycosaminoglycan production, and up-regulates PDGFα receptor expression in SSc skin fibroblasts, but not in normal skin fibroblasts (167). In contrast, TGFβ up-regulates βFGF receptor expression and the levels of COL2A1 mRNA to a much greater extent in normal skin fibroblasts than in SSc fibroblasts (162,164).

The Role of TGFβ in the Pathogenesis of SSc and Other Fibrotic Conditions

Elevated tissue expression of TGFβ mRNA, which precedes the accumulation of collagen, has been demonstrated in patients with idiopathic pulmonary fibrosis (168) and hepatic cirrhosis (169), as well as in animal models of pulmonary (170) and liver fibrosis (171). In patients with autologous bone marrow transplantation for breast cancer, elevated serum levels of TGFβ predicted the development of pulmonary and hepatic fibrosis

(172). The role of TGFβ in the fibrotic process of SSc has been studied extensively. Mononuclear cells in bronchoalveolar lavage fluid from patients with SSc and active lung disease show increased expression of TGFβ compared to cells from healthy individuals (173). SSc fibroblasts in monolayer culture display elevated TGFβ mRNA levels (20), and the expression of TGFβ1 and TGFβ2 in tissues from patients with localized and diffuse SSc (Fig. 7.7), fasciitis, and eosinophilia-myalgia syndrome is markedly elevated (29,71, 174). In these conditions, TGFβ epitopes were localized by immunofluorescence in the dermis, whereas, TGFβ mRNA transcripts were detected in infiltrating inflammatory cells as well as in der-mal fibroblasts, and were generally co-localized with fibroblasts expressing high levels of collagen mRNA. The synthesis of TGFβ in SSc dermal fi-broblasts suggests that TGFβ may function as a paracrine as well as an autocrine mediator of fi-broblast activation in these disorders. Taken to-gether, these observations indicate that in early SSc, TGFβ released by infiltrating mononuclear inflammatory cells in the lung and skin, as well as by fibroblasts in the skin, may be involved in up-regulation of collagen gene expression. In light of its remarkable profibrotic effects detailed above, and its ability to induce its own production, TGFβ has emerged as a critical molecule in the pathogenesis of fibrosis in SSc (175).

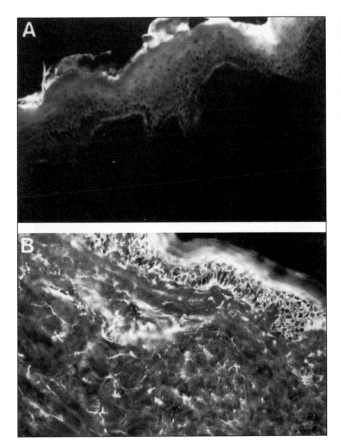

Figure 7.7. Immunodetection of TGFβ1 in SSc skin by indirect immunofluores-cence. Monoclonal antibodies for TGFβ1 were used. *A*, normal skin; *B*, SSc skin from a patient with early disease. Note intense immunofluorescence staining of TGFβ1 epitopes in SSc dermis (Courtesy of Dr. Ly-dia Rudnicka).

Other Growth Factors and Mediators

PLATELET-DERIVED GROWTH FACTOR (PDGF)

PDGF is a homo- or heterodimer of A and B chains that share 60% amino acid sequence identity (176). Originally isolated from platelets, PDGF is now known to be produced by activated macrophages, smooth muscle cells, endothelial cells, and fibroblasts as well. PDGF is associated with wound repair and other processes characterized by accumulation of connective tissue. The primary biological effect of PDGF is stimulation of proliferation and chemotaxis of fibroblasts, monocytes, and smooth muscle cells. *In vivo*, PDGF causes enhanced normal wound healing, and accelerates impaired healing induced by adriamycin (177). *In vitro*, PDGF has complex effects on connective tissue metabolism. Thus, it stimulates collagenase secretion and the synthesis of fibronectin and type V collagen, and decreases type II collagen synthesis but does not affect type I collagen (178–179).

The PDGF receptor, a dimer of α and β subunits, is expressed in low levels in normal, unstimulated fibroblasts. TGFβ induces the synthesis of PDGF A chain and α receptors, thereby increasing fibroblast responsiveness to PDGF (162). Expression of PDGF is elevated in the lungs of patients with idiopathic pulmonary fibrosis (180). The involvement of PDGF in the pathogenesis of SSc is suggested by the demonstration of PDGF and its receptors in both the clinically involved as well as macroscopically "uninvolved" skin in patients with SSc (174,181).

FIBROBLAST GROWTH FACTORS (FGFS)

The FGFs comprise a family of at least eight polypeptides, of which the 18 kD acidic and basic FGFs (aFGF and bFGF) are the best characterized (182). The FGFs bind to the same receptors, and have substantial amino acid homology. The binding of FGF to its receptors is followed by activation of protein kinase C and stimulation of the expression of the c-fos and c-jun oncogenes. The FGFs are produced by most cell types *in vivo* and *in vitro*, but unlike other polypeptide growth factors, lack conventional signal peptides. FGFs are secreted into the extracellular space via nontraditional pathways, and bind to pericellular heparin-like glycosaminoglycans. Thus, the FGFs can be considered as components of the extracellular matrix. The FGFs have been implicated in embryonic development and angiogenesis, and may play a role in the pathogenesis of cancer. *In vitro*, the FGFs exert potent effects on fibroblast proliferation, migration, and differentiation. Both aFGF and bFGF stimulate collagenase synthesis and inhibit collagen synthesis by normal skin fibroblasts at a pre-translational level (183,184). The biological effects of FGFs are markedly potentiated by binding to heparin, which protects the FGFs from proteolytic degradation. Accumulation of bFGF has been demonstrated in the skin of patients with SSc, and may contribute to vascular injury, but its role in the development of fibrosis remains to be clarified (185).

EPIDERMAL GROWTH FACTORS (EGF)

Epidermal growth factor (EGF) is a polypeptide detected in platelets and most human body fluids (186). Members of the EGF family bind to a common receptor present on most nonhematopoietic cells. The most prominent biological effect of EGF is stimulation of fibroblast and keratinocyte proliferation which may account for the acceleration of wound-healing induced by EGF (187). In osteoblastic cells and skin fibroblasts, EGF inhibits type I collagen gene expression via transcriptional modulation (188,189). EGF receptor affinity is decreased in dermal fibroblasts from SSc patients (22). Diminished responsiveness of SSc fibroblasts to EGF could result in impaired down-regulation of collagen synthesis, but a role for such an interaction in the pathogenesis of fibrosis has not been demonstrated.

PROSTAGLANDINS

Various products of cellular arachidonate metabolism are important autocrine and paracrine regulators of cellular functions. Prostaglandins of the E series exert potent inhibitory effects on collagen production *in vitro*, because of a combination of enhanced intracellular degradation of collagen and a transcriptionally-mediated decrease in type I collagen mRNA levels (190–192). Many inflammatory cytokines, including TNFα and IL-1, are potent stimuli for PGE_2 production in synovial, lung, and skin fibroblasts (193). TGFβ-induced endogenous PGE production in lung, but not in synovial, fibroblasts abrogates the stimulatory effects of TGFβ on collagen synthesis (193). Endogenous PGE also nullifies the stimulatory effects of IL-1 on collagen production in human synovial cells (194). Whether PGE-mediated down-regulation of collagen gene expression has a role in the physiologic or pathologic regulation of connective tissue remains to be established. In contrast to PGE, leukotriene C, another arachidonic acid metabolite, stimulates collagen synthesis *in vitro* (195).

Mast Cells and Eosinophils

In murine models of cutaneous fibrosis, such as chronic graft-versus-host disease, and the tight skin (Tsk) mouse, extensive degranulation of mast cells in the skin has been observed (196, 197). Infiltration by mast cells is prominent in affected tissues in SSc, keloids, and in tissue from patients with bleomycin- or irradiation-induced pulmonary fibrosis (198,199). Furthermore, evidence of extensive mast cell degranulation has been described in SSc skin (200–202). Mast cell-derived IL-4 stimulates collagen synthesis, but neither heparin nor histamine have a direct influence on connective tissue metabolism, and the role of mast cells in the pathogenesis of fibrosis remains speculative.

Cutaneous fibrosis is prominent in several conditions characterized by eosinophilia, such as the idiopathic hypereosinophilic syndrome, eosinophilic fasciitis, and eosinophilia-myalgia syndrome (202), and subepithelial bronchial fibrosis is prominent in patients with asthma (203). Conversely, tissue eosinophil infiltration is observed in wound healing and in localized fibrotic conditions, such as morphea and linear scleroderma, orbital pseudotumor, retroperitoneal fibrosis, idiopathic pulmonary fibrosis, and nodular sclerosing Hodgkin's disease (204–206). Although significant peripheral blood eosinophilia in patients with SSc is infrequent (207), eosinophil infiltration is prominent in the small intestine (208), and elevated numbers of eosinophils are found in bronchoalveolar lavage fluids (209). Serum levels of eosinophil granule proteins, which are indicative of eosinophil activation, and degranulation, are elevated in some SSc patients, and extracellular deposition of eosinophil cationic protein (ECP) has been reported in the affected skin (210).

Several studies have examined the effects of eosinophil-derived factors on fibroblasts. In some reports, conditioned media from cultured eosinophils were shown to stimulate fibroblast proliferation and glycosaminoglycan production *in vitro* (211–213). One recent study indicates that eosinophil cationic protein (ECP) enhanced proteoglycan accumulation in lung fibroblasts (214). Another important eosinophil product, major basic protein (MBP), induces platelet degranulation, which may result in the release of fibrogenic cytokines (215). In addition to granule proteins, activated eosinophils also secrete TGFβ (216–218). Therefore, eosinophils may be involved in the development of fibrosis, but their direct role in the pathogenesis of SSc has not been established conclusively.

The Role of Retroviral Proteins in Activation of Collagen Gene Expression

Autoantibodies that cross-react with retroviral antigens have been detected in the sera of many patients with SSc. Anti-Scl 70 autoantibodies, which are marker autoantibodies for the diffuse cutaneous form of SSc, recognize topoisomerase I. Topoisomerase I, which causes relaxation of supercoiled DNA, shares a six-amino acid sequence identity with the p30^{gag} protein of several retroviruses (219). Scl 70-positive sera from SSc patients recognize synthetic peptides containing these amino acids, and inhibit the activity of retroviral topoisomerase I *in vitro* (220). Another autoantibody present in the sera of some patients with SSc and Sjögren syndrome reacts with the p24^{gag} protein of the human retrovirus HTLV I (221). Cross-reactivity between cellular and retroviral epitopes raises the possibility that these autoantibodies arose in patients with SSc in response to retroviral infection, and cross-react with host tissue antigenic epitopes homologous to viral antigens.

The human immunodeficiency virus (HIV) encodes the transactivator protein tat, which is responsible for some of the altered host cell gene responses seen in HIV infection. Recent studies have shown that expression of the tat gene in human glial cells causes a marked increase in type I collagen and fibronectin mRNA levels as a result of the transcriptional activation of the genes (Fig. 7.8) (222). Furthermore, tat also induces the expression of TGFβ and other cytokines (223). These observations suggest that expression of retroviral proteins within immunocompetent and mesenchymal cells could cause persistent phenotypic activation of the host cell, resulting in alterations in cell-mediated immunity and exaggerated production of connective tissue macromolecules.

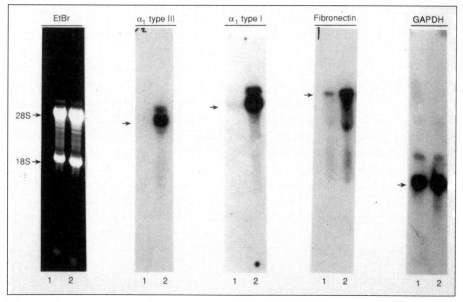

Figure 7.8. Stimulation of types I and III procollagen and fibronectin mRNA levels by the retrovirally encoded tat protein. Human glial cells were stably transfected with a tat expressor plasmid. Total cellular RNA from confluent cultures of tat-expressing glial cells was examined by Northern hybridization analysis. (Reproduced with permission from Taylor J, Cupp C, Diaz A, et al. Activation and expression of genes coding for extracellular matrix proteins in tat-producing glioblastoma cells. Proc Natl Acad Sci USA 1992;89:9617.)

Interaction of the Extracellular Matrix and Extracellular Signals and Their Effects on Fibroblast Connective Tissue Synthesis

In the normal milieu, fibroblasts are surrounded by abundant extracellular matrix, and during physiologic processes of tissue remodeling are exposed simultaneously or sequentially to several signal molecules. The extracellular matrix may directly modulate fibroblast function, or serve as a reservoir of informational molecules. The complex interaction of fibroblasts and the extracellular matrix is illustrated by the effects of decorin on connective tissue accumulation. Decorin, which is the most abundant interstitial proteoglycan, interacts with type I collagen and appears to play a role in fibril formation (224). Decorin also binds to TGFβ, and neutralizes its biological activities (225). Since TGFβ regulates the production of decorin in dermal fibroblasts (20, 226), decorin could be part of an autocoine regulatory loop modulating the tissue availability of active TGFβ, regulating collagen fiber formation, and its own synthesis.

Multiple cytokines interacting with fibroblasts simultaneously or sequentially may exert additive, synergistic, or antagonistic effects on fibroblast function. Indeed, it has been emphasized that the context of the signal determines how the target cell will respond to it (227). Furthermore, cytokines may modulate the expression of specific cytokine receptors on the surface of target cells, and mutually modulate their synthesis in inflammatory cells and fibroblasts. Therefore, in tissues undergoing physiologic or pathologic remodeling, complex and highly interactive extracellular matrix-cytokine networks exist and may be operative in the regulation of matrix protein biosynthesis.

Although much has been learned about cytokine regulation of fibroblast matrix biosynthesis employing tissue culture systems, most studies have examined fibroblast responses to isolated factors. Such observations often have limited applicability to the study of the complex biological responses occurring *in vivo*. An alternate approach involves the simultaneous or sequential study of several potentially relevant cytokines. The results from a limited number of such studies demonstrate that cytokines interact with each other and modulate collagen gene expression in a complex manner. For instance, IL-1, TNFα and IFNγ nullify the stimulatory effects of TGFβ on fibroblast collagen production (84,85,101,228), and can synergize with each other as inhibitors of collagen production (103, 104). Further *in vitro* studies will be necessary to fully characterize the interactions among a number of cytokines modulating collagen gene expression in fibroblasts. *In vivo* models of spontaneous or induced fibrosis offer several advantages for the study of regulation of connective tissue turnover. Analysis of affected tissues in models employing *in situ* hybridization and immunohistochemical methods should permit the identification of spatial and temporal expression of regulatory cytokines during normal and abnormal fibrogenesis.

Summary

It is now evident that persistent overproduction of collagen and other connective tissue macromolecules results in excessive tissue deposition, and is responsible for the progressive nature of fibrosis in SSc. Up-regulation of collagen gene expression in SSc fibroblasts appears to be a critical event in the development of tissue fibrosis. The coordinate transcriptional activation of a number of extracellular matrix genes suggests a fundamental alteration in regulatory control in SSc fibroblasts. Trans-acting nuclear factors which bind to cis-acting elements in enhancer and promoter regions of the collagen genes modulate their basal and inducible transcriptional activity. The identity of the nuclear transcriptional factors that regulate normal collagen gene expression remains to be firmly established. To date, no alterations in the level or in the activity of such DNA binding factors has been demonstrated in SSc fibroblasts.

In addition to important interactions between fibroblasts and the extracellular matrix, cytokines and other cellular mediators can positively and negatively influence fibroblast collagen synthesis. Some of these signaling molecules may have physiologic roles, and their aberrant expression, or altered responsiveness of SSc fibroblasts to them, may result in the acquisition of the activated phenotype. Other mediators may be relevant in the pathogenesis of SSc because of their inhibitory effects on collagen synthesis. The rapid expansion of knowledge regarding the effects of cytokines on extracellular matrix synthesis has led to an appreciation of the enormous complexity of regulatory networks that operate in the physiologic maintenance of connective tissue, and are responsible for the occurrence of pathologic fibrosis.

The ubiquitous growth factor TGFβ is the most potent inducer of collagen gene expression and connective tissue accumulation yet discovered. The expression of TGFβ in activated mononuclear cells infiltrating early SSc lesions suggests a role for this cytokine as a mediator of fibroblast activation in SSc. Furthermore, the recognition that TGFβ is capable of inducing its own expression in a variety of cell types, coupled with the demonstration that a subpopulation of SSc dermal fibroblasts produce TGFβ *in vivo*, indicates the existence of a possible autocrine loop whereby lymphocyte-derived TGFβ induces biosynthetic activation of fibroblasts and the endogenous production of TGFβ by the target fibroblasts themselves. Such autocrine loops involving TGFβ production may explain the persistent activation of collagen gene expression characteristic of SSc fibroblasts, and could be responsible for the chronic and frequently progressive nature of fibrosis in SSc. Numerous other cytokines, as well as cell-matrix interactions, also modify collagen gene expression in fibroblasts and can significantly influence the effects of TGFβ. While the physiological function of cytokines in tissue remodeling or involvement in abnormal fibrogenesis has not been demonstrated conclusively, the precise delineation of their biological effects, may provide important clues to understanding the pathogenesis of SSc. This information, in turn, will aid in the development of rational drug therapy aimed at interrupting the abnormal fibrogenic process.

ACKNOWLEDGMENTS

Supported by research grants from the National Institutes of Health, Public Health Service, U.S.A:AR-42309 (JV) and AR-19106 (SAJ). We are grateful for the expert secretarial assistance provided by Oanh Ma and Marlene Mills.

References

1. Krieg T, Hein R, Hatamochi A, et al. Molecular and clinical aspects of connective tissue. Eur J Clin Invest 1988;18:105.
2. Fleischmajer R, Dessau W, Timpl R, et al. Immunofluorescence analysis of collagen, fibronectin, and basement membrane protein in scleroderma skin. J Invest Dermatol 1980;75:270.
3. Perlish J, Lemlich G, Fleischmajer R. Identification of collagen in scleroderma skin. J Invest Dermatol 1988;90:48.
4. Rodnan G, Lipinski E, Luksick J. Skin thickness and collagen content in progressive systemic sclerosis and localized scleroderma. Arthritis Rheum 1979;22:130.
5. Fleischmajer R, Perlish J, Krieg T, et al. Variability in collagen and fibronectin synthesis by scleroderma fibroblasts in primary culture. J Invest Dermatol 1981;76:400.
6. Cooper S, Keyser A, Beaulieu A, et al. Increase in fibronectin in the deep dermis of involved skin in progressive systemic sclerosis. Arthritis Rheum 1979;22:983.
7. Fleischmajer R, Damiano V, Nedwich A. Scleroderma and the subcutaneous tissue. Science 1971;171:1019.
8. Fleischmajer R, Jacobs L, Schwartz E, et al. Extracellular microfibrils are increased in localized and systemic scleroderma skin. Lab Invest 1991;64:791.
9. Lovell C, Nicholls A, Duance V, et al. Characterization of dermal collagen in systemic sclerosis. Br J Dermatol 1979;100:359.

10. Seyer J, Kang A, Rodnan G. Investigation of type III collagen of the lung in progressive systemic sclerosis (scleroderma). Arthritis Rheum 1981; 24:625.

11. Herrmann K, Heckmann M, Kulozik M, et al. Steady-state mRNA levels of collagens I, III, fibronectin and collagenase in skin biopsies of systemic sclerosis patients. J Invest Dermatol 1991; 97:219.

12. Takeda K, Hatamochi A, Ueki H, Nakata M, Oishi Y. Decreased collagenase expression in cultured systemic sclerosis fibroblasts. J Invest Dermatol 1994;103:359.

13. Jimenez S, Martinez A. Fibroblasts. In: Roitt IM, Delves PJ, eds. Encyclopedia of Immunology. London: Saunders Scientific Publications, 1991;562.

14. LeRoy E. Connective tissue synthesis by scleroderma skin fibroblasts in cell culture. J Exp Med 1972;135:1351.

15. Kähäri VM, Vuorio T, Nanto-Salonen K, et al. Increased type I collagen mRNA levels in cultured scleroderma fibroblasts. Biochim Biophys Acta 1984;781:183.

16. Jimenez S, Feldman G, Bashey R, et al. Coordinate increase in the expression of type I and type III collagen genes in progressive systemic sclerosis fibroblasts. Biochem J 1986;237:837.

17. Bashey R, Millan A, Jimenez S. Increased biosynthesis of glycosaminoglycans by scleroderma fibroblasts in culture. Arthritis Rheum 1984;27:1040.

18. Kähäri VM, Multimaki P, Vuorio E. Elevated pro-α2(I) collagen mRNA levels in cultured scleroderma fibroblasts result from an increased transcription rate of the corresponding gene. FEBS Lett 1987;215:331.

19. Kähäri VM, Heino J, Larjava H, et al. Alterations in scleroderma fibroblast surface glycoproteins associated with increased collagen synthesis. Acta Derm Venerol 1987;67:199–205.

20. Vuorio T, Kähäri VM, Black C, et al. Expression of osteonectin, decorin, and transforming growth factor-β1 genes in fibroblasts cultured from patients with systemic sclerosis and morphea. J Rheumatol 1991;28:247.

21. Trojanowska M, Wu L, LeRoy E. Elevated expression of c-myc proto-oncogene in scleroderma fibroblasts. Oncogene 1988;3:477.

22. Tokiyama K, Yokota E, Niho Y. Epidermal growth factor receptor in fibroblasts from patients with scleroderma. J Rheumatol 1990;17:1453.

23. Abraham D, Lupoli S, McWhirter A, et al. Expression and function of surface antigens on scleroderma fibroblasts. Arthritis Rheum 1991;34:1164.

24. Majewski S, Hunzelmann N, Johnson J, et al. Expression of the intercellular adhesion molecule-1 (ICAM-1) in the skin of patients with systemic sclerosis. J Invest Dermatol 1991;97:667.

25. Sollberg S, Peltonen J, Uitto J, et al. Elevated expression of β1 and β2 integrins, endothelial adhesion molecule 1 and leukocyte adhesion molecule 1 in the skin of patients with systemic sclerosis of recent onset. Arthritis Rheum 1992;35:290.

26. Gruschwitz M, Driesch P, Kellner I, et al. Expression of adhesion proteins involved in cell-cell and cell-matrix interactions in the skin of patients with progressive systemic sclerosis. J Am Acad Dermatol 1992;27:169.

27. Kähäri VM, Sandberg M, Kalimo H, et al. Identification of fibroblasts responsible for increased collagen production in localized scleroderma by in situ hybridization. J Invest Dermatol 1988;90:664.

28. Peltonen J, Kähäri L, Jaakkola S, et al. Evaluation of transforming growth factor-β1 and type I procollagen gene expression in fibrotic skin diseases by in situ hybridization. J Invest Dermatol 1989; 94:365.

29. Kulozik M, Hogg A, Buttergeit B, et al. Co-localization of transforming growth factor β2 with α1(I) procollagen mRNA in tissue sections of patients with systemic sclerosis. J Clin Invest 1990;86:917.

30. Mauch C, Hatamochi A, Scharfetter K, et al. Regulation of collagen synthesis by fibroblasts within a three-dimensional collagen gel. Exp Cell Res 1988;178:493.

31. Gillery P, Bellon G, Coustry F, et al. Cultures of fibroblasts in fibrin lattices: Models for the study of metabolic activities of the cells in physiological conditions. J Cell Physiol 1989;140:483.

32. Eckes B, Mauch C, Huppe G, et al. Downregulation of collagen synthesis in fibroblasts within three-dimensional collagen lattices involves transcriptional and posttranscriptional mechanisms. FEBS Lett 1993;318:129.

33. Ivarsson M, McWhirter A, Black C, et al. Impaired regulation of collagen pro-α1(I) mRNA and change in pattern of collagen-binding integrins on scleroderma fibroblasts. J Invest Dermatol 1993;101:216.

34. Slack J, Liska D, Bornstein P. Regulation of expression of the type I collagen genes. Am J Med Gen 1993;45:140.

35. Rudnicka L, Varga J, Iozzo R, et al. Regulation of Type VII collagen by TGFβ and its expression in scleroderma. J Clin Invest 1994;93:1707.

36. Olsen D, Peltonen J, Jaakkola S, et al. Collagen

gene expression by cultured human skin fibroblasts: Abundant steady-state levels of Type VI procollagen mRNAs. J Clin Invest 1989;83:791.

37. Prockop D. Mutations in collagen genes as a cause of connective tissue disease. N Engl J Med 1992; 326:540.

38. Katayama K, Seyer J, Raghow R, et al. Regulation of extracellular matrix production by chemically synthesized subfragments of type I collagen carboxy propeptide. Biochemistry 1991;30:7097.

39. Perlish J, Timpl R, Fleischmajer R. Collagen synthesis regulation by the amino propeptide of procollagen I in normal and scleroderma fibroblasts. Arthritis Rheum 1985;28:647.

40. Chu ML, de Wet W, Bernard M, et al. Fine structural analysis of the human pro-α1(I) collagen gene. J Biol Chem 1985;260:2315.

41. Nehls M, Rippe R, Veloz L, Brenner D. Transcription factors nuclear factor I and Sp1 interact with the murine collagen α1(I) promoter. Mol Cell Biol 1991;11:4065.

42. Nehls M, Grapilon M, Brenner D. NF-1/Sp-1 switch elements regulate collagen α1(I) gene expression. DNA Cell Biol 1992;11:443.

43. Boast S, Su MW, Ramirez F, et al. Functional analysis of cis-acting DNA sequences controlling transcription of the human type I collagen genes. J Biol Chem 1990;265:13351.

44. Karsenty G, de Crombrugghe B. Two different negative and a positive regulatory factors interact with a short promoter segment of the α1(I) collagen gene. J Biol Chem 1990;265:9934.

45. Barsh G, Roush C, Gelinas R. DNA and chromatin structure of the human α1(I) collagen gene. J Biol Chem 1984;259:14906.

46. Rhodes K, Rippe RA, Umezawa A, Nehls M, Brenner DA, Breindle M. DNA methylation represses the murine α1(I) collagen promoter by an indirect mechanism. Mol Cell Biol 1994;14:5950.

47. Razin A, Cedar H. DNA methylation and gene expression. Microbiol Rev 1991;55:451.

48. Fleischmajer R, Perlish J, Reeves J. Cellular infiltrates in scleroderma. Arthritis Reum 1977;20: 775.

49. Jimenez S. Cellular immune dysfunction in the pathogenesis of scleroderma. Semin Arthritis Rheum 1983;13:104.

50. Roumm A, Whiteside T, Medsger T Jr. Lymphocytes in the skin of patients with progressive systemic sclerosis. Arthritis Rheum 1984;27:645.

51. Gruschwitz M, Sepp N, Kofler H, et al. Expression of class II-MHC antigens in the dermis of patients with progressive systemic sclerosis. Immunobiol 1991;182:234.

52. Ishikawa O, Ishikawa H. Macrophage infiltration in the skin of patients with systemic sclerosis. J Rheum 1992;19:1202.

53. Gustaffson R, Totterman T, Klareskog L, et al. Increase in activated T cells and reduction in suppressor inducer T cells in systemic sclerosis. Ann Rheum Dis 1990;49:40.

54. Ferrarini M, Steen V, Medsger T Jr, et al. Functional and phenotypic analysis of T-lymphocytes cloned from the skin of patients with systemic sclerosis. Clin Exp Immunol 1990;79:346.

55. Van de Water J, Haapanen L, Boyd R, et al. Identification of T cells in early lymphocytic infiltrates in avian scleroderma. Arthritis Rheum 1989;32: 1031.

56. Gruschwitz M, Moorman S, Kromer G, et al. Phenotypic analysis of skin infiltrates in comparison with peripheral blood lymphocytes, spleen and thymocytes in early avian scleroderma. J Autoimmun 1991;4:577.

57. Deguchi Y, Negoro S, Kishimoto S. Proto-oncogene expression and nuclear factor specifically bound to c-myc gene in peripheral blood mononuclear cells from progressive systemic sclerosis patients as indicator of clinical disease activity. J Clin Lab Immunol 1988;26:163.

58. Kahan A, Gerfaux J, Kahan A, et al. Increased proto-oncogene expression in peripheral blood T lymphocytes from patients with systemic sclerosis. Arthritis Rheum 1989;32:430.

59. Rudnicka L, Majewski S, Blaszczyk M, et al. Adhesion of peripheral blood mononuclear cells to vascular endothelium in patients with systemic sclerosis. Arthritis Rheum 1992;35:771.

60. Umehara H, Kumagai S, Ishida H, et al. Enhanced production of interleukin 2 in patients with progressive systemic sclerosis: Hyperactivity of CD4-positive T cells. Arthritis Rheum 1988;31:401.

61. Kantor T, Friberg D, Medsger T Jr, Buckingham R, Whiteside T. Cytokine production and serum levels in systemic sclerosis. Clin Immuno Immunopathol 1992;65:278.

62. Kahaleh M, LeRoy E. Interleukin-2 in scleroderma: Correlation of serum levels with extent of skin involvement and disease duration. Ann Intern Med 1989;1100:446.

63. Needleman B, Wigley F, Stair R. Interleukin-1, interleukin-2, interleukin-4, interleukin-6, tumor necrosis factor alpha and interferon-gamma levels in sera from patients with scleroderma. Arthritis Rheum 1992;35:67.

64. Reitamo S, Remitz A, Varga J, et al. Demonstration of interleukin-8 and antibodies to interleukin-8 in the serum of patients with systemic sclerosis and related disorders. Arch Dermatol 1993;129:189.

65. Sasaki T, Nakajima H. Serum adenosine deaminase activity in systemic sclerosis (scleroderma) and related disorders. J Am Acad Dermatol 1992;27:411.

66. Abraham D, Lupoli S, McWhirter A, et al. Expression and function of surface antigens on scleroderma fibroblasts. Arthritis Rheum 1991;34:1164.

67. Gillery P, Maquart FX, Le Corre Y, et al. Variability in the retraction of collagen lattices by scleroderma fibroblasts—relationship to protein synthesis and clinical data. Clin Exp Dermatol 1991;16:324.

68. Needleman B. Increased expression of intercellular adhesion molecule 1 on the fibroblasts of scleroderma patients. Arthritis Rheum 1990;33:1847.

69. Majewski S, Hunzelmann M, Schirren C, et al. Increased adhesion of fibroblasts from patients with scleroderma to extracellular matrix components: *In vitro* modulation by IFN-γ but not by TGF-β. J Invest Dermatol 1992;98:86.

70. Wantzin G, Ralfkiaer E, Steen L, Rothlein R. The role of intercellular adhesion molecules in inflammatory skin reactions. Br J Derm 1988;119:141.

71. Gruschwitz M, Muller P, Sepp N, et al. Transcription and expression of transforming growth factor beta in the skin of progressive systemic sclerosis: A mediator of fibrosis? J Invest Dermatol 1990;94:197.

72. Johnson R, Ziff M. Lymphokine stimulation of collagen accumulation. J Clin Invest 1976;58:240.

73. Krane S, Dayer JM, Simon L. Mononuclear cell-conditioned medium contains mononuclear cell factor (MCF) homologous with interleukin-1, stimulates collagen and fibronectin synthesis by adherent rheumatoid synovial cells. Coll Relat Res 1985;5:99.

74. Jimenez S, McArthur W, Rosenbloom J. Inhibition of collagen synthesis by mononuclear cell supernates. J Exp Med 1979;150:1421.

75. Neilson E, Phillips S, Jimenez S. Lymphokine modulation of fibroblast proliferation. J Immunol 1982;128:1484.

76. Postlethwaite A, Snyderman R, Kang A. The chemotactic attraction of human fibroblasts to a lymphocyte-derived factor. J Exp Med 1976;144:1188.

77. Pestka S, Langer J. Interferons and their actions. Annu Rev Biochem 1987;56:727.

78. Jimenez S, Freundlich B, Rosenbloom J. Selective inhibition of human diploid fibroblast collagen synthesis by interferons. J Clin Invest 1984;74:1112.

79. Duncan M, Berman B. Gamma interferon is the lymphokine and beta interferon the monokine responsible for inhibition of fibroblast collagen production and late but not early fibroblast proliferation. J Exp Med 1985;162:516.

80. Amento E, Bhan A, McCullagh K, et al. Influences of gamma interferon on synovial fibroblast-like cells. J Clin Invest 1985;76:837.

81. Rosenbloom J, Feldman G, Freundlich B, et al. Transcriptional control of human diploid fibroblast collagen synthesis by γ-interferon. Biochem Biophys Res Commun 1984;123:365.

82. Clark J, Dedon T, Wayner E, et al. Effects of interferon gamma on cell surface receptors for collagen and deposition of newly synthesized collagen by cultured human lung fibroblasts. J Clin Invest 1989;83:1505.

83. Goldring M, Sandell L, Stephenson M, et al. Immune interferon suppresses levels of procollagen mRNA and type II collagen synthesis in cultured human articular and costal chondrocytes. J Biol Chem 1986;261:9049.

84. Varga J, Olsen A, Herhal J, et al. Interferon-γ reverses the stimulation of collagen but not fibronectin gene expression by transforming growth factor-β in normal human fibroblasts. Eur J Clin Invest 1990;20:487.

85. Kähäri VM, Chen Y, Su M, et al. Tumor necrosis factor-α and interferon-γ suppress the activation of human type I collagen gene expression by transforming growth factor-β1. J Clin Invest 1990;86:1489.

86. Czaja M, Weiner F, Eghbali M, et al. Differential effects of γ-Interferon on collagen and fibronectin gene expression. J Biol Chem 1987;262:13348.

87. Duncan MR, Hasan A, Berman B. Pentoxifylline, pentifylline, and interferons decrease type I and III procollagen mRNA levels in dermal fibroblasts: Evidence for mediation by nuclear factor 1 downregulation. J Invest Dermatol 1995;104:282.

88. Rosenbloom J, Feldman G, Freundlich B, et al. Inhibition of excessive scleroderma fibroblast collagen synthesis by recombinant gamma interferon. Arthritis Rheum 1986;29:851.

89. Kähäri VM, Heino J, Vuorio T, et al. Interferon-γ and -α reduce excessive collagen synthesis and procollagen mRNA levels of scleroderma fibroblasts in culture. Biochem Biophys Acta 1988;968:45.

90. Gillery P, Serpier H, Polette M, et al. Gamma interferon inhibits extracellular matrix synthesis and remodelling in collagen lattice cultures of normal and scleroderma fibroblasts. Eur J Cell Biol 1992;57:244.

91. Duncan M, Berman B. Persistence of reduced collagen-producing phenotype in cultured scleroderma fibroblasts after short-term exposure to interferons. J Clin Invest 1987;79:1318.

92. Narayanan A, Whitey J, Souza A, et al. Effect of γ-interferon on collagen synthesis by normal and fibrotic human lung fibroblasts. Chest 1992;101:1326.

93. Prior C, Haslam P. *In vivo* levels and *in vitro* production of interferon-gamma in fibrosing interstitial lung diseases. Clin Exp Immun 1992;88:280.

94. Granstein R, Murphy G, Margolis R, et al. Gamma interferon inhibits collagen synthesis *in vivo* in the mouse. J Clin Invest 1987;1254.

95. Giri F, Hyde D, Marafino B. Ameliorating effect of murine interferon gamma on bleomycin-induced lung collagen fibrosis in mice. Biochem Med Metab Biol 1986;36:194.

96. Czaja M, Weiner F, Takahashi S, et al. Gamma-interferon treatment inhibits collagen deposition in murine schistosomiasis. Hepatology 1989;10:795.

97. Berman B, Duncan M. Short-term keloid treatment *in vivo* with interferon alfa-2b results in a selective and persistent normalization of keloidal fibroblast collagen, glycosaminoglycan and collagenase production *in vitro*. J Am Acad Dermatol 1989;21:694.

98. Stevens W, Vancheeswaran R, Black C. Alpha interferon-2a (Roferon-A) in the treatment of diffuse cutaneous systemic sclerosis: A pilot study. Br J Rheumatol 1992;31:683.

99. Freundlich B, Jimenez S, Steen V, et al. Treatment of systemic sclerosis with recombinant interferon-γ. Arthritis Rheum 1992;35:1134.

100. Vilcek J, Lee T. Tumor necrosis factor: New insights into the molecular mechanisms of its multiple actions. J Biol Chem 1991;266:7313.

101. Brenner D, O'Hara M, Angel P, et al. Prolonged activation of jun and collagenase genes by tumor necrosis factor. Nature 1989;348:661.

102. Solis-Herruzo J, Brenner D, Chojkier M. Tumor necrosis alpha inhibits collagen gene transcription and collagen synthesis in cultured human fibroblasts. J Biol Chem 1986;263:5841.

103. Mauviel A, Daireaux M, Dini F, et al. Tumor necrosis factor-α inhibits collagen and fibronectin synthesis in human dermal fibroblasts. FEBS Lett 1988;236:47.

104. Scharffetter K, Heckmann M, Hatamochi A, et al. Synergistic effects of tumor necrosis factor-α and interferon-γ on collagen synthesis of human skin fibroblasts *in vitro*. Exp Cell Res 1989;181:409.

105. Diaz A, Munoz E, Johnston R, et al. Regulation of human lung fibroblast α1(I) procollagen gene expression by TNF-α, IL-1β and prostaglandin E2. J Biol Chem 1993;268:10364.

106. Kähäri VM, Chen Y, Bashir M, et al. Tumor necro-

sis factor-α down-regulated human elastin gene expression: Evidence for the role of AP-1 in the suppression of promoter activity. J Biol Chem 1992;267:26134.

107. Weiner F, Shah A, Smith P, et al. Regulation of collagen gene expression in 3T3-L1 cells. Effects of adipocyte differentiation and tumor necrosis factor alpha. Biochemistry 1989;28:4094.

108. Piguet P, Collart M, Grau G, et al. Tumor necrosis alpha/cachectin plays a key role in bleomycin-induced pneumopathy and fibrosis. J Exp Med 1989;170:655.

109. Dinarello C, Wolff S. The role of interleukin-1 in disease. N Engl J Med 1993;328:106.

110. Duncan M, Berman B. Differential regulation of collagen, glycosaminoglycan, fibronectin and collagenase activity production in cultured human adult dermal fibroblasts by Interleukin-1 alpha and beta and Tumor Necrosis Factor alpha and beta. J Invest Dermatol 1989;92:699.

111. Armendariz-Borunda J, Katayama K, Seyer J. Transcriptional mechanisms of type I collagen gene expression are differenetially regulated by IL-1β, TNF-α, and TGFβ in Ito cells. J Biol Chem 1992;267:14316.

112. Harrison J, Vargas S, Petersen D, et al. Interleukin-1 and phorbol ester inhibits collagen synthesis in osteoblastic MC3T3-E1 cells by a transcriptional mechanism. Mol Endocrinol 1990;4:184.

113. Goldring M, Krane S. Modulation by recombinant interleukin 1 of synthesis of types I and III collagens and associated procollagen mRNA levels in cultured human cells. J Biol Chem 1987;262:16724.

114. Postlethwaite A E, Raghow R, Stricklin G P, et al. Modulation of fibroblast functions by interleukin 1: Increased steady-state accumulation of type I procollagen messenger RNAs and stimulation of other functions but not chemotaxis by human recombinant interleukin α1 and α. J Cell Biol 1988;106:311.

115. Mauviel A, Heino J, Kähäri VM, et al. Comparative effects of IL-1 and TNF-α on collagen production and corresponding procollagen mRNA levels in human dermal fibroblasts. J Invest Dermatol 1991;96:243.

116. Kawaguchi Y, Harigai M, Suzuki K, Hara M, Kobayashi K, Ishizuka T, Matsuki Y, Tanaka N, Nakamura H. Interleukin-1 receptor on fibroblasts from systemic sclerosis patients induces excessive functional responses to interleukin-1β. Biochem Biophys Res Commun 1993;190:154.

117. Dayer JM, de Rochemonteix B, Burrus B, et al. Human recombinant IL-1 stimulates collagenase

and PGE2 production by human synovial cells. J Clin Invest 1986;77:645.

118. Piguet P, Vesin C, Grau G, et al. Interleukin-1 receptor antagonist (IL-1ra) prevents or cures pulmonary fibrosis elicited in mice by bleomycin or silica. Cytokines 1993;5:57.

119. Kawaguchi Y. IL-1α gene expression and protein production by fibroblasts from patients with systemic sclerosis. Clin Exp Immunol 1994;97:445.

120. Paul W, Ohara J. B cell stimulatory factor/interleukin-4. Annu Rev Immunol 1987;429.

121. Postlethwaite A, Seyer J. Fibroblast chemotaxis induction by human recombinant interleukin-4. J Clin Invest 1991;87:2147.

122. Postlethwaite A, Holness M, Katai H, et al. Human fibroblasts synthesize elevated levels of extracellular matrix proteins in response to interleukin-4. J Clin Invest 1992;90:1479.

123. Gillery P, Fertin C, Nicolas J, et al. Interleukin-4 stimulates collagen gene expression in human fibroblast monolayer cultures. FEBS Lett 1992;302:231.

124. Van Snick J. Interleukin 6: An overview. Annu Rev Immunol 1990;8:253.

125. Romero L, Pincus S. *In situ* localization of interleukin-6 in normal skin and atrrophic cutaneous disease. Int Arch Allergy Immunol 1992;99:44.

126. Feghali C, Bost K, Boulware D, et al. Mechanisms of pathogenesis in scleroderma: Overproduction on interleukin 6 by fibroblasts cultured from affected skin sites of patients with scleroderma. J Rheumatol 1992;19:1207.

127. Lotz M, Guerne PA. IL-6 induces the synthesis of TIMP/erythroid potentiating activity (TIMP-1/EPA). J Biol Chem 1991;266:2017.

128. Duncan M, Berman B. Stimulation of collagen and glycosaminoglycan production in cultured human adult dermal fibroblasts by recombinant human interleukin 6. J Invest Dermatol 1991;97:686.

129. Ito A, Itoh Y, Sasaguri Y, et al. Effects of interleukin-6 on the metabolism of connective tissue components in rheumatoid synovial fibroblasts. Arthritis Rheum 1992;35:1197.

130. Oppenheim J, Zachariae C, Mukaida M, et al. Properties of the novel proinflammatory supergene intercrine cytokine family. Annu Rev Immunol 1991;9:617.

131. Koch A, Polverini P, Kunkel S, et al. Interleukin-8 as a macrophage-derived mediator of angiogenesis. Science 1992;258:1798.

132. Baggiolini M, Walz A, Kunkel S. Neutrophil activating peptide-1/interleukin-8, a novel cytokine

that activates neutrophils. J Clin Invest 1989;84:1045.

133. Unemori E, Amento E, Bauer E, et al. Melanoma growth stimulatory activity/GRO decreases collagen expression by human fibroblasts. J Biol Chem 1993;268:1338.

134. Idia N, Grotendorst G. Cloning and sequencing of a new gro transcript from activated human monocytes: Expression in leukocytes and wound tissue. Mol Cell Biol 1990;10:5596.

135. Carre P, Mortenson R, King T, et al. Increased expression of interleukin-8 gene by alveolar macrophages in idiopathic pulmonary fibrosis. J Clin Invest 1991;88:1802.

136. Howard M, O'Garra A. Biological properties of interleukin-10. Immunol Today 1992;13:198.

137. Reitamo S, Remitz A, Tamai K, Uitto J. Interleukin-10 modulates type I collagen and matrix metalloprotease gene expression in cultured human skin fibroblasts. J Clin Invest 1994;94:2489.

138. Sporn M, Roberts A. Transforming growth factor-β: Recent progress and new challenges. J Cell Biol 1992;119:1017.

139. Border W, Ruoslahti E. Transforming growth factor-β in disease: The dark side of tissue repair. J Clin Invest 1992;90:1.

140. Heine U, Munoz E, Flanders K, et al. The role of transforming growth factor-β in the development of the mouse embryo. J Cell Biol 1987;105:2861.

141. Roberts A, Sporn M, Assoian R, et al. Transforming growth factor type β: Rapid induction of fibrosis and angiogenesis and collagen formation *in vitro*. Proc Natl Acad Sci USA 1986;4167.

142. Ignotz R, Massague J. Transforming growth factor-β stimulates the expression of fibronectin and collagen and their incorporation into the extracellular matrix. J Biol Chem 1986;261:4337.

143. Ignotz R, Endo T, Massague J. Regulation of fibronectin and type I collagen mRNA levels by transforming growth factor-β. J Biol Chem 1987;262:6443.

144. Varga J, Rosenbloom J, Jimenez S. Transforming growth factor-β (TGFβ) causes a persistent increase in steady-state amounts of type I and Type III collagen and fibronectin mRNAs in normal human dermal fibroblasts. Biochem J 1987;247:597.

145. Raghow R, Postlethwaite A, Keski-Oja J, et al. Transforming growth factor-β increases the steady-state levels of type I procollagen and fibronectin mRNA posttranscriptionally in cultured human dermal fibroblasts. J Clin Invest 1987;79:1285.

146. Reed M, Vernon R, Abrass I, Sage E. TGF-β1 in-

duces the expression of type I collagen and SPARC, and enhances contraction of collagen gels by fibroblasts from young and aged donors. J Cell Physiol 1994;158:169.

147. Konig A, Bruckner-Tuderman L. Transforming growth factor-β stimulates collagen VII expression in cutaneous cells *in vitro*. J Cell Biol 1992; 117:679.

148. Heino J, Ignotz R, Hemler M, et al. Regulation of cell adhesion receptors by transforming growth factor-β: Concomitant regulation of integrins that share a common β subunit. J Biol Chem 1989;264:380.

149. Edwards D, Murphy G, Reynolds J, et al. Transforming growth factor-β modulates the expression of collagenase and metalloproteinase inhibitor. EMBO J 1987;6:1899.

150. Mustoe T, Pierce G, Thomason A, et al. Accelerated healing of incisional wounds in rats induced by TGFβ. Science 1987;237:1333.

151. Massague J. The transforming growth factor-β family. Annu Rev Cell Biol 1990;6:597.

152. Wrana J, Attisano L, Carcamo J, et al. TGFβ signals through a heteromeric protein kinase receptor complex. Cell 1992;71:1003.

153. Chakrabarty S. Role of protein kinase C in TGF-β1 induction of the CEA in human colon carcinoma cells. J Cell Physiol 1992;152:494.

154. Pertovaara L, Sistonen L, Bos T, et al. Enhanced jun gene expression is an early genomic response to TGFβ stimulation. Mol Cell Biol 1989;9: 1255.

155. Kim SJ, Angel P, Lafyatis R, et al. Autoinduction of transforming growth factor-β1 is mediated by the AP-1 complex. Mol Cell Biol 1990;10:1492.

156. Pentinnen R, Kobayashi S, Bornstein P. Transforming growth factor-β increases mRNA for matrix proteins both in the presence and in the absence of changes in mRNA stability. Proc Natl Acad Sci USA 1988;85:1105.

157. Rossi P, Karsenty G, Roberts A, et al. A nuclear factor 1 binding site mediates transcriptional activation of a type I collagen promoter by TGFβ. Cell 1988;52:405.

158. Ritzenthaler J, Goldstein R, Fine A, et al. Transforming growth factor-β activation elements in the distal promoter region of the rat α1 type I collagen gene. Biochem J 1991;280:157.

159. Ritzenthaler J, Goldstein R, Fine A, et al. Regulation of the α1(I) collagen promoter via a transforming growth factor-β activation element. J Biol Chem 1993;268:13625.

160. Inagaki Y, Truter S, Ramirez F. Transforming growth factor-β stimulates α2(I) collagen gene expression through a cis-acting element that con-

tains an Sp1-binding site. J Biol Chem 1994;269: 14828.

161. Jimenez SA, Varga J, Olsen A, Li L, Diaz A, Herhal J, Koch J. Functional analysis of human α1(I) procollagen gene promoter. J Biol Chem 1994;269: 12864.

162. Ishikawa O, LeRoy E, Trojanowska M. Mitogenic effect of transforming growth factor-β1 on human fibroblasts involves the induction of platelet-derived growth factor-β receptors. J Cell Physiol 1990;145:181.

163. Elias J, Lentz V, Cummings P. Transforming growth factor-β regulation of IL-6 production by unstimulated and IL-1-stimulated human fibroblasts. J Immunol 1991;146:3437.

164. Kikuchi K, Yamakage A, Smith E, et al. Differential modulation of bFGF receptors by TGF-β in adult skin, scleroderma skin, and newborn foreskin fibroblasts. J Invest Dermatol 1992;99:201.

165. Guerne P, Lotz M. Interleukin-6 and transforming growth factor-β synergistically stimulate chondrosarcoma cell proliferation. J Cell Physiol 1991;149:117.

166. Needleman B, Choi J, Burrows-Mezu A, et al. Secretion and binding of scleroderma and normal dermal fibroblasts. Arthritis Rheum 1990;18:241.

167. Yamakage A, Kikuchi L, Smith A, et al. Selective up-regulation of PDGFa receptors by TGF-β in scleroderma fibroblasts. J Exp Med 1992;175: 1227.

168. Broekelman T, Limper AHL, Coby T, et al. Transforming growth factor-β1 is present at sites of extracellular matrix expression in human pulmonary fibrosis. Proc Natl Acad Sci USA 1991; 88:6642.

169. Castilla A, Prieto J, Fausto, N. Transforming growth factor-β1 and α in chronic liver disease. N Engl J Med 1991;324:933.

170. Raghow R, Irish P, Kang A. Coordinate regulation of transforming growth factor-β gene expression and cell proliferation in hamster lungs undergoing bleomycin-induced pulmonary fibrosis. J Clin Invest 1989;84:1836.

171. Czaja M, Weiner F, Flanders K, et al. *In vitro* and *in vivo* association of transforming growth factor-β with hepatic fibrosis. J Cell Biol 1989;108: 2477.

172. Anscher M, Peters W, Reisenbichler H, et al. Transforming growth factor-β as a predictor of liver and lung fibrosis after autologous bone marrow transplantation for advanced breast cancer. N Engl J Med 1993;328:1592.

173. Deguchi Y. Spontaneous increase of transforming growth factor-β production by bronchoalveolar mononuclear cells of patients with systemic au-

toimmune diseases affecting the lung. Ann Rheum Dis 1992;51:362.

174. Gay S, Jones R, Huang G, et al. Immunohistologic demonstration of platelet-derived growth factor (PDGF) and cis-oncogene expression in scleroderma. J Invest Dermatol 1989;92:301.

175. Varga J, Jimenez SA. Modulation of collagen gene expression: Its relation to fibrosis in systemic sclerosis and other disorders. Ann Intern Med 1995; 122:60.

176. Heldin C, Westermark B. Platelet-derived growth factor: Mechanism of action and possible *in vivo* function. Cell Regul 1990;1:555.

177. Lynch S, Nixon J, Colvin R, et al. Role of platelet derived growth factor in wound healing: Synergistic effects with other growth factors. Proc Natl Acad Sci USA 1987;84:7696.

178. Bauer E, Cooper T, Huang J, et al. Stimulation of *in vitro* human collagenase expression by platelet-derived growth factor. Proc Natl Acad Sci USA 1985;82:4132.

179. Narayanan A, Page R. Biosynthesis and regulation of type V collagen collagen in diploid human fibroblasts. J Biol Chem 1983;258:11694.

180. Vignaud JM, Allam N, Martinet M, et al. Presence of platelet-derived growth factor in normal and fibrotic lungs is specifically associated with interstitial macrophages, while both interstitial macrophages and alveolar epithelial cells express c-sis protooncogene. Am J Resp Cell Mol Biol 1991;5:539.

181. Klareskog L, Gustaffson R, Scheyniu A, et al. Increased expression of platelet-derived growth factor type B receptors in the skin of patients with systemic sclerosis. Arthritis Rheum 1990;33:1534.

182. Gospodarowicz D. Biological activities of the fibroblast growth factors. Ann NY Acad Sci 1991; 638:1.

183. Tan E, Rouda S, Greenbaum S, et al. Acidic and basic fibroblast growth factors down-regulate collagen gene expression in keloid fibroblasts. Am J Pathol 1993;142:463.

184. Hurley M, Abreu C, Harrison J, et al. Basic fibroblast growth factor inhibits type I collagen gene expression in osteoblastic MC3T3 - E1 cells. J Biol Chem 1993;268:5588.

185. Gay S, Tranbadt A, Moreland L, et al. Growth factors, extracellular matrix, and oncogenes in scleroderma. Arhtritis Rheum 1992;35:304.

186. Carpenter C, Wahl M. The epidermal growth factor family. In: Sporn MB, Roberts AB, eds. Peptide growth factors and their receptors. Berlin: Springer-Verlag, 1990;227–238.

187. Laato M, Kähäri VM, Niinikoski J, et al. Epidermal growth factor increases collagen production in granulation tissue by stimulation of fibroblast proliferation and not by activation of procollagen genes. Biochem J 1987;247:385.

188. Hata R, Hori H, Nagai Y, et al. Selective inhibition of type I collagen synthesis in osteoblastic cells by epidermal growth factor. Endocrinology 1984; 115:867.

189. Hata H, Sunada H, Araki K, et al. Regulation of collagen metabolism and cell growth by epidermal growth factor and ascorbate in cultured human skin fibroblasts. Eur J Biochem 1988;173: 261.

190. Baum B, Moss J, Bruel S, Crystal R. Association in normal human fibroblasts of elevated levels of adenosine 3′5′-monophosphate with a selective decrease in collagen production. J Biol Chem 1978;253:3391.

191. Varga J, Diaz-Perez A, Rosenbloom J, et al. PGE2 causes a coordinate decrease in the steady-state levels of fibronectin and type I and III procollagen mRNAs in normal human dermal fibroblasts. Biochem Biophys Res Commun 1987;147:1282.

192. Fine A, Polick C, Donahue L, et al. The differential effects of prostaglandin E2 on transforming growth factor-β and insulin-induced collagen formation in lung fibroblasts. J Biol Chem 1989; 264:16988.

193. Diaz A, Varga J, Jimenez S. Transforming growth factor-β stimulation of lung fibroblast PGE2 production. J Biol Chem 1989;264:11554.

194. Mauviel A, Teyton L, Bhatnagar R, et al. Interleukin-1 α modulates collagen gene expression in cultured synovial cells. Biochem J 1988;252:247.

195. Phan S, McGarry B, Loeffler K, et al. Binding of leukotriene C4 to rat lung fibroblasts and stimulation of collagen synthesis *in vitro*. Biochemistry 1988;27:2846.

196. Lee Choi K, Giorno R, Claman H. Cutaneous mast cell depletion and recovery in murine graft-vs-host disease. J Immunol 1987;138:4093.

197. Walker M, Harley R, LeRoy E. Inhibition of fibrosis in Tsk mice by blocking mast cell degranulation. J Rheumatol 1987;14:299.

198. Fonseca E, Solis J. Mast cells in the skin: Progressive systemic sclerosis and the toxic oil syndrome. Ann Intern Med 1985;102:864.

199. Hawkins R, Claman H, Clark R, et al. Increased dermal mast cell populations in systemic sclerosis: A link in chronic fibrosis? Ann Intern Med 1985;102:182.

200. Seibold J, Giorno R, Claman H. Dermal mast cell degranulation in systemic sclerosis. Arthritis Rheum 1990;33:1702.

201. Irani A, Gruber B, Kaufman L, et al. Mast cell changes in scleroderma. Presence of MCt cells in

the skin and evidence of mast cell activation. Arthritis Rheum 1992;35:933.

202. Gleich G, Ottesen E, Leiferman K, et al. Eosinophils and human disease. Int Arch Allergy Appl Immunol 1989;88:59.

203. Roche W, Williams J, Beasley R, et al. Subepithelial fibrosis in the bronchi of asthmatics. Lancet 1989;i:520.

204. Noguchi K, Kephart G, Campbell R, et al. Tissue eosinophilia and eosinophil degranulation in orbital pseudotumor. Opthalmology 1991;98:928.

205. Noguchi H, Kephart G, Colby T, et al. Tissue eosinophilia and eosinophil degranulation in syndromes associated with fibrosis. Am J Pathol 1992;140:521.

206. Kadin M, Butmarc J, Elovic A, et al. Eosinophils are the major source of transforming growth factor-β1 in nodular sclerosing Hodgkin's disease. Am J Pathol 1993;142:11.

207. Gustaffson R, Fredens K, Nettelbladt O, et al. Eosinophil activation in systemic sclerosis. Arthritis Rheum 1991;34:414.

208. De Schryver K, Clouse R. Perineurial and intraneural infiltrates in the intestines of patients with systemic connective tissue disease. Arch Pathol Lab Med 1989;113:394.

209. Hallgren R, Bjermer L, Lundgren R, et al. The eosinophil component of the alveolitis in idiopathic pulmonary fibrosis. Am Rev Respir Dis 1989;139:373.

210. Varga J, Wright J, Earle L, et al. Eosinophil activation in diffuse cutaneous systemic sclerosis. Arthritis Rheum In press 1995.

211. Pincus S, Ramesh K, Wyler D. Eosinophils stimulate DNA synthesis. Blood 1987;70:572.

212. Shock A, Rabe K, Dent G, et al. Eosinophils adhere to and stimulate replication of lung fibroblasts *in vitro*. Clin Exp Immunol 1991;86:185.

213. Birkland T, Cheavens M, Pincus S. Human eosinophils (EOS) stimulate fibroblast (FIBRO) growth. Clin Res 1991;39:3A.

214. Hernas J, Sarnstrand B, Lindroth P, et al. Eosinophil cationic protein alters proteoglycan metabolism in human lung fibroblast cultures. Eur J Cell Biol 1992;59:352.

215. Rohrbach M, Wheatley C, Slifman N, et al. Activation of platelets by eosinophil granule proteins. J Exp Med 1990;1271.

216. Ohno I, Lea R, Flanders K, et al. Eosinophils in chronically inflamed human upper airway tissue express transforming growth factor-β1 gene. J Clin Invest 1992;89:1662.

217. Wong D, Elovic A, Matossian K, et al. Eosinophils from patients with blood eosinophilia express transforming growth factor-β. Blood 1991;78:2702.

218. Wong D, Donoff B, Yang J, et al. Sequential expression of transforming growth factors α and β1 by eosinophils during cutaneous wound healing in the hamster. Am J Pathol 1993;143:130.

219. Maul C, Jimenez S, Riggs E, et al. Determination of an epitope of the diffuse systemic sclerosis marker DNA topoisomerase-1: Sequence similarity with retroviral p30^{gag} protein suggests a possible cause for autoimmunity in systemic sclerosis. Proc Natl Acad Sci USA 1989;86:8492.

220. Priel E, Showalter S, Roberts M, et al. Topoisomerase I activity associated with human immunodeficiency virus (HIV) particles and equine infectious anemia virus core. EMBO J 1990;9:4167.

221. Dang H, Dauphinee M, Talal N, et al. Serum antibody to retroviral gag protein in systemic sclerosis. Arthritis Rheum 1991;34:1336.

222. Taylor J, Cupp C, Diaz A, et al. Activation and expression of genes coding for extracellular matrix proteins in Tat-producing glioblastoma cells. Proc Natl Acad Sci USA 1992;89:9617.

223. Cupp C, Taylor J, Khalili K, Amini S. Evidence for stimulation of the transforming growth factor-β1 promoter by HIV-1 Tat in cells derived from CNS. Oncogene 1993;8:2231–2236.

224. Fleischmajer R, Fisher L, MacDonald D, et al. Decorin interacts with fibrillar collagen in embryonic and adult human skin. J Struct Biol 1991;106:82.

225. Yamaguchi Y, Mann D, Ruoslahti E. Negative regulation of transforming growth factor-β by the proteoglycan decorin. Nature 1990;346:281.

226. Bassols A, Massague J. Transforming growth factor-β regulates the expression and structure of extracellular matrix chondroitin/dermatan sulfate proteoglycans. J Biol Chem 1988;263:3039.

227. Nathan C, Sporn M. Cytokines in context. J Cell Biol 1991;113:981.

228. Heino J, Heinonen T. Interleukin-1β prevents the stimulatory effects of transforming growth factor-β on collagen gene expression in human skin fibroblasts. Biochem J 1990;271:827.

MARCO MATUCCI-CERINIC
M. BASHAR KAHALEH
E. CARWILE LEROY

8

Vascular Involvement in Systemic Sclerosis

THE FIRST DESCRIPTION of vascular abnormalities in systemic sclerosis (SSc) was in 1862 by Maurice Raynaud (1). In 1875, the phenomenon described by Raynaud was definitively associated with SSc by Ball (2), who introduced the term sclerodactyly. In 1891, Dinkler suggested that skin involvement in SSc was associated with vascular disease (3). In addition, in 1925 Brown and O'Leary used capillaroscopic analysis to clearly depict abnormalities of the microvasculature in SSc (4). Although in its later stages SSc can be associated with vascular occlusion, thromboembolism, and peripheral gangrene/ischemia, it is the distinctive microvascular disruption and obliteration that links it to diabetes mellitus and distinguishes it from atherosclerosis and other large vessel disorders.

Although Raynaud's phenomenon (RP) is the early sign of SSc, frequently preceding other clinical features of the disease, vascular abnormalities were not emphasized until recently. Whereas the hypothesis of early vascular involvement in SSc was proposed during the middle of this century (5–7), the concept of fibrosis as primary in pathogenesis prevailed throughout this period. At the end of the 1960s, the vascular hypothesis was restarted. Norton et al (8) observed a microvascular injury in SSc and proposed to classify it as a vascular disease (9). In 1975, Campbell and LeRoy (10) described the morphological and functional features of vessel involvement and definitively proposed the vascular hypothesis for the pathogenesis of SSc. This view was confirmed by Fleischmajer et al in 1976 (11), who showed

that early events in SSc included destruction of capillaries, increased proliferation of endothelial cells, and plasma cell-lymphocyte infiltrates in the skin.

It is now clear that the rheumatic autoimmune diseases, including systemic lupus erythematosus (SLE), dermatomyositis/polymyositis, the systemic vasculitides, as well as SSc, are primarily vascular diseases (12), followed in time by different alterations of the connective tissue. These diseases share a common symptom complex of RP. In the last century, Maurice Raynaud elegantly depicted the triphasic color changes of the phenomenon (1), consisting in sequence of a vasospasm-induced pallor, followed in time by cyanosis, as a result of hypoxia, and rubor, from hyperemic reperfusion. The pathophysiology of RP remains unclear. It has been attributed both to overactivity of the sympathetic nervous system and to an exaggerated response to normal stimuli due to vascular wall changes; other pathogenetic mechanisms have been proposed as well (13). RP may be classified as primary or secondary (Table 8-1). A recent proposal for classification attempted to clarify the definition of patients with RP (14).

In SSc, RP is frequently (90%–95%) the first symptom of the underlying disease and is considered the most common clinical expression of vascular derangement (15). A variety of other vascular disorders are also associated with RP (13,14). For this reason, RP can be considered a diagnostic clue to SSc (Table 8-2) when the clinical findings in other systems do not permit the

Table 8.1. Conditions Associated with
Secondary Raynaud's Phenomenon

Connective tissue diseases:
  Systemic sclerosis (SSc)
  Systemic lupus erythematosus (SLE)
  Dermatomyositis (DM)
  Undifferentiated connective tissue disease (UCTD)
  Sjögren syndrome (SS)
Vascular diseases:
  Wegener's granulomatosis
  Behcet's syndrome
  Takayasu arteritis
  Kawasaki disease
  Schoenlein Henoch purpura
  Buerger's disease
  Polyarteritis nodosa
Occupational:
  Polyvinyl chloride
  Vibrations and percussion
  Nitrate workers
  Frozen food packers
  Trauma
Hematologic diseases:
  Cryoglobulinemia
  Paraproteinemia
  Polycytemia
  Thrombocythemia
  Intravascular coagulative states
Neurogenic factors:
  Reflex sympathetic dystrophy
  Thoracic outlet syndrome
  Carpal tunnel syndrome
  Hemiplegia
  Poliomyelitis
  Syringomyelia
Other diseases:
  Diabetes
  Neoplasms
  Hypothyroidism
  Primary pulmonary hypertension
  Atherosclerosis
  Uremia
Drugs:
  Beta blockers
  Ergot
  Bleomycin
  Estrogens and progesterones
  Cytotoxic drugs
  Methylsergide
  Cisplatinum

diagnosis of SSc and when other RP-associated disorders are not present. In these cases, the vascular nature of the process is demonstrated not only by the presence of RP but also by abnormalities observed with nailfold capillaroscopy. The detection of modifications of the nailfold capillaries by this simple technique provides a fundamental diagnostic tool (Table 8.2) (16) in the preclinical phase of SSc (17). In established SSc, sequential nailfold capillaroscopy often demonstrates a progression of microvascular changes (18). In the early stage of SSc, modifications of the microcirculation consist primarily of enlarged loops, one of the most characteristic features of microvascular involvement (19), and megacapillaries, an important abnormality which may antedate the development of other microvascular alterations (Fig. 8.1). Nailfold capillary abnormalities in patients with RP raise the strong suspicion of the future development of SSc (20). In fact, the capillary-positive pattern in an RP subject may be the most limited clinical pattern of the limited cutaneous SSc (lSSc) subset. In contrast, the absence of nailfold capillary abnormalities in the RP subject virtually ensures that SSc will not occur in the patient's lifetime.

Table 8.2. Proposed Criteria for Early Diagnosis of Systemic Sclerosis (in absence of taut skin proximal to the metacarpo-phalangeal joints or other definite organ involvement)

Major:
  1. Raynaud's phenomenon[a]
  2. Characteristic capillaroscopic pattern[b]
  3. Autoantibodies (ANA, Scl-70, ACA)[c]
  4. Nailfold bleeding[d]
Minor:
  1. Reduction of DLCO < 70%[e]
  2. Alteration of DTPA (in non-smokers)[f]

[a]Maricq HR, LeRoy EC, D'Angelo WA, et al. Diagnostic potential of in vivo capillary microscopy in scleroderma and related disorders. Arthritis Rheum 1980;23:183–189.
[b]Maricq HR, Weinberger AB, LeRoy EC. Early detection of scleroderma spectrum disorders by in vivo capillary microscopy: A prospective study of patients with Raynaud's phenomenon. J Rheumatol 1982;9:289–291.
[c]Chen, ZY, Silver RM, Ainsworth SK, et al. Association between fluorescent antinuclear antibodies, capillary patterns, and clinical features in scleroderma spectrum disorders. Am J Med 1984;77:812–822.
[d]Sato S, Takehara K, Soma Y, Tsuchida T, Ishibashi Y. Diagnostic significance of nailfold bleeding in scleroderma spectrum disorders. J Am Acad Dermatol 1993;28:198–203.
[e]Groen H, Wichers G, ter Borg EJ, et al. Pulmonary diffusing capacity disturbances are related to nailfold capillary changes in patients with Raynaud's phenomenon with and without an underlying connective tissue disease. Am J Med 1990;89:34–41.
[f]Matucci-Cerinic M, Pignone A, Iannone F, et al. Clinical correlations of plasma ACE activity in systemic sclerosis: A longitudinal study of plasma ACE levels, endothelial injury and lung involvement. Resp Med 1990;84:283–287.

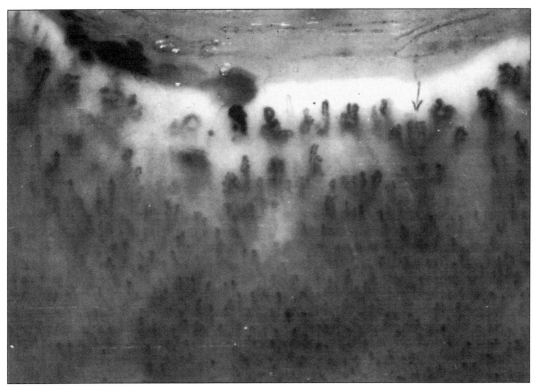

Figure 8.1. Enlarged capillaries associated with extensive avascular areas and "bushy" capillary formation (arrow). A characteristic SSc pattern.

The phenomenon of neoangiogenesis, consisting of the formation of new, "bushy" capillaries (Fig. 8.1) is also a feature of SSc capillary abnormalities (21). Recently, the presence of nailfold capillary bleeding has been proposed as a sensitive clinical sign for the early detection of SSc, in particular of the limited form (22).

As the disease progresses, SSc is characterized by: (*a*) architectural modification of the nailbed circulation, with alteration of both the distribution and the shape of capillaries; and (*b*) the loss of capillaries with the presence of avascular areas (17). The presence of these avascular areas at the onset of symptoms should be regarded as a marker of diffuse disease and possible rapid evolution (23).

Skin capillary abnormalities have been shown to be an indicator of internal organ involvement, thus predicting multisystem involvement in RP (24,25). When the disease is clinically apparent, nailfold capillary changes are not as useful in predicting organ involvement (26). It should be stressed that even at the onset of the disease, the presence of RP may already be indicative of organic obstructive arterial disease regardless of the presence or absence of skin involvement of the fingers (27).

Whether skin capillary abnormalities, which occur early and often before skin changes are clinically apparent, actually precede connective tissue changes or whether microscopic inflammatory and connective tissue changes influence vascular integrity remains to be distinguished conclusively. Nonetheless, the distinctive microvascular abnormalities of SSc are likely to be critical in both pathogenesis and prognosis.

Pathology

Vascular changes in SSc primarily involve small arteries (from 500 to 50 microns) and capillaries (9,28). In early SSc, perivascular mononuclear inflammatory infiltrates can be found in the subcutaneous tissue (28), accompanied by diffuse edema and the increased presence of glycosaminoglycans (29).

In small arteries, the internal elastic lamina and the tunica media are usually normal (10), while occurring adjacent to a mucoid and edematous concentric proliferation of the intima. This is the earliest histological evidence of vascular involvement in SSc (10). Proliferating intimal cells share ultrastructural features with smooth muscle cells, and are called myointimal cells. In more advanced disease, the most striking and consistent vascular finding is severe intimal fibrosis, consisting of extracellular matrix (mostly collagen) with varying degrees of intimal thickening associated with vessel narrowing, including obliteration (30,31). Fibrosis of the adventitia is a less consistent finding; interestingly, telangiectasia of the *vasa vasorum* may be seen (30), suggesting that the intimal lesion of SSc may have a microvascular basis. Luminal vascular narrowing provokes vasomotor instability, called RP, with the potential for hypoxia and reperfusion injury of the tissues.

SSc capillaries present a variety of morphological modifications (see previous). Ultrastructural observations include endothelial cell (EC) vacuolization, granular degeneration of the nucleus, cellular necrosis, gaps between endothelial cells, and reduplication of basal membranes. EC disruption is associated with vascular lumen obstruction. Altered permeability of vessel walls allows increased passage of plasma and mononuclear cells with formation of perivascular infiltrates (32), in which T lymphocytes and monocytes bearing macrophage markers predominate (33,34) with more CD4+ than CD8+ T cells (35). These studies emphasize that vascular wall involvement and tissue infiltration by inflammatory cells usually precede the development of fibrosis.

In SSc, widespread vascular involvement involving arterioles and capillaries of kidney, lungs, heart, skeletal muscle (36), and synovia (37) are well documented. In the kidney glomerulus, hyperplasia of interlobular arteries, fibrinoid necrosis of afferent arterioles, and "wire looping" of the glomerular basement membranes (38) are characteristic. The interlobular arteries may show marked concentric proliferation of intimal cells between an intact endothelium and internal elastic membrane (39). A further characteristic feature is adventitial fibrosis around arcuate and interlobular arteries (39,40). In the lung, in addition to interstitial changes, intimal hyperplasia, arteriolar thickening (41), and medial and intimal proliferation with mucinous degeneration of elastic arteries is noted (1000–5000 μ) (42). Muscular arteries demonstrate fibromuscular medial hyperplasia, concentric intimal proliferation, and obliteration of the lumen with fibrous thickening (42,43). Although vascular abnormalities are often observed in areas with parenchymal lung involvement (fibrosing alveolitis) (43), in the patient with early pulmonary hypertension, vascular changes may be seen in the virtual absence of interstitial changes.

Pathogenesis

THE INJURY OF THE ENDOTHELIUM

In the last twenty years there have been significant advances in the understanding of the mechanisms of vascular involvement in SSc. It was already clear that in SSc a distinct microvascular lesion is present (8). In SSc, this pattern indicated continuous chronic microvascular injury with morphologic characteristics different from the acute episodic microvascular injury of SLE and dermatomyositis (44). Figure 8.2 is a visual representation of factors potentially involved in the pathogenesis of SSc.

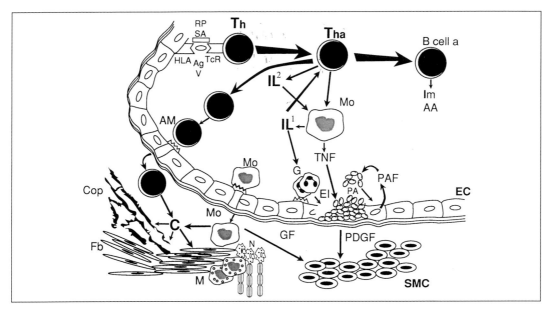

Figure 8.2. The hypothesis of the endothelial cell as antigen-presenting cell is visually depicted. EC presents antigen to T cells initiating a process that is sustained by endothelial injury, followed by platelet, B cell, and fibroblast activation. Tissue fibrosis is the natural conclusion of this process. (Courtesy of Professor Francesco Marongiu, University of Cagliari, Italy.)

SA	= superantigen	Mo	= monocyte
V	= virus	C	= cytokines
RP	= retroviral protein	GF	= growth factors
Th	= T helper lymphocyte	PDGF	= platelet derived growth factor (AA, AB, BB)
Tha	= T helper lymphocyte activated	M	= mast cells
B cell a	= B cell activated	Cop	= collagen production
Im	= immunoglobulins	N	= peripheral nerve
AA	= autoantibodies	PA	= platelet aggregation
PAF	= platelet aggregation factor	EC	= endothelial cells
TNF	= tumor necrosis factor	EI	= endothelial cell injury
IL 1	= interleukin 1	SMC	= smooth muscle cells
IL 2	= interleukin 2	Fb	= fibroblasts
G	= granulocyte	AM	= adhesion molecule expression

Changes observed in EC morphology indicated cellular derangement and dysfunction. In the last two decades, *in vitro* studies focused on the search and identification of a cytotoxic factor involved in the disease pathogenesis. Currie et al observed cythopathic destruction of different target cells cultured in the presence of peripheral blood monocytes from SSc patients (45). Cooper and Friou did not find cytotoxicity in the sera of SSc patients capable of inducing antibody dependent cell-mediated cytotoxicity against SSc

fibroblasts (46). In 1979, Kahaleh and LeRoy observed the capacity of the sera of SSc patients to kill human umbilical vein EC (47). Cytotoxic activity was nondializable, heat stable, eluted near albumin on gel filtration, and was inhibited by prior incubation with protease inhibitors (48). Other investigators found this activity only in 7% and 23% of SSc patients (49,50), or attributed this activity to circulating immune complexes and precipitating antibodies (51). Later, other authors confirmed the cytotoxicity of sera *in vivo* and *in vitro*, in 40% and 73%, respectively, of SSc patients (52,53). Recently, it was found that SSc serum was cytotoxic to venous and arterial EC when cocultured with peripheral blood mononuclear cells, suggesting that multiple immunological mechanisms (antiendothelial and anticardiolipin antibodies, antibody-dependent cell cytotoxicity, immunocomplexes) might be involved in the pathogenesis of vascular lesions (54). In contrast, Cifone et al recently demonstrated a normal level of lymphocyte and antibody-dependent cellular cytotoxicity in SSc (55). Of possible relevance, Evans et al found widespread deposition of IgM in the media and internal elastic lamina of small muscular arteries in SSc and suggested that the arteriopathy was mediated by complement-fixing antibodies (56).

The factor inducing EC cytotoxicity remains unidentified. There is a large body of evidence that a circulating soluble protease may be linked to the genesis of endothelial injury, and one candidate is granzyme from activated T cell granules. Granzyme A, identified in SSc sera (57) and expressed in SSc skin (58), is secreted by T lymphocytes in response to antigen or to stimuli that mimic antigen. Its activity may be potentiated by a state of functional deficiency of serum protease inhibitors in SSc serum (48). Clinically, plasmapheresis together with immunosuppression was shown to improve clinical status and reduce, *in vitro*, the cytotoxic activity of SSc sera (59).

LTB4 (60) and free radicals (61) have been proposed to be produced by local inflammation, but this hypothesis, although interesting, needs further documentation. Majewski et al showed that, depending on the methods of investigation used, the sera of limited SSc contained different serum factors inducing various types of endothelial cytotoxicity (62). Etoh et al showed that sera from SSc patients decreased significantly the survival of endothelial cells (EC); the fact that platelet-poor plasma did not affect EC survival prompted the authors to hypothesize that the EC survival was affected by platelet (63).

In SSc, monocytes can be localized to the sub-endothelium (11) where they may contribute, through the release of superoxide anions, cytokines or other substances, to endothelial injury, to endothelial cell proliferation, and to fibroblast growth stimulation (64). This peculiar activity of monocytes and macrophages, if expressed when resident in the vascular environment, may have a role in SSc pathogenesis because monocytes can function as antigen presenting cells, thereby perpetuating and amplifying the immune process. In particular, interleukin 1, produced in quantity by macrophages, may participate in fibroblast proliferation and fibrosis (65,66). Indeed, macrophage products, such as platelet-derived growth factor (PDGF) (AA, AB, BB) and IL-1, promote smooth muscle cell proliferation (66) and are expressed in the arterial wall during repair following experimental injury (67,68).

Many investigators have focused on alterations of immune mechanisms in the genesis of vascular damage in SSc, particularly the interaction of activated lymphocytes with the endothelium. Previous studies reported that CD8+ suppressor/cytotoxic T cells are decreased in the circulation (69). The ratio of circulating helper CD4+ to suppressor/cytotoxic CD8+ T cells is raised in patients with SSc (70). Also, a higher circulating count of HLA-DR positive, CD8+ and CD4+ T cells and a reduced number of CD45R+CD4+ (suppressor/inducer) cells has been described (70). Recently, the circulating proportion of T cells bearing activation markers has been found to be increased in SSc (71), and distinctive markers of helper T cell activation (memory T cells) have been detected in patients with rapidly evolving SSc (72). The presence of activated T cells implies a continuous T cell-dependent immune reaction throughout the pathologic process. Hypergammaglobulinemia and autoantibodies in SSc patients may be the result of polyclonal B cell activation (73), secondary to CD4+ helper activation.

In tissues, class II MHC antigens have been recognized on EC and on fibroblasts located in the vicinity of inflammation near blood vessels, usually in the acute phase of the disease (74).

Class II MHC expression is known to contribute to antigen presentation to T cells, to cytolytic T cell induction, to the amplification of helper-inducer T cell subsets, to the stimulation of autologous and allogeneic mixed lymphocyte reactions, and to endothelial cell-lymphocyte interactions. Thus, class II antigen expression is fundamental to both induction and/or perpetuation of autoimmunity (75).

The antigen(s) responsible for autoimmunity in SSc is(are) unknown. Viruses and, especially, retroviruses are potential etiologic candidates (76), and endogenous retroviruses have been particularly implicated in immune pathogenesis (77,78). A fascinating example of retroviral involvement has emerged in the MLR/1pr mouse, a model of several human autoimmune disorders (RA, SLE), in which lymphoid proliferation abounds. Mountz et al have shown that the integration of a retroviral long terminal repeat (5.1 kb) in the second intron of the fas gene, itself essential for lymphoid programmed cell death, disrupts fas expression, inhibits apoptosis, and results in uncontrolled lymphocyte proliferation (79).

Antibodies reacting with human retroviral proteins have been associated with severe skin lesions in SLE and MCTD (80). In atherosclerosis, where vascular pathology is similar to SSc, including smooth muscle activation and endothelial injury, a viral contribution to pathogenesis has been proposed (81), leading to endothelial activation and injury, alterations in extracellular matrix, enhancement of procoagulant factor synthesis, induction of monocyte and PMN adhesion receptor expression, activation of cytokine gene expression, and smooth muscle cell proliferation (81). Viruses can activate T and B cells to produce alloreactive T cells and antibodies. In the case of autoimmune diseases, such as SSc, virus may incorporate host antigens into the viral capsid or membrane and express them on the cell surface where they are recognized as nonself, leading to an immune response which cross reacts with self epitopes. A related mechanism for viral-mediated autoimmunity is that of molecular mimicry—the host and the infectious agent share the same structure. The resulting cross-reactive immune response directed against the virus reacts with self proteins, leading to injury (82).

In SSc, a retroviral agent could be involved in the pathogenesis of the disease. Maul et al found the major epitope of topoisomerase I to contain a 6-amino acid homology with the p30^{gag} retroviral protein (83). This led them to hypothesize that endothelial cells, T lymphocytes, and/or fibroblasts might be retrovirally transformed and present retroviral antigens to which T cells react. Garry et al found antibodies to p24^{gag} in 16.5% of SSc patients associated with diffuse cutaneous involvement, and suggested that these antibodies could account for antigen-independent B cell activation (84). This hypothesis needs confirmation.

Another possible explanation for autoimmune alterations in SSc is superantigens (85), which are microbial/viral molecules that trigger profound alterations in immune system without actually infecting lymphocytes or monocytes. Superantigens form complexes with MHC II. These complexes bind subsets of T cell receptor V β chains (86) and stimulate T cell function as if true antigens were presented (87), a mechanism suggested for graft versus host disease (85), whose pathology shares similarities with SSc (88).

Alternatively, EC may function as antigen presenting cells (89), presenting antigen epitopes to resting T cells and stimulating an allogeneic response, sustained largely by CD4+ T cells and directed against HLA-DR. Can EC initiate and sustain the immune response? Although human endothelial cells usually do not bear class II molecules, they may be induced *in vivo* on arterial EC during the vascular reaction of Kawasaki disease (90). The induction of MHC II antigens on EC may involve autologous T cells, perhaps through cytokine secretion (91). An EC hypothesis would highlight the role of lymphocytes in the induction of SSc, placing vascular involvement and damage as a consequence of cell-mediated immunity and the interrelationship between EC and T cells as key in disease progression (92,93). Cells capable of endothelial damage include natural killer (NK) and lymphokine activated killer cells (LAK). In SSc, circulating NK cell levels have been shown to be normal, decreased, or increased (55,94,95). A reduction of circulating NK cells could be explained by their disappearance resulting from IL-2-induced adhesion on EC (96). LAK cells can be directly involved in endothelial cytotoxicity, through the release of proteases (granzymes) (92). Critical for LAK activity is the expression on EC of adhesion molecules (ICAM-1, LAF-1) (93). Since NK cells can be precursors of LAK cells, an abnormality in LAK generation has been suggested to explain depressed LAK activity observed *in vitro* (97). Recently, Kantor et al demonstrated that SSc patients have normal circulating NK activity but deficient CD8+ and CD56+CD16+ levels associated with a deficiency in generating LAK cells in the presence of IL-2 (98). T cells can induce EC injury and death in two ways: first, via the "perforin" model in which T cells release lytic substances that directly damage the membrane; and second, by inducing EC cytolysis by a complement-dependent, antibody- dependent, cell-dependent mechanism.

In SSc, we do not know either the mechanism or the mediator of endothelial injury. Nonetheless, it has been demonstrated that even apparently uninvolved skin demonstrates metabolic and ultrastructural alterations of the endothelium (99) before the appearance of reduplicated basal lamina. This evidence of a generalized microangiopathy is confirmed by the increased expression of ELAM 1 and PC 1 on EC in both affected and unaffected skin (100).

Cytokines may have a role in endothelial activation and damage. Interleukin 1 (IL1) activates EC inducing the expression of both cellular adhesion molecules which enhance lymphocyte adhesion and PDGF, a potent activator of fibroblasts (101). *In vivo* IL1 has been linked with endothelial injury in the lung (102). It also has been demonstrated to be produced by circulating SSc monocytes (66,103), which inhibit endothelial

cell growth (65) and stimulate fibroblast proliferation (104). Conversely, Sandborg et al (105) and Wicher et al (106), demonstrated low levels of IL1 activity in SSc monocyte supernatants associated with a low molecular weight inhibitor. In a disease such as SSc characterized by hypoxia, EC could also be a source of IL1. In fact, it has been shown that hypoxia induces an increase of mRNA for IL1α and an increase in adhesion molecules on EC (ICAM-1)(107).

Tumor necrosis factor (TNF) is important in inflammation and inflammation-mediated fibrosis (101,108). Acutely, IL1 and TNF act synergistically to: activate the endothelium by inducing the expression of adhesion molecules such as ICAM-1 and ELAM, induce chemotaxis (together with IL8), and activate PMN (cyclooxygenase and nitric oxide (NO) synthase). Moreover, IL1 and TNF are mitogens for lymphocytes and stimulators of further cytokine production (possibly via activation of an AP-1 transacting pathway). TNFα is a potent inducer of IL1 in several cell types, so that many activities attributed to TNFα may be secondary to IL1-mediated effects and vice versa. TNFα and β (the latter originally called lymphotoxin) have the capacity to inhibit endothelial growth and to stimulate fibroblast growth (109); they are also important in the initial activation of T cells (110). Indeed, each induces EC morphological changes, the expression of ICAM-1 (111), and the release of PDGF, which is a smooth muscle cell and fibroblast mitogen (112). Currently, TNF is considered to be a principal cytokine responsible for the graft versus host reaction (113).

Gamma interferon (IFN) is a T cell product that induces the synthesis of HLA antigens on EC and fibroblasts (91), enhances lymphocyte adhesion to EC, and, in the presence of TNF, induces EC lysis and damage to the vascular wall (109). Particularly relevant to SSc is the hypothesis that IFN blocks the profibrotic effects of IL1 and TNF and that, in SSc, a deficiency in the production of IFN leaves the tissues unprotected from these two cytokines (114).

Interleukin 2 (IL2), synthesized by activated T

cells, plays a central role in the immune response. It promotes proliferation and differentiation of helper T cells, cytotoxic T cells, and B cells, and it stimulates cytokine expression in monocytes. IL2 is one of the immune mediators suspected to be a factor in T cell up-regulation in SSc (115). In 1988, Umehara et al (115) demonstrated that SSc lymphocytes were able to produce, when stimulated with PHA, increased quantities of IL2 (116). Later, Kahaleh and LeRoy showed that IL2 levels were positively correlated with the extent of skin involvement and inversely related to disease duration (117). Recently, the increased levels of circulating IL2 in SSc have been confirmed (73,118, 119) and IL2 receptors (sIL2) have been shown to be increased in both SSc sera (118,120) and on the surface of SSc T cells (121). Recombinant IL2 has been demonstrated to expand human NK cells selectively (122) and to induce rapid adhesion of NK cells to EC with subsequent injury (123). The expansion of NK cells may lead to increased LAK cell levels and to consequent LAK-induced cytotoxicity either directly or mediated by LAK-secreted products (i.e., granzymes). Recently, rIL2 has been shown to activate monocytes/macrophages and to increase 10- to 50-fold their production of the profibrotic cytokine, active TGFβ2. Increased levels of interleukin 4 (IL4), another T cell cytokine, have been reported in SSc sera (118,119).

IL4 is produced by Th2 cells that cooperate with B cells to generate vigorous immunoglobulin responses (124). In addition, IL4 mediates T cell growth, together with IL2 (125), and is a principal factor in the regulated differentiation of Th0 into Th2 cells (126). IL4 has the capacity to increase EC adhesion for T cells and to stimulate proliferation and extracellular matrix production by human fibroblasts *in vitro* (119).

Interleukin 6 (IL6) has recently been found to be the cytokine most frequently detected in SSc and to be overproduced by SSc fibroblasts (119,127). While capable of inducing IL1α and TNFα (128,129), IL6 also exerts both direct cell-cell stimulatory effects and can mediate T cell proliferation through soluble growth activity different from IL2 and IL4 (130). In SSc, IL6 has been shown to mediate enhanced expression of IL2 (121).

Interleukin 8 (IL8) displays homology to the connective tissue activating peptide III and is produced by fibroblasts, epithelial cells and endothelial cells (131). Recently, IL8 levels have been found to be increased in SSc sera together with specific anti-IL8 autoantibodies that might reflect a control mechanism to prevent prolonged chemotactic effect of IL8 (132).

Another potent cytokine, transforming growth factor beta (TGFβ), may have a role in the pathogenesis of SSc (133) because of its profibrotic effects up-regulating the matrix genes of several different collagens, fibronectin, and proteoglycans at the pretranslational level (134). TGFβ inhibits *in vitro* the proliferation of endothelial cells (135,136), being both cytostatic and cytotoxic for these and other epithelial cells (136). Recently, Sutton et al demonstrated that TGFβ effects upon EC depend on the cell phenotype, which, in turn, may be determined by extracellular matrix signals to these cells (136). Although TGFβ is interesting, more studies are needed to determine its real role in the pathogenesis of SSc.

It seems likely that the cytokine cascade induced by inflammatory stimuli has a role in the induction of endothelial activation and the loss of endothelial integrity. Several different mechanisms may be proposed (e.g., rearrangement of endothelial cytoskeleton, which could render EC susceptible to injury or, alternatively, poised to trigger immune activation), but the precise role of cytokines in the vascular involvement in SSc remains unclear. In SSc, involvement of endothelium may be evaluated both *in vitro* and *in vivo*, providing the opportunity for non-invasive monitoring of the state of EC perturbation in the intact patient. von Willebrand antigen has been proposed as a reliable marker for EC injury in SSc (137,138). It is well known that the von Willebrand factor is synthesized, stored, and released by EC and, for this reason, the circulating levels are considered to reflect endothelial "state-of-health." An endothelial protein, E92, reported to be increased in SSc, has been suggested as another marker of endothelial activation (139). Recently, angiotensin converting enzyme (ACE) levels have been found to be reduced in SSc (140,141) and in Kawasaki disease (142). The reduction of ACE levels provides major evidence for the argument that endothelial injury is more prominent than EC activation. *In vitro*, ACE increases during activation and decreases during injury while von Willebrand factor levels increase under both stimuli (142), indicating that ACE levels are a useful marker for the clinical monitoring of the endothelial derangement.

THE ENDOTHELIUM AND THE MODIFICATION OF ITS FUNCTIONS

Endothelium should be viewed as a tissue composed of single-cell thick EC, a complex basal lamina, and pericytes, all of which are likely to interact through cell-cell, matrix-cell, and soluble intercellular interactions. The endothelium has an active role as a barrier between the bloodstream and the connective tissue and to modulate the surrounding microenviroment. Nonthrombogenecity, permeability, and control of circulating cell trafficking are among its key functions. As mentioned above, the endothelium has a fundamental role in the pathogenesis of SSc and its alteration is an early event preceding fibrotic and organ insufficiency manifestations of the disease. It is now clear that in SSc the endothelium is unable to maintain its normal functions. Derangement of major aspects of endothelial function very likely contributes significantly to the development and progression of SSc. Altered EC may impair constitutive functions or may induce abnormal functions. These results are reflected in the perturbation of cell interactions such as adhesion or cell proliferation. The dysfunction may be reversible or may lead to more advanced injury and cellular death. Today, the definition of endothelial injury is controversial. In human diseases where endothelium is affected by different mechanisms, endothelial injury may be operationally defined as changes in metabolic and recognition functions of the

blood vessel leading to specific clinical and pathologic changes (143). Thus, distinctions between endothelial injury and endothelial activation are largely semantic. The main functions of the endothelium may be summarized as follows: angiogenesis; vascular tone control (vasomotion); fibrinolysis/coagulation; and inflammation and interactions with platelets, neutrophils, and lymphocytes. The following paragraphs will review selected physiological functions of the endothelium and the possible mechanisms by which alterations of these functions may contribute to the pathogenesis of SSc.

ANGIOGENESIS

Capillaroscopic observations suggest significant derangements of the microcirculation in SSc. Angiogenesis is a dynamic function of the endothelium with multiple steps to which different cell types probably contribute (144). In response to stimulus, EC retract from each other, exposing the basement membrane, which is digested by enzymes. This produces gaps through which endothelial cells migrate, divide, and form loops. The loops evolve into tubes around which basement membrane is secreted by these same EC, forming the new blood vessel.

In SSc, monocytes showed a decrease in angiogenic capability (145,146). Sera from patients with diffuse SSc markedly enhanced the production of angiogenic lymphokines by normal human peripheral blood mononuclear cells (147). The sera of limited SSc, however, were able to decrease angiogenesis further (147), strengthening the evidence that angiogenesis is decreased in SSc. In the healthy microenviroment, a balance of positive and negative factors probably maintains the physiological angiogenesis potential (148). Modulation of vascular cell migratory behavior is complex and involves multiple mechanisms, including protease-antiprotease systems, changes in selected matrix component synthesis, and organization of cell surface matrix binding proteins (integrins, selectins, and others), as well as changes in cytoskeletal organization. Usually EC exhibit high replication rates immediately after separation or displacement *in vivo* or *in vitro*. In SSc, microvessel injury is a pivotal event in the modification of endothelial behavior. Among the participating factors, FGF and TGFβ are candidates for the modification of angiogenesis in SSc. It is well known that after endothelial injury, smooth muscle cells migrate into the intima where they proliferate and synthesize matrix components that are deposited in close apposition to the endothelium (149). This results in the formation of a thickened intima with narrowed vessel lumen. The cellular contact of smooth muscle cells with EC activates TGFβ (150), which inhibits endothelial cell growth through two different mechanisms. The first is the direct inhibition of the angiogenic stimulatory effect of fibroblast growth factor by TGFβ (151); the second is the induction of fibronectin release that reduces endothelial proliferation (152). It is clear that the capacity of the endothelium to maintain angiogenesis is also influenced by interactions between EC and the ECM (153). Matrix composition and soluble factors may change the levels of both activators and inhibitors of plasminogen; furthermore, the addition of inhibitors of serine proteases decreases migration rates of endothelial cells (154). Still controversial is the role of TNFα in angiogenesis—while it has been shown to be cytotoxic toward EC and to inhibit their proliferation *in vitro*, it was conversely reported to induce angiogenesis in humans (155). Mast cells, another cell with a potential role in SSc pathogenesis (156), seem to stimulate endothelial cell migration and thus, together with platelets and monocytes, may actively participate in angiogenesis. In SSc, impaired angiogenesis linked to chronic endothelial injury is a principal event leading to the observed capillaroscopic observations. Putative positive and negative soluble factors in angiogenesis are listed in Table 8-3.

PLATELET ACTIVATION

Platelets do not adhere to intact endothelium but to basal lamina that is denuded of EC, or to the stroma surrounding interrupted basal lamina. Under particular conditions, platelets may also

Table 8.3. Reported Regulators of Angiogenesis

Enhancers	Inhibitors
FGF	TGFβ
EGF	TNFα
PD-ECGF	γIFN
Angiogenin	Thrombospondin
VEGF	Platelet factor IV
PDGF	Interferons
MDGF	MECIF

Abbreviations used: FGF = fibroblast growth factor; EGF = epidermal growth factor; PDGF = platelet-derived growth factor; MDGF = monocyte derived growth factor; TGFβ = transforming growth factor beta; γIFN = gamma interferon; TNFα = tumor necrosis factor alpha; PD-ECGF = platelet derived endothelial cell growth factor; MECIF = monocyte endothelial cell inhibiting factor.

adhere to injured endothelium without denudation. The absorption of von Willebrand factor released by EC facilitates adhesion. After adhesion, platelets aggregate and release the content of their granules (ADP, ATP, platelet factor 4, thromboxane A_2, PDGF, TGFβ). The presence of nitric oxide on endothelial surfaces seems to prevent unstimulated platelets from adhering to the endothelium (157,158). Prostacyclin (PGI_2) produced by the endothelium under various stimuli also inhibits adhesion of stimulated platelets (157).

Previous studies in SSc have found evidence of *in vivo* and *in vitro* activation of platelets. *In vitro*, the activation of SSc platelets has been shown by increased aggregation upon stimulation with adenosine diphosphate, adrenaline, collagen, and serotonin (158) and by enhanced adhesion to collagen (159). *In vivo*, increased plasma levels of β thromboglobulin, platelet factor 4, and platelet circulating aggregates have been described (160, 161). Elevated levels of β thromboglobulin before the development of fibrosis indicates early involvement of platelets in SSc pathogenesis (162), most likely a secondary event following activation and injury of the endothelium. The products released by platelets (e.g., PDGF and TGFβ) are capable of smooth cell and fibroblast activation.

The activated or damaged endothelium is itself able to produce substances which in turn activate platelets, such as platelet activating factor

(PAF) (163). PAF has not been investigated in SSc. It is involved in inflammation and leads to microvascular damage (163) through endothelial cell impairment both directly and through enhancement of neutrophil activation (164). It also increases pulmonary vascular permeability, promoting lung edema and injury of lung microcirculation (165). Studies of PAF in SSc are needed.

VASCULAR TONE CONTROL

The occurrence of Raynaud's phenomenon in early SSc represents an important modification of the vascular tone control. The endothelium contributes to the regulation of the contraction and relaxation of smooth muscle cells through the production and release of vasoactive substances, including prostacyclin (PGI), endothelial derived relaxing factor (EDRF), endothelial derived hyperpolarizing factor (EDHF), and endothelin (ET) (166). PGI and EDRF (the latter analogous in function to nitric oxide) induce smooth muscle cell relaxation and inhibit platelet aggregation, while ET is the most potent constrictor of smooth muscle cells (157). Recently, EDRF has been shown to participate in immune function and neurotransmission (167). Vasoactive substances released from perivascular nerves interact with the endothelium to modulate vessel tone (168). Neuropeptides derived from the peripheral nerve terminals may influence vascular relaxation or contraction through both direct or endothelium-mediated pathways. Two neuropeptides derived from the sensory system are particularly interesting: substance P acts on the endothelium inducing the release of EDRF, while a calcitonin gene related peptide relaxes smooth muscle cells directly (160).

The malfunction or functional absence of endothelium, induced by chronic injury, serves to aggravate vasospastic attacks characteristic of SSc (169). This mechanism seems to spare the release of PGI from EC (170). It has been demonstrated that the endothelium-mediated response to substance P is impaired more in the early phases, versus advanced phases, of SSc (171). The endothelial-independent vasodilation, induced by glycerol trinitrate, which is analogous to EDRF, was maintained early but became impaired later (171). These data indicate an early functional deficit of endothelial function already present before the onset of visceral and skin involvement. The impairment of endothelial-dependent relaxation has been recently confirmed by the evidence of reduced serum levels of nitric oxide in SSc (172). This state is probably worsened by increased ET levels that contribute to vasospasm and smooth muscle cell hypertrophy (173, 174). The role that neuropeptides have in the pathogenesis of the disease through their action on the endothelium and smooth muscle cells is still under investigation and remains uncertain (175). Particularly interesting is the fundamental contribution of neuropeptides to inflammation, to immune functions (176), and to endothelial activation (177). Further studies are needed to clarify the role of endothelium and its interacting systems in vascular tone dysfunction and SSc pathogenesis.

COAGULATION AND FIBRINOLYSIS

Vascular endothelial cells actively maintain antithrombotic and fibrinolytic capability. Perturbation or injury impairs both capacities, modifying:

1. Anticoagulant properties mediated by antithrombin III, heparin cofactor II, and protein C;
2. Fibrinolytic properties linked to the activity of plasminogen activators;
3. Procoagulant properties mediated by factor V, von Willebrand factor, thrombin, fibronectin, and tissue plasminogen activator inhibitor;
4. Antiplatelet properties (inhibition of adhesion and aggregation), mediated by PGI_2 and EDRF.

In general terms, procoagulant activities predominate in the arterial circulation while anticoagulant and fibrinolytic properties prevail in the capillary and venous circulations (178).

When vascular cells are deranged, these properties are altered, leading to increased expression of procoagulant activity, decreased expression of anticoagulant activity, and enhanced platelet adhesion and activation, due in large part to the conversion of the endothelial cells from their normal antithrombotic to a pathologic prothrombotic state. Consequent to exposure to cytokines such as IL1 (179) and TNFα (180), tissue factor activity and the protein C pathway are changed. After endothelial injury, enhanced procoagulant activity of factor V has been described (181). Injured EC also release von Willebrand factor multimers providing a substrate for platelet-vessel wall adhesion (138). Another major prothrombotic event is the increased secretion of plasminogen activator inhibitor. This seems to be sustained primarily by IL1, which also decreases tissue plasminogen activator production (182, 183). In response to IL1, EC synthesize platelet activating factor, which is a lipid mediator of inflammation that has prothrombotic properties (184) and is a potent activator of platelets, neutrophils, and basophils. There is wide agreement regarding the conversion to the prothrombotic state following EC injury (185).

There are discrepant views about fibrinolysis in SSc. Fibrin deposition has been described in arterioles and capillaries of patients with SSc (186). Also reported has been a decrease in plasminogen half life (187), reduced levels of antithrombin III, and increased plasminogen consumption (188). An alteration of fibrinolytic activity in SSc has been described by different authors. Cunliffe and Menon showed a decrease in plasma fibrinolytic activity (189); Furey et al showed that plasma fibrinolytic activity was normal, but thrombotic vessels showed a complete lack of fibrinolytic activity (190). Browse et al reported decreased fibrinolysis before venous stasis, but values after ten minutes of occlusion were not significantly different from controls (191). Holland and Jayson reported both impairment (192) and loss of diurnal variation of plas-

ma fibrinolytic activity (193). Our studies in SSc showed consistent fibrinolytic activity of dermal vessels (194), normal plasma plasminogen activation (195), and a normal circadian rhythm (195a). Godin-Ostro et al found increased levels of plasminogen activator (196); Kahan et al found plasma plasminogen activator/plasminogen inhibitor to be grossly normal (197). Falanga et al detected an increase in fibrin D-dimers, concluding that patients had evidence of both enhanced fibrin formation and enhanced degradation (198).

It seems likely that the prothrombotic changes observed in SSc are related to the injury of the endothelium. For the fibrinolytic system, because the venular endothelium is responsible for fibrinolysis and veins appear to be relatively unaffected in SSc, the relationship is less clear. At present, definitive conclusions about fibrinolysis in SSc would be premature. For the future, more accurate criteria in patient selection, in methods of sampling, and in assay choice and technique may improve the evaluation of fibrinolysis in SSc.

INFLAMMATION AND IMMUNE RESPONSE

Various overlapping phenomena involve EC during inflammation, including antigen presentation, leukocyte adhesion, and cytokine effects. Resting EC do not constituitively express MHC antigens. All three interferons and both TNFs induce HLA A, B, and C (Class I) expression, which present peptides primarily through CD8 T cells. In contrast, gamma interferon somewhat selectively induces HLA DR, DP, and DQ (Class II) expression, which enable EC to present peptides to CD4 (helper- inducer) T cells (91,199).

Leukocyte adhesion, a fundamental step in inflammation, is mediated by specific molecules expressed on the endothelial surface (199). Adhesion molecules may play important roles in SSc, mediating key steps in SSc pathogenesis (e.g., endothelial-lymphocyte interaction). ICAM 1, the ligand for LFA 1 (expressed by leukocytes and macrophages), has been demonstrated in inflammatory and immune reactions (111,199).

EC stimulated by IL 1, TNFs, and γIFN increase ICAM 1 expression, enhancing T cell adhesion (199,200). The number of adhesion molecules on EC is directly linked to the trafficking of T cells in the dermis (200). VCAM 1 also mediates the interaction between lymphocytes and endothelial cells, "driving" T cells to inflammatory sites. VCAM 1 is induced by IL1 and TNFα in inflammation associated with CD4+ activation (200). ELAM 1 is expressed on EC activated by IL1, TNFα, mast cells, and substance P (201). ELAM 1 expression seems to reduce the leukocyte rolling and favor interactions with the endothelium and their passage, through interaction with LFA 1 and VCAM 1, into the perivascular tissues (201).

An up-regulation of B1 and B2 integrins on lymphocytes (202), ICAM 1 on EC and fibroblasts, and ELAM 1 on EC (100,202,203) has been demonstrated in early diffuse SSc (100, 202). Increased serum levels of ICAM 1 were found in patients with diffuse progressive disease and in those with digital ulcers (204). In interstitial tissues, adhesion molecules have been demonstrated to be critical for fibroblast activation induced by lymphocytes (205,206). Cytokines influence the expression of adhesion molecules and the synthesis/release of various substances as prostacyclin, von Willebrand Factor, angiotensin converting enzyme, PDGF, and PAF (101).

Conclusion

A large body of evidence indicates that systemic sclerosis primarily affects the microvasculature, and secondarily affects the connective tissue. The disease targets the vasculature in key organs, including the lung, heart, kidney, gastrointestinal tract, and the skin, leading ultimately to fibrosis and functional insufficiency. The principal vascular pathological features of SSc make the disease unique: while it may share similarities with atherosclerosis, graft versus host disease and possibly microscopic polyangiitis, the main difference is that SSc affects arterioles and capillaries,

a characteristic that it shares with hypertension and diabetes mellitus. The knowledge that SSc chronically affects endothelium should spur the development of vascular therapeutic approaches to modify the disease. Thus, a long-range goal of SSc treatment might be the prevention of fibrosis in the early phase when Raynaud's phenomenon is the dominant symptom and skin and organ involvement is still limited. In this perspective, we should seek a drug, or a combination of drugs, having two effects: (*a*) to interfere with lymphocyte-endothelial and platelet-endothelial interaction, preventing lymphocyte homing and platelet adhesion and aggregation; and (*b*) to protect endothelium against chronic injury. Presently, the treatment of SSc is focused on the prevention of collagen secretion (D-penicillamine, griseofulvin, colchicine) and to relieve symptoms (vasodilators, angiotensin converting enzyme inhibitors). Recently, immunosuppression with drugs used in transplantation has generated some interest, in particular to inhibit IL2 production by lymphocytes (207), but a direct vascular approach to therapy is still lacking. We trust that the efforts of many investigators will improve the vascular future of our scleroderma patients.

References

1. Raynaud M. De la gangrene symetrique des extremites. Thesis, Université de Paris, 1862.
2. Ball P. Cas preséntation: " . . . un jeune homme atteinte de la sclerodactylie, avec tendence à l'invahissiment et à la sclérodermie generale." Bull Soc Med Hop Paris 1875;11:96.
3. Dinkler M. Zur lehre von der sklerodermie. Deutsch Arch Klin Med 1891;48:514–577.
4. Brown GE, O'Leary PA. Skin capillaries in scleroderma. Arch Intern Med 1925;36:73–88.
5. Banks BM. Is there a common denomination in scleroderma, dermatomyositis, disseminated lupus erythematosus, the Libmann-Sacks syndrome, and polyarteritis nodosa? N Engl J Med 1949;225:433–444.
6. Yardumian K, Kleinerman J. Pathogenesis of so-called diffuse vascular or collagen disease. Arch Intern Med 1949;83:1–26.

7. Ingram JT. Acrosclerosis and systemic sclerosis. Arch Dermatol 1958;77:79–85.

8. Norton WL, Hurd ER, Lewis DC, et al. Evidence of microvascular injury in scleroderma and systemic lupus erythematosus: Quantitative study of the microvascular bed. J Lab Clin Med 1968;71: 919–933.

9. Norton WL, Nardo JM. Vascular disease in progressive systemic sclerosis (scleroderma). Ann Intern Med 1970;73:317–324.

10. Campbell PM, LeRoy EC. Pathogenesis of systemic sclerosis: A vascular hypothesis. Semin Arthritis Rheum 1975;4:351–368.

11. Fleischmajer R, Perlish JS, Shaw KV, Pirozzi DJ. Skin capillary changes in early systemic scleroderma electron microscopy and *in vitro* autoradiography with tritiated thymidine. Arch Dermatol 1976;112:1553–1557.

12. Kahaleh MB. The role of vascular endothelium in the pathogenesis of connective tissue diseases: Endothelial injury, activation, participation and response. Clin Exp Rheumatol 1990;88:595–601.

13. Coffman JD. Raynaud's phenomenon. Oxford: Oxford University Press, 1989.

14. LeRoy EC, Medsger TA Jr. Raynaud's phenomenon: A proposal for classification. Clin Exp Rheumatol 1992;10:485–488.

15. Belch JJF. Raynaud's phenomenon: Its relevance to scleroderma. Ann Rheum Dis 1991;50:839–845.

16. Maricq HR, LeRoy EC, D'Angelo WA, et al. Diagnostic potential of in vivo capillary microscopy in scleroderma and related disorders. Arthritis Rheum 1980;23:183–189.

17. Maricq HR, Weinberger AB, LeRoy EC. Early detection of scleroderma spectrum disorders by in vivo capillary microscopy: A prospective study of patients with Raynaud's phenomenon. J Rheumatol 1982;9:289–291.

18. Wong ML, Highton J, Palmer DG. Sequential nailfold capillary microscopy in scleroderma and related disorders. Ann Rheum Dis 1988;47:53–61.

19. Engelhart M, Seibold JR. Cyanosis and Raynaud's phenomenon: The relation to underlying disease and venous abnormalities. Angiology 1990;41: 432–438.

20. Bollinger A, Jager K, Siegenthaler W. Microangiopathy of progressive systemic sclerosis: Evaluation by dynamic fluorescence videomicroscopy. Arch Intern Med 1986;146:1541–1545.

21. Maricq HR, Harper FE, Khan MM, Tan EM, LeRoy EC. Microvascular abnormalities as possible predictors of disease subsets in Raynaud phenomenon and early connective tissue disease. Clin Exp Rheumatol 1983;1:195–205.

22. Sato S, Takehara K, Soma Y, Tsuchida T, Ishibashi Y. Diagnostic significance of nailfold bleeding in scleroderma spectrum disorders. J Am Acad Dermatol 1993;28:198–203.

23. Chen, ZY, Silver RM, Ainsworth SK, et al. Association between fluorescent antinuclear antibodies, capillary patterns, and clinical features in scleroderma spectrum disorders. Am J Med 1984;77: 812–822.

24. Maricq HR, Spencer-Green G, LeRoy EC. Skin capillary abnormalities as an indicator of organ involvement in scleroderma (systemic sclerosis) Raynaud's syndrome and dermatomyositis. Am J Med 1976;61:862–870.

25. Groen H, Wichers G, ter Borg EJ, et al. Pulmonary diffusing capacity disturbances are related to nailfold capillary changes in patients with Raynaud's phenomenon with and without an underlying connective tissue disease. Am J Med 1990;89: 34–41.

26. Lovy M, MacCarter D, Steigerwald JC. Relationship between nailfold capillary abnormalities and organ involvement in systemic sclerosis. Arthritis Rheum 1985;28:496–501.

27. Dabich L, Bookstein JJ, Zweifler A, Zarafonetis JD. Digital arteries in patients with scleroderma. Arteriographic and plethysmographic study. Arch Intern Med 1972;130:708–714.

28. Fleischmajer R, Damiano V, Nedwick A. Scleroderma and the subcutaneous tissue. Science 1971; 171:1019–1021.

29. Fleischmajer R, Perlish J. Glycosaminoglycans in scleroderma and scleredema. J Invest Dermatol 1972;58:129–132.

30. Rodnan GP, Myerowitz RL, Justh GO. Morphologic changes in the digital arteries of patients with progressive systemic sclerosis (scleroderma) and Raynaud phenomenon. Medicine 1980;59: 393–408.

31. Matsui S. Uber die pathologie und pathogenese von Sklerodermia universalis. Mitt Med Fakult Univ Tokyo 1924;31:55–116.

32. Fleischmajer R, Perlish JS. Capillary alterations in scleroderma. J Am Acad Dermatol 1980;2:161–170.

33. Fleischmajer R, Perlish JS, Reeves JRT. Cellular infiltrates in scleroderma skin. Arthritis Rheum 1977;20:975–984.

34. Ishikawa O, Ishikawa H. Macrophage infiltration in the skin of patients with systemic sclerosis. J Rheumatol 1992;19:1202–1206.

35. Roumm AD, Whiteside TL, Medsger TA, Jr Rodnan GP. Lymphocytes in the skin of patients with progressive systemic sclerosis. Arthritis Rheum 1984;27:645–653.

36. Goetz RH. The pathology of progressive systemic sclerosis (generalized scleroderma) with special reference to changes in viscera. Clin Proc 1945;4: 337–392.

37. Schumacher RH Jr. The joint involvement in systemic sclerosis. Clin Dermatol 1994;12:277–282.

38. D'Angelo WA, Fries JF, Masi AT, Shulman LE. Pathologic observations in systemic sclerosis (scleroderma). A study of fifty-eight autopsy cases and fifty-eight matched controls. Am J Med 1969;46:428–440.

39. Cannon PJ, Hassar M, Case DB, et al. The relationship of hypertension and renal failure in scleroderma (progressive systemic sclerosis) to structural and functional abnormalities of the renal cortical circulation. Medicine 1974;53:1–46.

40. Henrichs KJ, Berry CL. Morphometry of intrarenal arteries in progressive sclerosis. Virchows Arch 1980;385:351–359.

41. Al-Sabbagh AR, Steen VD, Zee BC, et al. Pulmonary arterial histology and morphometry in systemic sclerosis: A case control autopsy study. J Rheumatol 1989;16:1038–1042.

42. Young RH, Mark GJ. Pulmonary vascular changes in scleroderma. Am J Med 1978;64:998–1004.

43. Harrison NK, Myers AR, Corrin B, et al. Structural features of interstitial lung disease in systemic sclerosis. Am Rev Respir Dis 1991;144:706–713.

44. Norton WL. Comparison of the microangiopathy of systemic lupus erythematosus, dermatomyositis, scleroderma and diabetes mellitus. Lab Invest 1970;22:301–308.

45. Currie S, Saunders M, Knowles M. Immunological aspects of systemic sclerosis. In vitro activity of lymphocytes from patients with the disorder. Br J Dermatol 1971;84:400–409.

46. Cooper SM, Friou GJ. Cytotoxicity in progressive systemic sclerosis. No evidence for increased cytotoxicity against fibroblasts of different origins. J Rheumatol 1979;6:25–29.

47. Kahaleh MB, Sherer GK, LeRoy EC. Endothelial injury in scleroderma. J Exp Med 1979;149:1326–1335.

48. Kahaleh MB, LeRoy EC. Endothelial injury in scleroderma: A protease mechanism. J Lab Clin Med 1983;101:553–560.

49. Shanahan WR, Jr, Korn JH. Cytotoxic activity of sera from scleroderma and other connective tissue diseases. Lack of cellular and disease specificity. Arthritis Rheum 1982;25:1391–1395.

50. Meyer O, Haim T, Dryll A, Lansaman J, Ryckewaert A. Vascular endothelial cell injury in progressive systemic sclerosis and other connective tissue diseases. Clin Exp Rheumatol 1983;1: 29–34.

51. Penning CA, Cunningham J, French MAH, et al. Antibody-dependent cellular cyotoxicity of human vascular endothelium in systemic sclerosis. Clin Exp Immunol 1984;57:548–556.

52. Cohen S, Johnson AR, Hurd E. Cytotoxicity of sera from patients with scleroderma. Effects on human endothelial cells and fibroblasts in culture. Arthritis Rheum 1983;26:170–178.

53. Drenk F, Deicher HRG. Pathophysiological effects of endothelial cytotoxic activity derived from sera of patients with progressive systemic sclerosis. J Rheumatol 1988;15:468–474.

54. Holt CM, Lindsey N, Moult J, et al. Antibody-dependent cellular cytotoxicity of vascular endothelium: Characterization and pathogenic associations in systemic sclerosis. Clin Exp Immunol 1989;78:359–365.

55. Cifone MG, Giacomelli R, Famularo G, et al. Natural killer cell activity and antibody-dependent cellular cytotoxicity in progressive systemic sclerosis. Clin Exp Immunol 80:360–365.

56. Evans DJ, Cashman SJ, Walport M. Progressive systemic sclerosis: autoimmune arteriopathy. Lancet 1987;1:480–482.

57. Kahaleh MB, Yin T. The molecular mechanisms of endothelial cell (EC) injury in scleroderma (SSc): Identification of Granzyme 1 (a product of cytolytic T cell) in SSc sera. Arthritis Rheum 1990;33:S21 (abstract).

58. Kahaleh MB, Fan PS. Cytotoxic T cell involvement in scleroderma: Detection of granzyme-a gene expression in systemic sclerosis skin. Arthritis Rheum 1992;35:S22 (abstract).

59. Dau PC, Kahaleh MB, Sagebiel RW. Plasmapheresis and immunosuppressive drug therapy in scleroderma. Arthritis Rheum 1981;24:1128–1136.

60. Deicher HRG, Drenk F, Hoffman G. Identification of an LTB4 protein complex as evidence of endothelial cell cytotoxicity activity (ECA) in progressive systemic sclerosis (PSS). Z Rheumatol 1987;46:196–197.

61. Murrell DF. A radical proposal for the pathogenesis of scleroderma. J Am Acad Dermatol 1993;28: 78–85.

62. Majewski S, Laszcyk M, Jablonska S, et al. Cytotoxic effect of sera from patients with systemic scleroderma: Comparison of three different in vitro methods. Rheumatol Int 1990;10:65–70.

63. Etoh T, Igarashi A, Iozumi K, Ishibashi Y, Takehara K. The effects of scleroderma sera on endothelial cell survival in vitro. Arch Dermatol Res 1990;282:516–519.

64. Kahaleh MB, DeLustro F, Bock W, LeRoy EC. Human monocyte modulation of endothelial cells and fibroblast growth: Possible mechanism for fi-

brosis. Clin Immunol Immunopathol 1988;39: 242–255.

65. Alcocer-Varela J, Martinez-Cordero E, Alarcon-Segovia D. Spontaneous production of and defective response to interleukin-1 by peripheral blood mononuclear cells from patients with scleroderma. Clin Exp Immunol 1985;59:666–672.

66. Kawaguchi Y, Harigai M, Hara M, et al. Increased interleukin-1 receptor, type 1, at messenger RNA and protein level in skin fibroblasts from patients with systemic sclerosis. Biochem Biophys Res Commun 1992;184:1504–1510.

67. Raines EW, Dower SK, Ross R. Interleukin-1 mitogenic activity for fibroblasts and smooth muscle cells is due to PGDF-AA. Science 1989;243: 393–396.

68. Wang AM, Doyle M, Mark DF. Quantitation of mRNA by the polymerase chain reaction. Proc Natl Acad Sci 1989;86:9717–9721.

69. Korn JH. Immunologic aspects of scleroderma. Curr Opin Rheumatol 1991;3:347–352.

70. Gustafsson R, Totterman TH, Klareskog L, Hallgren R. Increase in activated T cells and reduction in suppressor inducer T cell in systemic sclerosis. Ann Rheum Dis 1990;49:40–45.

71. Freundlich B, Jimenez SA. Phenotype of peripheral blood lymphocytes in patients with progressive systemic sclerosis: Activated T lymphocytes and the effect of D-Penicillamine therapy. Clin Exp Immunol 1987;69:375–384.

72. Fiocco U, Rosada M, Cozzi L, et al. Early phenotypic activation of circulating helper memory T-cells in scleroderma: Correlation with disease activity. Ann Rheum Dis 1993;52:272–277.

73. Famularo G, Giacomelli R, Alesse E, et al. Polyclonal B lymphocyte activation in progressive systemic sclerosis. J Clin Lab Immunol 1989;29: 59–63.

74. Gruschwitz M, Sepp N, Kofler H, Wick G. Expression of class II-MHC antigens in the dermis of patients with progressive systemic sclerosis. Immunobiology 1991;182:234–255.

75. Mellins ED. The role of the MHC in autoimmunity: An overview. J Rheumatol 1992;19(suppl 33):63–69.

76. Krieg AM, Steinberg AD. Retroviruses and autoimmunity. J Autoimmun 1990;3:137–166.

77. Abraham GN, Khan AS. Human endogenous retroviruses and immune diseases. Clin Immunol Immunopathol 1990;56:1–8.

78. Krieg AM, Gourley MF, Perl A. Endogenous retroviruses: Potential etiologic agents in autoimmunity. FASEB J 1992;6:2537–2544.

79. Jian Y, Zhou T, Wu J, Mountz J. The fas-ligand and apoptosis in LPR and GLD mice. Arthritis Rheum 1993;36:R25 (abstract).

80. Ranki A, Kurki P, Rriepponen S, Stephansson E. Antibodies to retroviral proteins in autoimmune connective tissue disease. Relation to clinical manifestations and ribonucleoprotein autoantibodies. Arthritis Rheum 1992;35:1483–1491.

81. Hajjar DP. Viral pathogenesis of atherosclerosis. Impact of molecular mimicry and viral genes. Am J Pathol 1991;139:1195–1211.

82. Barnett LA, Fujinami RS. Molecular mimicry: A mechanism for autoimmune injury. FASEB J 1992;6:840–844.

83. Maul GG, Jimenez SA, Riggs E, Ziemnicka-Kotula D. Determination of an epitope of the diffuse systemic sclerosis marker antigen DNA topoisomerase I: Sequence similarity with retroviral p30^{gag} protein suggests a possible cause for autoimmunity in systemic sclerosis. Proc Natl Acad Sci 1989;86:8492–8496.

84. Dang H, Dauphinee MJ, Talal N, et al. Serum antibody to retroviral gag proteins in systemic sclerosis. Arthritis Rheum 1991;34:1336–1337.

85. Friedman SM, Posnett DN, Tumang JR, Cole BC, Crow MK. A potential role for microbial superantigens in the pathogenesis of systemic autoimmune diseases. Arthritis Rheum 1991;34:468–480.

86. Gascoigne NRJ, Ames KT. Direct binding of secreted T cell receptor beta chain to superantigen associated with class II major histocompatibility complex protein. Proc Natl Acad Sci 1991;88: 613–616.

87. Herman A, Kappler JW, Marrack P, Pullen AM. Superantigens: Mechanism of T cell stimulation and role in immune responses. Annu Rev Immunol 1991;9:745–772.

88. Jaffee BD, Claman HN. Chronic graft-versus-host disease (GVHD) as a model for scleroderma. I. Description of models. Cell Immunol 1983;77: 1–12.

89. Jaffe EA. Cell biology of endothelial cells. Hum Pathol 1987;18:234–239.

90. Terai M, Kohno Y, Namba M, et al. Class II major histocompatibility antigen expression of coronary arterial endothelium in a patient with Kawasaki disease. Human Pathol 1990;21:231–234.

91. Pober JS, Gimbrone MA, Jr, Cotran RS, et al. Ia expression by vascular endothelium is inducible by activated T cells and by human gamma interferon. J Exp Med 1983;157:1339–1353.

92. Kahaleh MB, Yin T. Enhanced lymphocyte endothelial cell (EC) interaction in scleroderma (SSc). Arthritis Rheum 1990;33:S63.

93. Kahaleh MB. The vascular disease in scleroderma: Endothelial T lymphocyte-fibroblast interactions. Rheum Dis Clin North Am 1990;16:53–73.

94. Miller EB, Hiserodt JC, Hung LE, Steen VD, Medsger TA, Jr. Reduced natural killer cell activity in patients with systemic sclerosis. Correlation with clinical disease type. Arthritis Rheum 1988;31:1515–1523.

95. Wright JK, Hughes P, Rowell NR. Spontaneous lymphocyte-mediated (NK cell) cytotoxicity in systemic sclerosis: A comparison with antibody-dependent lymphocyte (K cell) cytotoxicity. Ann Rheum Dis 1982;41:409–413.

96. Rudnicka L, Majewski S, Blaszczyk M et al. Adhesion of peripheral blood mononuclear cells to vascular endothelium in patients with systemic sclerosis (scleroderma). Arthritis Rheum 1992;35:771–775.

97. Silver RM. Lymphokine activated killer (LAK) cell activity in the peripheral blood lymphocytes of systemic sclerosis (SSc) patients. Clin Exp Rheumatol 1990;8:481–486.

98. Kantor TV, Whiteside TL, Friberg D, Buckingham RB, Medsger TA Jr. Lymphokineactivated killer cell and natural killer cell activities in patients with systemic sclerosis. Arthritis Rheum 1992;35:694–699.

99. Freemont AJ, Hoyland J, Fielding P, Hodson N, Jayson MIV. Studies of the microvascular endothelium in uninvolved skin of patients with systemic sclerosis: Direct evidence for a generalized microangiopathy. Br J Dermatol 1992;126:561–568.

100. Claman HN, Giorno RC, Seibold JR. Endothelial and fibroblastic activation in scleroderma. The myth of the uninvolved skin. Arthritis Rheum 1991;34:1495–1501.

101. Dinarello C. Interleukin one and tumor necrosis factor: Effector cytokines in autoimmune disease. Semin Immunol 1992;4:133–145.

102. Goldblum SE, Yoneda K, Cohen DA, McClain CJ. Provocation of pulmonary vascular endothelial injury in rabbits by human recombinant interleukin-1 beta. Infect Immunol 1988;56:2255–2263.

103. Umehara H, Kumagai S, Murakami M, et al. Enhanced production of interleukin-1 and tumor necrosis factor alpha by cultured peripheral blood monocytes from patients with scleroderma. Arthritis Rheum 1990;33:893–897.

104. Korn JH, Halushka PV, LeRoy EC. Monuclear cell modulation of connective tissue function: Suppression of fibroblast growth by stimulation of endogenous prostaglandin production. J Clin Invest 1980;65:543–559.

105. Sandborg CI, Berman MA, Andrews BS, Friou GJ. Interleukin-1 production by mononuclear cell from patients with scleroderma. Clin Exp Immunol 1985;60:294–302.

106. Whicher JT, Gilbert AM, Westacott C, Hutton C, Dieppe PA. Defective production of leukocytic endogenous mediator (interleukin-1) by peripheral blood leukocytes of patients with systemic sclerosis, systemic lupus erythematosus, rheumatoid arthritis and mixed connective tissue disease. Clin Exp Immunol 1986;65:80–89.

107. Shreeniwas R, Koga S, Karakurum M, et al. Hypoxia-mediated induction of endothelial cell interleukin-1 α. An autocrine mechanism promoting expression of leukocyte adhesion molecules on the vessel surface. J Clin Invest 1992;90:2333–2339.

108. Ruddle N. Tumor necrosis factor a and lymphotoxin (TNF-β). Curr Opinions Immunol 1992;4:327–332.

109. Kahaleh MB, Smith EA, Soma Y, LeRoy EC. Effect of lymphotoxin and tumor necrosis factor on endothelial and connective cell tissue growth and function. Clin Immunol Immunopathol 1988;49:261–267.

110. Bendtzen K. Tumor necrosis factor alfa and tumor necrosis factor beta/lymphotoxin are essential growth factors for human T lymphocytes. Clin Rheumatol 1990;6:120–129.

111. Wertheimer SJ, Myers CL, Wallace RW, Parks TP. Intercellular adhesion molecule-1 gene expression in human endothelial cells: Differential regulation by tumor necrosis factor-alfa and phorbol myristate acetate. J Biol Chem 1992;267:12030–12035.

112. Hajjar KA, Hajjar DP, Silverstein RL, Nachman RL. Tumor necrosis factor-mediated release of platelet-derived growth factor from cultured endothelial cells. J Exp Med 1987;166:235–245.

113. Piguet PF, Grau GE, Allet B, Vassalli P. Tumor necrosis factor/cachectin is an effector of skin and gut lesions of the acute phase of graft-vs-host disease. J Exp Med 1987;166:1280–1289.

114. Elias JA, Freundlich B, Kern JA, Rosenbloom J. Cytokine networks in the regulation of inflammation and fibrosis in the lung. Chest 1990;97:1439–1445.

115. Alcocer-Varela J, Laffon A, Alarcon-Segovia D. Differences in the production of and/or the response to interleukin-2 by T lymphocytes from patients with the various connective tissue diseases. Rheumatol Int 1984;4:39–44.

116. Umehara H, Kumagai S, Ishida H, et al. Enhanced production of interleukin-2 in patients with progressive systemic sclerosis. Hyperactivity of CD4-positive T cells. Arthritis Rheum 1988;31:401–407.

117. Kahaleh BM, LeRoy EC. Interleukin-2 in sclero-

derma: Correlation of serum level with extent of skin involvement and disease duration. Ann Intern Med 1989;110:446–450.

118. Needleman BW, Wigley FM, Stair RW. Interleukin-1, interleukin-2, interleukin-4, interleukin-6, tumor necrosis factor α and interferon gamma levels in sera from patients with scleroderma. Arthritis Rheum 1992;35:67–72.

119. Postlethwaite AE, Holness MA, Katai H, Raghow R. Human fibroblasts synthesize elevated levels of extracellular matrix proteins in response to interleukin-4. J Clin Invest 1992;90:1479–1485.

120. Degiannis D, Seibold JR, Czarnecki M, Raskova J, Rask K Jr. Soluble interleukin-2 receptors in patients with systemic sclerosis. Clinical and laboratory correlations. Arthritis Rheum 1990;33:375–380.

121. Kahaleh MB, Yin TG. Enhanced expression of high-affinity interleukin-2 receptors in scleroderma: Possible role for interleukin-6. Clin Immunol Immunopathol 1992;62:97–102.

122. Caligiuri MA, Murray C, Robertson MJ, et al. Selective modulation of human natural killer cells in vivo after prolonged infusion of low dose recombinant interleukin-2. J Clin Invest 1993;91:123–132.

123. Aronson FR, Libby P, Brandon EP, Janicka MW, Mier JW. Interleukin-2 rapidly induces natural killer cell adhesion to human endothelial cells. A potential mechanism for endothelial injury. J Immunol 1988;141:158–163.

124. Tonkonogy S, McKenzie D, Swain S. Regulation of isotype production by IL-4 and IL-5: Effects of lymphokines on Ig production depend on the state of activation of the responding B cells. J Immunol 1989;142:4351–4360.

125. Or R, Renz H, Terada N, Gelford E. IL-4 and IL-2 promote human T cell proliferation through symmetrical but independent pathways. Clin Immunol Immunopathol 1992;64:210–217.

126. Abehsira-Amar O, Gibert M, Joliy M, Theze J, Jankovic D. IL-4 plays a dominant role in the differential development of Tho into Th1 and Th2 cells. J Immunol 1992;148:3820–3829.

127. Feghali C, Bost K, Boulware D, Levy L. Mechanisms of pathogenesis in scleroderma. 1) Overproduction of IL-6 by fibroblasts cultured from affected skin sites of patients with scleroderma. J Rheumatol 1992;19:1207–1211.

128. Sironi M, Breviario F, Proserpio P, et al. IL-1 stimulates IL-6 production in endothelial cells. J Immunol 1989;145:549–553.

129. Walther Z, May LT, Sehgal PB. Transcriptional regulation of the interferon-B$_2$/B cell differentiation factor BSF-2/hepatocyte-stimulating factor gene in human fibroblasts by other cytokines. J Immunol 1985;140:974–977.

130. Endler-Jobst B, Schraven B, Hutmacher B, Meuer SC. Human T cell responses to IL-1 and IL-6 are dependent on signals mediated through CD2. J Immunol 1991;146:1736–1743.

131. Baggiolini M, Walz A, Kunkel SL. Neutrophil activating peptide 1 interleukin 8, a novel cytokine that activates neutrophils. J Clin Invest 1989;84:1045–1049.

132. Reitamo S, Remitz A, Varga J, Ceska M, Effenberger F, Uitto J. Demonstration of interleukin 8 and autoantibodies to interleukin 8 in the serum of patients with systemic sclerosis and related disorders. Arch Dermatol 1993;129:189–193.

133. LeRoy EC, Smith EA, Kahaleh MB, Trojanowska M, Silver RM. A strategy for determining the pathogenesis of systemic sclerosis. Is transforming growth factor beta the answer? Arthritis Rheum 1989;32:817–822.

134. Rossi P, De Crombrugghe B. Identification of a cell-specific transcriptional enhancer in the first intron of the mouse α2 (type I) collagen gene. Proc Natl Acad Sci 1987;84:5590–5594.

135. Baird A, Durkin T. Inhibition of endothelial cell proliferation by type β transforming growth factor: Interactions with acidic and basic fibroblast growth factors. Biochem Biophys Res Commun 1986;138:476–482.

136. Sutton AB, Canfield AE, Schor SL, et al. The response of endothelial cells to TGFβ-1 is dependent upon cell shape, proliferative state and the nature of the substratum. J Cell Sci 1991;99:777–787.

137. Kahaleh MB, Osborn I, LeRoy EC. Increased factor VIII/von Willebrand factor antigen and von Willebrand factor activity in scleroderma and in Raynaud's phenomenon. Ann Intern Med 1981;94:482–484.

138. Mannucci PM, Lombardi R, Lattuada A, Perticucci E, Valsecchi R, Remuzzi G. Supranormal von Willebrand factor multimers in scleroderma. Blood 1987;73:1586–1591.

139. Carson CW, Hunder GG, Kaplan KL, Johnson CM. Detection of circulating endothelial antigen. J Rheumatol 1991;18:379–383.

140. Matucci-Cerinic M, Pignone A, Lotti T, et al. Reduced angiotensin converting enzyme plasma activity in scleroderma. A marker of endothelial injury? J Rheumatol 1990;17:328–330.

141. Matucci-Cerinic M, Pignone A, Iannone F, et al. Clinical correlations of plasma ACE activity in systemic sclerosis: A longitudinal study of plasma ACE levels, endothelial injury and lung involvement. Resp Med 1990;84:283–287.

142. Matucci-Cerinic M, Jaffa A, Kahaleh BM. Angiotensin converting enzyme: An *in vivo* and *in vitro* marker of endothelial injury. J Lab Clin Med 1992;120:428–433.

143. Kahaleh BM, Matucci Cerinic M. Endothelial injury and its implications. In: Neri Serneri GG, Gensini GF, Abbate R, Prisco D, eds. Thrombosis: An update. Florence: Scientific Press, 1992;649–658.

144. Klagsbrun M, Folkman J. Angiogenesis. In : Sporn MB, Roberts AB, eds. Handbook of experimental pharmacology, peptide growth factors and their receptors II. Berlin: Springer Verlag, 1990;95:549–586.

145. Kaminski MJ, Majewski S, Jablonska S, Pawinska M. Lowered angiogeneic capability of peripheral blood lymphocytes in progressive systemic sclerosis (scleroderma). J Invest Dermatol 1984;82:239–243.

146. Koch AE, Litvak MA, Burrows JC, Polverini PJ. Decreased monocyte mediated angiogenesis in scleroderma. Clin Immunol Immunopathol 1992;64:153–160.

147. Majewski S, Skopinska-Rozewska E, Jablonska S, et al. Modulatory effect of sera from scleroderma patients on lymphocyte-induced angiogenesis. Arthritis Rheum 1985;28:1133–1139.

148. Klagsbrun M, D'Amore P. Regulators of angiogenesis. Annu Rev Physiol 1991;53:217–239.

149. Clawes AW, Reidy MA, Clawes MM. Kinetics of cellular proliferation after arterial injury I. Smooth muscle growth in the absence of endothelium. Lab Invest 1983;49:327–333.

150. Sato Y, Rifkin DB. Inhibition of endothelial cell movement by perycites and smooth muscle cells: Activation of a latent TGF beta 1 like molecule by plasmin derived co-culture. J Cell Biol 1989;109:309–315.

151. Bird D, Durkin T. Inhibition of endothelial cell proliferation by type eta TGF: Interactions with acidic and basic FG factors. Biochem Biophys Res Commun 1986;138:476–482.

152. Madri JA, Reidy MA, Kocher O, Bell L. Endothelial cell behaviour after denudation injury is modulated by TGF beta 1 and fibronectin. Lab Invest 1989;60:755–765.

153. Ingber DE, Folkman J. Mechanochemical switching between growth and differentiation during fibroblast growth factor-stimulated angiogenesis in vitro: Role of extracellular matrix. J Cell Biol 1989;109:317–330.

154. Madri SA, Merwin JR, Bell L, et al. Interactions of soluble factors in vascular response to injury. Modulation of cell phenotype. In: Simionescu N, Simionescu M, eds. Endothelial cell dysfunctions. New York: Plenum Press, 1992;11–19.

155. Fajardo LF, Kwaan HH, Kowalski J, Prionas SD, Allison AC. Dual role of tumor necrosis factor alfa in angiogenesis. Am J Pathol 1992;140:539–544.

156. Claman HN. On scleroderma: Mast cells, endothelial cells, and fibroblasts. JAMA 1989;262:1206–1209.

157. Vane JR, Anggard EE, Botting RM. Regulatory functions of the vascular endothelium. N Engl J Med 1990;323:27–36.

158. Friedhoff LT, Seibold JR, Kim HC, Simestet KS. Serotonin induced platelet aggregation in systemic sclerosis. Clin Exp Rheumatol 1984;2:119–123.

159. Kahaleh BM, Scharstein KK, LeRoy EC. Enhanced platelet adhesion to collagen in scleroderma: Effect of scleroderma plasma and scleroderma platelets. J Rheumatol 1985;12:468–471.

160. Kahaleh BM, Osborn I, LeRoy EC. Elevated levels of circulating platelet aggregates and beta-thromboglobulin in scleroderma. Ann Intern Med 1982;96:610–613.

161. Lima J, Fonnolosa V, Fernandez-Cortuo J, et al. Platelet activation, endothelial cell dysfunction in the absence of anticardiolipin antibodies in systemic sclerosis. J Rheumatol 1991;18:1833–1836.

162. Seibold JR, Harris JN. Plasma beta thromboglobulin in the differential diagnosis of Raynaud's phenomenon. J Rheumatol 1985;12:99–103.

163. Zimmerman G, Prescott SM, McIntyre TM. PAF: A fluid phase and cell-associated mediator of inflammation. In: Gallin JI, Goldstein IM, Snyderman R, eds. Inflammation: Basic principles and clinical correlates, ed. 2. New York: Raven Press, 1992.

164. Kubes P, Suzuki M, Granger N. PAF-induced microvascular dysfunction: role of adherent leucocytes. Am J Physiol 1990;258:G158–163.

165. Chung KF. PAF in inflammation and pulmonary disorders. Clin Sci 1992;83:127–138.

166. Nagao T, Vanhoutte P. Endothelium-derived hyperpolarizing factor and endothelium-dependent relaxations. Am J Resp Cell Mol Biol 1993;8:1–6.

167. McCall M, Vallance P. Nitric oxide takes centrestage with newly defined roles. TIPS 1992;13:1–6.

168. Burnstock G. Local mechanisms of blood flow control by perivascular nerves and endothelium. J Hypertens 1990;8(suppl 7):S95–S106.

169. Vanhoutte P. Could the absence or malfunction of vascular endothelium precipitate the occurrence of vasospasm? J Mol Cell Cardiol 1986;18:679–689.

170. Holt CM, Moult J, Lindsay N, Hughes P, Greaves M, Rowell NR. Prostacyclin production by human umbilical vein endothelium in response to

serum from patients with systemic sclerosis. Br J Rheumatol 1989;28:216–220.

171. Matucci-Cerinic M, Pietrini U, Marabini S. Local venomotor response to intravenous infusion of substance P and glyceryl trinitrate in systemic sclerosis. Clin Exp Rheumatol 1990;8:561–565.

172. Kahaleh BM, Fan PS, Matucci-Cerinic M, Stefanovic-Racic M, Ignarro L. Study of endothelial dependent relaxation in scleroderma. Arthritis Rheum 1993;36(suppl):b233.

173. Kahaleh BM. Endothelin, an endothelial-dependent vasoconstrictor in scleroderma. Enhanced production and profibriotic action. Arthritis Rheum 1991;34:978–983.

174. Yamane K, Miyouchi T, Suzuki N, et al. Significance of plasma endothelin 1 levels in patients with systemic sclerosis. J Rheum 1992;19:1566–1571.

175. Matucci-Cerinic M. Sensory neuropeptides and rheumatic diseases. Rheum Dis Clin North Am 1993;19:975–991.

176. Payan D. The role of neuropeptides in inflammation. In: Gallin JI, Goldstein IM, Snyderman R, eds. Inflammation, basic principles and clinical correlates. New York: Raven Press, 1992;177–192.

177. Matis WL, Lavker RM, Murphy GF. Substance P induces the expression of ELAM by microvascular endothelium. J Invest Dermatol 1990;94:492–496.

178. Speiser W, Anders E, Preissner KT, Wagner O, Muller-Berghaus G. Differences in coagulant and fibrinolytic activities of cultured human endothelial cells derived from omental tissue microvessels and umbilical veins. Blood 1987;69:964–967.

179. Bevilacqua MP, Pober JS, Majeau GR, Cotran RS, Gimbrone MA Jr. IL 1 induces biosynthesis and cell surface expression of procoagulant activity in human vascular endothelial cells. J Exp Med 1984;163:740–745.

180. Nawroth PP, Stern DM. Modulation of endothelial cell hemostatic properties by tumor necrosis factor. J Exp Med 1986;163:740–745.

181. Annamalai AE, Stewart GJ, Hansel B, et al. Expression of factor V on human umbilical vein endothelial cells is modulated by cell injury. Arteriosclerosis 1986;6:196–202.

182. Bevilacqua MP, Schleef RR, Gimbrone MA Jr, Loskutoff DJ. Regulation of the fibrinolytic system of cultured human vascular endothelium by interleukin 1. J Clin Invest 1986;78:587–591.

183. Schleef RR, Bevilacqua MP, Sawdey M, Gimbrone MA Jr, Loskutoff DJ. Cytokine activation of vascular endothelium. Effects on tissue type plasminogen activator and type 1 plasminogen activator inhibitor. JBC 1988;263:5797–5803.

184. Dejana E, Breviario F, Erroi A, et al. Modulation of endothelial cell functions by different molecular species of interleukin 1. J Clin Invest 1986;78:587–591.

185. Lee P Norman C, Sukenik S, Alderdice CA. The clinical significance of coagulation abnormalities in systemic sclerosis (scleroderma). J Rheumatol 1985;12:514–517.

186. Norton W. Comparison of the microangiopathy of systemic lupus eryhtematosus, dermatomyositis, scleroderma and diabetes mellitus. Lab Invest 1970;22:301–308.

187. Gratwick GM, Klein R, Sergent J, et al. Fibrinogen turnover in progressive systemic sclerosis. Arthritis Rheum 1978;21:343–347.

188. Rothschild B, Thompson LD, Chesney M, et al. Perturbation of fibrinolysis inhibitors in progressive systemic sclerosis. Med Hypotheses 1985;16:253–260.

189. Cunliffe WJ, Menon IS. Blood fibrinolytic activity in diseases of small blood vessels and the effect of low molecular weight dextran. Br J Dermatol 1969;81:220–229.

190. Furey NL, Schmid FR, Kwaan HC, et al. Arterial thrombosis in scleroderma. Br J Dermatol 1975;93:683–687.

191. Browse NI, Gray L, Jarrett PEM, et al. Blood and vein fibrinolytic activity in health and vascular diseases. Br Med J 1977;1:478–483.

192. Holland CD, Jayson MIV. Venous blood fibrinolysis and fibrinolytic potential in primary Raynaud's phenomenon and systenic scleroderma associatcd Raynaud's phenomenon. In: Black C, Myers AR, eds. London: Gower Med Publ Lmtd, 1985;267–274.

193. Keegan AC, Holland CD, Jayson MIV. Loss of diurnal variation in fibrinolytic activity in systemic sclerosis. Br J Rheumatol 1985;24:21.

194. Lotti T, Matucci-Cerinic M, Marmugi D, Fabbri P. Cutaneous fibrinolytic activity in scleroderma. Clin Exp Rheumatol 1985;3:248–251.

195. Matucci-Cerinic M, Lotti T, Lombardi A, et al. Cutaneous and plasma fibrinolytic activity in systemic sclerosis. Evidence of normal plasminogen activation. Int J Dermatol 1990;29:644–648.

195a. Pignone A, Lombardi A, Matucci-Ceninic M, Lotti T. Chronobiology, fibrinolysis and systemic sclerosis (letter, comment). J Amer Acad 1994;31(2 Part 1):297–298.

196. Godin-Ostro E, Mitrane M, Heller I, et al. Plasma plasminogen activator in systemic sclerosis. Arthritis Rheum 1985;28:80.

197. Kahan A, Awada H, Sultan Y, Menkes C, Amor B. Tissue plasminogen activator activity and tPA inhibition (PAI) in systemic sclerosis. Arthritis Rheum 1988;31:S101.

198. Falanga V, Kruskal J, Franks JJ. Fibrin and fibrinogen related antigens in systemic sclerosis (scleroderma). J Am Acad Dermatol 1991;25:771–775.

199. Cotran RS. New roles for the endothelium in inflammation and immunity. Am J Pathol 1987; 129:407–413.

200. Zimmerman GA, Prescott SM, McIntyre TM. Endothelial cell interactions with granulocytes: Tethering and signaling molecules. Immunol Today 1992;13:93–100.

201. Shimizu Y, Newman W, Tanaka Y, Shaw S. Lymphocyte interactions with endothelial cells. Immunol Today 1992;13:106–112.

202. Sollberg S, Peltonen J, Uitto J, Jimenez SA. Elevated expression of beta 1 and beta 2 integrins, intercellular adhesion molecules 1, and endothelial leukocyte adhesion molecule 1 in the skin of patients with systemic sclerosis of recent onset. Arthritis Rheum 1992;35:290–298.

203. Majewski S, Hunzelmann N, Johnson JP, et al. Expression of intercellular adhesion molecule 1 in the skin of patients with systemic scleroderma. J Invest Dermatol 1991;97:667–671.

204. Sfikakis PP, Tesar J, Baraf H, et al. Circulating intercellular adhesion molecules 1 in patients systemic sclerosis. Clin Immunol Immunopathol 1993;68:88–92.

205. Abraham D, Lupoli S, McWhirter A, et al. Expression and function of surface antigens on scleroderma fibroblasts. Arhritis Rheum 1991;34:1164–1172.

206. Smith TH, Korn JH. Lymphocyte modulation of fibroblasts function in systemic sclerosis. Clin Dermatol 1994;12:369–377.

207. Clements P, Lachenbruch P, Sterz A, et al. Cyclosporine in systemic sclerosis. Results of a 48-week open study. Arthritis Rheum 1993;36: 75–83.

ANGELINE DOUVAS

9

Pathogenesis: Serologic Correlates

Overview

Humoral autoimmunity in scleroderma is expressed as a series of antibodies reacting with certain defined nuclear and cytoplasmic (n/c) structures. The n/c structures have some interesting and essential regulatory functions in normal cells that include unwinding supercoiled DNA, splicing nuclear RNA, transporting and assembling ribosomal components, regulating transcription, and segregating chromosomes during mitosis. This chapter summarizes a wealth of current data bearing on two key questions regarding the pathologic significance of autoantibodies in scleroderma. The first question is whether the autoantibodies, autoantigens, or their genes have a direct role in initiating or mediating pathophysiologic events. The second question is whether the autoantibodies are elicited by direct stimulation by the identified n/c antigens or by an indirect mechanism such as molecular mimicry (to be defined later in the chapter). These inquiries are supported by significant recent advances in the following areas: in associating antigen/antibody (ag/ab) reactivities with specific alleles of the HLA gene complex; in correlating ag/ab specificities with clinical and prognostic patterns; in elucidating the functions, regulatory roles and molecular structures of some of the major nuclear/cytoplasmic (n/c) antigens; in identifying specific epitopes within the gross molecular structures; and in recognizing structural similarities between these epitopes and other molecules with potential pathologic significance.

One of the concepts which finds support in recent studies is that the regulatory functions of some of the n/c antigens may be directly linked to pathogenesis. For example, certain signs and symptoms in polymyositis/dermatomyositis (PM/DM) are associated with antibodies to a discrete cluster of tRNA synthetases, in what has been identified as an "anti-synthetase syndrome" (1). Other examples, in which a mechanistic connection may be inferred between the function of the antigen and clinical manifestations, are discussed in this chapter.

Another concept that is supported by current studies is that "molecular mimicry" may play an important role in immunopathogenesis. The term "molecular mimicry," coined by Damian in 1964, is defined as the sharing of epitopes in proteins having otherwise different structures and functions (2). Progress in characterizing specific epitopes and epitope regions (ER) in the major n/c antigens has led to the recognition that their amino acid sequences are not unique, but occur in other molecules that are more exposed to the immune system. Therefore, autoantibodies specific for n/c antigens may cross-react with these structures. Conversely, antibodies resulting from immunization with these structures may cross-react with n/c antigens. Examples of such similarities, or homologies, which may be relevant to immunopathology in scleroderma include sequence similarities between the major scleroderma nuclear antigens and: (a) HLA class I and II molecules (3); (b) neuromuscular proteins and adrenergic and cholinergic receptors (4,5); and

(c) immunopathic viruses, including HIV-1 (3, 6), murine leukemia virus (7), type C retroviruses (8), adenoviruses (6,9,10), and rhabdoviruses (11). Thus, the immunologic cross-reactivities resulting from molecular mimicry (2,12) may play a direct role in the pathogenesis of scleroderma. The extrapolation of this concept beyond the protein level, to DNA sequences, suggests that regulatory functions expressed by exogenous pathogens may activate n/c antigen expression, which in turn may have regulatory effects on the pathogen. This cycle is suggested by the effects of the La/SS-B antigen on both the transcription and translation of poliovirus functions (13).

Further discussion of some of these provocative concepts rests on new findings on autoimmune reactivities in scleroderma per se, and in associated or overlapping disorders. The next section of this chapter (*Auto-AG/AB Reactivities in SSc and CREST*) undertakes a survey of ag/ab reactivities in scleroderma *per se*, where the prevalence of autoantibodies in all forms of the disorder, excluding morphea and linear scleroderma, is 90% to 96% (14,15). The two major clinical subsets of scleroderma, accounting for 90% of the cases of cutaneous thickening (15), are diffuse cutaneous sclerosis, synonymous with systemic sclerosis (SSc), and limited cutaneous sclerosis (16), also referred to as CREST syndrome (an acronym for calcinosis, Raynaud's phenomenon, esophageal dysfunction, sclerodactyly, and telangiectasias) (17). Auto-ag/ab reactivities in SSc and CREST are discussed in the next section and in Tables 9.1 and 9.2. This discussion covers the molecular and functional characteristics of the n/c antigens, antibody prevalence and HLA associations, clinical and prognostic correlations, and epitope characterization. The remaining 10% of clinical subsets, representing the overlapping or associated syndromes, include mixed connective tissue disease (MCTD), dermatomyositis (DM), polymyositis (PM) and Sjögen's syndrome (SS). These are discussed in the section titled *Auto-AG/AB Reactivities in Associated Syndromes* and in Tables 9.2 and 9.4. For current interest and future reference,

the chromosomal locations of the genes encoding a few of the major n/c antigens are presented in Table 9.3. The *Summary and Conclusions* section describes some of the direct pathogenetic roles suggested for autoantibodies and n/c antigens in scleroderma, and also discusses the possible immunogenic and etiologic contributions of other factors, including viruses and molecular mimicry.

Auto-AG/AB Reactivities in SSc and CREST

Three types of auto-ab/ag reactivities were originally discerned in scleroderma by indirect immunofluorescence (IF) on rat or mouse tissue sections: (*a*) an antibody type giving a diffuse pattern of staining of nuclei, reacting with a soluble and precipitable nuclear antigen originally called Scl-1 (18). The antigen was found to be a 70kD, chromatin-associated protein, which was given the clinical designation Scl-70 (19), and later shown to be a DNA topoisomerase I (20–22); (*b*) an antibody reactivity which binds to a series of centromere proteins, designated CENP-A to -F (23,24); and (*c*) an antibody reactivity localizing to nucleoli in IF assays (18). The discussion of these three reactivities begins with Scl-70/ topo I. Some of the auto-ag/ab reactivities have been named after the antigen, whereas some have been named after the associated clinical syndrome, the patient in which they were first described, or combinations thereof.

SCL-70/TOPO I

Molecular and Functional Characteristics

Scl-70/topo I is a nuclear protein that has been isolated from mammalian tissues in forms ranging from 100 kD to 60kD (Table 9.1). It is a basic polypeptide (pI = 10.7), which is phosphorylated both *in vivo* and *in vitro* by a casein kinase type II (25). Its sequence reveals asymmetry between the NH_2 and COOH-terminal ends. The highly charged amino acids are concentrated at the

Table 9.1. Autoantigens in SSc and CREST Syndrome

Clinical Designation	Molecular Description	Functional Association	Prevalence	Reference
Sci-70	100 kD polypeptide; 70kD cleavage product	DNA topoisomerase 1	28–70% of SSc[a]	18, 19–22, 25–54
Centromere	CENP-A (17kD), -B (80kD), -C (140kD), -D (50kD), -E (300kD) and -F (400kD)	Segregation of chromosomes during mitosis and meiosis	55–96% in CREST[b]	23, 24, 45, 57–96
Nucleolar	*multiple structures*		8–20%	15, 16, 97–109
	14 to 210 kD subunits	RNA polymerase 1	4%	98
	Fibrillarin	U[3] snRNP	8%	99, 100
	Th	Endoribonuclease	10% OF CREST[b]	100, 101
	NOR-90	Nucleolar organizer	Rare	102
	nucleolin(110KD)	Multiple functions	Unknown	103

[a]SSc = diffuse cutaneous scleroderma.
[b]CREST = usually meant to connote limited cutaneous scleroderma.

NH_2-end, unlike the centromere proteins and U1 snRNP protein 70K (discussed below), which have the opposite polarity.

The antigenic polypeptide is an enzyme, a DNA topoisomerase I (topo I) (20–22), which catalyzes relaxation of supercoiled DNA by breaking one of the strands, unwinding the helix to a lower torsional strain, and repairing the break (26,27). DNA unwinding is essential for gene expression. Topo I breaks and unwinds genes at specific DNA base sequences (26). The collagen genes, which contain multiple copies of these base sequences, may be selectively activated by increases in topo I activity, thereby contributing to collagen overexpression in scleroderma (28).

Topo I has two pharmacologic inhibitors: an alkaloid, camptothecin (27), and zinc (29). Antibodies occurring in scleroderma also inhibit catalytic activity (30–35). The active site is located between amino acids 658 and 750 in the carboxy-terminal end of the protein (34).

Antibody Prevalence, Ethnic Variability and HLA Associations

In the United States, the overall prevalence of antibodies to Scl-70/topo I in scleroderma is approximately 26%, whereas in the diffuse form of the disease (SSc) the prevalence is 34% or higher (16,36,37). In comparisons of African-Americans and Caucasians in the US, the reported prevalence in African-Americans is slightly higher (25%–37%) than that in Caucasians (17%–29%) (38,39). More striking differences were reported in a comparison of Caucasian Australians with SSc to Thai patients with SSc (6% and 70%, respectively) (37). Similarly, Japanese scleroderma patients have a considerably higher prevalence (65%) than Caucasian American patients (29%) (38).

Although several factors may account for the variable prevalence of anti-Scl-70/topo I (abbreviated topo I) antibodies in different populations, one likely explanation is the variable distribution of HLA class II alleles (Table 9.2). In both American Caucasians and Japanese, genetic predisposition to topo I reactivity is associated with the DQB1 locus. In Japanese patients who are topo I(+), there is a 100% association with the DQB1*0601 and DQB1*0301 alleles (38). These two alleles are detected in 25% and 14% of the general population, respectively. In American Caucasians, however, the DQB1* 0601 allele is detectable in only 2% of the general population, and the primary association with topo I antibodies is with the DQB1*0301 allele, detectable in 14% of the population (39). Interestingly, one study found that the DQB1*0301 allele, and other DQB1 alleles having tyrosine at position 30, were present in 100% of Caucasian patients who were topo I antibody positive (40). In Japanese

gen-driven mechanism (14,30,49). The alternative is that the antibodies arise initially from a more restricted response, which is activated by a molecular mimic. The discovery of monoclonal reactivities to the same hydrophilic region of Scl-70/topo I in both humans and TSK mice, and perhaps to the same epitope (54), suggests that B cell clones specific for this region exist in the autoimmune repertoire and may be activated by a homologous microbial sequence. Similarly, Kato et al identified a broad region of Scl-70/topo I (amino acids 349–570) reported to contain a "universal epitope" reacting with all Scl-70/topo I(+) sera (51). The authors suggest activation of a response to this epitope by molecular mimicry and subsequent development of an antigen-driven response. Other homologies to potential mimics presented above are the **EKYINK** sequence, which is homologous to p30^{gag} (6), and the **FLEDR** homology to certain HLA DRB alleles (38) (see Table 9.2).

Based on other models of autoimmunity, it is possible for a single T cell clone activated by a microbial epitope to stimulate multiple clones of B cells, resulting in a polyclonal antibody response (55,56). However, this model is relevant only if the initial epitope has a demonstrated pathologic role. Unlike the well-established paradigms of ankylosing spondylitis and myasthenia gravis, cross-reactivities associated with pathogenesis have not been demonstrated in scleroderma. Furthermore, pathogenetic inferences based on single homologies between Scl-70/topo I and microbial proteins should be regarded with caution. We surveyed eight n/c antigens (including Scl-70/topo I) and 41 normal human proteins for homologies to 61 proteins belonging to viruses that are human pathogens (6). The result was that at least one in three normal proteins has an exact 6-amino acid homology to a viral protein. However, three of the n/c antigens, including Scl-70/topo I, each had multiple homologies to immunoinfective viruses. This finding suggests that molecular mimicry may be the driving mechanism behind autoantibody production in some instances. However, because there are mul-

tiple homologies (17 in Scl-70/topo I), it is unnecessary to postulate a broadening mechanism for generating a polyclonal response. The pathophysiologic significance of multiple homologies is discussed further in relation to the U1 snRNP protein 70K.

THE CENTROMERE PROTEINS CENP-A, -B, -C, -D, -E, AND -F

Molecular and Functional Characteristics

The centromere is the primary constriction of mitotic chromosomes. The kinetochore, situated on either side of the centromere, is a trilaminar, disc-shaped structure which serves as the attachment site for spindle microtubules. The microtubules facilitate chromosome alignment and separation during mitosis (57,58). The centromere antigen, a major target of antibodies in the CREST variant of scleroderma (59), is a complex of at least six polypeptides: CENP-A through CENP-F (see Table 9.1). The specific localization of the individual proteins, as inferred from immunoelectron microscopy, is depicted graphically in reference 59 and other sources that will be cited in following paragraphs. More than 90% of ACA-positive sera from scleroderma patients react with CENP-A, -B, and -C (60). Because of the size of CENP-C, it was thought to be a possible precursor of CENP-A and -B (60). However, despite some crossreactivity between antibodies to the latter proteins and CENP-C (60), the primary sequence of this polypeptide is not appreciably homologous to CENP-A and -B.

Injection of antibodies specific for anti-A-, B-, or -C into nuclei disrupts mitosis (61). Although the CENP polypeptides have similar clinical associations, each has distinctive structural and functional characteristics (as discussed in the following paragraphs). The highly unusual epitopes in this cluster of proteins, which are homologous to sequences in other cellular organelles, receptors, and microbial proteins, have pathogenetic implications, which are discussed later in the chapter.

CENP-A (17-19 kD). CENP-A was first described as a 19.5 kD protein that reacted with nearly all ACA-positive scleroderma sera (62). This basic protein is so similar to histone H3 of the H3/H4 nucleosomal core that it is sometimes referred to as a histone (63). Although it co-purifies with H3/H4 (63,64), it is centromere specific, owing to a distinctive centromere binding domain (62). Moreover, it is retained in chromatin during mammalian spermatogenesis, whereas histones H3 and H4 are replaced by protamines (65). It has been difficult to define the distribution of CENP-A in the centromere, because purified antibodies to this protein cross-react with CENP-B (57) (also discussed later in this section under *Epitopes and Homologies*).

CENP-B (80 kD). This fascinating and anomalous DNA-binding protein of 594 amino acids is the major component of the centromere antigen, reacting with 100% of ACA (+) sera (66,67). Its acidic character derives from two domains in the COOH-end, one of nearly uninterrupted glutamic acid residues and the other a mixture of glutamic and aspartic acid (66). It has been suggested that the acidic domains serve to "capture" the basic NH_2-ends of histones (66). The DNA-binding domain is in the NH_2-terminal 134 amino acids (67), which form alpha-helical structures (68,69). The helical domains bind to alpha-satellite, also called alphoid DNA, which is one of the repetitive families of DNA occurring in the centromere (70–72). A 17 base-pair tandemly repeating sequence within the alphoid DNA, referred to as the CENP-B box, constitutes the specific binding site for individual CENP-B molecules (73), which dimerize to form higher order structures (67).

The primary role of CENP-B thus appears to be in organizing the formation of centromeric heterochromatin. This conclusion is supported by immunoelectron microscopic studies, which show that >95% of CENP-B is distributed throughout this heterochromatin (74). Unlike CENP-A and -C, levels of CENP-B vary widely among human chromosomes in proportion to the amount of alpha-satellite DNA in the chromosomes (66,70,73).

As summarized in Table 9.3, the gene encoding CENP-B has been localized to chromosome 20, as has the gene encoding Scl-70/topo I (75, 76). The gene for CENP-C, discussed in the next paragraph, is on chromosome 12. Other genes encoding major n/c antigens in scleroderma are also shown.

CENP-C (140 kD). Unlike CENP-B, this protein is present in approximately equal amounts in all human chromosomes (24,74) and is essential for normal centromere function (77). Immunoelectron microscopy reveals that CENP-C is a component of the inner kinetochore plate (77). Its amino acid sequence reveals short hydrophilic stretches dispersed relatively evenly throughout the polypeptide without the asymmetry that is characteristic of Scl-70/topo I and CENP-B. Like Scl-70/topo I, it is basic with a calculated pI of 9.4 (77).

CENP-C is far less abundant in nuclei than -A and -B, and there are correspondingly lower titers of antibodies in scleroderma sera. Given its restricted localization in the inner kinetochore plate, it seems more likely that antibodies to this protein are generated by cross-reactivity rather than primary immunization.

Table 9.3. Chromosome Localization of Some n/c Antigens

n/c Antigen	Chromosome	Locus	Reference
CENP B	20		75
CENP C	12		75
Scl-70/topo I	20	q11.2–13.1	76
U1 RNA	1	p36.3	119
U1 snRNP 70K	19	q13.3	120
snRNP A	19		121
snRNP B	15	q11–13	122
snRNP B'	15	q11–14	122
snRNP E	1	q25–43	123
Ro/SSA 52kD	11		155
Ro/SSA 60kD[a]	19		156
Ro/SSA 60kD[a]	1	q31	157

[a]The gene encoding this polypeptide has been assigned to chromosome 19 and chromosome 1 by McCauliffe et al. (160) and Chan et al. (161), respectively.

CENP-D (50 kD), -E (300 kD), and -F (400 kD). CENP-D is only found in mitotically active chromosomes (79,80). It is very homologous to a product of the RCC1 gene, which is involved in regulating the onset of chromosome condensation (81). CENP-E is identifiable in centromeres only in the early stages of mitosis (82) and is degraded in the later stages (82,83). It becomes redistributed to the spindle midzone during anaphase, which suggests a role in chomatid separation (83). CENP-F is homogeneously distributed in nuclei during G2, but during mitosis is localized to the outer kinetochore plate (84). Autoimmune sera that recognize CENP-F also react with determinants in the central helical rod of CENP-E (84).

Of considerable relevance to the question of how antibodies to the centromere proteins are generated are calculations demonstrating that they are all present in low copy number in nuclei. The most abundant of the proteins, CENP-B, is estimated to be present in 20,000 to 50,000 copies per cell (66,71). Moreover, with the exception of CENP-B, which is distributed throughout the central domain of the centromere, the CENP molecules are highly restricted in their localization, as noted previously (66,70,73). Thus, the most plausible mechanism by which these recondite proteins become targets of the most prevalent autoantibodies in scleroderma is some form of cross-reactivity. An exploration of the types of molecules that bear substantial homology to major CENP epitopes, and which in principal may be involved in cross-reactivities, is attempted later in this section under *Epitopes and Homologies.*

Antibody Prevalence, Ethnic Variability, and HLA Associations

The overall reported prevalence of ACA in scleroderma is between 19% and 41% (36,39,45,59, 85). In African-Americans, the reported prevalence ranges from 4% to 11% (38,39) and in Japanese, ranges from 12% to 16% (38,86). In patients whose disease meets the criteria for the CREST variant (16), the reported prevalence ranges from 55% to 96% (36,45,59,85). ACA

have been reported in 11% of patients with primary biliary cirrhosis (59), 5% of morphea patients (59), 19% to 34% of Raynaud's patients (36,85), 3% of systemic lupus erythematosus (SLE) patients (85), and 0% to 3% of normals (59,85). The presence of ACA and anti-topo I antibodies is mutually exclusive (45). All anti-centromere sera have antibodies to CENP-B (60, 87), while 50% have antibodies to CENP-C (87).

ACA are associated with HLA class II types DR1, DR5, and the Dw 13 subtype of DR4 (45, 88). Further, a DQB1 allele having a polar amino acid at position 26, rather than leucine, was found in 100% of ACA(+) patients in one study (88). The presence or absence of a leucine at position 26 of DQB1 appears to be important in autoantibody reactivities associated with scleroderma including antibodies to Ro, which are discussed later in this chapter. A subgroup of ACA(+) patients is defined by the presence of one or more of alleles of DR1, DR4, or DRw8 (43). This group consists of patients with rheumatoid arthritis (RA).

Clinical and Prognostic Associations

Owing to the association between ACA and CREST, the clinical manifestations most often present are those represented by the CREST acronym. The frequency of pulmonary fibrosis is significantly lower in ACA(+) patients than in Scl-70/topo I(−) or ANA(−) scleroderma patients (36,45). Other manifestations that occur in significantly lower frequency include heart involvement (6% of ACA(+) versus 16% with Scl-70/topo I antibodies) (45), renal involvement (45), facial skin involvement (36), and arthritis (36). Occurring in significantly higher frequency are telangiectasias and calcinosis (36,37,45). Raynaud's phenomenon (RP) occurs with high frequency in all scleroderma patients (45,60). However, in a prospective study of patients with primary Raynaud's, two thirds of those becoming ANA(+) developed ACA associated with telangiectasias (37). Despite the commonality of clinical features in ACA(+) and (−) scleroderma patients, the lack of overlap between ACA and

Scl-70/topo I antibodies has led to the suggestion that these are two distinct disease entities (45), a view for which there is some support in the HLA associations (see Table 9.2). ACA(+) sera are heterogeneous with respect to their reactivity to four different CENP-B epitopes; however, epitope preference does not correlate with clinical presentation (89).

Among CREST patients, Weiner et al (36) found no correlation between disease severity score and the presence of ACA (36). However, in a Japanese study, the 10-year survival of ACA(+) patients was 93% versus 66% for Scl-70/topo I(+), 72% for anti-U1 snRNP(+), and 30% for anti-RNP polymerases I, II, and III (86).

An interesting study by Jabs et al analyzed chromosome breaks and aneuploidy in ACA(+) and (−) scleroderma patients and attempted to correlate the findings with disease classification (87). A type I, II, III disease classification was employed: I = sclerodactyly, II = skin stiffness proximal to the MCP joints but sparing the trunk, and III = skin stiffness including the trunk. Reactivities to individual CENP proteins in the sera of ACA(+) patients were analyzed by immunoblot analysis. All ACA(+) sera reacted to CENP-B and 50% also to CENP-C. Cytogenetic analysis of the PBMC revealed that aneuploidy was significantly higher in ACA(+) scleroderma patients than in ACA(−) patients or normal controls. Type I patients, which were predominantly ACA(+), had significantly more aneuploidy and chromatid breaks than type III patients. Interestingly, the presence of aneuploidy in cells from the 50% of ACA(+) patients who were CENP-C(+) was 2-fold higher than in the CENP-B(+) and CENP-C(−) patients. These results were interpreted as suggesting that the presence of ACA may directly lead to centromere dysfunction (87). The potential role of autoantibodies in pathogenesis is discussed further in *Summary and Conclusions.*

Epitopes and Homologies

In view of the restricted localization and low copy number of the CENP polypeptides (as re-viewed in the previous section) the question arises as to how their epitopes, if unique, have sufficient contact with the immune system to elicit any type of immunologic reaction. As part of a review of epitope distribution and structure, this section discusses the multiplicity of homologies between the CENP proteins and proteins that are far more abundant and immunologically accessible. The existence of these homologies lends support to molecular mimicry as the mechanism whereby ACA are generated. However, like the Sm/U1RNP antigens in SLE and the Ro-SSA/La-SSB antigens, the centromere complex defines a "cluster" of reactivities, which is regarded as evidence for an antigen-driven mechanism (90). The term "clustering" describes the occurrence in a particular syndrome of antibodies to two or more distinct molecules (e.g., a polypeptide and nucleic acid, two or more polypeptides, or two or more loosely associated particles such as U1 and U2 snRNP). However, what appears to be clustering may actually be cross-reactivity to homologous epitopes or to conformational epitopes, which may include molecular configurations from both a protein and its associated nucleic acid. Thus, the anti-centromere reactivities, as analyzed at the level of epitopes, may contain important clues pertaining to the generation of autoantibodies in scleroderma and related autoimmune disorders.

CENP-A is unique among the centromere proteins because of its structural relationship to histone 3. However, there are several regions in CENP-A that are non-homologous to histones (65). In particular, the amino acid sequence **EGEGEEEGEE** is homologous to alpha tubulin and also to an epitope in CENP-B. Antibodies to this sequence may therefore account for some of the cross-reactivity to CENP-B.

Affinity purified antibodies to **CENP-B** bind to both CENP-A and -C (24,91). Two dominant epitopes (I and II) have been identified in the acidic COOH-end of CENP-B and two epitopes (III and IV) in the extreme NH_2 end (66,67,70, 92). The NH_2-terminal epitopes occur in the helix-loop-helix (HLH) region which binds to

DNA, and antibodies to these epitopes disrupt DNA binding (67,70). CENP-B is a highly conserved protein in mammals, although some divergence between humans and mice has been detected in the epitope II region (92). The dominant epitope regions in the acidic COOH-end of CENP-B have multiple homologies to a variety of proteins with seemingly unrelated functions. Homologies to DNA viruses include the sequences **EEEGE** (in HSV-1) and **DEDDDD** (in HSV-1 and CMV) (6). Homologies to HIV-1 include the sequence **EEEGGE**, which is an epitope in the HIV-1 envelope glycoprotein gp41 (2,6). In addition, homologous acidic sequences are found in several human intracellular and extracellular proteins. Earnshaw (93) notes that anionic (A−) regions, defined as local high concentrations of acidic residues, occur in the nucleus in the high-mobility group (HMG) proteins, in nucleoplasmin, and Scl-70/topo I. Suggested functions for these regions include unfolding condensed chromatin, binding to histones, and stabilizing enzyme complexes (93).

In addition to the homology to tubulin, we have found that acidic configurations occur in a family of calcium-binding proteins, which may be relevant to the pathophysiology of CREST (94). These include calcium ion channels in both cholinergic and adrenergic autonomic receptors (e.g., the acetylcholine receptor), which are of possible relevance to the physiology of RP. Calcium binding sites consisting of stretches of glutamic acid also occur in thrombin, troponin (both smooth and skeletal muscle), and in bone sialoprotein. Also, the sequence **EEEEEAEEGGEE** occurs in the triplet neurofilament protein. In an ELISA analysis of ACA from 24 CREST patients, we found that subgroups of patients reacted with one or more of these proteins. Serum from a patient with sensoryneural hearing loss reacted uniquely with a 150 kD neurofilament polypeptide (94). The pathogenetic significance of these reactivities will be discussed further in the concluding section *Summary and Conclusions*. It is apparent that antibodies are not only able to en-

ter living cells (95,96), but they also can clear viruses and viral RNAs from cells of the nervous system (96).

CENP-C has at least two separate epitope regions (24, 78). Rabbits immunized with CENP-C produce antibodies cross-reacting with CENP-A and -B (78). Although the basis for this cross-reactivity has not been fully explored, CENP-C shares the sequence **DDDDEE** with CENP-B. As mentioned previously, **CENP-D** is extensively homologous to RCC1, which is a regulator of chromosome condensation (81). Autoimmune sera that recognize the central helical rod of **CENP-E** also react with determinants in **CENP-F** (84).

This synopsis of the CENP polypeptides has focused on properties that may help to understand how antibodies to these proteins are generated. Reactivity to the CENP proteins nearly fulfills the criteria for an antigen-driven response (90), namely:

The response is polyclonal.
Discontinuous epitopes are present.
There is clustering of antigens and antibodies.
There are antigenic sites that are exposed to the surface and occur in hypermobile sites or in active sites.

However, the CENP proteins are recondite antigens. Although some of the intensely hydrophilic epitopes may be on the surface, their functions suggest that they may be masked by proteins of the opposite charge. Furthermore, their low copy number and localization in centromeres renders it much less likely that they will come in contact with the immune system than their homologous counterparts in viruses, muscle, bone, microtubules, and neurofilaments. Nevertheless, it is possible that some etiologic agent may greatly alter the expression of the CENP genes, resulting in quantitative or qualitative changes which may provide direct antigen stimulation to the immune system. This interesting scenario, which might result in clinically significant cross-reactivities to external proteins, is discussed further in *Summary and Conclusions*.

THE NUCLEOLAR ANTIGENS

To date, five nucleolar structures have been identified as the targets of antibodies in scleroderma (see Table 9.1) (97–103). A sixth, PM-Scl, is an antigen in the associated syndrome polymyositis, which is discussed in the next major section titled *Auto-AG/AB Reactivities in Associated Syndromes*. Among the rheumatic syndromes, antinucleolar antibodies are restricted to scleroderma (97). They also appear following exposure to silica and other agents inducing a sclerodermatous clinical pattern (104), and following exposure of laboratory animals to silver and mercury (105,106). Antibodies to fibrillarin, Nor-90, and other nucleolar polypeptides are also associated with hepatocellular carcinoma (107).

Molecular and Functional Characteristics

As revealed by electron microscopy, the nucleolus is organized into three distinct regions: (*a*) a granular component, composed of 15 to 20 nm particles; (*b*) a fibrillar component of 5 to 10 nm fibrils; and (*c*) a denser fibrillar component surrounding the 5 to 10 nm fibrils (108). These levels of organization are reflected in the different IF patterns seen with anti-nucleolar antibodies from scleroderma patients. The genes for mammalian 28S, 18S, and 5.8S ribosomal RNA are clustered in the nucleolus and are transcribed as a 45S precursor by RNA polymerase I. The precursor is then spliced by U3 snRNP, which is located in the dense fibrillar region (109).

Antibodies to **RNA polymerase I** characteristically give a speckled nucleolar staining pattern (98). Sera with this type of staining pattern immunoprecipitate several polypeptide subunits of RNA polymerase I, with molecular weights ranging from 14,000 to 210,000 kD. Microinjection of these antibodies into nuclei results in marked reduction in the accumulation of newly synthesized 28S and 18S RNA (98). **Fibrillarin** is a 34-36 kD component of the U3 snRNP particle (109) and is also found associated with other nucleolar snRNP. This polypeptide is the major target of anti-U3 antibodies, which are highly specific for scleroderma (16,99,100). It localizes to the dense fibrillar region of the nucleolus. Fibrillarin is thought to play a role in maturation and methylation of pre-ribosomal RNA and in ribosome assembly (99). Whether or not fibrillarin is an RNA binding protein has not been determined, although it has an 8-amino acid sequence resembling the RNA binding site of other proteins in the snRNP family (99) (see also the discussion of U1 snRNP in the section titled *Auto-AG/AB Reactivities in Associated Syndromes*).

Anti-**Th** antibodies recognize a 40kD protein component of the **Th RNP** particle (100,101). This interesting particle, located in the granular compartment of the nucleolus, is an endoribonuclease (100). Anti-Th antibodies have been found in scleroderma, primary Raynaud's syndrome, and SLE (101). **NOR-90** is a 90kD polypeptide found in the nucleolus-organizer regions (NOR) located at the distal ends of chromosomes 13, 14, 15, 21, and 22 (102). Nucleoli reform around these regions after mitosis, but the exact role of NOR-90 and other NOR proteins in this process is unknown.

Nucleolin is a 92 to 110 kD protein with multiple functions, including regulating RNA polymerase I transcription of pre-ribosomal RNA and nucleocytoplasmic transport of ribosomal components (103). Antibodies to this protein are generally of the IgM isotype and occur in SLE as well as scleroderma. Antibodies have also been detected in patients with acute hepatitis A and infectious mononucleosis, but have not been detected in normal sera.

Nucleolin belongs to a family of proteins having lengthy stretches of >25 amino acids consisting almost entirely of glutamic acid. Other proteins in this family are CENP-B, the glutamic acid rich protein (GARP) of *Plasmodium falciparum*, and the high mobility group protein HMG1. Because of their unbroken acidity, these stretches in nucleolin cross-react with anti-single stranded DNA antibodies occurring in SLE.

Antibody Prevalence, Ethnic Variability, and HLA Associations

The overall prevalence of anti-nucleolar antibodies in scleroderma is estimated to be 8% to 20% (45,97,98,100). Antibodies to RNA polymerase I are restricted to scleroderma. In one series that examined 208 scleroderma patients, these antibodies were found in 4% of the patients (98). Anti-fibrillarin (U3 RNP) antibodies occur primarily in scleroderma, but are also detected in SLE, DLE, RA, and myositis (100). Antibodies to Th are most prevalent in scleroderma but are also found in SLE (16,100,101). The prevalence of antibodies to nucleolin is difficult to estimate because of cross-reactivity to other proteins containing glutamic acid stretches and to single-stranded DNA (103). Antibodies to the NOR of nucleoli are rare. In one study, only 9 of 254 patients with rheumatic diseases were found to have antibodies recognizing the NOR, of which five patients had scleroderma and the remainder had unknown diagnoses (102). These prevalences seem to apply to both Caucasians and Japanese (86,97,98,103). No HLA associations have been reported.

Clinical and Prognostic Associations

As a group, patients with anti-RNA polymerase antibodies (I, II, or III) have been reported to have the lowest 10-year survival (30%) of all scleroderma patients that have been grouped according to antibody specificity (86). Antibodies to RNA polymerase I are associated with a high prevalence of organ involvement including cardiac and renal, and particularly renal, crisis (86, 97,98). There is an association with diffuse scleroderma (98), with arthritis, arthralgias, and tendon involvement as presenting signs and symptoms (97). Conversely, anti-U3 antibodies are associated with a significantly lower prevalence of arthritis (99). Anti-Th antibodies are associated with primary Raynaud's syndrome and diffuse scleroderma (16,100), although in one study

this specificity was found in 10% of CREST patients (101).

Epitopes and Homologies

There is little that can be inferred about specific epitopes in the polypeptide structure of the nucleolar antigens. Th and fibrillarin are rarely detected on immunoblots, suggesting that the epitopes are discontinuous (100). Fibrillarin has a distinctive NH_2-terminal glycine-arginine rich domain (GAR), which has the repetitive, charged characteristics of other epitope domains with alternating basic amino acids (e.g., the 70K protein of the U1 snRNP particle, discussed in the following section). The polypeptide is highly conserved; mouse and human forms are 94% homologous (99). The structural similarity between the acidic domains of nucleolin and CENP-B was referred to earlier in this section. Minota et al (103) have suggested that the repeating glutamic configuration **EEEEEE . . .** may be of special significance in the generation of n/c antibodies.

Auto-AG/AB Reactivities in Associated Syndromes

The associated syndromes (Table 9.4) are clinical entities that occur concurrently with cutaneous sclerosis in some scleroderma patients. These entities include the overlap syndrome **mixed connective tissue disease** (MCTD), which combines features of scleroderma, SLE, and **PM**. Other major associated syndromes are **Sjögren's syndrome** (SS), **primary biliary cirrhosis**, and PM, which may be combined with **dermatomyositis** (DM) in a PM/DM syndrome (110). Whereas the three primary ag/ab reactivities in SSc and CREST are mutually exclusive, it is not uncommon to find more than one of the reactivities shown in Table 9.4 in the same individual. The prevalence of these reactivities in all forms of scleroderma is estimated to be 5% to 20% (16). The antigens represent a diversity of essential regulatory functions that may mediate pathophysiologic events. Interestingly, the majority of the antigens listed in Table 9.4 are associated with RNA polymerase III transcripts. Several examples are discussed in the following paragraphs.

MCTD AND THE U1 snRNP PARTICLE

The U1 snRNP Particle and Anti-RNP Antibodies

So-called anti-RNP antibodies, reacting with the nuclear RNA splicing particle U1 snRNP, are the defining serologic characteristic of MCTD and, by definition, are present in 100% of patients with this diagnosis (110–114). The particle consists of a U1 RNA core and the polypeptides 70K, A, B, B', C, D, E, F, and G, of which only 70K, A, and C are antigenic in MCTD (114–118). As summarized in Table 9.3, the gene for U1 RNA is located on chromosome 1 (119), and the genes for polypeptides 70K, A, B, B', and E are located

on chromosomes 19, 19, 15, 15, and 1, respectively (120–123).

The U1 snRNP particle is part of the apparatus involved in removing intervening sequences from pre-mRNA as a step in producing functional mRNA (113). The U1 RNA interacts with the 5' splice site. Both the 70K and A splicing proteins belong to the family of RNA-binding proteins that bind to U1 via a consensus sequence of roughly eight amino acids (124–129). As discussed in *Epitopes and Homologies*, later in this section, the consensus sequence of 70K is a major epitope for anti-RNP antibodies (130–133), which are potent inhibitors of RNA splicing (111,112). Thus, the functions of Scl-70/topo I, the centromere proteins, and the U1 snRNP particle are inhibited by their respective antibodies, as are the functions of the Ro/SS-A and La/SS-B antigens and the tRNA synthetases (discussed later in this section).

Table 9.4. Auto-AG/AB Reactivities in Associated Syndromes

Syndrome	Clinical Designation	Molecular Description(Ag)	Function(Ag)	Reference
Mixed Connective Tissue Disease	U1snRNP	U1RNA and polypeptides A, C and 70kD	RNA splicing	110–146
Sjögren's Syndrome	RO/SS-A	60 and 52 kD proteins	Ro-RNP (YRNAs)	147–161 177–183, 185–187
	LA/SS-B	48 kD protein	Transcription termination factor (RNA pol III)	162–183 185–187
Primary Biliary Cirrhosis	AMA[a]	Multienzyme complexes	pyuvate-DH[b] α-ketoacid-DH α-ketoglutarate-DH	188–192
Polymyositis/ Scleroderma	PM-Scl	Nucleolar multi-subunit particle (20–100kD)	Unknown	193–198
			tRNA *Synthetases*	1, 199–206
Polymyositis/ Dermatomyositis	Jo-1	55/60 kD protein	Histidyl	199–200
	PL-7	80kD protein	Threonyl	199, 201
	PL-12	110 kD protein	Alanyl	201, 202
	EJ	Unknown	Glycyl	202–203
	OJ	Multiple synthetases	Isoleucyl	204

[a]anti-mitochondrial antibodies
[b]DH = dehydrogenase

Antibody Prevalence, Ethnic Variability, and HLA Associations

Anti-RNP antibodies occur in approximately 10% of patients with scleroderma (16). Like Scl-70/topo I, their prevalence in Asians with scleroderma is higher than it is in Caucasian SSc patients (38). There are also ethnic differences in HLA associations (see Table 9.2). In American Caucasians with connective tissue disease, the presence of anti-RNP antibodies is significantly associated with DR4, DRw53, and DQB1*0302 alleles (134,135). In African-Americans, there is an association with the DQB1*0501 allele (135).

Clinical and Prognostic Associations

Early studies noted that the presence of anti-RNP antibodies correlated with a low frequency of renal disease and a relatively favorable prognosis in connective tissue disease patients (110). In a series of patients having antibodies of either the Sm or U1 snRNP specificity, the latter were associated with arthritis, arthralgias, and RP (136). However, there was no temporal correlation between antibody titers, which remained relatively constant, and disease activity, which fluctuated markedly. A comparison of 10-year survival rates in scleroderma patients with either anti-centromere, anti-RNP, or anti-Scl-70/topo I antibodies reported rates of 93%, 72%, and 66%, respectively (86). The presence of anti-RNP antibodies, in this study, correlated significantly with arthritis, pulmonary arterial hypertension, cerebral hemorrhage, and sicca complex.

Epitopes and Homologies

The largest of the antigenic U1 snRNP polypeptides, 70K (68-70kD), has two major epitope domains (A and B) reacting with 85% and 95% to 100% of anti-RNP sera, respectively (118,132, 133,137,138). Domain B contains the hydrophobic epitope **GRAFIEYE**, which has three significant associations:

(1) This sequence is a T cell as well as a B cell epitope (139,140).

(2) It belongs to the family of consensus binding sequences which bind to stem-loop I of U1 RNA (125).

(3) It is homologous to a dominant epitope of the HIV-1 envelope protein gp120, which is also a T and B cell epitope in HIV infected individuals (3).

Thus anti-RNP antibodies not only cross-react with this important sequence on gp120 (5), but also block the infectivity of HIV-1 *in vitro* (141).

The A domain of 70K (not to be confused with the A polypeptide) is located within a short region containing two hydrophilic motifs: **ETPEER** and **ERKRR**. These motifs are homologous to a sequence in the type C retroviral protein, p30[gag] (8), and to a sequence in the influenza B virus matrix protein, M1, respectively (130). Anti-RNP antibodies cross-react with the repetitive viral sequences, but unlike the HIV-1 homology, no impairment of viral functions has been demonstrated.

The A protein (33 kD), like 70K and the C protein, is present exclusively on U1 snRNP (115). However, A is extensively homologous to the B" protein found on U2 snRNP (142), and also has one cross-reactive epitope with A', which is also found on U2 snRNP (90,114). Thus, the A protein is recognized by both anti-RNP and anti-Sm sera. At least four distinct epitope regions have been identified in A (90). This protein has the additional interesting property of inhibiting its own production by suppressing the polyadenylation of its own mRNA (143). Nearly all anti-RNP sera reacting with 70K also have antibodies to A (90).

The C protein (22kD) demonstrates little homology to other n/c antigens (144). Approximately two thirds of anti-U1 snRNP sera recognize epitopes on this polypeptide (90,144). The C protein has a high proline and methionine content and lacks the consensus RNA-binding sequence present in the 70K and A polypeptides (145). Nevertheless, it has an essential role in the assembly of the U1 snRNP particle and its binding to the 5' splice site (146).

SJÖGREN'S SYNDROME (SS) AND THE Ro/SS-A AND La/SS-B ANTIGEN/ANTIBODY SYSTEMS

Sjögren's syndrome (dry eyes, dry mouth, and parotid gland enlargement) is present in approximately 30% of scleroderma patients, of which 50% have anti-Ro/SS-A and/or La/SS-B antibodies (147). These antibodies also occur in MCTD and in an estimated 30% of SLE patients, suggesting a common immunogenic link in these disorders. The antigens have been given different names by different groups of investigators, hence Ro, or SS-A, and La, or SS-B, are represented here as Ro/SS-A and La/SS-B.

Structure, Functions, Epitopes, and Homologies

Ro/SS-A. The Ro/SS-A antigen is composed of nucleocytoplasmic particles containing RNA and two antigenic polypeptides, 52kD and 60kD (148–154). The gene encoding 52kD has been localized to chromosome 11 (see Table 9.3) (155), whereas the 60kD gene has been assigned to chromosomes 19 and 1 by two different groups (156,157). The RNA moiety consists of a family of small RNAs designated Y1 Y5 (150), which are pol III transcripts. The function of these RNAs, which are non-covalently associated with the polypeptides, is unknown.

The 60kD polypeptide contains a zinc finger, capable of binding to DNA, and also has two RNA-binding sequences (152). The dual DNA/RNA binding capacity suggests a role in transcription. The 52kD protein also contains DNA/RNA binding motifs, including a zinc finger and a leucine zipper (153). By immunofluorescence, both proteins are detectable in nuclei and in the cytoplasm of cells. There is no appreciable homology between 60kD and 52kD, and antibodies to the two polypeptides do not cross-react (153). Antibodies to 60kD are heterogeneous, reacting predominantly to conformational, rather than linear, epitopes (158). Sera from most patients who are positive for anti-Ro/SS-A antibodies react with both 60kD and 52kD, although there is a predominance of reactivity to 60kD (153, 159,160).

Detailed analyses of epitopes of 60kD and 52kD are presented in references 160 and 161, respectively. The 60 kD polypeptide contains six small regions, including a dominant epitope, that are homologous to the nucleocapsid protein of vesicular stomatitis virus (VSV) (11). This relationship is analogous to that between the 70K protein of U1 snRNP and the HIV-1 envelope complex gp120/41 (3).

La/SS-B. The La/SS-B antigen is an example of an initially elusive molecule, detected first in the cytoplasm using antibodies from SLE patients, and subsequently identified as a nuclear protein (162,163). Originally thought to be a small RNP component (164–166), the antigen was later characterized as a 48kD polypeptide, which is a transcription termination factor for pol III (167–173). Because of the association of the 48kD protein with pol III transcripts, anti-La/SS-B antibodies immunoprecipitate precursors of 5S ribosomal and tRNAs (166), as well as pol III transcripts induced by adenovirus and EB-V (164). The 48kD protein also associates with apparent sequence specificity with the leader RNA of VSV, although it is a pol II transcript (168).

The function of the 48kD protein in nuclei is to facilitate termination of transcription by pol III, and thus increase the efficiency of re-initiation (171–173). Under some conditions, including viral infection, the 48kD protein redistributes to the cytoplasm, where it may facilitate translation (13). *In vitro* experiments demonstrate that the 48kD polypeptide not only stimulates translation of poliovirus RNA, but also corrects aberrant translation (13).

Similar to the 70K U1 snRNP protein, the dominant epitope region of 48kD includes its RNA-binding site (167). Several epitopes have been identified in non-overlapping peptides spanning the entire length of the protein (174–176).

Prevalence, Clinical Correlates in Scleroderma, and HLA Associations

The majority of patients with primary SS (>90%) produce Ro/SS-A and/or La/SS-B antibodies, although anti-Ro/SS-A alone are more prevalent than anti-La/SS-B alone (161,177). In scleroderma, SS is associated with the CREST variant (147). In CREST patients with SS, the prevalence of anti-Ro/SS-A and La/SS-B antibodies is 29% and 41%, respectively, with 53% having either or both of these antibodies (147). As seen also in MCTD and SLE, there is a significant correlation in scleroderma between the presence of either antibody and rheumatoid factor (147). In primary SS, as in scleroderma, the presence of anti-Ro/SS-A antibodies correlates with glandular dysfunction and a positive lip biopsy (147,178).

HLA associations with primary SS and anti-Ro/SS-A and anti-La/SS-B antibodies are presented in Table 9.2. DR3 and DRw8 alleles correlate with the presence of anti-Ro/SS-A antibodies in Caucasians, and DR3 also associates with anti-La/SS-B (179–181). However, studies in Greek patients with SLE show an association between the presence of both antibody specificities and B8, but not DR3 (182,183). Also associated with anti-Ro/SS-A antibodies are DQB1 alleles with leucine at position 26 (184–187).

PRIMARY BILIARY CIRRHOSIS, MITOCHONDRIAL ANTIGENS, AND ANTI-MITOCHONDRIAL ANTIBODIES

The occurrence of primary biliary cirrhosis (PBC) in conjunction with scleroderma has been widely reported. Anti-mitochondrial antibodies (AMA) are the hallmark of PBC, occurring in >90% of patients (188–192).

Structure, Functions, and Epitopes of Mitochondrial Antigens

AMAs react with multienzyme complexes of the 2-oxo-acid dehydrogenase (DH) family, residing on the inner mitochondrial membrane. These antigens were previously referred to as M2. Four antigens have been identified: protein X (54 kD) and components of the three enzyme complexes pyruvate DH, alpha-ketoacid DH, and alpha-ketoglutarate DH (188). Each DH complex is composed of subunits, which are designated E1,

E2, and E3. The acetyltransferase subunits (E2) contain the lipoic acid binding sites, which are major epitopes for AMAs (188,192). These subunits range in size from 40kD to 70kD. The 70kD polypeptide was initially recognized as a major component of M2 (189). In addition, the E1 subunits of both pyruvate DH and alpha-ketoglutarate DH, composed of alpha and beta chains, react with AMA antibodies (188,192).

Prevalence and Clinical Associations in Scleroderma

AMAs have been reported in 7% to 25% of scleroderma patients (189). However, only a fraction of those with AMAs have concurrent PBC. In one study, 3 of 19 scleroderma patients with AMA had PBC, and AMA were most frequently seen in the CREST variant (189). The role of AMAs in pathogenesis and immunogenesis is unclear. In some cases, a concurrent myopathy, with alterations in muscle mitochondria, has been reported (191). Environmental, geographic, and HLA class II associations have been described (192).

POLYMYOSITIS/SCLERODERMA AND THE PM/SCL AG/AB SYSTEM

Structure, Function, and Epitopes of the PM-Scl Antigen

PM-Scl is a nucleolar complex of 11 to 16 proteins, ranging from 20 to 110 kD (193–195). Although its function is unknown, immunoelectron microscopy studies localize the antigen to the granular portions of nucleoli, suggesting that it is a component of pre-ribosomes (194). There is no RNA associated with the immunoprecipitated antigen. The predominant epitopes are in the 100 to 110kD and 70 to 75kD polypeptides (193). The two polypeptides are not immunologically related, but both contain highly charged amino acids in their COOH-terminal regions (195).

Prevalence, Clinical Correlates in Scleroderma, and Ethnic and HLA Associations

Anti-PM-Scl antibodies are associated with inflammatory muscle disease in scleroderma.

Among patients with anti-PM-Scl antibodies, 41% to 92% are reported to have scleroderma-myositis overlap, and 3% to 5% have scleroderma without myositis (43,193). In scleroderma, these antibodies are seen in patients with diffuse, limited, and atypical disease (43,193). Overall, approximately 8% of myositis patients have anti-PM-Scl antibodies (196). There is one report of a patient presenting with renal hypertension and anti-PM-Scl antibodies, who subsequently developed sclerodermatous skin changes (197). A diagnosis of scleroderma renal crisis was made by biopsy. A suggestion, confirmed by retrospective studies, is that scleroderma renal crisis, associated with ANAs, may precede skin changes in a subset of individuals (197).

There is strong evidence for ethnic and racial variations in the prevalence of anti-PM-Scl antibodies. Two major studies of Japanese patients with inflammatory myopathies failed to detect any anti-PM-Scl antibodies (38,196) and none were detected in African-Americans (38). Thus, this antibody specificity may be restricted to Caucasians. There is a strong association of anti-PM-Scl antibodies with HLA DR3 (43,198).

POLYMYOSITIS/DERMATOMYOSITIS (PM/DM) AND THE tRNA SYNTHETASE AG/AB SYSTEMS

Antibodies to five aminoacyl-tRNA synthetases (referred to here as the synthetases) have been identified in a PM/DM syndrome (the anti-synthetase syndrome), which is highly associated with interstitial lung disease (1). These synthetases, and their clinical significance, are discussed in this section.

Structures, Functions, Epitopes, and Homologies

Four soluble tRNA synthetases are the targets of anti-synthetase antibodies, as shown in Table 9.4. The antibody/tRNA synthetase pairs are: Jo-1/histidyl (199,200), PL-7/threonyl (201), PL-12/alanyl (202), and EJ/glycyl (203). In addition, OJ antibodies precipitate an insoluble complex containing isoleucyl-tRNA synthetase (204).

The complex also contains several other tRNA synthetases (including those for glutamine, leucine, lysine, arginine, and methionine), but the activity of these enzymes is not inhibited by OJ antibodies (204). The function of aminoacyl-tRNA synthetases is to catalyze binding of specific amino acids to their respective tRNAs for incorporation of the amino acids into polypeptides on the ribosomes.

Using highly purified antigen, Jo-1 antibodies have been reported in 31% of "pure" myositis patients, 4.5% of "pure" dermatomyositis patients, and 4.5% of those with overlap syndromes, including scleroderma (199). In overlap syndromes, Jo-1 antibodies occur in conjunction with other specificities, including anti-RNP and anti-La/SS-B (200). The Jo-1 antigen is a 50kD subunit of histidyl tRNA synthetase (199). Jo-1 antibodies inhibit the enzyme. Antibodies of the PL-7 specificity block an 80kD protein, thereby inhibiting threonyl tRNA synthetase (201). Although PL-7 and Pl-12 (antibodies to alanyl-tRNA synthetase) may occur in the same serum, they bind independently to their antigens (202). Also, EJ antibodies do not cross-inhibit histidyl or glycyl tRNA synthetases (203).

A study of OJ antibodies, which was directed against a multienzyme complex of synthetases, provides evidence that anti-synthetase antibodies react primarily with conformational determinants (204). It is further suggested in this study that an antibody reaction to isoleucyl tRNA synthetase may appear first, followed by extension to other synthetases, which is consistent with an antigen driven mechanism (204). Homologies between alanyl and histidyl tRNA synthetase and myosin and the viruses EB-V, influenza, and adenovirus, have been presented in support of a molecular mimicry mechanism of immunogenesis and pathogenesis (4). The mechanisms are compatible if one postulates that a myopathic virus (coxsackievirus B and picornaviruses have been suggested in reference 200) utilizing host tRNA synthetase mechanisms causes cell damage, thereby releasing the enzyme complexes and overcoming immunological tolerance.

Prevalence, Clinical Correlates,
and HLA Association

Anti-synthetase antibodies occur in 25% to 30% of PM/DM patients (1, 204). Jo-1 antibodies are the most prevalent, occurring 5 to 10 times more frequently than any other specificity, and 2 to 4 times more often than the other four specificities combined (1). There is no direct evidence for pathogenesis. Although capillary loss and ischemic damage are important in DM, findings of antibody deposition are inconsistent and uncommon (1).

Despite the lack of direct evidence for antibody pathogenicity, there are some strong correlations with specific clinical findings, which as a group define an "anti-synthetase syndrome" (1, 204). One of these is interstitial lung disease, which is present in 50% to 75% of patients with anti-synthetase antibodies, as compared to 10% to 12% of others with myositis (1). Others are increased frequencies of severe and deforming arthritis, present in >90%, and RP, present in 60% (205,206). Another interesting association is with the cutaneous feature of "mechanic's hands," which involves hyperkeratosis, fissuring, and hyperpigmentation along both radial and palmar aspects of the fingers, giving the appearance of dirty horizontal lines (205).

There is a strong association between Jo-1 antibodies and the DR3 allele in Caucasians, and an even stronger association with the DR52 allele in both Caucasians and African-Americans (198). Data on associations between HLA alleles with other anti-synthetase antibodies are few at present; however, preliminary data do not suggest an association with DR3 (198).

Summary and Conclusions

The familiar and most prevalent pattern of humoral autoimmune reactivity in scleroderma is that of autoantibodies to Scl-70/topo I, centromeres or nucleoli, as summarized in Table 9.1. However, to understand the relationship between autoantibody expression and the etiology of cutaneous sclerosis, it is also important to consider the broader and more diverse pattern of reactivities included in Table 9.4. Thus, rather than emphasizing a hierarchy of autoantibodies based on prevalence, this chapter has attempted to summarize a wealth of data which contribute to the search for mechanisms.

The central questions addressed are: (*a*) whether autoantibodies, antigens, or their genes contribute directly to any of the pathophysiologic manifestations of scleroderma, including cutaneous sclerosis; and (*b*) whether autoantibody production results from direct stimulation by the identified n/c antigens, or by indirect mechanisms such as molecular mimicry. Most of the hypotheses and supporting data relevant to these two questions were presented and discussed in the text. This section provides a synopsis.

EVIDENCE FOR A ROLE FOR AUTOANTIBODIES, ANTIGENS, OR THEIR GENES IN PATHOGENESIS

It is evident from the studies summarized in Tables 9-1 and 9-4 that those n/c antigens whose functions have been identified have critical roles in nuclear and/or cytoplasmic regulation. In many of the examples presented, a link to pathogenesis has been hypothesized, although not definitively proven. The claim that antibodies have pathologic effects by inhibiting the essential functions of intracellular antigens immediately raises the objection that antibodies cannot effectively penetrate cells. Contrary to this view, there are reports of autoantibodies penetrating viable cells, perhaps via a facilitated mechanism, and binding to their target antigens (95,96). It is also possible that antibodies exert pathologic effects by binding to cell surface molecules and receptors with epitopes that mimic those of nuclear antigens. An example involving acidic epitopes of CENP-B having homologous counterparts in the acetylcholine receptor and other surface molecules was discussed in the section titled *Auto-AG/AB Reactivities in SSc and CREST* and in reference (94). A prediction based on this specific example is that there may be a relationship between scleroderma and myasthenia gravis. To date, there is a published report of a case of myasthenia gravis which evolved into scleroderma (207), and an unpublished case, which was referred to this laboratory, of a scleroderma patient who later developed myasthenia gravis. A second example is the association between anti-CENP-C antibodies and a high frequency of aneuploidy and chromosome breaks in patients with CREST (87). In general, however, there is insufficient experimental evidence that autoantibodies exert major pathologic effects by inhibiting the functions of intracellular n/c targets *in vivo*.

This chapter provides several examples in which the function of a n/c antigen is linked to a pathogenetic mechanism, or in which a function, rather than a molecular structure, is linked to a specific clinical syndrome. What is implied in these examples is that some disturbance in the function of the antigen, rather than the antibodies *per se*, is involved in pathogenesis. These examples include: (*a*) the hypothesized role of the topo I function of Scl-70/topo in hyperactivating collagen genes, thereby contributing to collagen overproduction (28); and (*b*) the association of tRNA synthetases with an "anti-synthetase" syndrome (1,203,205). More generally, any n/c antigen whose function is essential to an infecting virus is subject to major alterations in its rate of production and distribution during infection. An example is the La/SS-B antigen, which is a pol III-associated transcription termination factor (discussed in the section titled *Sjögren's syndrome (SS) and the Ro/SS-A and La/SS-B Antigen/Antibody Systems*). During viral infection, this protein redistributes to the cytoplasm, where it facilitates translation of viral mRNAs (13). The U1 snRNP particle is utilized to splice viral RNAs, as discussed in reference (3). Interestingly, pol III transcripts, which include U1, 5S, t, and the Y RNAs, are either structural components or substrates of the U1 snRNP, Ro/SS-A, La/SS-B, Jo-1, PL-7, PL-12, EJ, and OJ n/c antigens. Thus, viruses that activate pol III promoters can potentially affect the quantities or functions of any or all of these n/c antigens.

If multiple n/c antigens are rendered immunogenic by a viral infection, the specificity of autoantibodies would depend on the HLA type of the host, as well as on the type of virus. The autoimmune response induced by HIV-1 which cross-reacts with U1 snRNP may result from a combination of circumstances, including utilization and amplification of host cell splicing mechanisms, as well as from homologies between the viral surface and the 70K protein (3).

ANTIGEN-DRIVEN VERSUS INDIRECT MECHANISMS OF AUTOANTIBODY PRODUCTION

The rationale for presenting detailed analyses of epitopes and homologies in this chapter is to emphasize the complexity of factors which may trigger a polyclonal antibody reaction to a cluster of antigens. Polyclonality and a clustering of antigens and antibodies are two key characteristics of an antigen-driven mechanism, as outlined in the sub-section titled *The Centromere Proteins CENP-A, -B, -C, -E, and -F*. In the narrowest sense, an antigen-driven mechanism implies that the n/c antigens found to react with a patient's serum are the same molecules as those that triggered the initial autoimmune response. This hypothesis has at least two significant limitations. First, it fails to explain how certain antigens present in very low copy number, and with a restricted distribution (e.g., the centromere polypeptides) can become immunogens without some amplifying mechanism (*Epitopes and Homologies* sub-section to *The Centromere Proteins CENP-A, -B, -C, -E, and -F*). Moreover, even intensely hydrophilic sequences that may be exposed to the surface in these recondite proteins are masked by proteins of the opposite charge. The second limitation is that molecular mimics may have multiple epitope homologies to a n/c antigen (6), thereby directly eliciting a polyclonal antibody response without the need for a mechanism of broadening the initial reaction (55,56). Two examples are the multiple epitope homologies between: (*a*) the U1 snRNP polypeptide 70K and the HIV-1 envelope complex gp120/41 (3); and (*b*) the 60kD Ro/SS-A polypeptide and the nucleocapsid protein of VSV (11).

Thus, an exogenous stimulus, such as a virus, can both mimic and amplify n/c antigens, which are required to complete its life cycle. The possibility of amplifying clusters of n/c antigens by a virus that activates pol III promoters was mentioned previously. In this regard, it is interesting that antibody reactivities to pairs of n/c antigens containing pol III transcripts (e.g., U1 snRNP and Ro/SS-A) occur frequently in the scleroderma-associated syndromes.

References

1. Targoff IN. Humoral immunity in polymyositis/dermatomyositis. J Invest Dermatol 1993;100:116S–123S.

2. Damien RT. Moleculer mimicry: Parasite evasion and host defense. Microbiol Immunol 1989;145:101–115.

3. Douvas A, Takehana Y. Cross-reactivity between autoimmune anti-U1 snRNP antibodies and neutralizing epitopes of HIV-1 gp120/41. AIDS Res Hum Retroviruses 1994;10:253–262.

4. Walker EJ, Jeffrey PJ. Polymyositis and molecular mimicry, a mechanism of autoimmunity. Lancet 1986;13:605–607.

5. Douvas A, Takehana Y, Duffin M, Ehresmann G. Calcium receptors and anti-centromere antibodies in the pathogenesis and treatment of CREST. Arthritis Rheum 1993;36:181S.

6. Douvas A, Sobelman S. Multiple overlapping homologies between viral and nuclear antigens. Proc Natl Acad Sci USA 1991;88:6328–6332.

7. Maul GG, Jimenez SA, Riggs E, Ziemricka-Kotula D. Determination of an epitope of the diffuse systemic sclerosis marker antigen DNA topoisomerase I: Sequence similarity with retroviral P30gag protein suggests a possible cause for autoimmunity in systemic sclerosis. Proc Natl Acad Sci USA 1989;86:8492–8496.

8. Query CC, Keene JD. A human autoimmune protein associated with U1 RNA contains a region of homology that is cross-reactive with a retroviral p30gag antigen. Cell 1987;51:211–220.

9. Catalano MS, Carson DA, Slovin SF, Richman DD, Vaughan JH. Antibodies to Epstein-Barr virus-determined antigens in normal subjects and in patients with seropositive rheumatoid arthritis. Proc Natl Acad Sci USA 1979;76:5825–5828

10. Shillitoe JE, Daniels TE, Whitcher JP, Strand CV, Talal N, Greenspan JS. Antibody to cytomegalovirus in patient with Sjögren's syndrome. Arthritis Rheum 1982;25:260–265.

11. Scofield RH, Harley JB. Autoantigenicity of Ro/SSA antigen is related to a nucleocapsid protein of vesicular stomatitis virus. Proc Natl Acad Sci USA 1991;88:3343–3347.

12. Oldstone MBA. Molecular mimicry as a mechanism for the cause and as a probe uncovering etiologic agent(s) of autoimmune disease. Curr Top Microbiol Immunol 1989;145:127–135.

13. Meerovitch K, Svitkin YV, Lee HS, Leibkowitz F, Kenan DJ, Chan EK, et al. La autoantigen enhances and corrects aberrant translation of poliovirus RNA in reticulocyte lysate. J Virol 1993;67:3798–3807.

14. Tan EM, Rodnan GP, Garcia I, Moroi Y, Fritzler MJ, Peebles C. Diversity of antinuclear antibodies in progressive systemic sclerosis. Arthritis Rheum 1980;23:617–625.

15. Bernstein RM, Steigerwald JC, Tan EM. Association of antinuclear and antinucleolar antibodies in progressive systemic sclerosis. Clin Exp Immunol 1982;48:43–51.

16. Medsger TA Jr. Systemic sclerosis (scleroderma), localized forms of scleroderma, and calcinosis. In: McCarty DJ, Koopman WJ, eds. Arthritis and allied conditions, 12th ed. Philadelphia: Lea and Febriger, 1993.

17. Varga J, Jimenez SA. Cutaneous sclerosis localized to one limb after immobilization in a patient with CREST syndrome. J Rheumatol 1987;14:637–638.

18. Tan EM, Rodnan GP. Profiles of antinuclear antibodies in progressive systemic sclerosis (PSS). Arthritis Rheum 1975;18:S430.

19. Douvas AS, Achten M, Tan EM. Identification of a nuclear protein (Scl-70) as a unique target of human antinuclear antibodies in scleroderma. J Biol Chem 1979;254:10514–10522.

20. Shero JH, Bordwell B, Rothfield NF, Earnshaw WC. Autoantibodies to topoisomerase I are found in sera from scleroderma patients. Science 1986;231:737–740.

21. Maul GG, French BT, Van Venrooij WJ, Jimenez SA. Topoisomerase I identified by scleroderma 70 antisera: Enrichment of topoismerase I at the centromere in mouse mitotic cells before anaphase. Proc Natl Acad Sci USA 1986;83:5145–5149.

22. Guldner HH, Szostecki C, Vosberg HP, Lakomek HJ, Penner E, Bautz FA. Scl-70 autoantibodies from scleroderma patients recognize a 95KD protein identified as DNA topoisomerase I. Chromosoma 1986;94:132–138.

23. Steen VD, et al. Clinical and laboratory associations of anti-centromere antibody (ACA) in patients with progressive systemic sclerosis (scleroderma). Arthritis Rheum 1984;27:125–131.

24. Earnshaw WC, Rothfield N. Identification of a family of human centromere proteins using autoimmune sera from patients with scleroderma. Chromosoma 1985;9:313–321.

25. Turman MA, Douvas A. A casein kinase type II (CK-II)-like nuclear protein kinase associates with, phosphorylates, and activates topoisomerase I. Biochem Med Metab Biol 1993;50:210–225.

26. Champoux JJ, Dulbecco R. An activity from mammalian cells that untwists superhelical DNA-a possible swivel for DNA replication. Proc Natl Acad Sci USA 1992;69:143–146.

27. Liu LF, Miller KG. Eukaryotic DNA topoisomerases: Two forms of type I DNA topoisomerases from HeLa cell nuclei. Proc Natl Acad Sci USA 1981;78:3487–3491.

28. Douvas A. Does Scl-70 modulate collagen production in scleroderma? Lancet 1988;ii:475–477.

29. Douvas A, Lambie PB, Turman MA, Nitahara K, Hammond L. Negative regulation of Scl-70/70 topoismerase I by zinc and an endogenous macromolecule. Biochem Biophys Res Commun 1991;178:414–421.

30. D'Arpa P, Cooper-White H, Cleveland DW, Rothfield NF, Earnshaw WC. Use of molecular cloning methods to map the distribution of epitopes on topoisomerase-I (Scl-70) recognized by sera of scleroderma patients. Arthritis Rheum 1990;33:1501–1511.

31. Hildebrandt S, Weiner ES, Senecal J-L, Noell GS, Earnshaw WC, Rothfield NF. Autoantibodies to topoisomerase-I (Scl-70): Analysis by gel diffusion, immunoblot and enzyme-linked immunosorbent assay. Clin Immunol Immunopathol 1990;57:399–410.

32. Heck MM, Hittleman WN, Earnshaw WC. Differential expression of DNA topoisomerases I and II during the eurkaryotic cell cycle. Proc Natl Acad Sci USA 1988;85:1086–1090.

33. Hoffman A, Heck MM, Bordwell B, Rothfield NF, Earnshaw WC. Human autoantibody to topoisomerase I. Exp Cell Res 1989;180:409–418.

34. Oddou P, Schmidt UT, Knippers R, Richter A. Monoclonal antibodies neutralizing mammalian DNA topoisomerase I activity. Eur J Biochem 1988;177:523–529.

35. Juarez C, Vila JL, Glepi C, Agusti M, Amengual MJ, Martinez MA, Rodriguez JL. Characterization of the antigen reactive with anti-Scl-70 antibodies and its application in an enzyme-linked immunosorbent assay. Arthritis Rheum 1988;31:108–115.

36. Weiner ES, Earnshaw WC, Senecal J-L, Bordwell B, Johnson P, Rothfield NR. Clinical association of anticentromere antibodies and antibodies to topoisomerase I. Arthritis Rheum 1988;31:378–385.

37. Weiner E, Hilderbrandt S, Senecal J-L, Daniels I, Noell GS, Earnshaw WC, Rothfield NF. Prognostic significance of anticentromere antibodies and antitopoismerase I antibodies in Raynaud's Disease. Arthritis Rheum 1991;34:68–77.

38. Kuwana M, Okano Y, Kaburaki J, Tojo T, Medsger TA Jr. Racial differences in the distribution of systemic sclerosis-related serum antinuclear antibodies. Arthritis Rheum 1994;37:902–906.

39. Reveille JD, Durban E, Goldstein R, Moreda R, Arnett FC. Racial differences in frequencies of scleroderma-related autoantibodies. Arthritis Rheum 1992;35:216–218.

40. McNeilage LJ, Youngchaiyud U, Whittingham S. Racial differences in antinuclear antibody patterns and clinical manifestations of scleroderma. Arthritis Rheum 1989;32:54–60.

41. Kuwana M, Kaburaki J, Okano Y, Inoko H, Tsuji K. The HLA-DR and DQ genes control the autoimmune response to DNA topoisomerase I in systemic sclerosis (scleroderma). J Clin Invest 1993;92:1296–1301.

42. Briggs D, Stephens C, Vaughan R, Welsh K, Black C. A molecular and serologic analysis of the major histocompatibility complex and complement component C4 in systemic sclerosis. Arthritis Rheum 1993;36:943–954.

43. Genth E, Mierau R, Genetzky P, vonMuhlen CA, Kaufmann S, von Wilmowsky H, Meurer M, et al. Immunogenetic associations of scleroderma-related antinuclear antibodies. Arthritis Rheum 1990;33:657–664.

44. Reveile JD, Durban E, MacLeod-St Clair MJ, Goldstein R, Moreda R, Altman RD, Arnett FC. Association of amino acid sequences in HLA-DQB1 first domain with the antitopoisomerase I autoantibody response in scleroderma (progressive systemic sclerosis). J Clin Invest 1992;90:973–980.

45. Steen VD, Powell DL, Medsger TA Jr. Clinical correlations and prognosis based on serum autoantibodies in patients with systemic sclerosis. Arthritis Rheum 1988;31:196–203.

46. Catoggio LJ, Bernstein RM, Black CM, Hughes

GRV, Maddison PJ. Serological markers in progressive systemic sclerosis: Clinical correlations. Ann Rheum Dis 1983;42:23–27.

47. Kuwana M, Kaburaki J, Mimori T, Tojo T, Homma M. Autoantigenic epitopes on DNA topoisomerase I: Clinical and immunogenetic associations in systemic sclerosis. Arthritis Rheum 1993; 36:1406–1413.

48. Weiner ES, et al. Prognostic significance of anticentromere antobodies and anti-topoisomerase I antibodies in Raynaud's disease. Arthritis Rheum 1991;34:68–77.

49. Cram DS, Fisicaro N, McNeilage LJ, Coppel RL, Harrison LC. Antibody specificities of Thai and Australian scleroderma sera with topoisomerase I recombinant fusion proteins. J Immunol 1993; 151:6872–6881.

50. Meesters TM, van-den-Hoogen FH, Verheijen R, Habets WJ, van-Venrooij WJ. Analysis of an immunodominant epitope of topoisomerase I in patients with systemic Sclerosis. Mol Biol Rep 1992;16(2):117–123.

51. Kato T, et al. Identification of a universal B cell epitope on DNA topoisomerase I, an autoantigen associated with scleroderma. Arthritis Rheum 1993;36:1580–1587.

52. D'Arpa P, Machlin PS, Ratrie H, Rothfield NF, Cleveland DW, Earnshaw WC. cDNA cloning of human DNA topoisomerase-I: Catalytic activity of a 67.7-kDa carboxyl-terminal fragment. Proc Natl Acad Sci USA 1988;85:2543–2547.

53. Verheijen R, et al. A recombinant topoisomerase I used for autoantibody detection in sera from patients with systemic sclerosis. Clin Exp Immunol 1990;80:38–43.

54. Muryoi T, et al. Antitopoisomerase I monoclonal autoantibodies from scleroderma patients and tight skin mouse interact with similar epitopes. J Exp Med 1992;175:1103–1109.

55. Milch DR, McLachian A, Thornton GB, Hughes JL. Antibody production to the nucleocapsid and envelope of the hepatitis B virus primed by a single synthetic T cell site. Nature 1987;329:8.

56. Adams TE, Alpert S, Hanahan D. Non-tolerance and autoantibodies to a transgenic self antigen expressed in pancreatic β cells. Nature 1987;325 (6101):223–228.

57. Pluta AF, Cooke CA, Earnshaw WC. Structure of the human centromere at metaphase. Trends Biochem Sci 1990;15:181–185.

58. Rieder CL. The formation structure and composition of the mammalian kinetochore and kinetochore fiber. Int Rev Cytol 1982;79:1–58.

59. Powell FC, Winkelmann RK, Venencie-Lemarchand F, Spurbeck JL, Schroeter AL. The anticentromere antibody: Disease specificity and clinical significance. Mayo Clin Proc 1984;59:700–706.

60. Earnshaw W, Bordwell B, Marino C, Rothfield N. Three human chromosomal autoantigens are recognized by sera from patients with anticentromere antibodies. J Clin Invest 1986;77: 426–430.

61. Bernat RL, Borisy GG, Rothfield NF, Earnshaw WC. Injection of anticentromere antibodies in interphase disrupts events required for chromosome movement at mitosis. J Cell Biol 1990;111: 1519–1533.

62. Guldner HH, Lakomek H-J, Bautz FA. Human anti-centromere sera recognise a 19.5kD non-histone chromosomal protein from HeLa cells. Clin Exp Immunol 1984;58:13–20.

63. Palmer DK, O'Day K, Trong LH, Charbonneau H, Margolis RL. Purification of the centromere-specific protein CENP-A and demonstration that it is a distinctive histone. Proc Natl Acad Sci USA. 1991;88:3734–3738.

64. Billings PB, Martinez A, Haselby JA, Hoch SO. Protein blot assays specific for the discrimination of the centromere autoantigen, CENP-A, from human cells. Electrophoresis 1993;14:909–916.

65. Palmer DK, Margolis RL. A 17-kD centromere protein (CENP-A) copurifies with nucleosome core particles and histones. J Cell Biol 1987;104: 805–815.

66. Earnshaw WC, et al. Molecular cloning of cDNA for CENP-B the major human centromere autoantigen. J Cell Biol 1987;104:817–829.

67. Sugimoto K, Muro Y, Himeno M. Anti-helix-loop-helix domain antibodies: Discovery of autoantibodies that inhibit DNA binding activity of human centromere protein B (CENP-B). J Biochem 1992;111:478–483.

68. Masumoto H, Masukata H, Muro Y, Nozaki N, Okazaki T. A human centromere antigen (CENP-B) interacts with a short specific sequence in alphoid DNA, a human centromeric satellite. J Cell Biol 1989;109:1963–1973.

69. Yoda K, Kitagawa K, Masumoto H, Muro Y, Okazaki T. A human centromere protein, CENP-B, has a DNA binding domain containing four potential alpha helices at the NH2 terminus, which is separable from dimerizing activity. J Cell Biol 1992;119:1413–1427.

70. Sullivan KF, Glass CA. CENP-B is a highly conserved mammalian centromere protein with homology to the helix-loop-helix family of proteins. Chromosoma 1991;100:360–370.

71. Wevrick R, Earnshaw WC, Howard-Peebles PN, Willard HF. Partial deletion of alpha satellite DNA associated with reduced amounts of the

centromere protein CENP-B in a mitotically stable human chromosome rearrangement. Mol Cell Biol 1990;10:6374–6380.

72. Pluta AF, Saitoh N, Goldberg I, Earnshaw WC. Identification of a subdomain of CENP-B that is necessary and sufficient for localization to the human centromere. J Cell Biol 1992;116:1081–1093.

73. Muro Y, Masumoto H, Yoda K, Nozaki N, Ohashi M, Okazaki T. Centromere protein B assembles human centromeric alpha-satellite DNA at the 17-bp sequence, CENP-B box. J Cell Biol 1992; 116:585–596.

74. Cooke CA, Bernat RL, Earnshaw WC. CENP-B: A major human centromere protein located beneath the kinetochore. J Cell Biol 1990;110:1475–1488.

75. Sugimoto K, Yata H, Himeno M. Mapping of the human CENP-B gene to chromosome 20 and the CENP-C gene to chromosome 12 by a rapid cycle DNA amplification procedure. Genomics 1993; 17:240–242.

76. Kunze N, et al. Localization of the active type I DNA topoisomerase gene on human chromosome 20q11.2-13.1, and two pseudogenes on chromosomes 1q23-24 and 22q11.2-13.1. Hum Genet 1989;84(1):6–10.

77. Saitoh H, Tomkiel J, Cooke CA, Ratrie H 3rd, Maurer M, Rothfield NF, Earnshaw WC. CENP-C, an autoantigen in scleroderma, is a component of the human inner kinetochore plate. Cell 1992; 70:115–125.

78. Tomkiel J, Cooke CA, Saitoh H, Bernat RL, Earnshaw WC. CENP-C is required for maintaining proper kinetochore size and for a timely transition to anaphase. J Cell Biol 1994;125:531–545.

79. Kingwell B, Rattner JB. Mammalian kinetochore/centromere composition: A 50 kDa antigen is present in the mammalian kinetochore/centromere. Chromosoma 1987;95:403–407.

80. Hadlaczky G, Praznovszky T, Rasko I, Kereso J. Centromere Proteins: I. Mitosis specific centromere antigen recognized by anti-centromere autoantibodies. Chromosoma 1989;97:282–288.

81. Bischoff FR, Maier G, Tilz G, Ponstingl H. A 47-kDa human nuclear protein recognized by antikinetochore autoimmune sera is homologous with the protein encoded by RCCI, a gene implicated in onset of chromosome condensation. Proc Natl Acad Sci USA 1990;87:8617–8621.

82. Yen TJ, et al. CENP-E, a novel human centromere-associated protein required for progression from metaphase to anaphase. EMBO J 1991;10:1245–1254.

83. Liao H, Li G, Yen TJ. Mitotic regulation of micro-tubule cross-linking activity of CENP-E kinetochore protein. Science 1994;265:394–398.

84. Rattner JB, Rao A, Fritzler JJ, Valencia DW, Yen TJ. CENP-F is a .ca 400 kDa kinetochore protein that exhibits a cell-cycle dependent localization. Cell Motil Cytoskeleton 1993;26:214–216.

85. Rothfield N, Whitaker D, Bordwell B, Weiner E, Scnecal J-L, Earnshaw W. Detection of anticentromere antibodies antibodies using cloned autoantigen CENP-B. Arthritis Rheum 1987;30: 1416–1419.

86. Kuwana M, Kaburaki J, Okano Y, Tojo T, Homma M. Clinical and prognostic associations based on serum antinuclear antibodies in Japanese patients with systemic sclerosis. Arthritis Rheum 1994;37: 75–83.

87. Jabs EW, Tuck-Muller CM, Anhalt GJ, Earnshaw W, Wise RA, Wigley F. Cytogenetic survey in systemic sclerosis: Correlation of aneuploidy with the presence of anticentromere antibodies. Cytogenet Cell Genet 1993;63:169–175.

88. Reveille JD, Owerbach D, Goldstein R, Moreda R, Isern RA, Arnett FC. Association of polar amino acids at position 26 of the HLA-DQB1 first domain with anticentromere autoantibody response in systemic sclerosis (scleroderma). J Clin Invest 1992;89:1208–1213.

89. Muro Y, Sugimoto K, Himeno M, Ohashi M. The clinical expression in anticentromere antibody-positive patients is not specified by the epitope recognition of CENP-B antigen. J Dermatol 1992; 19:584–591.

90. Habets WJ, Hoet MH, van Venroij WJ. Epitope patterns of anti-RNP antibodies in rheumatic disease. Arthritis Rheum 1990;33:834–841.

91. Earnshaw WC, Machlin PS, Bordwell BJ, Rothfield NF, Cleveland DW. Analysis of anticentromere autoantibodies using cloned autoantigen CENP-B. Proc Natl Acad Sci USA 1987;84: 4979–4983.

92. Sugimoto K, Migita H, Hagishita Y, Yata H, Himeno M. An antigenic determinant on human centromere protein B (CENP-B) available for production of human-specific anticentromere antibodies in mouse. Cell Struct Func 1992;17: 129–138.

93. Earnshaw WC. Anionic regions in nuclear proteins. J Cell Biol 1987;105:1479–1482.

94. Douvas A, Takehana Y, Duffin MD, Ehresmann GE. Calcium receptors and anti-centromere antibodies in the pathogenesis and treatment of CREST. Arthritis Rheum 1993;36(9)S:181.

95. Ma J, Chapman GV, Chen S-L, Melick G, Penny R, Breit SN. Antibody penetration of viable human cells, I. Increased penetration of human lympho-

cytes by anti-RNP IgG. Clin Exp Immunol 1990;
84:43–91.

96. Levine B, Hardwick JM, Trapp BD, Crawford TO, Bollinger RC, Griffin DE. Antibody-medicated clearance of alphavirus infection from neurons. Science 1991;254:856–860.

97. Reimer G, Stein VO, Penning CA, et al. Correlates between autoantibodies to nucleolar antigens and clinical, feature in patients with systemic sclerosis (scleroderman). Arthritis Rheum 1988;31:525–532.

98. Reimer G, Rose KM, Scheer U, Tan EM. Autoantibody to RNA polymerase I in scleroderma sera. J Clin Invest 1987;79:65–72.

99. Turley SJ, Tan EM, Pollard KM. Molecular cloning and sequence analysis of U3 snRNA-associated mouse fibrillarin. Biochim Biophys Acta 1993;1216:119–122.

100. Verheijen R, et al. Screening for autoantibodies to the nucleolar U3-and Th(7-2) ribonucleoproteins in patients' sera using antisense riboprobes. J Immunol Methods 1994;169:173–182.

101. Okano Y, Mesger TA Jr. Antibody to Th ribonucleoprotein (nucleolar 7.2 RNA protein particle) in patients with systemic sclerosis (scleroderma). Arthritis Rheum 1990;33:1822–1828.

102. Rodriguez-Sanchez J, Gelpi C, Juarez C, Hardin JA. A new autoantibody in scleroderma that recognizes a 90-kDa component of the nucleolus organizing region of chromatin. J Immunol 1987;139:2579–2584.

103. Minota S, et al. Autoantibodies to nucleolin in systemic lupus erythematosus and other diseases. J Immunol 1991;146:2249–2252.

104. Sanchez-Roman J, Wichmann I, Salaberri J, Varela JM, Nunez-Roldan A. Multiple clinical and biological autoimmune manifestations in 50 workers after occupational exposure to silica. Ann Rheum Dis 1993;52:534– 538.

105. Hultman P, Enestrom S, Turley SJ, Pollard KM. Selective induction of anti-fibrillarin autoantibodies by silver nitrate in mice. Clin Exper Immunol 1994;96(2):285–291.

106. Monestier M, Losman MJ, Novick KE, Aris JP. Molecular analysis of mercury-induced antinucleolar antibodies in H-2S mice. J Immunol 1994;152(2):667–675.

107. Imai H, Ochs RL, Kiyosawa K, Furuta S, Nakamura RM, Tan ME. Nucleolar antigens and autoantibodies in hepatocellular carcinoma and other malignancies. Am J Pathol 1992;140:859–870.

108. Sadava DE. Cell biology: Organelle structure and function. Boston: Jones and Bartlett, 1993.

109. Tyc K, Steitz JA. U3, U8 and U13 comprise a new class of mammalian snRNPs localized in the cell nucleolus. EMBO J 1989;8:3113–3119.

110. Reichlin M. Introduction to systemic rheumatic diseases: Nosology and overlap syndromes. In: McCarty DJ, Koopman WJ, eds. Arthritis and allied conditions, 12 ed. Philadelphia: Lea and Febriger, 1993.

111. Lerner MR, Steitz JA. Antibodies to small nuclear RNAs complexed with proteins are produced by patients with systemic lupus erythematosus. Proc Natl Acad Sci USA 1979;76:5495–5499.

112. Lerner MR, Boyle JA, Mount SM, Wolin SL, Steitz JA. Are snRNPs involved in splicing? Nature 1980;283:220–224.

113. Luhrmann R, Kastner B, Bach M. Structure of spliceosomal snRNPs and their role in pre-mRNA splicing. Biochim Biophys Acta 1990;1087:267–292.

114. Reuter R, Luhrmann R. Immunization of mice with purified U1 small nuclear ribonucleoprotein (RNP) induces a pattern of antibody specificities characteristic of the anti-Sm and anti-RNP autoimmune response of patients with lupus erythematosus, as measured by monoclonal antibodies. Proc Natl Acad Sci USA 1986;83:8689–8693.

115. Bringmann P, Luhrmann R. Purification of the individual snRNPs U1, U2, U5 and U4/U6 from HeLa cells and characterization of their protein constituents. EMBO J 1986;5:3509–3516.

116. Theissen H, et al. Cloning of the human cDNA for the U1 RNA-associated 70K protein. EMBO J 1986;5:3209–3217.

117. Spritz RA, Strunk K, Surowy CS, Hoch SO, Barton ED, Francke U. The human U1-70K snRNP protein: cDNA cloning, chromosomal localization, expression, alternative splicing and RNA-binding. Nucleic Acids Res 1987;15:10373–10391.

118. Netter HJ, Guldner HH, Szostecki C, Lakomek H, Will H. A recombinant autoantigen derived from the human (U1) small nuclear RNP-specific 68-kd protein. Arthritis Rheum 1988;31:616–622.

119. Naylor SL, Zabel BU, Manser T, Gesteland R. Localization of human U1 small nuclear RNA genes to band p36.3 of chromosome 1 by in situ hybridization. Somat Cell Mol Genet 1984;10:307–313.

120. Spritz RA, Strunk K, Surowy CS, Mohrenweiser HW. Human U1-70K ribonucleoprotein antigen gene: Organization, nucleotide sequence, and mapping to locus 19q13.3. Genomics 1990;8:371–379.

121. Nelissen RL, Sillekens PT, Beijer RP, Geurts-van-Kessel AH, van-Venrooij WJ. Structure, chromosomal localization and evolutionary conservation

of the gene encoding human U1 snRNP-specific A protein. Gene 1991;102:189–196.

122. Glenn CC, Proter KA, Jong MT, Nicholls RD, Driscoll DJ. Functional imprinting and epigenetic modification of the human snRNP gene. Hum Mol Genet 1993;2:2001–2005.

123. Neiswanger K, et al. Assignment of the gene for the small nuclear ribonucleoprotein E (snRNPE) to human chromosome 1q25-q43. Genomics 1990;7:503–508.

124. Hamm J, van Santen VL, Spritz RA, Mattaj IW. Loop I of U1 small nuclear RNA is the only essential RNA sequence for binding of specific U1 small nuclear ribonucleoprotein particle proteins. Mol Cell Biol 1988;8:4787–4791.

125. Surowy CS, van Santen VL, Scheib-Wixted SM, Spritz RA. Direct, sequence-specific of the human U1-68K ribonucleoprotein antigen protein to loop I of U1 small nuclear RNA. Mol Cell Biol 1989;9:4179–4186.

126. Query CC, Bentley RC, Keene JD. A specific 31-nucleotide domain of U1 RNA directly interacts with the 70K small nuclear ribonucleoprotein component. Mol Cell Biol 1989;9:4872–4881.

127. Krainer AR, Mayeda A, Kozak D, Binn G. Functional expression of cloned human splicing factor SF2: Homology to RNA-binding proteins, U1 70K, and Drosophila splicing regulators. Cell 1991;66:383–394.

128. Bandziulis RJ, Swanson MS, Dreyfuss G. RNA-binding proteins as developmental regulators. Genes Dev 1989;3:431–437.

129. Query CC, Bentley RC, Keene JD. A common RNA recognition motif identified within a defined U1 RNA binding domain of the 70K U1 snRNP protein. Cell 1989;57:89–101.

130. Guldner HH, Netter HJ, Szostecki C, Jaeger E, Will H. Human anti-P68 autoantibodies recognize a common epitope of U1 RNA containing small nuclear ribonucleoprotein and influenza B virus. J Exp Med 1990;171:819–829.

131. Francoeur A. Anti-Sm and anti-U1-RNP lupus antibody fine specificities. J Clin Immunol 1989; 9:256–263.

132. Netter HJ, Guldner HH, Szostecki C, Will H. Major autoantigenic sites of the (U1) small nuclear ribonucleoprotein-specific 68-kDa protein. Scand J Immunol 1990;32:163–176.

133. Cram DS, Fisicaro N, Coppel RL, Whittingham S, Harrison LC. Mapping of multiple B cell epitopes on the 70-Kilodalton autoantigen of the U1 ribonucleoprotein commplex. J Immunol 1990; 145:630–635.

134. Hoffman RW, Rettenmaier LJ, Takeda Y, Hewett JE, Pettersson I, Nyman U, Luger AM, et al. Hu-

man autoantibodies against the 70kd polypeptide of U1 small nuclear RNP are associated with HLA-DR4 among connective tissue disease patients. Arthritis Rheum 1990;33:666–674.

135. Olsen ML, Arnett FC, Reveille JD. Contrasting molecular patterns of MHC class II alleles associated with the anti-Sm and anti-RNP precipitin autoantibodies in systemic lupus erythematosus. Arthritis Rheum 1993;36:94–104.

136. Lundberg I, Nyman U, Petterson I, Hedfols E. (1992). Clinical manifestations and anti-U1 snRNP antibodies: A prospective study of 29 anti-RNP antibody positive patients. Br J Rheumatol 1992;31:811–817.

137. Guldner HH, Netter HJ, Szostecki C, Lakomek HJ, Will H. Epitope mapping with a recombinant human 68-kDa (U1) Ribinucleoprotein antigen reveals heterogeneous autoantibody profiles in human autoimmune sera. J Immunol 1988;141: 469–475.

138. Netter HJ, Will H, Szostecki C, Guldner HH. Repetitive P68-Autoantigen specific epitopes recognized by Human anti-(U1) small nuclear ribonucleoprotein autoantibodies. J Autoimmun 1991;4:651–663.

139. O'Brien RM, Cram DS, Coppel RL, Harrison LC. T cell epitopes on the 70-kDa protein of the (U1) RNP complex in autoimmune rheumatologic disorders. J Autoimmun 1990;3:747–757.

140. Okubo M, et al. Detection and epitope analysis of autoantigen-reactive T cells to the U1-small nuclear ribonucleoprotein a protein in autoimmune disease patients. J Immunol 1993;151:1108–1115.

141. Douvas A, Daar ES, Takehana Y, Ehresmann G. (1995). In vitro inhibition of HIV-1 strains by uninfected autoimmune sera. 1995, submitted.

142. Sillekens PTG, Habets WJ, Beijer RP, van Venrooij WJ. cDNA cloning of the human U1 snRNA-associated A protein: Extensive homology between U1 and U2 snRNP-specific protein. EMBO J 1987;6:3841– 3848.

143. Booelens WC, Jansen EJR, van Venrooij WJ, Stripecke R, Mattaj IW, Gunderson SI. The human U1 snRNP-specific U1A protein inhibits polyadenylation of its own pre-mRNA. Cell 1993; 72:881–892.

144. Yamamoto K, Miura H, Moroi Y, Yoshinoya S, Goto M, Nishioka K, Miyamoto T. Isolation and characterization of a complementary DNA expressing human U1 small nuclear ribonucleoprotein C polypeptide. J Immunol 1988;140:311–317.

145. Sillekens P, Beijer RP, Habets WJ, van VenroiJ WJ. Human U1 snRNP-specific C protein: Complete-c DNA and protein sequence and identification of

a multigene family in mammals. Nucleic Acids Res 1988;16:8307–8321.

146. Heinrichs V, Bach M, Winkelmann G, Luhrmann R. U1-specific protein C needed for efficient complex formation of U1 snRNP with a 5' splice site. Science 1990;247:69–72.

147. Osial TA, Whiteside TL, Buckingham RB, Singh G, Barnes EL, Pierce JM, Rodnan GP. Clinical and serologic study of Sjögren's syndrome in patients with systemic sclerosis. Arthritis Rheum 1983;26: 500– 508.

148. Clarke G, Reichlin M, Tomasi TB. Characterization of a solid cytoplasmic antigen reactive with sera from patients with systemic lupus erythematosus. J Immunol 1969;102:117–122.

149. Alspaugh MA, Talal N, Tan EM. Differentiation and characterization of autoantibodies and their antigens in Sjögren's syndrome. Arthritis Rheum 1976;19:216–222.

150. Wolin SL, Steitz JA. The Ro small cytoplasmic ribonucleoproteins: Identification of the antigenic protein and its binding site on the Ro RNAs. Proc Natl Acad Sci USA 1984;81:1996–2000.

151. Lieu T-S, Newkirk MM, Capra JD, Sontheimer RD. Molecular characterization of human Ro/SS-A antigen. J Clin Invest 1988;82:96–101.

152. Ben-Cherit E, Gandy BJ, Tan EM, Sullivan KF. Isolation and charaterization of a cDNA clone encoding the 60-kD component of the human SS/Ro ribonucleoprotein autoantigen. J Clin Invest 1989;83:1284–1292.

153. Chan KL, Hamel JC, Buyon JP, Tan EM. Molecular definition and sequence motifs of the 52-kD component of human SS-S/Ro autoantigen. J Clin Invest 1991;87:68-76.

154. Lieu T-S, Jiang M, Steigerwald JS, Tan EM. Identification of the SS-A/Ro intracellular antigen with autoimmune sera. J Immunol Methods 1984;71:217–228.

155. Frank MB, Itoh K, Fujisaku A, Pontarotti P, Mattei MG, Neas BR. The mapping of the human 52-kD Ro/SSA autoantigen gene to human chromosome 11, and its polymorphisms. Am J Hum Genet 1993;52:183–191.

156. McCauliffe DP, et al. Molecular cloning, expression, and chromosome 19 localization of a human Ro/SS-A autoantigen. J Clin Invest 1990;85: 1379–1391.

157. Chan KL, Tan M, Ward C, Matera AG. Human 60-kDa SS-A/Ro ribonucleoprotein autoantigen gene (SSA2) localized to 1q31 by fluorescence in situ hybridization. Genomics 1994;23:298–300.

158. Boire G, Lopez-Longo F-J, Lapointe S, Menard H-A. Sera from patients with autoimmune disease recognize conformational determinants on the 60-kd Ro/SS-A protein. Arthritis Rheum 1991;34: 722–730.

159. St. Clair WE, Burch JA Jr, Saitta M. Specificity of autoantibodies for recombinant 60-kD and 52-KD Ro autoantigens. Arthritis Rheum 1994;37: 1373–1379.

160. Saitta MR, Arnett FC, Keene JD. 60-kDa Ro protein autoepitopes identified using recombinant polypeptides. J Immunol 1994;152:4192–4202.

161. Bozic B, Prujin GJM, Rozman B, van Venrooij WJ. Sera from patients with rheumatic diseases recognize different epitope regions on the 52kDa Ro/SS-A protein. Clin Exp Immunol 1993;94:227–235.

162. Mattioli M, Reichlin M. Heterogeneity of RNA protein antigens reactive with sera of patients with systemic lupus erythematous. Arthritis Rheum 1974;17:421–429.

163. Akizuki M, Powers R Jr, Holman HR. A soluble acidic protein of the cell nucleus which reacts with serum from patients with systemic lupus Erythematosus and Sjögren's syndrome. J Clin Invest 1977;59:264– 272.

164. Lerner MR, Andrews NC, Miller G, Steitz JA. Two novel classes of small ribonucleoproteins detected by antibodies associated with lupus erythematous. Science 1981;211:400–402.

165. Lerner MR, Andrews NC, Miller G, Steitz JA. Two small RNAs encoded by Epstein-Barr virus and complexed with protein are precipitated by antibodies from patients with systemic lupus erythematosus. Proc Natl Acad Sci USA 1981;78:805– 809.

166. Rinke J, Steitz JA. Precursor molecules of both human 5S ribosomal RNA and transfer RNA are bound by a cellular protein reactive with anti-La lupus antibodies. Cell 1982;29:149–159

167. Chambers JC, Keene JD. Isolation and analysis of cDNA clones expressing human lupus La antigen. Proc Natl Acad Sci USA 1985;82:2115–2119.

168. Kurilla MG, Keene JD. The leader RNA of vesicular stomatitis virus is bound by a cellular protein reactive with anti-La lupus antibodies. Cell 1983; 34:837–845.

169. Madore SG, Weiben ED, Pederson T. Eukaryotic small proteins, anti-La human autoantibodies react with U1 RNA-protein complexes. J Biol Chem 1984;259:1929–1933.

170. Francoeur AM, Chan EKL, Garrels JI, Mathews MB. Characterization and purification of lupus antigen La, an RNA-binding protein. Mol Cell Biol 1985;5:586–590.

171. Gottlieb E, Steitz JA. Function of the mammalian La protein: Evidence for its action in transcription termination by RNA polymerase III. EMBO J 1989;8:851–861.

172. Gottlieb E, Steitz JA. The RNA binding protein La influence both the accuracy and the efficiency of RNA polymerase III transcription in vitro. EMBO J 1989;8:841–850.

173. Maraia RJ, Kenan DJ, Keene JD. (1994). Eukaryotic transcription termination factor la mediates transcript release and facilitates reinitiation by RNA polymerase III. Mol Cell Biol 1994;14:2147–2158.

174. St. Clair EW, Pisetsky DS, Reich CF, Keene JD. Analysis of autoantibody binding to different regions of the human La antigen expressed in recombinant fusion proteins. J Immunol 1988;141:4173–4180.

175. Sturgess AD, Peterson MG, McNeilage LJ, Whittingham S, Coppel RL Characteristics and epitope mapping of a cloned human autoantigen La. J Immunol 1988;140:3212–3218.

176. McNeilage LJ, Macmillan EM, Whittingham SF. Mapping of epitopes on the La(SS-B) autoantigen of primary Sjögren's syndrome: Identification of a cross-reactive epitope. J Immunol 1990;145:3829–3835.

177. Tan EM. Autoantibodies to nuclear antigens. Adv Immunol 1992;33:167–240.

178. Tsuzaka K, et al. (1994). Clinical significance of antibodies to native or denatured 60-kd or 52-kd Ro/SS-A proteins in Sjögren's syndrome. Arthritis Rheum 1994;37:88–92.

179. Garcia PR, et al. Immunogenetics of the Sjögren's syndrome in southern Spain. Ann Medicina Interna 1994;11:56–61.

180. Fei H, Scharf S, Erlich H, Peebles C, Tan E, Fox R. Relationship between HLA D region gene and primary Sjögren's syndrome. Chung Hua I Hsueh Tsa Chih 1991;71:555–559.

181. Lulli P, et al. HLA antigens in Italian patients with systemic lupus erythematosus: Evidence for the association of DQw2 with the autoantibody response to extractable nuclear antigens. Clin Exp Rheum 1991;9:475–479.

182. Drosos AA, Dimou GS, Siamopoulou MA, Hatzis J, Moutsopoulos HM. Subacute cutaneous lupus erythematosus in Greece. A clinical, serological and genetic study. Ann Medecine Interne 1990;141:421–424.

183. Andonopoulos AP, Papasteriades CA, Drosos AA, Dimou GS, Moutsopoulos HM. HLA alloantigens in Greek patients with systemic lupus erythematosus. Clin Exp Rheum 1990;8:47–50.

184. Reveille JD, MacLeod MJ, Whittington K, Arnett FC. Specific amino acid residues in the second hypervariable region of HLA-DQA1 and DQB1 chain genes promote the Ro (SS-A)/La (SS-B) autoantibody responses. J Immunol 1991;146:3871–3876.

185. Hamilton RG, et al. Two Ro (SS-A) autoantibody responses in systemic lupus erythematous. Arthritis Rheum 1988;31:496.

186. Harley JB, et al. Anti-Ro (SS-A) and anti-La (SS-B) in patients with Sjögren's syndrome. Arthritis Rheum 1986;29:196.

187. Harley JB, et al. Gene interaction at HLA-DQ enhances autoantibody production in primary Sjögren's syndrome. Science 1986;232:1145.

188. Fregeau DR, Roche TE, Davis PA, Coppel R, Gershwin ME. Inhibition of pyruvate dehydrogenase complex activity by autoantibodies specific for EIα, a non-lipoic acid containing mitochondrial enzyme. J Immunol 1990;144(5):1671–1676.

189. Fregeau DR, et al. Autoantibodies to mitochondria in systemic sclerosis. Arthritis Rheum 1988;31:386–392.

190. Gershwin ME, Mackay LR, Sturgess A, Coppel RL. Identification and specificity of a cDNA encoding the 70 KD mitochondrial antigen recognized in primary biliary cirrhosis. J Immunol 1987;138:3525–3531.

191. Varga J, Heiman-Patterson T, Munoz S, Love LA. Myopathy with mitochondrial alterations in patients with primary biliary cirrhosis and antimitochondrial antibodies. Arthritis Rheum 1993;36:1468–1475.

192. Caldwell SH, et al. Antimitochondrial antibodies in kindreds of patients with primary biliary cirrhosis: Antimitochondrial antibodies are unique to clinical disease and are absent in asymptomatic family members. Hepatology 1992;16:899–905.

193. Targoff IN. Autoantibodies in polymyositis. Rheum Disease Clin North Am 1992;18(2):455–482.

194. Reimer G, Scheer U, Peters J-M, Tan EM. Immunolocalization and partial characterization of a nucleolar autoantigen (Pm-Scl) associated with polymyositis/scleroderma overlap syndromes. J Immunol 1986;137:3802–3808.

195. Ge Q, Frank MB, O'Brien C, Targoff IN. Cloning of a complementary DNA coding for the 100-kD antigenic protein of the PM-Scl autoantigen. J Clin Invest 1992;90:559–570.

196. Hirakata M, Mimori T, Akizuki M, Craft J, Hardin JA, Homma M. Autoantibodies to small nuclear and cytoplasmic ribonucleoproteins in Japanese patients with inflammatory muscle disease. Arthritis Rheum 1992;35:449–456.

197. Zwettler U, Andrassy K, Waldherr R, Ritz E. (1993). Scleroderma renal crisis as a presenting feature in the absence of skin involvement. Am J Kidney Dis 1993;22(1):53–56.

198. Garlepp MJ. Immunogenetics of inflammatory myopathies. Baillieres Clin Neurol 1993;2:579–597.
199. Nishikai M, Reichlin M. Heterogeneity of precipitating antibodies in polymyositis and dermatomyositis: Characterization of the Jo-1 antibody system. Arthritis Rheum 1980;23:881–888.
200. Mathews MB, Bernstein RM. Myositis autoantibody inhibits histidyl-tRNA synthetase: A model for autoimmunity. Nature 1983;304:177–179.
201. Mathews MB, Reichlin M, Hughes GR, Bernstein RM. Anti-threonyl-tRNA synthetase, a second myositis-related autoantibody. J Exp Med 1984;160:420–434.
202. Bunn CC, Bernstein RM, Mathews MB. Autoantibodies against alanyl-tRNA synthetase and tRNA Ala co-exist and are associated with myositis. J Exp Med 1986;163:1281–1291.
203. Targoff IN, Trieu EP, Plotz PH, Miller FW. Anitbodies to glycyl-transfer RNA synthetase in patients with myositis and interstitial lung disease. Arthritis Rheum 1992;35:821–830.
204. Targoff IN. Reaction of anti-OJ autoantibodies with components of the multi-enzyme complex of aminoacyl-tRNA synthetases in addition to isoleucyl-tRNA synthetase. J Clin Invest 1993;91(6):2556–2564.
205. Love LA, Leff RL, Fraser DD, Targoff IN, Dalakas MC, Plotz PH, Miller FW. A new approach to the classification of idiopathic inflammatory myopathy: Myositis specific autoantibodies define useful homogeneous patient groups. Medicine 1991;70:360–374.
206. Miller FW, Waite KA, Biswas T, Plotz PH. The role of an autoantigen, histidyl-tRNA synthetase, in the induction and maintenance of autoimmunity. Proc Natl Acad Sci USA 1990;87:9933–9937.
207. Bhalla R, Swedler WI, Lazarevic MB, Ajamani HS, Skosey JL. Myasthenia gravis and scleroderma. J Rheumatol 1993;20:1409–1410.

ESTHER M. STERNBERG

10

Pathogenesis: Environmental

THE FIRST PART of this chapter will outline basic principles of the etiology and pathogenesis of environmental sclerodermas. It will also provide definitions of the term "environmental scleroderma," and the concepts of etiology, pathogenesis, and proof of cause and effect of illnesses associated with environmental exposure. The dual role played in such diseases by the environmental trigger and the host responses to exposure to that trigger will also be discussed.

The second part of the chapter will provide specific examples of environmental sclerodermas, their clinical characteristics, and characteristics of the environmental agents associated with development of the illness. The relative role of host versus environmental factors, and the strength of the evidence for specific environmental agents will be discussed in specific cases.

Environmental Sclerodermas: General Principles of Etiology and Pathogenesis

ENVIRONMENTAL SCLERODERMA: DEFINITION

Environmental sclerodermas can be defined as any form of skin sclerosis or scleroderma that develops in association with exposure to an environmental agent. Such forms of scleroderma can be classified according to the nature of the environmental agent or according to the pattern of disease that develops in the host. Because the development of inflammatory and autoimmune diseases, including scleroderma, depends on both the specific characteristics of the pro-inflammatory stimulus and the host's responses to that stimulus, both approaches to classification of environmental sclerodermas are valid.

The term systemic sclerosis (SSc), or scleroderma, is a clinical and pathological definition that is based on the presence of proliferative responses of fibrous connective tissue in skin and other organs. Many different agents in the environment, including chemicals, drugs, and physical injury, have been associated with the development of different clinical forms of scleroderma (Tables 10.1 and 10.2). Most forms of SSc have no known cause, and are thus called idiopathic. There are many patterns of expression: localized versus systemic forms, or forms restricted to skin versus those including major organ involvement such as lung, heart, or kidneys. It is likely that many different etiologic agents are capable of inducing fibrous connective tissue to proliferate and produce increased collagen. Clues to the etiology of clinically similar forms of idiopathic scleroderma may be gleaned from understanding the nature of the environmental agents that have been associated with the development of "hard skin" syndromes, and by defining the different patterns of disease, whether local or systemic sclerosis, which develop after exposure to different environmental agents.

Table 10.1. Therapeutic Agents Associated with Scleroderma Syndromes

Drug	Chemical Structure	Pharmacologic Action	Clinical Features	P450	HLA
Bleomycin	polypeptide mixture	antineoplastic/ antibiotic	pulmonary fibrosis	a	
Methysergide	amine alkaloid	serotonin antagonist partial agonist, potent antagonist tryptaminergic receptors	retroperitoneal fibrosis		
Pentazocine	benzomorphan derivative	analgesic/ opioid μ antagonist κ agonist	hyperpigmented local ulcers, symmetric myopathy	a	
Ethosuximide	succinimide	anticonvulsant	eosinophilia	a	
Cocaine	benzoylmethyl-ecgonine (amino alcohol base related to atropine)	sympathomimetic	sclerodactyly, skin ulcers	a	
Appetitie suppressents			sclerodactyly, skin ulcers		
diethylproprion HCl	β-phenylethylamine derivative	sympathomimetic	"		
phenmetrazine	β-phenylethylamine derivative	sympathomimetic	"		
amphetamine	β-phenylethylamine derivative	sympathomimetic	"		
dexamphetamine	D-isomer amphetamine	sympathomimetic	"		
metaqualone		sympathomimetic	"		
Amino acids and derivatives					
L-tryptophan	amino acid	weak serotonin agonist/precursor	eosinophilia, myalgias, fasciitis, SSc[b]		weak DR4[c]
L-5-hydroxy-tryptophan	a.a. metabolite	serotonin agonist/precursor	eosinophilia, myalgias, fasciitis, SSc[b]		
Penicillamine	D-ββ dimethyl-cysteine	metal chelator	SSc[b]; morphea		
Therapeutic Devices					
Silicone	dimethylpolysil-oxane polymers	cosmetic, reconstructive	fatigue, SSc[b], Raynaud's		DQAI [a]0102
Paraffin	paraffin		SSc[b]		

[a]Agents known to be substrates for P450 cytochrome. [b]Some combination of features of systemic sclerosis, including generalized skin sclerosis, sclerosis of major organs including heart, lungs, liver, GI. [c]Weak association with progression to chronic disease.

ETIOLOGY AND PATHOGENESIS: DEFINITIONS

A clear distinction must be made between the terms "etiologic agent" and the "pathogenesis of disease." An etiologic agent is the agent responsible for initiating the pathological reaction. The pathogenesis of disease depends not only on exposure to the etiologic agent, but also on the subsequent pathologic responses of the host. Identi-

fying an environmental agent and proving that it is responsible for causing disease are separate issues from identifying the cascade of events that ensues in the host after exposure to that agent, and which ultimately leads to full expression of pathology (i.e., the pathogenesis of the illness).

While the term "environmental scleroderma" implies a cause-and-effect relationship between an environmental exposure and the development of illness, in most cases of scleroderma developing in conjunction with an environmental exposure, cause and effect is difficult to prove definitively. The resulting pathology is relatively less difficult to define. The following discussion will focus on etiologic agents.

JOINT CONTRIBUTION OF ENVIRONMENTAL ETIOLOGIC AGENT AND HOST FACTORS TO PATHOGENESIS OF ENVIRONMENTAL SCLERODERMAS

As in any environmentally-induced inflammatory or autoimmune disease, the overall severity and pattern of expression of disease in the exposed individual can be viewed as the sum of an equation resulting from the balance of the dose, potency, and nature of the environmental toxicant to which the host has been exposed and the host's responses to such agents. These host responses include the entire cascade of the inflammatory, immune, and genetic responses, which allow the host's immune system to recognize and react to the toxicant, as well as the counterbalancing hormonal, neuronal, and biochemical responses which can either amplify or suppress the resultant inflammation and scarring (1). Variations in host responses play a role in variable expression of any environmental disease, ranging from the absence of symptoms to the manifestation of severe symptoms. The fact that variable host responses can result in variable disease severity in exposed hosts does not, however, nullify the role played by the environmental agent in initiating the disease.

PROOF OF THE ETIOLOGIC ROLE OF THE ENVIRONMENTAL AGENT IN CAUSING THE DISEASE VERSUS DEFINITION OF PATHOGENESIS

Central to defining the etiology of environmental sclerodermas is an appreciation of the

Table 10.2. Non-therapeutic Environmenral Exposures Associated with Scleroderma Syndromes

Exposure	Chemical Structure	Clinical Features	P450	HLA
Organic Solvents				
Aromatic hydrocarbon	non-chlorinated	morphea, SSc[b]	a	
Aliphatic hydrocarbon	non-chlorinated			
Vinyl chloride	chlorinated	Raynaud's, clubbing, distal sclerosis	a	DR3 DR3/B8
Trichlorethylene/ Perchlorethylene	chlorinated	Raynaud's, clubbing, distal sclerosis	a	
Epoxy resins	BAMM[d]	generalized morphea-like skin sclerosis, muscle weakness, fascial thickening, total body erythrma myalgias, arthralgias fatigue		
Inorganic occupational exposures				
Silica	inorganic silica	SSc[b]		
Unknown toxins				
Toxic oil syndrome	?aniline derivative in adulterated cooking oil ?oleylanilide	pulmonary infiltrates, eosinophilia, SSc[b]		DR4[c]
Physical exposure				
Vibration injury		Raynaud's saclerodactyly		

[a]Agents known to be substrates for P450 cytochrome. [b]Some combination of features of systemic sclerosis, including generalized skin sclerosis, sclerosis of major organs including heart, lungs, liver, GI. [c]Weak association with progression to chronic disease. [d]Possible causative agent: BAMM, bis(4-amino-3-methylcyclohexyl)methane.

principles of proof of causation of environmental disease. In this definition, it is important to distinguish between criteria necessary for proof of causation and those necessary for definition of pathogenic mechanism of disease. Proof, in its most definitive form according to Koch's postulates, requires reproduction of the characteristic features of the illness in an animal or human after exposure to the putative environmental agent, followed by resolution of the disease after removal of the agent. Proof that a given exposure causes a particular pattern of disease does not necessarily require a full definition of the mechanisms by which the toxicant causes the disease.

In contrast, defining the pathogenesis of environmental diseases requires elucidation of the molecular, biochemical, and cellular events that occur in the host and which, in the case of scleroderma-like illnesses, lead to fibrosis and increased collagen production. Definition of the pathogenesis of disease does not necessarily provide proof of the etiology of the illness, and proof of causation does not require that mechanisms of pathogenesis be defined.

WEIGHT OF SCIENTIFIC EVIDENCE PROVIDING PROOF OF CAUSE AND EFFECT IN ENVIRONMENTAL ILLNESS

Evidence that a particular environmental agent causes disease can be considered on a continuum from the weak evidence of simple association to the stronger evidence of direct proof of cause and effect. While anecdotal reports associating a particular environmental exposure with development of scleroderma may provide valuable indications for directions for future study, such associations do not constitute proof that a given environmental agent actually causes the disease. Full proof requires cumulative evidence from a variety of disciplines, including epidemiological, chemical, biochemical, animal, and *in vitro* studies.

Distinct clinical patterns of disease after exposure to related compounds may provide clues that a related group of compounds can cause scleroderma, and may suggest mechanisms by which the etiologic agent might cause disease. Such similar clinical patterns of illness still do not provide definitive evidence that a particular agent causes disease. Evidence that an environmental agent acts at a cellular or molecular level indicates that such a compound is biologically active. If in the whole animal the compound also causes disease, such *in vitro* biological activity provides further evidence for its etiologic role. Ultimately, however, proof of cause and effect requires reproduction of the characteristic features of the disease in an animal exposed to the implicated environmental agent. The availability of animal models also provides a powerful tool for defining the pathologic events and mechanisms of induction of disease, which occur over time after exposure to the putative toxicant at the tissue, cellular, and molecular levels. Animal models provide controllable complex systems in which to define the relative input of environmental agents and host factors in the pathogenesis of disease.

Difficulties and pitfalls are numerous in proving cause and effect, even in initial recognition of possible environmental toxins. In a chronic illness such as scleroderma, development of symptoms may not occur acutely after exposure to the etiologic agent, making identification or suspicion of the etiologic agent difficult. Similarly, initial symptoms, which do develop early, may not resemble scleroderma and may only evolve into scleroderma at a much later point in time making identification of associations difficult. If a clinical association is noted, several cases may be necessary to establish epidemiological evidence that an environmental exposure is associated with disease. Variations in dose, route, and duration of exposure in different individuals, as well as genetic differences in host responses, may result in variable expression of disease even if an environmental agent clearly is responsible for causing disease. Thus, if the potency of the environmental toxin is low, or if the number of persons exposed is low, an association greater than that which would occur by chance alone may be difficult to establish. Finally, even if an association is noted and strongly suspected on the basis of statistical association in large populations, it may be difficult to prove cause and effect by reproducing the disease in animals for several reasons. Species differences in expression of disease, which are related to differences in metabolism of the toxicant and immune, inflammatory, and fibrotic responses, make it likely that animals exposed to a putative toxicant will develop some but not all of the characteristic features of the illness seen in humans.

Thus, the conclusion that exposure to a particular environmental agent causes scleroderma requires an integrated and weighted analysis of all pieces of evidence along the continuum of proof of cause and effect: from simple association to reproduction of many features of the disease in animals exposed to the putative toxin. The more pieces of evidence which point in the same direction, the stronger the case for a cause-and-effect relationship between an environmental exposure and development of disease.

Understanding these principles is critical for valid scientific and medical evaluation of the effects of a given environmental exposure, as well for development of potential new treatments for scleroderma. Insights and principles derived from defining the etiology and pathogenesis of environmental sclerodermas can also be extrapolated to defining the etiology and pathogenesis of idiopathic sclerodermas. In addition, a clear understanding of these principles is increasingly important in legal, industrial, and societal decisions, where proof that an environmental exposure causes a chronic, debilitating, and sometimes lethal disease such as scleroderma may have far-reaching impact in the courts or in legislative arenas. The clearer the proof that an environmental agent causes disease, the stronger the basis for implementation of environmental modifications to reduce continued exposure to potentially harmful agents (2).

Variables Related to Environmental Agents and to Host Factors Which Could Contribute to Variations in Clinical Disease Expression

Both the characteristics of the environmental agent and the host's responses to exposure play a role in the pattern and severity of the scleroderma-like disease which results. Some of the general principles contributing to disease variability related to the environmental agent and host responses are outlined in the following paragraphs.

CHEMICAL CHARACTERISTICS, ROUTE OF EXPOSURE, DOSE AND DURATION OF EXPOSURE TO PUTATIVE ENVIRONMENTAL TOXIN

Many environmental agents have been associated with the development of scleroderma (see Tables 10.1 and 10.2). Variation in chemical characteristics, route, dose, and duration of exposure can contribute to variable disease outcomes.

Chemical Characteristics

Within each larger category of exposure (i.e., drugs and organic solvents) there are sub-categories of chemically related compounds which are associated with different patterns of disease (see Tables 10.1 and 10.2, Figs. 10.1 and 10.2). In some cases, chemical structures within these sub-categories resemble each other; in other cases, chemical structures differ but pharmacological or physicochemical properties are similar.

Thus, cocaine, appetite suppressants, and vasoconstrictive agents are associated with different patterns of scleroderma than are organic solvents. The former, all vasoconstrictive agents, have similar pharmacological effects, even though their chemical structures are unrelated. The latter share physicochemical properties of solubility and volatility, although their chemical structures

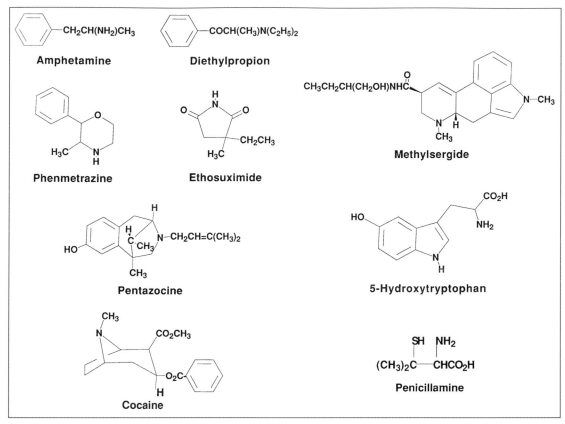

Figure 10.1. Chemical structures of some drugs associated with SSc. For further details see text and Table 10.1.

differ. Vasoconstrictive agents initially produce ulcers suggestive of ischemia, while organic solvents are associated with non-ulcerative fibrotic changes. Such differences in disease patterns suggest differences in mechanism of induction of scleroderma-like changes. Furthermore, such groupings suggest that many environmental agents, some related to each other, may produce different forms of scleroderma-like illness. Thus, it is unlikely that a single overriding cause of scleroderma will be found.

Route of Exposure

Different routes of exposure of the same compound, such as absorption through the skin versus inhalation or parenteral injection, may also be associated with differences in patterns of organ fibrosis. Some substances may be inert under some circumstances, but produce intense fibrotic reactions if exposure occurs through different routes. Thus, some have postulated that direct injection of silicone intramuscularly may induce fibrosis, whereas if it is applied as in an intact silicone implant, and therefore protected from leakage, silicone may be less likely to cause disease. Such differences in individual exposure may be difficult to quantitate and detect, leading to difficulties in proof of association and cause and effect between a particular environmental exposure and development of scleroderma.

Dose, Potency, and Duration of Exposure

The combination of dose, potency, and duration of exposure to environmental chemicals should also be taken into consideration as variables in causing disease. Low doses of potent chemicals are more likely to induce disease than low doses of weak etiologic agents. Similarly, prolonged exposure to weak toxicants is more likely to cause disease than shorter durations of exposure. Many of these variables are difficult, if not impossible, to quantitate in human populations exposed to putative environmental agents associated with environmental sclerodermas. In the case of compounds with low potency, proof of cause and effect in animals may require prolonged duration of exposure before even mild symptoms develop.

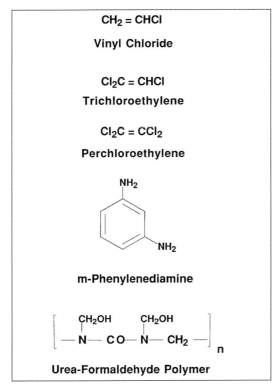

Figure 10.2. Chemical structures of some environmental chemicals associated with SSc. For further details see text and Table 10.2.

NATURE OF HOST FACTORS

Variations in individual host responses to environmental exposure can alter the final severity and pattern of disease which results after uniform exposure to a known environmental toxicant. Host factors can be considered at the clinical, cellular, immunological, biochemical, and molecular levels.

Clinical Patterns of Disease

Table 10.3 summarizes scleroderma-like syndromes according to overall pattern of disease, and lists environmental exposures which have been associated with them. From this point of view, similarities in clinical manifestations of disease may suggest similarities in mechanism of induction of scleroderma. Alternately, clinical similarities may simply reflect the limited ways in which skin and connective tissue react to a variety of types of injuries.

Table 10.3. Clinical Patterns of Scleroderma-like Illness Associated with Environmental Exposures

Clinical Pattern	Reported Associated Exposures
Raynaud's, acrocyanosis	vibration; VC, PCE, TCE
Sclerodactyly	vibration; VDC, PCE, TCE
Local ulcers	pentazocine; appetite suppressants
Morphea	organic solvents
Hyperpigmentation	bleomycin
Fasciitis	L-5-HTP; L-TRP; TOS
Generalized scleroderma	TOS; silicone implant; L-TRP; L-5-HTP
Pulmonary fibrosis	bleomycin; VC, PCE, TCE; silica
Retroperitoneal fibrosis	methysergide
Renal involvement	cocaine; TCE (rare)
Cardiac involvement	L-TRP; TOS
GI involvement	VC, PCE, TCE; TOS;L-TRP
Peripheral neuropathy	VC, PCE, TCE; L-TRP; L-5-HTP; TOS
Eosinophilia	L-5-HTP; L-TRP; TOS
Thrombocytopenia	VC, PCE, TCE; TOS; L-TRP
Thrombocytosis	TOS; L-TRP

VC= vinyl chloride; PCE= perchlorethylene; TCE= trichloroethylene; L-5-HTP= L-5-hydroxytryptophan; L-TRP= L-tryptophan; TOS= toxic oil syndrome.

Tissue and Cellular Responses

Idiopathic scleroderma is characterized by vascular, immune, and fibrotic features (3–5) and are thoroughly reviewed in Chapters 7–9 and 11–13. Similarly, environmental sclerodermas are also characterized by varying degrees of this triad of features, suggesting that, depending on the environmental agent and also perhaps the route and intensity of exposure, the initiating pathogenic event may be primarily vascular endothelial damage, primarily immune activation, or primarily induction of collagen synthesis. Some discussion, additional to that in the following paragraphs, may be found in Chapter 5.

The cascade of cellular, inflammatory, and immune events, which occur after exposure to a variety of environmental agents, have been defined in varying degrees depending on the environmental agent involved. Initial exposure may be associated with cellular responses suggestive of ischemia, as after exposure to cocaine and appetite suppressants. In other cases, initial exposure is associated with inflammatory cell infiltrates. Whether the initial event is ischemia or inflammation, fibrosis and collagen deposition appear late in the sequence of events—in the repair phase of tissue responses.

Variations in degree of autoimmune and allergic phenomena are also reported in association with exposure to different environmental agents. Differences in initial infiltrating cellular type are associated with different environmental exposures and scleroderma-like illnesses. A particular category of scleroderma-like syndrome, the eosinophilia-myalgia syndrome (EMS), is associated with initial blood eosinophilia, although the presence of tissue eosinophils is low, and lymphocytes and mononuclear cells predominate (see Chapter 5). In other forms of scleroderma, mast cells have been reported to be among the earliest infiltrating cells, while in others monocytes predominate. Such cellular differences suggest differences in mechanism of induction of subsequent fibrosis by different etiologic agents. In the case of EMS, it is not clear whether the initial eosinophilia plays a pathologic role in the subsequent fibrotic features of the syndrome, or whether the etiologic factor induces both early eosinophilia and later fibrosis independently. Animal studies, in which there is no eosinophilia in the context of presence of fibrosis, suggest that eosinophils do not play an important etiologic role in the development of fibrosis. Tissue presence of eosinophil granule products, such as eosinophil-derived neurotoxin (EDN) and major basic protein (MBP), suggest that some secondary pathologic features of the syndrome may be induced by eosinophil degranulation products (6).

Immune Responses

Specific antibodies, patterns of cytokine, and cellular responses have been characterized in environmental sclerodermas, and provide further insights into similarities and differences between environmental and idiopathic sclerodermas. Variations in immune responses, including genetically determined differences in the recognition of antigens, may affect variations in patterns and severity of scleroderma-like changes which develop after environmental exposures.

Genetic Factors

The degree to which genetic factors contribute to development of environmental sclerodermas has been addressed in some cases by the evaluation of associations of major histocompatibility antigens with development of disease, and are discussed in depth in Chapter 2. Associations have been found with certain HLA types (7–10). In some cases, these associations are weak; in other cases, they are more definite. Such variations in relative strength of HLA associations are consistent with variations in the relative input of the environmental agent versus host factors. One possible explanation of weak HLA associations is that the nature and dose of the environmental agent may play a relatively greater role in development of acute symptoms, while HLA type, or other associated genetic factors, may play a relatively greater role in the tendency to progression to chronic disease.

Growth Factors and Adhesion Molecules

The expression of specific mRNAs, as well as the protein content of collagen, TGFβ, adhesion, and other molecules, have been defined and quantitated in many environmental sclerodermas. Collagen metabolism has also been extensively studied in scleroderma and related illnesses. Findings generally indicate that collagen metabolism, TGFβ, and adhesion molecules are increased with increased production and increased turnover of new collagen. While these studies suggest that increased collagen synthesis is secondary to increased production of growth factors such as TGFβ and cytokines such as IL-1, the etiologic agents causing such growth factor increases may be multifactorial.

Biochemical Responses and Potential Toxicity of Secondary Metabolites

Exposure to environmental chemicals that can be metabolized, either through endogenous detoxification systems (see discussion of P450 microsomal enzymes, below) or through natural metabolic pathways, presents the potential for toxicity not only of the parent compound to which the individual is exposed, but also of toxicity of secondary metabolites. Variations in host metabolic pathways as a result of the presence or absence of detoxifying enzymes, differences in rates of enzyme activity, or inducibility of enzymes may lead to further variations in the final expression of disease due to differences in resultant levels of toxic secondary metabolites.

Two examples of endogenous metabolic systems that may contribute to the presence of potentially toxic intermediate metabolites in environmental sclerodermas are tryptophan metabolism (Fig. 10.3) and chlorinated hydrocarbon metabolism (Fig. 10.4).

Tryptophan metabolism is altered in a variety of autoimmune and inflammatory illnesses, including scleroderma and scleroderma-like ill-

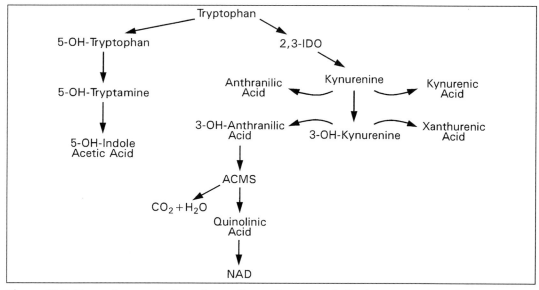

Figure 10.3. Tryptophan metabolic pathways. Tryptophan is metabolized via two major pathways, the serotonin (5-OH-tryptamine) and kynurenine pathways. 2,3-IDO = indoleamine-2,3 dioxygenase, the rate-limiting enzyme in the kynurenine pathway, which is induced by inflammatory mediators, including interferon γ. Increases in the levels of both kynurenine and quinolinic acid can result from induction of 2,3-IDO by inflammatory mediators. ACMS = 2-amino-3-carboxy-muconic semialdehyde. NAD = nicotinamide adenine dinucleotide.

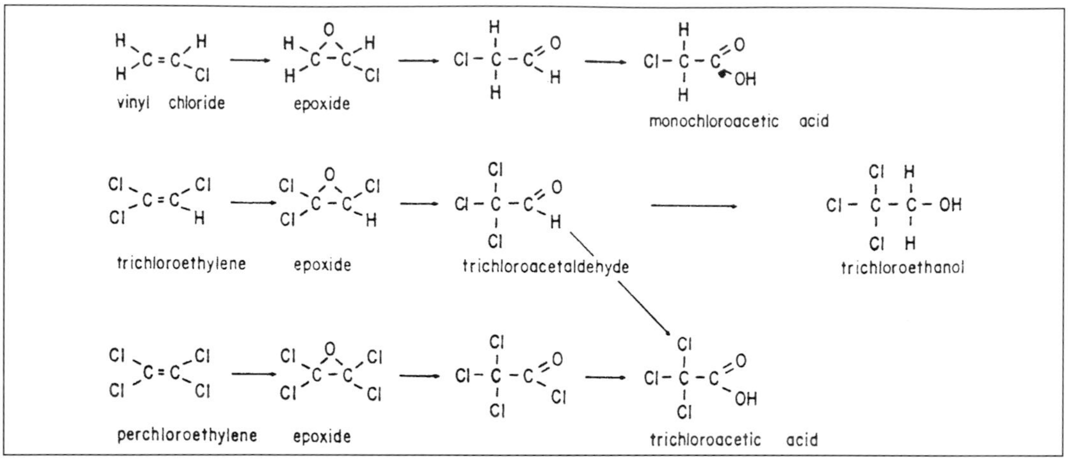

Figure 10.4. Vinyl chloride, perchloroethylene, and trichloroethylene metabolic pathways. (Lockey JE, Kelly CR, Cannon GW, et al. Progressive systemic sclerosis associated with exposure to trichloroethylene. J Occupation Med 1987;29:495, with permission.)

nesses. Levels of kynurenine, a metabolite of L-tryptophan (L-TRP), increase in these illnesses. It is clear that increased tryptophan metabolism via the kynurenine pathway is not the primary cause of scleroderma, nor is it the result of an inborn error of metabolism; rather, it is secondary to induction by gamma interferon of the rate limiting enzyme in the kynurenine pathway of tryptophan metabolism—indoleamine 2,3 dioxygenase (see Fig. 10.3). Nonetheless, the resultant elevated levels of L-TRP metabolites may also exert some toxicity. Thus, quinolinic acid is known to be neurotoxic, and kynurenic acid has vasoconstrictive properties. The increased levels of such metabolites could contribute to, or amplify, neurotoxic or vasoconstrictive features of the illness.

Other endogenous metabolic pathways may also produce toxic intermediates that could play a pathogenic role in environmental sclerodermas. Although vinyl chloride, perchloroethylene, and trichloroethylene are not endogenous compounds, they are all detoxified through similar metabolic pathways via highly reactive epoxide intermediates to a common metabolic product. In some studies, these metabolites have been shown to have greater toxicity than the parent compound (11).

Detoxification Systems:
Cytochrome P450 Enzymes

In any analysis of disease resulting from exposure to a potentially toxic agent, one must include an evaluation of the body's major drug detoxification system—the cytochrome P450 enzyme system. The P450 cytochromes are a family of drug-detoxifying isoenzymes found mainly in the hepatic microsomal system. Increased activity of cytochrome P450 2D6 has been associated with a greater tendency to bladder cancer (12), and idiopathic scleroderma has been associated with decreased activity of cytochromes P450 $2C_{MP}$ and P450 3A4 (13). Table 10.1 identifies drugs associated with development of scleroderma-like syndromes, which are known to be substrates for various P450 cytochromes. In some cases, such as vinyl chloride disease (14), P450 cytochrome activities have been evaluated. In one such study comparing a small sample of vinyl chloride exposed workers who developed scleroderma-like illness to those who had not, no difference was found in drug metabolizing activity. However, in most cases in which a putative environmental toxin is known to be detoxified by the P450 system, such studies have not been performed. Therefore, there is no direct evidence that the

P450 system plays a role in development of scleroderma after environmental exposure.

Specific Examples of Drug-Related Sclerodermas

The categories of compounds that have been associated with development of scleroderma-like syndromes include drugs, organic solvents, and inorganic exposures. Tables 10.1 and 10.2 summarize the compounds that have been associated with development of scleroderma-like syndromes. Included in this list is scleroderma associated with: (*a*) adulterated food products, such as the toxic oil syndrome; (*b*) amino acids and amino acid-derivatives, such as L-tryptophan and L-5-hydroxytryptophan; and (*c*) the non-pharmacologic therapeutic agent silicone used for breast implants. In addition to chemical exposures, there have also been reports of the development of sclerodactyly and Raynaud's phenomenon (RP) in association with physical occupational exposure to vibration. While in some cases the evidence for these associations is strong, in others evidence is at this time still anecdotal. Selected examples from each category are discussed in detail in the body of this chapter.

Several recent reviews have discussed the environmental agents that have been associated with the development of scleroderma-like illnesses (15–19). Some studies of the epidemiology of scleroderma have shown that the prevalence of scleroderma associated with environmental exposure is high in populations of patients with scleroderma of all causes. The following paragraphs describe specific examples of compounds within each category of environmental agents that have been associated with a variety of sclerosing syndromes. Scleroderma-like syndromes that develop in relation to selected environmental agents in each chemical category will be described in detail according to their clinical characteristics, pathophysiology, immune, biochemical, and molecular changes.

THERAPEUTIC AGENTS

Therapeutic agents that have been associated with development of scleroderma syndromes include drugs, amino acids, and non-ingested chemical therapeutic agents used in devices such as silicone implants. Examples of scleroderma-like illnesses associated with these categories of compounds are listed in Table 10.1 and selected examples are discussed in the following paragraphs (see also Chapters 2 and 5).

ANTI-NEOPLASTIC AGENTS

Bleomycin

Bleomycin is an anti-neoplastic antibiotic composed of a mixture of polypeptides isolated from the bacteria *Streptomyces verticillus*. It has been associated with the development of pulmonary fibrosis and skin changes resembling scleroderma, including hyperpigmentation, infiltrated plaques and nodules, dermal bands, edema, and hair loss (20). Development of symptoms appears to be dose-related, with skin changes occurring at lower cumulative doses and pulmonary changes occurring at higher doses (21, 22). Skin changes may be spontaneously reversible upon discontinuation of the drug and have been reported to regress with high-dose steroids (23).

Evidence that the reported clinical association of bleomycin and scleroderma is a causal one is provided by induction of the characteristic features of the illness in mice (24) and rats (25) after chronic parenteral administration of the drug. Availability of such animal models allows further analysis of the histopathology of the illness, which evolves over time. Initial endothelial cell edema of the intima of the pulmonary arteries and veins is followed by lymphocyte and plasma cell infiltration, multifocal necrosis of type 1 alveolar epithelial cells with fibrinous exudation, and, finally, repair with proliferation and metaplasia of type 2 alveolar epithelial cells and fibrosis of the interstitium (24). Biochemical analyses of human skin and lung fibroblasts from bleomycin scleroderma patients have shown increased procollagen synthesis, with a predominance of type 1 procollagen synthesis (26). More recent studies have indicated that bleomycin induces chromosomal damage (27).

SYMPATHOMIMETICS, APPETITE SUPPRESSANTS

A group of drugs sharing common pharmacologic actions have been associated in case reports, and in some cases confirmed in animal studies, with scleroderma-like changes ranging from local sclerosis at sites of injection, to regional or symmetric sclerosis and indurated myopathies, to more general features of scleroderma. These drugs include cocaine and appetite suppressants that are structurally related to amphetamine. It is not known whether the sclerosis-inducing effects of these compounds are related to their pharmacologic actions. One feature that these agents share in common is their vasoconstrictor property, and it may be that vasoconstriction with ischemia and subsequent repair underlies some of their sclerosis-inducing effects. The clinical pattern of the sclerosing syndromes related to this group of compounds share features suggestive of ischemia, with ulcers and necrosis at the sites of injection and regional sclerosis more prominent than generalized sclerosis. Histopathology is also suggestive of a pattern of ischemia followed by endothelial damage and subsequent repair and fibrosis.

Cocaine

Cocaine is a sympathomimetic, which acts by blocking norepinephrine presynaptic re-uptake. Recent case reports have associated scleroderma renal crisis (28) and diffuse scleroderma (29) with cocaine use. Initial reports (30) described two patients with acral vasospasm, atrophic depressed finger pad scars, and diffuse skin sclerosis extending above the wrists, without systemic involvement. In one case, the patient had used both amphetamines and cocaine. A single case

has been reported fulfilling the preliminary criteria for systemic sclerosis (31). Cocaine-induced skin lesions in rats show vascular damage and scarring in healing areas. Although cocaine-induced hepatotoxicity has been shown to be caused by reactive metabolic intermediates of cocaine formed by a cytochrome P450 dependent pathway (32), similar studies have not been performed in skin or fibroblasts.

Appetite Suppressants

These drugs are β-phenylethylamine derivatives with sympathomimetic activity. Included in this category are diethylpropion HCl, mazindol, amphetamine, dexamphetamine, and metaqualone. Several case reports have associated chronic use of appetite suppressants with development of RP, hand swelling, sclerodactyly, and dysphagia (33, 34). Most of these involved diethylpropion HCl, and some subjects had also ingested other appetite suppressants including mazindol, amphetamine, dexamphetamine, and metaqualone. A direct causal link between appetite suppressants and scleroderma-like changes has not been established in animal studies.

OPIOID DERIVATIVES

Pentazocine

Pentazocine is a benzomorphan derivative (see Table 10.1), which produces morphine-like opioid effects including analgesia, sedation, and respiratory depression. Chronic subcutaneous or intramuscular injections of pentazocine have been associated in both humans and rats with the development of indurated ulcers surrounded by a halo of hyperpigmentation at the sites of injection (35–37). Fibrous myopathy (38) and symmetric myopathy have also been reported in several case reports. Histopathological changes in animal studies showed vessel occlusion with infarction of the dermis and epidermis, suggesting that subsequent sclerotic changes resulted from vasoconstriction and ischemia (35).

AMINO ACIDS AND
RELATED COMPOUNDS

Prior to 1989, circumstantial evidence and isolated case reports had linked tryptophan, the tryptophan-derived compound L-5-hydroxytryptophan (L-5-HTP) (39), and serotonin-related compounds with various forms of fibrosing illness. None of these associations had been reported on a large scale, and the mechanism of the relationship between fibrosis and such tryptophan derivatives was not known. The fact that structurally unrelated serotonergic compounds, such as methysergide and serotonin itself, when injected repeatedly subcutaneously in animals, were associated with fibrosis, initially suggested that such associations might occur through serotonin-related mechanisms. The subsequent large scale epidemic of eosinophilia-myalgia and fasciitis, which occurred in 1989 in persons ingesting L-tryptophan (L-TRP) manufactured by a single company, suggested that the etiology of this syndrome was related to exposure to impure L-tryptophan. Further studies have indicated that while impure L-TRP causes many of the characteristic features of the syndrome in animals, pure L-tryptophan is also associated with significant scarring in other organs, primarily the pancreas, and may have contributed to the pathogenesis of the syndrome.

It is important to note that the diagnosis of EMS is a clinical and pathological definition. Thus, the retrospective identification of cases with similar symptoms in patients not exposed to L-tryptophan does not rule out L-tryptophan, impure L-tryptophan, or impurities, such as 1,1′-ethylidene bis L-tryptophan (EBT), as etiological agents in EMS. In fact, this syndrome may represent an example of similar pathological changes in fascial tissue caused by several related etiological agents.

L-Tryptophan (L-TRP)

In the summer and fall of 1989, patients across the United States developed eosinophilia, myalgias, and fever (40,41), which eventually evolved in many patients to a chronic illness characterized by fasciitis, scleroderma-like skin changes often sparing the hands, neuropathies, and pulmonary and cardiac fibrosis (42) (see also Chapter 5). This syndrome, termed L-tryptophan-related eosinophilia-myalgia syndrome (L-TRP EMS), occurred in persons taking L-tryptophan for insomnia, depression, and pre-menstrual syndrome. L-TRP EMS was clinically very similar or identical to the syndrome reported in association with L-5-hydroxytryptophan (see following) and to the toxic oil syndrome, which occurred in Spain in 1981 in persons ingesting adulterated cooking oil (see following). L-TRP EMS closely resembled idiopathic eosinophilic fasciitis (Shulman's syndrome), differing from the latter in the degree of internal organ system involvement (43), which, in EMS, included pulmonary and cardiac fibrosis and neuropathies, in addition to the fasciitis and peripheral blood eosinophilia reported in Shulman's syndrome. L-TRP EMS ultimately affected up to 6000 individuals in the United States and was associated with 38 deaths.

Epidemiological studies at first indicated a case association with certain lots of L-TRP manufactured by a single company: Showa Denko K.K. [41]. Subsequent chemical studies indicated that these lots showed a fingerprint pattern on high performance liquid chromatography (HPLC) and contained over 60 different impurities (44–46). Two of these impurities, EBT (45) and 3-(phenylamino)-L-alanine (PAA) (46), have been identified (Fig. 10.5) and synthesized, making direct toxicological testing possible. Initial epidemiological studies suggested a strong case-association with EBT (44). More recent analysis, which took time factors into account, suggests a weaker association with EBT and greater association with other impurities (47). The association with PAA is particularly interesting, because this impurity structurally resembles one of the possible contaminants in the TOS, 3-phenylamino-1,2-propanediol (see following and Fig. 10.6).

Figure 10.5. Chemical structures of impurities found in L-tryptophan associated with EMS and in oils associated with TOS. 1,1′-ethylidenebis [tryptophan] (EBT), and 3-[phenylamino]-L-alanine are impurities found in EMS case-associated L-tryptophan, and oleylanilide is found in TOS case-associated oils.

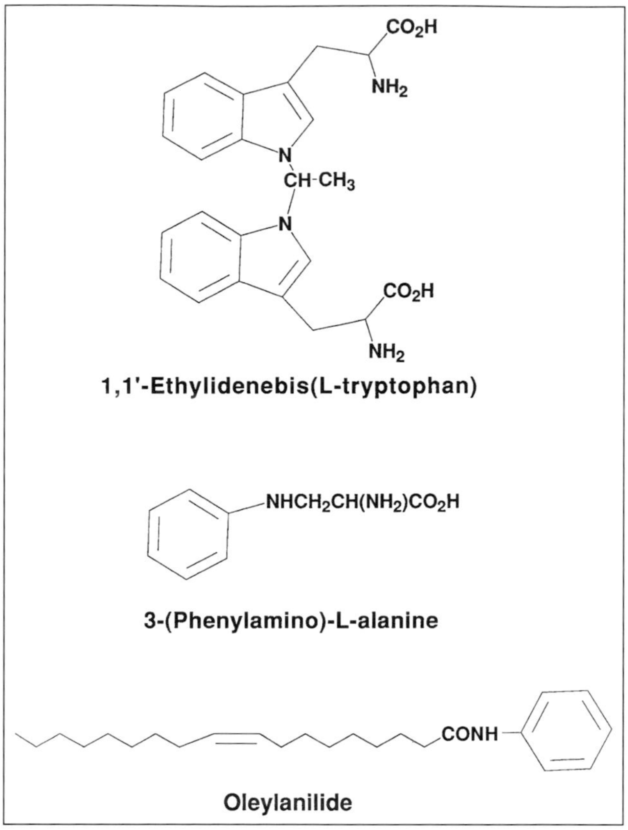

1,1′-Ethylidenebis(L-tryptophan)

3-(Phenylamino)-L-alanine

Oleylanilide

Figure 10.6. Chemical structures of 3-phenyl-amino-1,2-propanediol and 3-phenylamino alanine. (Philen RM, Posada M. Toxic oil syndrome and eosinophilia-myalgia syndrome: May 8–9, 1991, World health meeting report. Semin Arthritis Rheum 1993;23:117, with permission.)

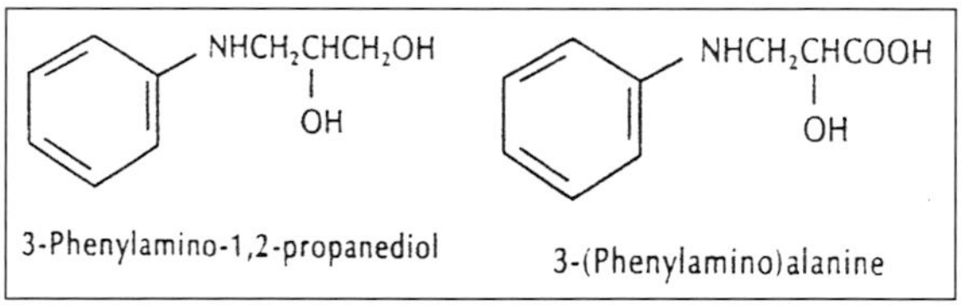

3-Phenylamino-1,2-propanediol

3-(Phenylamino)alanine

Subsequent studies addressed the etiology and pathogenesis of the L-tryptophan eosinophilia myalgia syndrome. Animal studies in rats (48,49) and mice (50) support the hypothesis that impure L-TRP and at least one of the impurities, EBT, are important etiologic agents in causing many of the fascial scarring and inflammatory features of the syndrome. These studies, comparing the effects of impure L-TRP or EBT to pure L-TRP, also suggest that pure L-TRP, while not causing the syndrome, may contribute

to its scarring features, because treatment of animals with doses equivalent to the median doses taken by patients is associated with severe pancreatic acinar hyperplasia and with some mild increased collagen and adhesion molecule expression in tissues. Eosinophilia has not been reproduced in any animal systems to date.

Interactions between environmental agent and host responses are numerous in this syndrome. Initial studies of host factors involved in the pathogenesis of EMS focused on tryptophan metabolism. More recent studies have examined the role of P450 enzymes, HLA type, and immune and tissue responses in EMS.

Tryptophan metabolism is altered compared to non-inflamed controls in patients with L-TRP EMS, as in L-5-HTP-related scleroderma. This pattern of tryptophan metabolites, which includes elevated plasma quinolinic acid in parallel with elevated plasma kynurenine, is consistent with activation of the enzyme indoleamine 2,3-dioxygenase (IDO). Because IDO can be activated by inflammatory mediators, these findings are consistent with initiation of the syndrome by an inflammatory stimulus, indicating that the elevated plasma kynurenine is secondary to inflammation and is not related to an inborn error of metabolism. Regardless of the mechanism of induction of inflammation, subsequent elevated tryptophan metabolites could still play a role in amplifying or producing some of the pathological features of the syndrome. Because quinolinic acid is an excitatory amino acid known to be neurotoxic, it could potentially contribute to some of the neuropathic features of the illness.

Genetic HLA factors may play only a weak role, and have been reported to show only a trend to association with progression to chronic disease (7).

Impure L-TRP and EBT have also been shown to affect neuroendocrine host responses, which are important in modulating the severity of inflammation (48,51). Treatment of rats with case-associated impure L-TRP or EBT, in contrast to pure L-TRP or vehicle control, was associated with suppression of hypothalamic corticotrophin releasing hormone (CRH) mRNA expression. It is not clear whether this suppression was a direct neurotoxic or pharmacologic effect of the impurity or was secondary to the chronic inflammation. *In vitro* studies suggest that neurotoxicity is possible, because one of the tetrahydrobetacarboline isomers of the acid breakdown product of EBT is toxic to mature murine spinal cord neurons in culture. This toxicity is both maturation-and interleukin-1-dependent (52). Regardless of the mechanism, interruptions of

the hypothalamic-pituitary-adrenal axis have been shown to be associated with exacerbations of inflammatory disease (1). This suggests yet another potential mechanism of toxicity of environmental agents: that of HPA axis interruption with enhanced susceptibility to inflammation.

Other host responses that have been examined in this syndrome include cellular, tissue growth factor, and cytokine responses. Peripheral blood eosinophilia is an important defining feature of the syndrome, although eosinophils are only rarely found in tissues. On the other hand, eosinophil degranulation products, such as eosinophil-derived neurotoxin (EDN) and major basic protein (MBP), are increased in affected EMS tissues, suggesting that eosinophil products may play a role in amplifying some features of the syndrome. Lung biopsies show infiltration of CD8+ lymphocytes, suggesting a possible immune cytotoxic/suppressor lymphocyte role in pathogenesis. Cytokines, such as IL-8 (53), and growth factors, such as TGFβ (54), have also been reported to be elevated. Classic allergic phenomena are unlikely to play a role, because in most cases there is no elevation of IgE, although mast cells are increased in some patients (55). Increases in the eosinophil and mast cell maturation factor IL-5 have also been reported (56,57), and are consistent with and could explain the increased mast cells, eosinophilia, and hyperplasia of bone marrow eosinophil precursors (58).

L-5-Hydroxytryptophan (L-5-HTP)

Since the initial case report and biochemical study of L-5-HTP related scleroderma (39), several similar cases have been reported throughout the world: most recently, a family in Canada whose members developed either full-blown EMS, or partial manifestations, after exposure to L-5-HTP (59). The mother in this family developed the characteristic features of EMS while administering L-5-HTP to her two infant sons for treatment of their GTP cyclohydrolase deficiency. The children showed eosinophilia and thrombocytosis, but no clinical evidence of EMS. Previous reports of EMS in an L-TRP-exposed infant also indicated only a partial form of the illness, with eosinophilia and thrombocytosis. Because the L-5-HTP was life-sustaining in these cases and could not be discontinued, HPLC evaluation of the family's L-5-HTP as well as all available sources of L-5-HTP was undertaken. An additional peak, co-eluting with one of the impurities found in the case-associated L-tryptophan, was identified in the L-5-HTP used by this family. Although the identity of this peak has not been determined, substitution of a source of L-5-HTP which did not contain this peak was associated with resolution of clinical signs in the children. This case is an example of the difficulty of fully establishing cause and effect in environmental illness, even when the putative toxicant is available for study and when removal of the environmental agent is associated with resolution of symptoms, because not all children who had been treated with the implicated lot of L-5-HTP developed symptoms. Such variable expression of disease could be related to variations in routes of exposure, dosing, or variable host factors.

Penicillamine

Penicillamine is a derivative of cysteine, D-$\beta\beta$ dimethyl cysteine, which is used as a chelating agent in the treatment of Wilson's disease, as well as an agent in the treatment of idiopathic scleroderma. There have been scattered case reports of development of scleroderma or morphea in patients treated for Wilson's disease with high-dose penicillamine (60,61).

OTHER THERAPEUTIC DEVICES

Included in the category of therapeutic devices are silicone implants used in cosmetic surgery (see also Chapter 2). Scleroderma-like syndromes have been reported in patients who had previously undergone cosmetic surgery, primarily augmentation mammoplasty, with silicone or paraffin. The earliest case reports were in the Japanese literature (62) of patients who had received either paraffin or silicone by direct injection. In an initial series of patients (63), scleroderma-like illness was observed primarily in patients who had undergone cosmetic surgery with paraffin, while rheumatoid arthritis-like and human adjuvant disease symptoms were associated with cosmetic surgery with silicone. Subsequent studies have reported scleroderma-like syndromes in association with silicone, the chemical currently used in such cosmetic surgery. Most such reports are collections of case reports representing relatively few patients; therefore, although they are strongly suggestive, these reports do not prove conclusively a cause-and-effect relationship between silicone and autoimmune disease. Most recently, a large scale retrospective population-based study did not find an excess of autoimmune disease in breast implant patients (64). However, this study represented a 10-year follow-up, in contrast to the reported greater than 12-year mean duration of exposure associated with the onset of symptoms in earlier case reports.

Silicone

Silicone is a general term used for a group of organic fluids, gels, and rubbers that are derived from dimethylpolysiloxane polymers in which silicon has been substituted for carbon. The larger the polymer, the more solid the silicone product (65). Silicone in the form of a gel enclosed in silastic envelope is used in cosmetic surgery, primarily for augmentation mammoplasty, but also for chin implants. Solid silicone rubber, termed silastic, is manufactured by polymerization and cross-linking with a catalyst, and is used in arthroplastic replacement surgery.

The possible development of connective tissue disease after silicone exposure illustrates several general principles of environmental illness related to variables in both the environmental agent and the host, which make the etiology and pathogenesis of these syndromes difficult to define conclusively.

The lag time between initial exposure and reported onset of symptoms is long (mean time approximately 12 years), making recognition of a connection between exposure and illness difficult. Further complicating proof of association is the large variety of connective tissue syndromes that have been reported in relation to cosmetic surgery with silicone. Most commonly reported are systemic sclerosis-like syndromes, with an estimated 3- to 8-fold increase in incidence of scleroderma in patients undergoing augmentation mammoplasty (63,65). Also reported are rheumatoid arthritis, systemic lupus erythematosus (SLE), Sjögren's syndrome, Hashimoto's thyroiditis, mixed connective tissue disease, inflammatory arthritis, and a poorly defined syndrome of fever and polyarthralgias termed human adjuvant disease (63,65,66).

The precise chemical make-up of silicone is variable, and synthetic purity standards may have changed over time, raising the possibility that contaminants in the silicone, rather than the silicone itself, may have contributed to some illness. Finally, the physicochemical form of the silicone (i.e., liquid versus solid), degree of polymerization, and variations in polymer size, as well as variable availability to systemic dissemination via leakage may also play a role in the pattern of development of symptoms.

Different routes of exposure (direct injection versus silicone contained in silastic envelope of breast prostheses) may contribute to the degree of host reaction and thus final expression of disease. Acuteness versus chronicity of exposure, ranging from accidental direct injection into the blood stream to slow leakage from a damaged implant, or gradual foreign body reaction to damaged arthroplastic implants, may all further contribute to variable host responses and final disease expression.

Host tissue handling of silicone, such as degree of dissemination to regional lymph nodes, and resultant variations in degree of immune system activation may also contribute to final pattern and severity of illness. Other host factors, including HLA type [10] and concurrent or previous infection with tuberculosis (63), have been postulated as possible variables in development of these illnesses in much the same way that adjuvant induces autoimmune diseases in susceptible animals.

Patients who develop scleroderma-like illness develop a pattern of disease resembling SSc, with chronic fatigue, myalgias, RP, skin sclerosis, arthralgias, arthritis, pulmonary, and neurologic symptoms. In addition, lymphadenopathy, local inflammatory reactions, and breast discomfort are reported. Variable improvement has been reported after removal of implants, with few patients completely remitting, some partially or transiently improving, and others showing no effect (10,63,65).

Evidence of immune activation in these patients is derived from the presence of autoantibodies including rheumatoid factor (RF), antinuclear antibodies (ANAs), anti-DNA, snRNP, and anti-thyroid antibodies. In addition, specific anti-silicone antibodies have been detected by enzyme-linked immunoabsorbent assay (ELISA), and an as yet undefined antibody to a large molecular weight protein has also been detected in women with breast implants and associated connective tissue symptomatology. Histopathological changes include evidence of foreign body reactions with granulomata: clear spaces sometimes containing refractile material, surrounded by inflammation and foreign body giant cells.

Attempts to reproduce the syndrome in animals have included studies of subcutaneous injection of silicone fluid in mice (67) and intra-articular injection of particulate silastic in rabbits (68). In both cases, inflammatory responses were noted—in the latter, in the knee injected with silastic particles but not in the contralateral control knee joint. In mice, an initial polymorphonuclear infiltration was followed by lymphocyte and fibroblast infiltration and subsequent subsiding of inflammation, followed by increased extracellular material. The presence of vacuolized macrophages and multinucleated giant cells was suggestive of phagocytosis of silicone.

Hypotheses regarding pathogenesis of these syndromes involve systemic or lymphatic exposure to the silicone polymer via either direct injection or gradual leakage from a damaged implant. Phagocytosis by macrophages, as evidenced by vacuolization and giant cell formation, then allows systemic dissemination to organs and the lymphatic system with resultant immune system activation. Support for this hypothesis is provided by recent studies showing silicon, as identified by electron probe microanalysis, within the fibrous breast capsule, inflammatory cell infiltrate, and in chronically inflamed and fibrotic distal tissues, including skin, synovium, and alveolar macrophages. Circumstantial evidence that genetic host factors may play a role in susceptibility to development of symptoms is suggested by the increased prevalence of the HLADQAI*0102 haplotype in women with implant-related dermatomyositis (10).

Non-Therapeutic Exposures to Environmental Chemicals

Scleroderma-like illnesses have been reported not only in relation to exposure to therapeutic agents, but also in association with non-therapeutic environmental chemicals. Exposure to potentially toxic environmental chemicals is ubiquitous; however, because of frequency, duration, and dose of exposure, it is particularly prevalent in industrial situations and occupational exposures. Typical exposures include organic solvents, pesticides, and inorganic chemicals such as silica dust. These and other examples of environmental sclerodermas are listed in Table 10.2, and discussed in the following paragraphs.

ORGANIC SOLVENT-RELATED SCLERODERMA-LIKE ILLNESS

A variety of scleroderma-like syndromes, ranging from RP and morphea to SSc with pulmonary involvement and esophageal dysfunction, have been associated in case reports with exposure to organic solvents (see following and Chapters 2 and 5). Solvents can be grouped according to chemical category: (a) aromatic hydrocarbons, such as benzene, toluene, white spirits, xylene, and dieselene; (b) aliphatic hydrocarbons, such as hexane; and (c) chlorinated solvents such as perchloroethylene, trichloroethylene, and vinyl chloride.

Most cases occur as a result of industrial exposures and are difficult to associate definitively with a single solvent, because in many cases mixtures of solvents are used. Furthermore, because the solvents are often used in industrial degreasing, it is possible that the etiologic agent may be a chemical or chemicals dissolved in the solvent, rather than the solvent itself. Exposure to aromatic hydrocarbons typically occurs through occupational exposures to dry-cleaning fluids or paint thinners (69). The primary sites of absorption are the lungs and unprotected skin. Vinyl chloride disease, and the closely related trichloroethylene toxicity, have been studied in most detail.

NON-CHLORINATED HYDROCARBONS

The aromatic and aliphatic hydrocarbons are widely used solvents, applied as paint thinners, used in dry cleaning, and used for other household and industrial purposes. Case reports have associated scleroderma, RP, morphea, and sometimes systemic illness with exposure to the petroleum-derived solvents benzene, toluene, and xylene, as well as to the aromatic mixes white spirits and dieselene (69–71). The etiologic role of some of these solvents has been tested in animals. Skin sclerosis has been reported in one study in mice receiving chronic intraperitoneal injections of a variety of aliphatic hydrocarbons (71) and epoxy resins (72).

CHLORINATED HYDROCARBONS

The chlorinated hydrocarbons are chemically related, and the clinical syndromes associated with them resemble each other. Compounds in this category include vinyl chloride, trichlorethylene, and perchlorethylene.

Vinyl Chloride (PVC) Scleroderma

Vinyl chloride is a chlorinated hydrocarbon; its chemical formula is CH_2CHCl. The monomer resin is mixed with other chemicals to produce the polymer $(CH_2CHCl)_x$ used in plastics and other synthetic products. Vinyl chloride disease, first described in 1963 by Suciu et al (73), is characterized by early numbness and tingling of the fingers, cold sensitivity, RP, pseudoclubbing of the fingers, edema, skin thickening of the fingers, hands, forearms (74), and chest x-ray changes. Prevalence of symptoms has been reported to increase with duration of exposure, and is greatest after 5, 10 or 20 years of exposure (75), depending on the symptom reported. In a single industrial facility (75), abnormal Allen tests, indicating poor hand circulation, occurred in 26% of all workers, RP in 6%, and skin changes in 6% of workers. Others have reported lower prevalences: 31 out of 3,000 personnel (76) and 25 out of 5,011 workers in 32 industrial facilities across the US and Canada (77). Development of symptoms appears to be related to work practices and overall cumulative exposures over time.

Histopathological changes of the skin resemble morphea, with swelling of collagen bundles, fragmented elastic fibers, lymphocyte infiltration, and atrophy in hair follicles. The presence of vascular changes including luminal narrowing of digital arteries, stenosis, and subtotal occlusion (74), suggest a vascular component in the pathogenesis of the illness. The associated prevalence of thrombocytopenia and splenomegaly with lack of bone marrow involvement suggest a potential relationship between the observed vascular changes and altered platelet function. Both the vascular and platelet alterations are reminiscent of such abnormalities in idiopathic scleroderma.

Host factors that have been evaluated include HLA type (9) and cytochrome P450 activity (14). As in idiopathic scleroderma, an increased prevalence of DR3 and DR3/B8 haplotypes in patients with PVC disease was found. Although cytochrome P450s are substrates for vinyl chloride, no differences in P450 activity were found in patients with this syndrome compared to the general population.

One hypothesis for the pathogenesis of this syndrome suggests that vinyl chloride combines with host proteins rendering them antigenic (78). Others have suggested that the toxicants are mixtures of partially polymerized material left in the industrial scrapings (77), and thus mixtures of different size polymers rather than vinyl chloride itself may be the initiating factors in this illness.

Trichloroethylene/Perchloroethylene Scleroderma

The structural similarity between trichloroethylene, perchloroethylene, and vinyl chloride, and the observation that these compounds are also associated with development of clinically similar scleroderma-like syndromes, strengthens the possibility that these compounds play an etiologic role in environmental sclerodermas. The relationship, however, is still defined in terms of "association," because these compounds also share physico-chemical properties as solvents. Therefore, common solutes(s), rather than the solvents, may be the etiological agents primarily responsible for the illness. Similarly, their related metabolic pathways (see Fig. 10.4) may indicate that the etiologic agent is a common metabolite or intermediate rather than the parent compounds.

INORGANIC EXPOSURE

Silica (see also Chapters 2 and 5)

Exposure to silica dust occurs primarily in gold and coal miners, but it also occurs in other occupations in which rock particles and silica dust may be aerosolized, such as sand-blasters and cement, pottery factory, and foundry workers (79). In addition to the well-known pulmonary fibrosis among workers exposed to silica dust, these workers also exhibit a significantly increased incidence of a systemic disease that is clinically indistinguishable from SSc (79–81). One study reported a calculated incidence of SSc of 81.8 per million in silica-exposed men, compared to 3.4 per million in the general population ($p < .001$) (80).

Clinical features of this illness include RP, limited dermal sclerosis with necrosis of finger tip pulp, and esophageal involvement. There appears to be a higher incidence of bibasilar pulmonary fibrosis in silica-related SSc than in idiopathic SSc. Less often, there is generalized dermal sclerosis, and only rarely is renal involvement reported.

Studies addressing the pathogenesis of this syndrome have postulated that phagocytosis of silica crystals by pulmonary alveolar macrophages, and subsequent systemic spread of these crystals with phagocytosis by endothelial cells, may set up a cycle of endothelial and macrophage activation (81). Such endothelial cell activation and damage coupled with resultant release of cytokines, such as interleukin-1, could induce both the vascular and immune features of the illness.

Evidence for both vascular endothelial damage and immune activation in silica-related SSc includes increased levels of von Willebrand factor and circulating immune complexes, elevated immunoglobulins, ANAs, and anti-Scl-70 antibody. That the endothelial damage occurs early, before systemic symptoms appear, and therefore may be a primary pathogenic event, is suggested by elevated levels of von Willebrand factor and circulating immune complexes not only in silica-related scleroderma patients but also in healthy silica-exposed co-workers. Further support for this hypothesis is provided by animal studies showing enhanced interleukin-1 production by alveolar macrophages in silica-exposed rats (82).

Table 10.4. Clinical Signs and Symptoms of TOS and EMS

Symptoms	TOS			EMS
	Acute Phase	Intermediate Phase	Chronic Phase	
Fever	+++	–	–	+++
Asthenia	+++	–	–	?
Cough	+++	–	–	+++
Dyspnea	++	–	–	+++
Myalgia	++	++	+++	++++
Pruritus	++	–	–	++
Headache	+++	–	–	+++
Rash	++	–	–	+++
Confusion	+	–	–	++
Arthralgia	+	+	–	++
Weight loss	–	++	–	+++
Sensory neuropathy	–	++	++	++
Motor neuropathy	–	+	++	+
Edema	–	++	–	+++
Scleroderma	–	–	++	+++
Alopecia	–	+	+	++
Hepatopathy	+	++	++	–
Pulmonary hypertension	–	++	+	+
Thrombosis	–	+	–	+
Sicca syndrome	–	++	++	++
Dysphagia	+	++	+	–
Cramps	+	–	+++	+++

TOS, toxic oil syndrome; EMS, eosinophilia-myalgia syndrome.
NOTE. Percentage of patients with sign or symptom: + + + +, 100 to 76%; + + +, 75 to 51%; + +, 50 to 26%; +, 25 to 1%; –, 0%.
(From Philen RM, Posada M. Toxic oil syndrome and eosinophilia-myalgia syndrome: May 8–10, 1991, World health organization meeting report. Semin Arthritis Rheum 1993;23:110, with permission.)

UNKNOWN TOXINS

In some cases of environmental sclerodermas, the scleroderma-like illness clearly develops in relation to an environmental exposure, but the toxin has remained unidentified. This category of illness includes the clinically well-defined Spanish toxic oil syndrome (TOS).

Toxic Oil Syndrome (TOS)

The term TOS refers to an epidemic that occurred in Spain in 1981 in persons who had ingested adulterated cooking oil. Over 20,000 persons were ultimately affected, with over 800 deaths (see also Chapter 5).

The syndrome was characterized by acute onset atypical pneumonia with diffuse pulmonary infiltrates, myalgias, and eosinophilia (83). A more complete listing of symptoms and lab findings is shown in Tables 10.4 and 10.5. Clinically, TOS resembles L-TRP EMS, which occurred in the United States 10 years later (see Table 10.4),

as well as L-5-HTP scleroderma (39) (see section on amino acid derivatives). TOS differed from EMS in the acuteness and fulminance of its onset and the more prominent early pulmonary infiltration and atypical pneumonia. EMS, in contrast, had a more gradual onset, characterized by more general constitutional symptoms, such as myalgias and fever. Both illnesses were characterized by acute, intermediate, and chronic phases. Acute symptoms evolved into chronic sclerodermatous changes and associated neuropathies in both syndromes.

Both illnesses exhibited epidemiological features of environmental sclerodermas. TOS cases were clustered geographically in the environs of Madrid. In contrast, relatively few cases of EMS occurred in any one geographic location, but were widespread, occurring in every state throughout the United States. The geographic distribution of both illnesses was consistent with the geographic distribution of the implicated agent to which the at-risk population was exposed (83).

Table 10.5. Laboratory Findings in Patients with TOS and EMS

| Finding | TOS | | | |
	Acute Phase	Intermediate Phase	Chronic Phase	EMS
Eosinophilia	+++	++++	+++++	++++
Thrombocytopenia	−	++	−	+/−
Thrombocytosis	−	++	−	+/−
Elevated transaminases	+	+++	++	+
Elevated aldolase	++	−	−	+
Creatinine phosphokinase	—	—	—	—
Elevated triglycerides	−	−	−	−
Hyperglycemia	−	+	−	−
Hypoalbuminemia	−	++	−	+
Elevated alkaline phosphatase	−	−	−	−
DL CO	+	++	−	
Elevated IgE	++	−	−	−
Elevated T4/T8	++	−	−	−
Presence of HLA DR3, DR4	−	−	++	−
Elevated C3 complement	−	−	−	−
Antinuclear antibody	++	+	+	−

TOS, toxic oil syndrome; EMS, eosinophilia-myalgia syndrome.
NOTE. Percentage of patients with sign or symptom: + + + +, 100 to 76%; + + +, 75 to 51%; + +, 50 to 26%; +, 25 to 1%; −, 0%.
(From Philen RM, Posada M. Toxic oil syndrome and eosinophila-myalgia syndrome: May 8–10, 1991, World health organization meeting report. Semin Arthritis Rheum 1993;23:110.)

Furthermore, the incidence of disease in both cases fell dramatically after the implicated product was removed from the market.

The primary pathological feature of TOS was a vascular lesion characterized by endothelitis, lymphohistiocytic infiltrates, sub-endothelial edema, and eosinophil and mononuclear cell infiltrates. Later, this evolved to intimal proliferation and fibrosis, which involved not only vessel intima, but also dermis, perineurium, GI submucosa, salivary and thyroid glands, breasts, pancreas, and cardiac conducting system.

Host factors that may have some association with progression to chronic illness include HLA DR3 and DR4 (84). In addition, there is a female preponderance in the illness of 1.5:1, and some age associations have been noted. Virtually no infants developed the syndrome. Both the sex and age association, however, may be related to exposure rather than host factors in these groups.

The primary risk factor was exposure to the adulterated cooking oil. The etiologic agent responsible for initiation of TOS has never been identified. However several contaminants in the adulterated cooking oil have been implicated. Since the adulterated cooking oil was rapeseed oil denatured for industrial use with aniline, aniline derivatives have been considered candidates, particularly oleylanilide (see Fig. 10.5). Although it is not clear whether the latter is itself an etiologic agent, or whether it is simply a strong marker for case-related oils, oleylanilide also exhibits a strong dose-effect (83). The structural similarity between aniline and anthranilic acid, the starting product for production of L-TRP by bacterial fermentation, suggests that families of such compounds might represent a group of environmental agents which could induce certain forms of environmental sclerodermas. Most recently, chemical analysis show the presence of fatty acid esters of the oleylanilide and 3-(N-phenylamino)-1,2-propanediol in the case-associated oils, but not in non-case associated oils (85). This finding is significant, because 3-(phenylamino)-1,2 propanediol is chemically related to 3-(phenylamino)alanine, one of the impurities found in impure case-associated L-tryptophan (83).

Another hypothesis suggests that unknown toxic industrial chemicals previously transported in the clandestine tanker trucks in which the oil was transported may be responsible for the illness. Again, as in the case of environmental scleroderma related to organic solvents (see previous), the issue of solvent versus solute as etiological agent is difficult to resolve.

Animal studies have not yielded a clear-cut animal model for TOS. The main difficulty in such studies is that an etiologic agent has not been identified, and duration of time and storage conditions of the implicated oils make identification of a putative toxicant increasingly less likely. Thus, attempts have been made to reproduce the denaturation/renaturation process of the fraudulently produced oils. Preliminary reports indicate *in vitro* toxicity in rat neuroblastoma and rat hepatocyte cultures of such synthetic oils compared to controls (86).

PHYSICAL INJURY

In addition to the many chemical environmental exposures described above, which have been associated with development of scleroderma-like illnesses, repeated vibration injury has been associated with RP and sclerodactyly (87,88). Such illness can occur in workers who operate jackhammers or chain saws. An increased incidence of RP and sclerodactyly is reported in chain-saw workers compared to non-exposed controls, with dose and duration of exposure contributing factors (87).

Summary

The plethora of environmental agents described to be associated with various clinical forms of scleroderma-like illness suggest that many different agents may, through several different pathogenic mechanisms, initiate fibrosing syndromes. These mechanisms may initially be primarily vascular, as in relation to the sympathomimetic agents, initially primarily immune, as in silicone implant disease, but all, by definition, evolve to include some form of increased synthesis of collagen and connective tissue elements. That host factors are clearly also involved in final expression and outcome of the disease response to such environmental insults is evidenced by the variable expression, frequent HLA associations, variable severity, and relatively low incidence of these illnesses even in populations known to have been exposed to putative toxins. Such variable host responses do not, however, mean that the environmental agent in question does not play an etiologic role in initiating development of disease.

The potential for development of such chronic, debilitating, and potentially life-threatening diseases after exposure to many agents ubiquitously present in today's environment leads to a dilemma of social responsibility. Because it is not possible to completely remove all potential environmental toxins, our aim in the future should be to apply all available scientific tools to clearly identify and characterize the environmental agents capable of initiating such illnesses, and at the same time to define the factors that render some hosts more susceptible to development and perpetuation of disease. Only with clear definition of all variables involved can appropriate measures be taken to remove the implicated environmental agents or minimize susceptible hosts' exposure to them.

References

1. Sternberg EM, Chrousos GP, Wilder RL, Gold PW. The stress response and the regulation of inflammatory disease. Ann Intern Med 1992;117:854–866.
2. Hadler NM. Managing toxicopathic rheumatic diseases in the current legal climate. Editorial. Arthritis Rheum 1991;34:634–637.
3. Kahaleh MB, Osborn I, LeRoy EC. Increased factor VII/von Willebrand factor antigen and von Willebrand factor activity in scleroderma and Raynaud's phenomenon. Ann Intern Med 1981;94:482–484.
4. Miossec P, Cavender D, Ziff M. Production of interleukin I by human endothelial cells. J Immunol 1986;136:2486–2491.
5. Alcocer-Varela J, Martinez-Cordero E, Alarcon-Segovia D. Spontaneous production of, and defective response to, interleukin-I by peripheral blood mononuclear cells from patients with scleroderma. Clin Exp Immunol 1985;59:666–672.
6. Hertzman PA, Maddoux GL, Sternberg EM, Heyes MP, Mefford IN, Kephart GM, Gleich GJ. Repeated coronary artery spasm in a young woman with the eosinophilia myalgia syndrome. JAMA 1992;267:2932–2934.
7. Kaufman LD, Gruber BL, Gregersen PK. Clinical follow-up and immunogenetic studies of 32 patients with eosinophilia-myalgia syndrome. Lancet 1991;337:1071–1074.
8. Silman AJ. Epidemiology of scleroderma. Ann Rheum Dis 1991;50:846–853.
9. Black CM, Welsh KI, Walker AE, Bernstein RM, Catoggio LJ, McGregor AR, Lloyd Jones JK. Genetic susceptibility to a scleroderma-like syndrome induced by vinyl chloride. Lancet 1983;i:53–55.
10. Fenske NA, Vasey FB. Silicone-associated connective tissue disease. Arch Dermatol 1993;129:97–98.
11. Smith GF. Trichlorethylene: A review. Br J Ind Med 1966;23:249.
12. Kaisary A, Smith P, Jacqz E. Genetic predisposition to bladder cancer, ability to hydroxylate debrisoquine and mephenytoin as risk factors. Cancer Res 1987;47:5488–5493.
13. May DG, Black CM, Olsen NJ. Scleroderma is associated with differences in individual routes of drug metabolism: A study with dapsone, debrisoquine and mephenytoin. Clin Pharmacol Ther 1990;48:286–295.
14. Black C, May G, Csuka ME, Lupoli S, Wilkinson GR, Branch RA. Activity of oxidative routes of metabolism of debrisoquin, mephenytoin, and dapsone is unrelated to the pathogenesis of vinyl chloride-induced disease. Clin Pharmacol Ther 1992;52:659–667.
15. Silman AJ, Jones S. What is the contribution to occupational environmental factors to the occurrence of scleroderma in men. Ann Rheum Dis 1992;51:1322–1324.
16. Bourgeois P, Aeschlimann A. Drug-induced scleroderma. Baillieres Clin Rheumatol 1991;5:13–20.
17. Haustein UF, Ziegler V. Environmentally induced systemic sclerosis-like disorders. Int J Dermatol 1985;24:147–151.
18. Owens GR, Medsger TA Jr. Systemic scleroderma secondary to occupational exposure. Am J Med 1988;85:114–116.

19. Fishman SJ, Russo GG. The toxic pseudoscleroder-mas. Int J Dermatol 1991;30:837–842.
20. Luna MA, Bedrossian CWM, Lichtiger B. Intersti-tial pneumonitis associated with bleomycin thera-py. Am J Clin Pathol 1972;58:501–510.
21. Finch W, Rodnan G, Buckingham R, Prince RK, Winkelstein A. Bleomycin induced scleroderma. J Rheumatol 1980;7:651–659.
22. Kiefer O. Uber die nebenwirkungen der bleomy-cintherapie auf der haut. Dermatologica 1973;146: 229–243.
23. Kerr LD, Spiera H. Scleroderma in association with the use of bleomycin: A report of 3 cases. J Rheu-matol 1992;19:294–296.
24. Adamson IYR, Bowden DH. The pathogenesis of bleomycin-induced pulmonary fibrosis in mice. Am J Pathol 1974;77:185–198.
25. Mountz JD, Downs Minor MB, Turner R, Thomas MB, Richards F, Pisko E. Bleomycin-induced cuta-neous toxicity in the rat: Analysis of histopatholo-gy and ultrastructure compared with progressive systemic sclerosis (scleroderma). Br J Dermatol 1983;108:679–686.
26. Clark JC, Starcher BC, Uitto J. Bleomycin-induced synthesis of type I procollagen by human lung and skin fibroblasts in culture. Biochim Biophys Acta 1980;631:359–370.
27. Wolff DJ, Needleman BW, Wasserman SS, Schwartz S. Spontaneous and clastogen induced chromosomal breakage in scleroderma. J Rheuma-tol 1991;18:837–840.
28. Lam M, Ballou SP. Reversible scleroderma renal crisis after cocaine use. N Engl J Med 1992;326: 1435.
29. Kilaru P, Kim W, Sequeira W. Cocaine and sclero-derma: Is there an association. J Rheumatol 1991; 18:1753–1755.
30. Trozak DJ, Gould WM. Cocaine abuse and con-nective tissue disease. J Am Acad Dermatol 1984; 10:525.
31. Kerr HD. Cocaine and scleroderma. South Med J 1989;82:1275.
32. Boelsterli UA, Goldin C. Biomechanisms of co-caine-induced hepatocyte injury mediated by the formation of reactive metabolites. Arch Toxicol 1991;65:351–360.
33. Tomlinson IW, Jayson MIV. Systemic sclerosis after therapy with appetite suppressants. J Rheumatol 1984;11:254.
34. Aeschlimann A, de Truchis P, Kahn MF. Scleroder-ma after therapy with appetite suppressants. Re-port of four cases. Scand J Rheumatol 1990;19: 87–90.
35. Parks DL, Perry HO, Muller SA. Cutaneous com-plications of pentazocine injections. Arch Derma-tol 1971;104:231–235.
36. Swanson DW, Weddige RL, Morse RM. Hospital-ized pentazocine abusers. Mayo Clin Proc 1973;48: 85–93.
37. Schlicher JE, Zuehlke RL, Lynch PJ. Local changes at the site of pentazocine injections. Arch Derma-tol 1971;104:90–91.
38. Oh SJ, Rollins JL, Lewis I. Pentazocine-induced fi-brous myopathy. JAMA 1975;231:271–273.
39. Sternberg EM, Van WM, Young SN, Magnussen I, Baker H, Gauthier S, Osterland CK. Development of a scleroderma-like illness during therapy with L-5-hydroxytryptophan and carbidopa. N Engl J Med 1980;303:782–787.
40. Hertzman PA, Blevins WL, Mayer J, Greenfield B, Ting M, Gleich GJ. Association of the eosinophil-ia-myalgia syndrome with the ingestion of trypto-phan. N Engl J Med 1990;323:357–365.
41. Swygert LA, Maes EF, Sewell LE, Miller L, Falk H, Kilbouren EM. Eosinophilia-myalgia syndrome. JAMA 1990;264:1698–1703.
42. Silver RM, Heyes MP, Maize JC, Quearry B, Vion-net FM, Sternberg EM. Scleroderma, fasciitis, and eosinophilia associated with the ingestion of tryp-tophan. N Engl J Med 1990;322:874–81.
43. Shulman LE. The eosinophilia myalgia syndrome associated with ingestion of L-tryptophan. Arthri-tis Rheum 1990;33:913–917.
44. Belongia EA, Hedberg CW, Gleich GJ, White KE, Mayeno AN, Loegering DA. An investigation of the cause of the eosinophilia-myalgia syndrome asso-ciated with tryptophan use. N Engl J Med 1990; 323:357–365.
45. Smith MJ, Mazzola EP, Farrell TJ. 1,1′-Ethyli-denebis (L-tryptophan), structure determination of contaminant "97"—implicated in the eosino-philia-myalgia syndrome (EMS). Tetrahedron Lett 1991;32:991–994.
46. Goda Y, Suzuki J, Maitani T. 3-Anilino-L-alanine, structural determination of UV-5, a contaminant in EMS-associated L-tryptophan samples. Chem Pharm Bull 1992;40:2236–2238.
47. Hill RHJ, Caudill SP, Philen RM. Contaminants in L-tryptophan associated with eosinophilia-myal-gia syndrome (EMS). Arch Environ Contam Toxi-col 1993;25:134–142.
48. Crofford LJ, Rader JL, Dalakas MC, Hill RHJ, Brady LS, Page SW, Needham LL, et al. L-tryptophan im-plicated in human eosinophilia-myalgia syndrome causes fascitis and perimyositis in the Lewis rat. J Clin Invest 1990;86:1757–1763.
49. Love LA, Rader JL, Crofford LJ, Raybourne RB, Principato MA, Page SW, Trucksess MW, et al.

Pathological and immunological effects of ingesting L-tryptophan (L-TRP) and 1,1′-ethylidene bis[tryptophan] in Lewis rats. J Clin Invest 1993; 91:804–811.

50. Silver RM, Ludwicka A, Hampton M, Ohba T, Bingel SA, Smith T, Harley RA, et al. A murine model of eosinophilia-myalgia syndrome induced by 1,1′-ethylidenebis(L-tryptophan). J Clin Invest 1994;93:1473–1480.

51. Brady LS, Page SW, Thomas FS, Rader JL, Lynn AB, Polterak B, Zelazowski E, et al. 1,1′-ethylidenebis(L-tryptophan) (EBT), a contaminant implicated in L-tryptophan eosinophilia-myalgia syndrome, suppresses mRNA expression of hypothalamic corticotropin-releasing hormone in Lewis (LEW/N) rat brain. Neuroimmunomodulation 1994;1:59–65.

52. Brenneman DE, Page SW, Schultzberg M, Thomas FS, Zelazowski P, Burnet P, Avidor R, et al. A decomposition product of a contaminant implicated in L-tryptophan eosinophilia-myalgia syndrome affects spinal cord neuronal cell death and survival through stereospecific, maturation and partly IL-1-dependent mechanisms. J Pharmacol Exp Ther 1993;266:1029–1035.

53. Reitamo S, Remitz A, Varga J. Demonstration of interleukin-8 and autoantibodies to interleukin-8 in the serum of patients with systemic sclerosis and related disorders. Arch Dermatol 1993;129:189–193.

54. Tazelaar HD, Myers JL, Strickler JG. An immunophenotypic, immunofluorescent, and electron microscopic study. Mod Pathol 1993;6:56–60.

55. Kaufman LD, Seidman RJ, Phillips ME. Cutaneous manifestations of the L-tryptophan-associated eosinophilia-myalgia syndrome: A spectrum of sclerodermatous skin disease. J Am Acad Dermatol 1990;23:1063–1069.

56. Owen WFJ, Petersen J, Scheff DM, Folkerth RD, Anderson RJ, Corson JM, et al. Hypodense eosinophils and interleukin-5 activity in the blood of patients with eosinophilia-myalgia syndrome. Proc Natl Acad Sci USA 1990;87:8647–8651.

57. Yamaoka KA, Miyasaka N, Inuo G, Saito I, Kolb JP, Fujita K, Kashiwazaki S. 1,1′-ethylidenebis(tryptophan) (peak E) induces functional activation of human eosinophils and interleukin-5 production from T lymphocytes: Association of eosinophilia-myalgia syndrome with a L-tryptophan contaminant. J Clin Immunol 1994;14:50–60.

58. Philen RM, Eidson M, Kilbourne EM. Eosinophilia-myalgia syndrome: A clinical case series of twenty-one patients. Arch Intern Med 1991;151:533–537.

59. Michelson D, Page SW, Casey R, Trucksess M, Love L, Milstein S, Wilson C, et al. Eosinophilia-myalgia syndrome and related disorders associated with exposure to L-5-hydroxytryptophan. J Rheumatol (In press).

60. Bernstein RM, Ann Hall M, Gostelow BE. Morphea-like reaction to D-penicillamine therapy. Ann Rheum Dis 1981;40:4244.

61. Miyagawa S, Yoshioka A, Hatoko M. Systemic sclerosis-like lesions during long-term penicillamine therapy for Wilson's disease. Br J Dermatol 1987; 116:95–100.

62. Miyoshi K, Miyaoka T, Kobayashi Y, Itakura T, Nishijo K, Higashibara M, Shiragami H, et al. Hypergammaglobulinemia by prolonged adjuvanticity in man: Disorders developed after augmentation mammoplasty. Ijishimpo 1964;2122:9–14.

63. Kumagai Y, Shiokawa Y, Medsger TA, Rodnan GP. Clinical spectrum of connective tissue disease after cosmetic surgery. Arthritis Rheum 1984;27:1–12.

64. Gabriel SE, O'Fallon WM, Kurland LT, Beard CM, Woods JE, Melton W. Risk of connective tissue diseases and other disorders after breast implantation. N Engl J Med 1994;330:1697–1702.

65. Endo LP, Edwards NL, Longley S, Corman LC, Panush RS. Silicone and rheumatic diseases. Semin Arthritis Rheum 1987;17:112–118.

66. Spiera H, Kerr LD. Scleroderma following silicone implantation: A cumulative experience of 11 cases. J Rheumatol 1993;20:958–961.

67. Andrews JM. Cellular behavior to injected silicone fluid: A preliminary report. Plast Reconstruct Surg 1966;38:581–583.

68. Worsing RA, Engber WD, Lange TA. Reactive synovitis from particulate silastic. J Bone Joint Surg 1982;64A:581–585.

69. Walder BK. Solvents and scleroderma. Lancet 1965;2:436.

70. Walder BK. Do solvents cause scleroderma. Int J Dermatol 1983;22:157–158.

71. Yamakage A, Ishikawa H. Generalized morphea-like scleroderma occurring in people exposed to organic solvents. Dermatologica 1982;165:186–193.

72. Yamakage A, Ishikawa H, Saito Y, Hattori A. Occupational scleroderma-like disorder occurring in men engaged in the polymerization of epoxy resins. Dermatologica 1980;161:3344.

73. Suciu I, Drejman I, Valeskai M. Investigation of the diseases caused by vinyl chloride. Med Intern 1963; 15:967–978.

74. Veltman C, Lange CE, Juhe S, Stein G, Bachner V. Clinical manifestations and course of vinyl chloride disease. N Y Acad Sci 1975;246:6–17.

75. Lilis R, Anderson H, Nicholson WJ, Daum S, Fischbein AS, Selikoff LJ. Prevalence of disease among vinyl chloride and polyvinyl chloride workers. Ann NY Acad Sci 1975;246:22–41.

76. Wilson RH, McCormick WE, Tatum CF, Creech JL. Occupational acroosteolysis. JAMA 1967;201:577–581.

77. Dinman BD, Cook WA, Whitehouse WM, Magnuson HJ, Ditcheck T. Occupational acroosteolysis. An epidemiological study. Arch Environ Health 1971;22:61.

78. Ward AM. Evidence of an immune complex disorder in vinyl chloride workers. Proc R Soc Med 1976;69:289–290.

79. Rodnan GP, Benedek TG, Medsger TA Jr, Cammarata RJ. The association of progressive systemic sclerosis (scleroderma) with coal miners pneumoconiosis and other forms of silicosis. Ann Intern Med 1967;66:323–334.

80. Cowie RL. Silica-dust-exposed mine workers with scleroderma (systemic sclerosis). Chest 1987;92:260–262.

81. Rustin MHA, Bull HA, Ziegler V, Melhorn J, Haustein U-F, Maddison PJ, James J, et al. Silica-associated systemic sclerosis is clinically, serologically and immunologically indistinguishable from idiopathic systemic sclerosis. Br J Dermatol 1990;123:725–734.

82. Oghiso Y, Kubota Y. Enhanced interleukin I production by alveolar macrophages and increase in Ia-positive lung cells in silica-exposed rats. Microbiol Immunol 1986;30:1189–1198.

83. Philen RM, Posada M. Toxic oil syndrome and eosinophilia-myalgia syndrome: May 8–10, 1991, World Health Organization Meeting Report. Semin Arthritis Rheum 1993;23:104–124.

84. Vicario JL, Serrano-Rios M, San Andres F. HLA-DR3, DR4 increase in chronic stage of Spanish oil disease. Lancet 1982;1:236.

85. Hill RH, Schurz H, Posada M, Borda IA, Philen RM, Kilbourne EM, Head SL, et al. Possible etiologic agents for toxic oil syndrome: Fatty acid esters of 3-(N-phenylamino)-1,2-propanediol. Arch Environmental Contam Toxicol 1995;28:259.

86. Slack PT, Wood GM, Mallinson CB. Toxic oil disaster. Nature 1990;345:583.

87. Nagata C, Yoshida H, Mirbod SM, Komura Y, Fujita S, Inaba R, Iwata H, et al. Cutaneous signs (Raynaud's phenomenon, sclerodactylia and edema of the hands) and hand-arm vibration exposure. Int Arch Occup Environ Health 1993;64:587–591.

88. Blair HM, Headington IT, Lynch PJ. Occupational trauma, Raynaud's phenomenon and sclerodactylia. Arch Environ Health 1974;28:80–81.

BARBARA WHITE

11

Pathogenesis: Immune Aspects

Activation of the immune system is an early event in humans with systemic sclerosis (SSc). T cells, plasma cells, macrophages, mast cells, eosinophils, and basophils are found in increased numbers and an activated state in tissues of SSc patients. These cells are capable of modifying fibroblast and endothelial cell functions through the production of soluble mediators or cytotoxic effects. By these means, activated immune system cells may promote the fibrosis and vascular damage that characterize involved tissues in SSc patients.

Recent advances in the understanding of basic immunologic processes have been applied to extend our knowledge about the immune system in SSc patients. Compared to 5 years ago, more complete descriptions are available of types of immune cells, T cell antigen receptor (TCR) gene use, human leukocyte antigen (HLA) alleles, autoantibody targets, cytokines, and adhesion molecules in SSc patients. Despite our burgeoning capacity to describe immune abnormalities in SSc patients, it remains a mystery whether activation of the immune system is an initiating or secondary event in the pathogenesis of this disease. The answer to this enigma is a crucial clue to the cause of SSc.

T Cell Abnormalities in SSc Patients

T cells appear to be central to the development of tissue damage in SSc patients. They provide specificity to the immune response, they dominate the inflammatory infiltrates in tissues of SSc patients, and they regulate functions of many hematopoietic and non-hematopoietic cells, including fibroblasts and endothelial cells.

T CELLS IN TISSUES

In a meticulous analysis of sequential skin biopsies from SSc patients, Prescott et al [1] observed that one of the earliest abnormalities is a collapse of vimentin intermediate filaments around the nucleus of endothelial cells. Next, both $CD4^+$ and $CD8^+$ T cells migrate into the skin, where they scatter throughout the subcutaneous tissue and dermis or localize to areas around the vessels, nerves, and skin appendages [1–8]. γ/δ T cells are sparse in the skin of SSc patients (White B, unpublished data). Expression of HLA class II molecules indicates that the infiltrating T cells have been recently activated [1,3,6,7]. Coincident with T cell infiltration, additional morphologic and functional changes are noted in the endothelial cells [1]. Tissue fibrosis follows [1]. Those fibroblasts that are actively producing $pro\alpha1(I)$ and $pro\alpha1(III)$ collagen mRNAs are located next to the area of T cell infiltration [8], which suggests that activated T cells may have a causal relationship to fibrosis.

Because cytoskeletal alterations of endothelial cells precedes lymphocytic infiltration in the skin, the argument could be made that activation of T cells occurs in response to changes in the endothelial cells. It is equally possible, however, that the changes in endothelial cell cytoskeleton occur in response to circulating soluble mediators produced by T cells. Of note, interleukin (IL)-4 induces a collapse in vimentin intermediate filaments in cultured endothelial cells (9).

Both CD4$^+$ and CD8$^+$ T cells are found in the skin of patients with idiopathic SSc, but CD4$^+$ T cells are the major subpopulation (1,6). In contrast, CD8$^+$ T cells are more frequent in the skin of patients who develop an SSc-like illness during chronic human graft-versus-host disease (GVHD) (10). CD8$^+$ T cell infiltration of tissues has also been observed in a patient with HTLV-I associated myelopathy who developed limited scleroderma (11).

A potential role for CD8$^+$ T cells in SSc is underscored by findings in bronchoalveolar lavage (BAL) of patients with active lung disease. SSc patients with interstitial lung disease have increased numbers and percentages of lymphocytes in the interstitium on biopsy (12) and frequently in BAL (12–19). T cells, rather than B cells, are the predominant lymphocyte seen within BAL from SSc patients, and 85% to 90% of these cells bear the memory marker CD29 (19). Analyses of the T cells within BAL of SSc patients with alveolitis show increased CD8$^+$, reduced CD4$^+$, and normal γ/δ T cells, compared to peripheral blood from the same patients or blood and BAL from normal patients (19). Relevant to the finding of increased CD8$^+$ T cells in the lungs of SSc patients is the observation by Kahaleh and Yin (20) that endothelial cell cytotoxicity in SSc patients is mediated in part by granzyme A, which is released by cytotoxic T cells. The dominance of distinct T cell subpopulations in the skin (CD4$^+$) and lungs (CD8$^+$) of SSc patients suggests that different T cells may contribute to the disease process in different organs.

T CELLS IN BLOOD

Reports of immunologic testing of the blood of SSc patients frequently contradict each other. The clinical expression of SSc is heterogeneous, and the disease has different stages and levels of activity. Disagreement in results may be caused by the selection of different patient populations and analyses of small numbers of patients. Moreover, results from peripheral blood may not reflect disease processes in the tissues of SSc patients, so care should be taken in the interpretation of any results not confirmed by analysis of tissues.

Absolute lymphocyte counts, absolute numbers and percentages of T cells, and absolute numbers and percentages of CD8$^+$ T cells are all reported to be normal or decreased in peripheral blood mononuclear cells (PBMC) of patients with SSc (21–30). Percentages of CD4$^+$ T cells are reported to be increased (30), normal (22,25, 26,29), or decreased (25). The ratio of CD4$^+$ to CD8$^+$ T cells is increased (22,23,26,27,29,30) or normal (25,27). Percentages of γ/δ T cells are normal (19). CD29$^+$CD3$^+$, CD29$^+$CD4$^+$, and CD45RA$^-$ memory T cells are increased (24,25, 31) or normal (21,26). CD26 levels are increased on memory CD4$^+$CD45RA$^-$ T cells (31). CD8$^+$ T cells bearing the memory marker CD29 are reportedly decreased (31).

Evidence of activation of circulating T cells in SSc patients comes from their cell surface expression of HLA-DR molecules and IL-2 receptors (R) (21–23, 31), but even these findings are disputed (26,29). Soluble IL-2R levels are increased (21,32–36), and the levels either correlate (33), or do not correlate (32), with disease activity. Soluble CD4 levels are increased (35), and soluble CD8 levels are increased (33) or decreased (35). As another marker of T cell activation, serum adenosine deaminase levels are increased in SSc patients (37).

ABNORMALITIES OF T CELL ANTIGEN RECEPTOR (TCR) GENE EXPRESSION

A change in the number or percentage of CD4$^+$, CD8$^+$, or γ/δ T cell subpopulations provides a crude indication of T cell selection. Better evidence for T cell selection comes from the finding of restriction in the T cell repertoire, as estimated through analyses of the diversity of expressed TCR. Two types of analyses of TCR diversity are commonly performed: one determines the relative use of different TCR variable (V) gene families, and the other determines the diversity of the rearranged V-diversity (D)-joining (J) junctional regions. The junctional region of the TCR, which is analogous to the complementarity determining region 3 of immunoglobulin (19), determines conventional peptide antigen specificity of the T cell (38). The finding of increased expression of a given V gene family, without any limitation in the diversity of the TCR junctional regions that use the same V gene family, is more compatible with T cell selection through superantigen stimulation (39,40). In contrast, the finding of limited diversity in TCR junctional regions that use a given V gene family is more compatible with T cell selection through stimulation by classical peptide antigens (38,41).

Analyses of relative use of different TCR V gene families in SSc patients have begun. White and coworkers (19) found an increase in the percentages of CD3$^+$ T cells and total γ/δ T cells that express the Vδ1 gene, in both peripheral blood and BAL cells (19). This increase in Vδ1$^+$ γ/δ T cells did not correlate with disease type or duration.

Sakamoto et al (42) found restricted use of Vβ 5/7, 5, or 17 gene families among CD4$^-$CD8$^-$ α/β T cells in the blood of three SSc patients. Williams et al (43) tested TCR V gene expression in the skin of SSc patients and found little difference from controls. Multiple Vα and Vβ gene families were expressed, with no difference in the major V gene families expressed in SSc and normal skin. The Vβ6 and Vβ8 gene families and the Vα3C, Vα7, Vα14, Vα15, Vα16, and Vα28 gene families were the dominant ones expressed. In SSc biopsies, there was slightly higher expression of Vα12 and lower expression of Vα3B gene families. Southcott et al (44) found similar numbers and patterns of Vα gene family expression in lung tissue from SSc patients, patients with tumors, and patients with idiopathic pulmonary fibrosis.

In an analysis of TCR junctional region diversity, Yurovsky et al (45) found evidence for a selected expansion of these Vδ1$^+$ γ/δ T cells in both peripheral blood and BAL cells from SSc patients, when compared to controls. There was more restriction in the nucleotide lengths of Vδ1$^+$ junctional regions in SSc patients. In addition, more repeated Vδ1$^+$ junctional region sequences were isolated from blood of SSc patients than controls. Identical Vδ1 chains were cloned from multiple sites of individual SSc patients, including the blood, lungs, and gut. Identical Vδ1 sequences were also isolated from different specimens obtained from an individual patient over a 6-month period. Vδ1$^+$ junctional regions from different SSc patients, while never identical, could be grouped into several clusters of sequences with amino acid homology. The findings of an increased expression of the Vδ1 gene (19) in association with restricted diversity of Vδ1$^+$ junctional region sequences (45) suggests an antigen-driven selection of Vδ1$^+$ γ/δ T cells in SSc patients.

T CELL STIMULATORY ANTIGENS

Attempts have been made to identify soluble and cellular antigens that stimulate T cells in SSc patients. Lymphocytes from SSc patients respond in a migration inhibition assay to skin extracts (2), which contain collagen. Purified collagen (46), including type I (47) and type IV collagen (48), all activate T cells from SSc patients. Cellular antigens on fibroblasts, epithelial cells, and muscle cells stimulate cytotoxic T cell responses (49), although not all investigators have found this to be the case (2,50). Of interest, some patients with morphea and linear scleroderma have elevated antibodies and lymphoproliferative responses to *Borrelia burgdorferi* (51).

FUNCTIONAL STUDIES OF T CELLS

In vivo T cell responses in SSc patients are normal. Lupoli et al (52) reported that SSc patients have a normal response to primary immunization and recall antigens with T-dependent antigens, with normal cutaneous delayed type hypersensitivity and antibody production. Results of *in vitro* testing of T cells in SSc patients have been contradictory, with increased, normal, and decreased T cell proliferative, helper, or suppresser responses to activation with a variety of stimuli (24,29,30,47,48,53–63).

IMMUNOGENETIC STUDIES IMPLICATE A ROLE FOR T CELLS IN SSC

Recent immunogenetic studies of SSc patients indirectly implicate T cells as playing a role in the clinical subsets of SSc associated with production of anticentromere, anti-topoisomerase 1, and anti-PM-Scl antibodies (64–69). The anticentromere antibody response is tightly associated with HLA-DQ alleles, with a polar glycine or tyrosine at position 26 of the DQβ chain (64). The anti-topoisomerase 1 antibody response in Caucasian Americans and Black Americans is associated with HLA-DQ alleles, with a tyrosine residue at position 30 or the TRAELDT sequence of the DQβ chain (65). In Japanese patients, anti-topoisomerase I antibodies are associated with a tyrosine residue at position 30 of the DQβ chain, with HLA-DR alleles with the amino acid sequence FLEDR at position 67–71 of the DRβ chain, and with the serologically defined HLA-DR52 antigen (66). In English (67), but not North American (68), Caucasians, the anti-topoisomerase I antibody response is associated with an acidic residue at position 69 in the DPβ chain. Autoantibodies to PM-Scl correlate with the presence of the HLA-DRB1*0301, DQA1-*0501, DQB1*0201 haplotype (69).

These reports associate HLA-DP, DQ, and DR alleles with autoantibody production. HLA molecules do not restrict B cell recognition of antigen. Instead, T cell activation is restricted by recognition of antigenic peptides bound to HLA molecules. Thus, an explanation for the association of HLA alleles with autoantibody production in SSc patients is that these particular HLA alleles are required to activate T cells, which provide the help necessary for B cells to make anti-centromere, anti-topoisomerase 1, and anti-PM-Scl antibodies. Distinct subsets of T cells may be activated by antigenic peptides associated with these different HLA alleles. These subsets of T cells may be responsible for the differences in disease manifestations in patients with limited cutaneous SSc, diffuse cutaneous SSc, and SSc overlap with polymyositis.

IMMUNOMODULATORY THERAPIES

No agent has been shown to be effective in improving survival or in reducing the development of organ damage in SSc patients via double-blind, placebo-controlled studies (70). However, a number of unblinded or non-placebo-controlled trials hint at potential efficacy of interventions that suppress immune function. Silver et al (71) reported that patients with cellular BAL who were treated with prednisone and cyclophosphamide had improvement in forced vital capacity, whereas a study by Crystal and coworkers (16) found no improvement in active lung disease with prednisone therapy alone. Plasmaphoresis and cyclophosphamide therapy is reported to be associated with some improvement in skin ulcers and internal organ involvement (72). Extracorporeal photochemotherapy is a form of immunotherapy that particularly affects T cells. A non-placebo-controlled trial suggested mild, transient improvement in skin involvement at 6 months, but not at 10 months, in SSc patients who were treated with photochemotherapy when compared to patients who were treated with D-penicillamine (73). Three SSc patients have improved with anti-thymocyte globulin therapy (74,75). Clements et al (76) gave cyclosporin in open label to 10 SSc patients for 48 weeks, with improvement in skin score, although significant renal toxicity occurred.

T CELLS IN ANIMAL MODELS

T cells are a central component of several animal models of SSc. Chronic GVHD is induced in mice by T cell allorecognition of major or minor histocompatibility complex-encoded molecules (77). Histologically, skin changes of murine chronic GVHD are similar to those of human SSc, with a mononuclear cell infiltrate present deep within the dermis early in the disease, as well as loss of dermal fat, increased collagen deposition, and drop-out of dermal appendages. Chronic GVHD in mice is initiated by, and dependent upon, CD8$^+$ T cell allorecognition of MHC-encoded molecules.

In hereditary avian scleroderma, University of California at Davis line-200 (L200) chickens have a defect in thymic maturation of T cells. Consequently, they develop severe perivascular T cell infiltration of the skin and internal organs (78). Lymphocytes in the deep dermis and subcutaneous tissues are enriched for CD4$^+$ α/β T cells, whereas lymphocytes in the papillary dermis are enriched for γ/δ T cells, 20% of which are CD8$^+$. Expression of MHC class II molecules indicates that these T cells are activated. As a result of this infiltration with activated T cells, fibrosis and vascular occlusion develop in L200 chickens.

In a third animal model, the tight skin (TSK/$^+$) mouse, thickened skin is tightly bound to the subcutaneous tissues and, unlike SSc, to deep muscular tissue (79). Disease expression is determined by an autosomal dominant gene, which affects connective tissue almost exclusively (79). The usefulness of TSK/$^+$ mice as a model of SSc has been questioned, because these mice do not have vascular changes nor lymphocytic infiltration of their skin. ANAs occur late, at 8 months, and only in 50% of TSK/$^+$ animals (80). Despite these late and variable immunologic abnormalities, dermal fibrosis can be transferred from TSK/$^+$ mice to normal CD57Bl/6 Pa/Pa littermates by infusion of bone marrow or, to a lesser extent, by a combination of T and B cells (81). This fibrosis follows an infiltration of the skin with mononuclear cells, which is not a characteristic of the original TSK/$^+$ donor. Potential stimulatory T cell antigens in TSK/$^+$ mice are being sought. CD4$^+$ T cells proliferate in an MHC class II-restricted manner to the basement membrane heparin sulfate proteoglycan, which is a critical cell surface and extracellular matrix component (82).

To increase immunologic abnormalities in TSK/$^+$ mice, a new animal model of SSc has been made by breeding TSK and NZB mice (83). The TSK/NZB progeny have skin changes characteristic of the TSK/$^+$ parent and immunological abnormalities more like the NZB parent. T cell proliferation is decreased in response to autologous stimulators. Autoantibodies occur earlier (3 months) in TSK/NZB than in TSK/$^+$ mice, with a pattern of specificities similar to that seen in the NZB parent.

B Cell Abnormalities in SSc

Autoantibody production is an early, nearly universal finding in SSc patients. Identification of the antigens that are specific for SSc and delineation of the B cell epitopes on these targets provide clues about the etiology of the disease. Evidence that autoantibodies cause significant tissue damage in SSc patients is limited.

B CELLS IN TISSUES

Increased plasma cells are seen within the skin of SSc patients (1,3,5,6) and in lung biopsies of SSc patients with alveolitis (12).

B CELLS IN BLOOD

Hypergammaglobulinemia and autoantibodies are found in the sera of SSc patients. Hypergammaglobulinemia results from polyclonal B cell activation in SSc patients (3,84,85), with increases in IgG, IgA, IgM, and IgE. IgG levels also increased in BAL of SSc patients (13,15), where there is no correlation with disease activity as defined by abnormal BAL cellularity (15). ANAs occur early and uniformly (90%–98%) in patients with SSc (86,87). The isotype of the ANA is usually IgG, especially the IgG3 subclass, although IgM, IgE, and IgA ANAs are also seen

(88,89). Titers of the auto-antibodies for topoisomerase 1 (90) and anti-centromere antibodies (91) remain relatively stable for years. ANAs may (87) or may not (92) be detected more frequently in the blood of relatives and spouses of SSc patients than in the blood of controls; nevertheless, ANAs in relatives and spouses do not bind targets specific for scleroderma (87).

B CELL STIMULATORY ANTIGENS

Multiple autoantigens are recognized by autoantibodies from SSc patients. Some autoantibody targets that are quite specific for SSc include the topoisomerase 1 (93,94); centromeric proteins (95,96); chromosomal antigens (97); RNA polymerases I, II, and III (98–102); U3 (98,103) and U11 (104) small nRNPs; and the PM-Scl antigen in SSc overlap with polymyositis (105). Many other autoantigens that are not specific for SSc include endothelial cells (106); fibroblasts; smooth muscle; thyroid tissue; salivary gland tissue; red blood cells; platelets; heat shock protein (107); types l, lll, and IV collagen (108); laminin (109); interleukin-6 (110); interleukin-8 (111); IgG (84); cardiolipin (112); FcγR, including FcγRI (CD64), FcγRII (CD32), and FcγRIII (CD16) (113); histones (114); mitochondria (115); single-stranded RNA; nuclear ribonucleoproteins (nRNP) (116); Th ribonucleoproteins (117,118); the 92-kDa UBF (NOR-90) antigen (119); and the Ku antigen (120). Antibody responses to retroviral gag proteins have been demonstrated on Western blots (121,122).

Autoantibodies against self antigens may arise through several mechanisms (123). In molecular mimicry, an immune response that is initially directed against unrelated exogenous antigens will cross-reactively recognize sequences in self antigens. Molecular mimicry may play a role in the development of the anti-topoisomerase I and anti-PM-Scl antibody responses in SSc patients. Sera from some (124), but not all (125–127), SSc patients bind a region in the carboxyterminus of the topoisomerase 1 molecule that includes amino acids 741–746, an area that is homologous

to the p30^{gag} protein from feline sarcoma virus. Anti-topoisomerase 1 antibodies also bind a region of topoisomerase 1 that contains five sequential amino acid residues (residues 121–126), which are shared with UL70 protein of human cytomegalovirus (128). Anti-PM-Scl antibodies bind to a 138-amino acid fragment of PM-Scl containing regions that are homologous to the nuclear localization signal of SV-40 large T antigen and a molecular signal found in the HIV tat protein (129). The finding of areas of homology between SSc autoantigens and viruses suggests that the induction of autoimmunity in SSc patients may be caused by agents that are capable of infecting target cells or cells of the immune system.

If molecular mimicry were the sole mechanism underlying the production of autoantibodies in SSc patients, it would be unexpected to find that many SSc-specific antigens are involved in similar cellular processes. Thus, it is curious that many SSc-specific antigens are involved in the regulation of gene transcription. Autoantibodies against centromeres recognize four centromeric proteins (CENPs), CENP-A, -B, -C, and -D (130–132), which are components of the centromeric heterochromatin. Both CENP-A and CENP-B are thought to play a role in packing of centromeric DNA, which regulates DNA availability for transcription. The role of CENP-C, which is located at the inner plate of the kinetochore, is unknown, but it is present at functional centromeres and absent at inactive centromeres (133). CENP-D has been implicated in the onset of chromosome condensation because of its homology to the cell cycle regulatory protein RCC1 (134). Ten to 15% of patients with anti-centromere antibodies also have antibodies to 23–25 kDa chromosomal antigens, including the chromo domain, which is thought to be involved in the down-regulation of transcription (97). Topoisomerase 1 catalyzes the relaxation of negatively supercoiled DNA prior to transcription and is necessary for elongation of RNA transcripts (135,136). RNA polymerase I synthesizes ribosomal RNA precursors in the nucleoli; RNA polymerase II synthesizes mRNA precursors and small nuclear RNAs, which are components of ribonucleoprotein particles that mediate pre-mRNA splicing; and RNA polymerase III synthesizes small RNAs, including 5S ribosomal and transfer RNAs (123). A heptapeptide repeat is the B cell target in the carboxyterminal domain of the 220 and 145kDa subunits of RNA polymerase II (137). This domain is a prerequisite for normal responses to activation signals at some promoters. As such, this domain has an essential role in gene transcription.

An alternative mechanism to molecular mimicry for the production of autoantibodies is the presentation of self proteins that are altered in some way or exposed to the immune system in greater amounts, so that tolerance is broken. Under these circumstances, the self proteins are the actual antigens that provoke the autoantibody response. Of interest, topoisomerase 1 is expressed in greater amounts and its degradation is increased during T cell activation (138). Centromeric proteins and RNA polymerases I, II, and III occur in multi-unit complexes (123). More than one member of each of these complexes is recognized by SSc sera, which might occur if the entire complex were processed and presented by antigen presenting cells. RNA polymerases consist of 8 to 14 polypeptide subunits, with some subunits unique to the particular RNA polymerase and other subunits shared among RNA polymerases I, II, and III. Both the unique and shared subunits serve as targets for anti-RNA polymerase antibodies in SSc patients (101,102). Anti-RNA polymerase II antibodies bind to the carboxyterminal domain of the unique 220 and 145 kilodalton subunits and to the 42 and 25 kilodalton subunits, which are shared with RNA polymerases I and III (101, 102). Autoantibody recognition of multiple subunits within a protein complex suggests that the complex itself served as a stimulating antigen.

Other results which suggest that the targets of SSc-specific autoantibodies may be stimulating antigens are the findings that multiple B cell epitopes are present on a given protein target. There

are multiple B cell epitopes on CENP-B (139). Sera from individual SSc patients recognize multiple B cell epitopes on topoisomerase 1, which are scattered throughout the molecule (124–128, 140) and which include the active site of the enzyme, a tyrosine at position 723 (141).

Hardin (142) and Tan (143) have appreciated that many autoantibodies bind multiple subunits of macromolecular complexes, with different components of the complexes recognized by individual sera. They suggest that a polyclonal and multifocal nature of an autoantibody response suggests that the response is antigen-driven, rather than arising solely through molecular mimicry. However, molecular mimicry may play a role in initiating these responses, with the first antibody response directed against an epitope on a foreign antigen that is homologous to a self antigen. The subsequent antibody response may spread to include other epitopes on the self antigen (144,145).

ANTIBODY-MEDIATED TISSUE DAMAGE

Antibodies against endothelial cells may cause damage through antibody-dependent cellular cytotoxicity (146,147). Many of the autoantibodies in SSc patients do not activate the complement cascade (148), and serum complement levels are normal (3,149). Immune complexes are present in the sera of approximately 25% of SSc patients (14,15,150–156), although they are not typically deposited in tissues (1). Patients with high levels of circulating immune complexes are more likely to have pulmonary fibrosis (151, 152), although less correlation has been found in other studies (14,155). Silver et al (14) found more immune complexes in BAL fluids from SSc patients than in BAL fluids from normal patients; however, there was no correlation of immune complex level with disease activity in the SSc patients (15). Patients with circulating immune complexes are also more likely to have abnormal echocardiogram (155).

Another way that autoantibodies might contribute to pathology in SSc patients is through the inhibition of function of the antibody targets. Antibodies against centromeric proteins, topoisomerase 1, and RNA polymerases all inhibit the function of their respective targets (99, 101,102,141,157). For example, anticentromere antibodies can disrupt the assembly of the centromere, inhibit normal chromosomal segregation, and cause aneuploidy and multinucleated cells (157). This inhibition may have some clinical consequences. Jabs et al (158) found a correlation between anti-centromeric antibodies, especially anti-CENP-C antibodies and aneuploidy, in SSc patients. An association was also found between increased chromatid breaks, especially centromeric breaks, and anticentromeric antibodies. Anticentromeric antibodies may disrupt the functional centromere and allow for malsegregation of chromosomes during mitoses (158).

B CELLS IN ANIMAL MODELS

TSK/$^+$ mice produce anti-FCγR antibodies (159) and ANA (80). ANA production occurs in only half of old animals greater than 8 months of age (80). Targets of the ANA include antinucleolar antigens (160), including anti-topoisomerase I (161,162) and RNA polymerase I (163). Production of anti-topoisomerase I and anti-RNA polymerase I antibodies can be transferred by bone marrow into normal littermates (81). Human and mouse anti-topoisomerase 1 antibodies share a cross-reactive idiotope, which indicates that this antibody response is conserved during phylogeny (128). It is important to note, however, that others have not found an increase in topoisomerase 1 antibodies in TSK/$^+$ mice (164). In TSK$^+$/NZB animals, there is an early (3 months) appearance of autoantibodies (83). University of California at Davis L200 chickens also make ANA, with a progressive increase in autoantibodies to histones, ssDNA, dDNA, poly(l), poly(CG), and cardiolipin (165). Antibodies to centromeric proteins or topoisomerase 1 are rarely observed in these chickens (165).

Abnormalities of Other Cells of the Immune System in SSc Patients

MAST CELLS

The skin, lungs, and heart are all reported to be sites of increased mast cell numbers and degranulation in SSc patients. In the skin, numbers of mast cells have been reported across a range from decreased (166), to normal (3,166), to increased (167–169). Increased mast cells are found in other fibrotic disorders, such as toxic oil syndrome (170), eosinophilic fasciitis (171), and bleomycin-induced pulmonary fibrosis (172). Mast cells containing tryptase, which are the predominant mast cells in the gastrointestional mucosa and alveolar walls of the lung, and mast cells containing both tryptase and chymase, which are the predominant mast cell in the skin and gastrointestinal tract submucosa, are both present (166). The finding of this latter type of mast cells in the skin is compatible with mast cell activation. Degranulation of mast cells provides direct evidence for mast cell activation within the skin of SSc patients (166,169,173). Mast cell degranulation is also noted in chronic murine GVHD (174,175) and in TSK/$^+$ mice (176). Increased levels of nerve growth factor, a neurotrophic factor that induces an increase in mast cells and histamine release, is found in the dermis of SSc patients (177). This finding raises the possibility that nerve growth factor contributes to the increase in mast cell numbers and degranulation that is seen in SSc skin (177).

Mast cell numbers in BAL fluids of SSc patients with alveolitis are increased, and levels of histamine, tryptase, and hyaluronic acid are elevated, which are compatible with mast cell activation within the lungs of SSc patients (178). These mast cell abnormalities are more pronounced in patients with abnormal chest x-rays, suggesting a correlation with disease severity. Nonetheless, mast cells remain relatively rare within BAL fluids of SSc patients and constitute only 0.6 ± 0.6% of all cells, compared to 0.002 ±

0.04% in normal patients (178). Myocardial mast cell infiltration has been reported in two cases of SSc with fatal heart involvement, and evidence of mast cell degranulation was found in a third patient (179).

NATURAL KILLER (NK) CELLS

The numbers and activity of NK cells in SSc patients are reported to be increased (26,180,181), normal (26), or decreased (22,23,182,183). IL-2-activated killer cell activity is decreased in SSc patients (26), which may result from reduction in numbers of CD8$^+$ T cells. Lymphokine activated killer cell activity is reported to be increased (180) or decreased (26,183).

EOSINOPHILS

Numbers of eosinophils are increased in peripheral blood (184,185), BAL fluids (12–16,184, 185), and clinically unaffected, but not fibrotic, skin from SSc patients (184). Eosinophils have been activated, because major basic protein levels are increased in the blood (185). Major basic protein has been found in one lung biopsy and 1 of 11 skin biopsies (185). Eosinophil cationic protein is present in increased levels in BAL fluids (184).

MACROPHAGES

One report has described an intense accumulation of macrophages around blood vessels and hair follicles in skin biopsies of SSc patients (186), although others have generally not found a predominance of macrophages, even in early disease (1). Langerhans cells, a specialized antigen presenting cell in the skin, are present in increased numbers in SSc skin early in the disease (1). On lung biopsy, patients with interstitial disease have macrophages in the interstitium and on alveolar epithelial surfaces (12). Total numbers of macrophages in BAL fluids are increased, although the percentage of macrophages is decreased (14,15). Cultures of alveolar macro-phages from BAL fluids from SSc patients with alveolitis contain higher levels of fibronectin (12,15) and alveolar-macrophage-derived growth factor (12) than BAL fluids from patients without alveolitis or controls. Monocyte-mediated angiogenesis is decreased in SSc patients, whose monocytes are less responsive to activation by interferon-γ (IFN-γ), with decreased HLA-DR expression (187).

BASOPHILS

Evidence for the possible involvement of basophils in SSc comes from the report of De Paulis et al (188), who found increased spontaneous histamine release from peripheral blood basophils from SSc patients, as well as increased basophil reactivity (maximal percent histamine secretion) or basophil sensitivity (concentration of stimulant required for submaximal histamine secretion). Basophil numbers are normal in BAL fluids from SSc patients (12).

NEUTROPHILS

Neutrophils do not infiltrate involved tissues in SSc patients, with exception of the lungs. Neutrophils are increased in lung biopsies (12) and in BAL (12–16,189). In BAL, neutrophilic alveolitis correlates with the development of greater restrictive lung disease over time (15,16,189). Neutrophils from SSc patients have an increased spontaneous release of hydrogen peroxide (190).

Cytokine Abnormalities in SSc Patients

Cytokines may contribute to extracellular matrix deposition and vascular activation/damage in SSc patients. Cathcart et al (191) and Gonzalez-Amaro et al (192) showed that PBMC from SSc patients produce soluble factors *in vitro* that stimulate fibroblast proliferation, protein synthesis, and collagen production to a greater degree than do lymphocytes from controls. This capacity to stimulate fibroblast anabolic activity may not be a property unique to SSc Iymphocytes, but rather a matter of degree, and may reflect their heightened state of activation. Exposure to supernatants from stimulated normal PBMC can induce an SSc-like phenotype in normal fibroblast lines (193–195). Cytokines capable of altering endothelial cell function are found in SSc sera or tissues, including IL-1, IL-2, IL-4, IL-6, IL-8, lymphotoxin, TNFα, transforming growth factor-β (TGFβ), and platelet-derived growth factor (PDGF) (196–204). Granzyme 1 (20), a lysosomal protein released by cytotoxic T cells, leukotriene B_4 (205), and endothelin (206) are other circulating factors that may damage or alter function of fibroblasts or endothelial cells in SSc patients.

TRANSFORMING GROWTH FACTOR-β

TGF-β may be one of the cytokines involved in a network leading to fibrosis. It induces fibrosis and angiogenesis *in vivo* and stimulates collagen formation *in vitro* (207). Activated TGF-β1 has been found in the sera of six of 25 SSc patients but not in the sera of controls, with no associations with clinical parameters (208). TGF-β mRNAs or proteins have been found in the skin of SSc patients (203,204,209–211). There is disagreement whether the source of the TGF-β is mononuclear cells, fibroblasts, or endothelial cells (204,210,211); whether TGF-β1 mRNA is present in the skin (209–211); and whether TGF-β2 mRNA is present in the dermis of patients with fibrotic stages (203,211). Increased levels of TGF-β2 mRNA and proα1(I) and proα(lll) collagen mRNA co-localize within inflammatory infiltrates in skin from SSc patients in the early phase of disease (212).

Several observations question a causal relationship of increased TGF-β expression to dermal fibrosis. Gabrielli et al (211) found intracellular TGF-β more commonly than extracellular TGF-β in endothelial cells in patients with SSc, and found extracellular TGF-β in the papillary dermis, but this was not different from individuals with primary Raynaud's disease. Because primary Raynaud's disease is not associated with fibrosis, this finding indicates that TGF-β deposition does not necessarily lead to dermal fibrosis. Sfikakis et al (210) found intense immunohistochemical staining for TGF-β2 protein in the extracellular matrix of involved areas, but not in uninvolved skin or controls. Because TGF-β binds to fibronectin (213), proteoglycans (214), and collagen IV (215), all of which are overexpressed in SSc skin, these authors raised the issue that increased TGF-β expression may be secondary to increased matrix deposition.

A ten-fold increase in transcription of TGF-β has been found in BAL cells from SSc patients with lung involvement, with TGF-β mRNA levels correlating with TGF-β protein levels (216). In contrast to this report, Moreland et al (217) found higher levels of TGF-β in normal lungs than in SSc lungs, with no association between TGF-β levels and cellularity of BAL fluids.

Majewski et al (218) found that SSc fibroblasts are more adherent to extracellular matrix than are control fibroblasts, and that exposure to TGF-β increases the adhesion of control fibroblasts to extracellular matrix, mimicking the adhesive properties of SSc fibroblasts. TGF-β causes SSc fibroblasts, but not normal fibroblasts, to increase their synthesis of type-α PDGF receptor, which is necessary to allow a proliferative response to PDGF isoform AA (219). PDGF, PDGF AA, and PDGF type β receptors are all increased in scleroderma skin (219–221). Given that scleroderma fibroblasts have a normal number of, and affinity for, TBF-β receptors (222) and do not produce increased amounts of TGF-β (222, 223), an unusual behavior in response to TGF-β may reflect intracellular events. Of note, *in vitro* exposure of fibroblasts to TGF-β does not induce an SSc phenotype (223).

INTERLEUKIN-1

Monocyte production of IL-1, including IL-1α and IL-1β (224,225), is increased in SSc patients, although there is not uniform agreement on this point (226,227). Increased serum levels of IL-1α and IL-1β are seen in no, or a few, SSc patients (32,36,196), although one study found that up to 50% of SSc patients have increased levels (35). PBMC from SSc patients spontaneously produce more IL-1β than do control PBMC (36). IL-1β levels are similar in BAL fluids from SSc patients and controls (228). Scleroderma fibroblasts, which express more IL-1R (229), are reported to be 10 to 100 times more sensitive to IL-1 stimulation of IL-6, prostaglandin E2, and IL-1β mRNA (230).

TUMOR NECROSIS FACTOR α

Similar to the findings with IL-1, TNFα levels have been reported to be normal (196,225) or increased (32,35,36). Production of TNFα by SSc PBMC (36) and monocytes (225) is increased.

INTERLEUKIN-6

Elevated IL-6 levels are found more frequently in SSc patients than controls (196), although smaller studies do not confirm this (231,232). Stimulated PBMC from SSc patients release 10 to 20 times more IL-6 than do control PBMC (233). There is no difference between SSc patients and normals in IL-6 levels in BAL fluids (228) or in spontaneous or stimulated IL-6 production by alveolar macrophages (234). IL-6 may be responsible for a two-fold increase in IL-2R expression on PBMC from SSc patients (233). Because binding of IL-2 to high affinity IL-2R regulates T cell and B cell growth, an IL-6-mediated increase in high affinity IL-2R might alter immune processes in SSc patients, in the presence of elevated levels of IL-2.

INTERLEUKIN-2

Interleukin-2 levels have been reported to be normal (27), increased in a small number of patients (32,34,36,196) without relationship to disease duration or type (32), or increased in most patients, with levels correlating with an index of disease activity (235). Elevated levels of IL-2 mRNA have been found in the blood and BAL of only a small number of SSc patients, and at a rate no greater than controls (236).

INTERLEUKIN-4

IL-4, which is produced by activated T cells, mast cells, and basophils, is present in the sera of SSc patients (196). In SSc patients, IL-4 protein production by activated PBMC is increased (34), and levels of IL-4 mRNA in mononuclear cells from the blood and BAL are increased (236). This increase in IL-4 protein and mRNA, with little change in IL-2 and IFN-γ proteins and mRNAs, suggests a Th2 pattern of T cell activation in SSc patients. Elevated IL-4 levels may contribute to the disease process, given the capacity of IL-4 to promote fibroblast proliferation, chemotaxis, and extracellular matrix production (237–239) and to induce changes in vimentin intermediate filaments in endothelial cells (9).

INTERFERON-γ

Interferon-γ protein has not been detected in peripheral blood of SSc patients (196,240). Secretion of IFN-γ by SSc PBMC, either unfractionated (36,240,241) or enriched for non-adherent cells (242), is lower than that from control PBMC. Similarly, IFN-γ protein is not found in BAL from SSc patients (240) and IFN-γ mRNA levels in BAL from SSc patients are not different from those in controls (236).

INTERLEUKIN-8

Compared to controls, elevated serum levels of IL-8 are found in SSc patients with both limited and diffuse SSc (111). This finding is not specific for SSc, because serum IL-8 levels are also increased in patients with eosinophilic fasciitis and Raynaud's phenomenon (111). Elevated IL-8 mRNA and protein levels are found in some BAL fluids from SSc patients with pulmonary fibrosis (228, 243), but are also found in BAL fluids from patients with idiopathic interstitial fibrosis (243). Because IL-8 is a neutrophil chemotractant, the question can be raised whether IL-8 is responsible for some of the neutrophilia seen in SSc patients with alveolitis (228).

Adhesion Molecule Abnormalities in SSc

Cell surface expression of adhesion molecules is necessary for lymphocyte trafficking through the blood vessels and subsequent adherence in tissue. Migration and adherence of lymphocytes in the skin of SSc patients may be facilitated by an increased expression of adhesion molecules on vascular endothelium, lymphocytes, and fibroblasts.

ADHESION MOLECULE EXPRESSION ON ENDOTHELIAL CELLS

Increased cell surface expression of HLA class II molecules, β_1 integrins, and endothelial cell adhesion molecule-1 (ECAM-1) indicates activation of the endothelial cells in SSc patients (1,7, 173,244,245). Endothelial leukocyte adhesion molecule-1 (ELAM-1) is a member of the selectin family that appears on the endothelial cell surface during inflammation and mediates endothelial cell interactions with neutrophils, granulocytes, monocytes, and CD4$^+$ T cells (246). ELAM-1 levels are elevated in SSc patients, but levels do not correlate with disease activity and are not SSc-specific, being present in patients with temporal arteritis, polyarteritis nodosa, and systemic lupus erythematosus (247). ELAM-1 and intercellular adhesion molecule-1 (ICAM-1) expression are both increased on endothelial cells in SSc patients (7,173,244,245), where levels correlate with the amount of mononuclear cell infiltration (7). Dermal endothelial cells of SSc patients also have increased expression of very late antigen-2 (VLA-2) and VLA-4 (7).

ADHESION MOLECULE EXPRESSION ON LYMPHOCYTES

Once T cells migrate through the endothelium into tissue, adhesion to fibroblasts is mediated in part by interactions between lymphocyte function associated antigen-1 (LFA-1) on T cells and ICAM-1 on the fibroblasts (248). Serum ICAM-1 levels are elevated two-fold in SSc patients (249). Dermal perivascular lymphocytes in SSc skin show increased expression of β_1, β_2, β_3 integrins (7,244,245), with β_2 and β_3 expression occurring in acute skin (7,244). There is no difference in β_4 integrin expression from normals (244). The $\alpha 1$ chain expression is increased on inflammatory cell infiltrates in acute and chronic SSc skin, as is expression of VLA-1, -2, -3, -4, and -6 (7). SSc patients have reduced numbers of circulating T cells capable of adhering to endothelial cells *in vitro*, which is thought to be the result of depletion of T cells by increased adherence to vascular endothelium *in vivo* (250).

ADHESION MOLECULE EXPRESSION ON FIBROBLASTS

Surface expression of ICAM-1 on SSc fibroblasts is increased (7,244,245,251,252), a property which increases their binding of T cells (248). Expression of $\alpha 1$ and $\alpha 3$ integrin chains are increased on fibroblasts in SSc skin (7).

References

1. Prescott RJ, Freemont AJ, Jones CJP, et al. Sequential dermal microvascular and perivascular changes in the development of scleroderma. J Pathol 1992;166:255.
2. Kondo H, Rabin BS, Rodnan GP. Cutaneous antigen-stimulating lymphokine production by lymphocytes of patients with progressive systemic sclerosis (scleroderma). J Clin Invest 1976;58:1388.
3. Fleischmajer R, Perlish JS, Reeves JRT. Cellular infiltrates in scleroderma skin. Arthritis Rheum 1977;20:975.

4. Andrews BS, Friou GJ, Barr RJ, et al. Loss of epidermal Langerhans' cells and endothelial cell HLA-DR antigens in the skin in progressive systemic sclerosis. J Rheumatol 1986;13:314.

5. Jimenez SA. Cellular immune dysfunction and the pathogenesis of scleroderma. Semin Arthritis Rheum 1983;13:104.

6. Roumm AD, Whiteside TL, Medsger TA Jr, Rodnan GP. Lymphocytes in the skin of patients with progressive systemic sclerosis: Quantification, subtyping and clinical correlations. Arthritis Rheum 1984;27:645.

7. Gruschwitz M, Von Den Driesch P, Kellner P, et al. Expression of adhesion proteins involved in cell-cell and cell-matrix interactions in the skin of patients with progressive systemic sclerosis. J Am Acad Dermatol 1992;27:169.

8. Kahari VM, Sandberg M, Kalimo H, et al. Identification of fibroblasts responsible for increased collagen production in localized scleroderma by *in situ* hybridization. J Invest Dermatol 1988; 90:664.

9. Klein NJ, Rigley KP, Callard RE. IL-4 regulated the morphology, cytoskeleton, and proliferation of human umbilical vein endothelial cells: Relationship between vimentin and IL-4. Int Immunol 1992;5:293.

10. Lampert IA, Switters AJ, Janossy G, et al. Lymphoid infiltrates in skin in graft-versus-host disease. Lancet 1981;2:1352.

11. Kuroda Y, Fukuoka M, Endo C, et al. Occurrence of primary biliary cirrhosis, CREST syndrome and Sjögren's syndrome in a patient with HTLV-1-associated myelopathy. J Neurol Sci 1993; 116:47.

12. Rossi GA, Bitterman PB, Rennard SI, et al. Evidence for chronic inflammation as a component of the interstitial lung disease associated with progressive systemic sclerosis. Am Rev Respir Dis 1985;131:612.

13. Silver RM, Metcalf JF, Stanley JH, LeRoy EC. Interstitial lung disease in scleroderma. Analysis by bronchoalveolar lavage. Arthritis Rheum 1984; 27:1254.

14. Silver RM, Metcalf JF, LeRoy EC. Interstitial lung disease in scleroderma. Immune complexes in sera and bronchoalveolar lavage fluid. Arthritis Rheum 1986;29:525.

15. Silver RM, Miller KS, Kinsella MB, et al. Evaluation and management of scleroderma lung disease using bronchoalveolar lavage. Am J Med 1990;88:470.

16. Wallaert B, Hatron PY, Grosbois JM, et al. Subclinical pulmonary involvement in collagen-vascular diseases assessed by bronchoalveolar lavage. Relationship between alveolitis and subsequent changes in lung function. Am Rev Respir Dis 1986;133:574.

17. Edelson JD, Hyland RH, Ramsden M, et al. Lung inflammation in scleroderma: Clinical, radiographic, physiologic and cytopathological features. J Rheumatol 1993;12:957.

18. Gustafsson R, Fredens K, Nettelbladt O, Haligren R. Eosinophil activation in systemic sclerosis. Arthritis Rheum 1991;34:414.

19. White B, Wigley FM, Wise R, et al. Increased expression of CD8 and $V\delta 1^+$ γ/δ T cells in the lungs of systemic sclerosis patients. Arthritis Rheum, submitted.

20. Kahaleh MB, Yin T. The molecular mechanism of endothelial cell (EC) injury in scleroderma (SSc). Arthritis Rheum 1990;33:S21.

21. Degiannis D, Seibold J, Czamecki M, et al. Soluble and cellular markers of immune activation in patients with systemic sclerosis. Clin Immunol Immunopathol 1990;56:259.

22. Freundlich B, Jimenez SA. Phenotype of peripheral blood lymphocytes in patients with progressive systemic sclerosis: Activated T lymphocytes and the effect of D-penicillamine therapy. Clin Exp Immunol 1987;69:375.

23. Frieri M, Angadi C, Paolano A, et al. Altered T cell subpopulations and lymphocytes expressing natural killer cell phenotypes in patients with progressive systemic sclerosis. J Allergy Clin Immunol 1991;87:773.

24. Inoshita T, Whiteside TL, Rodnan GP, Taylor FH. Abnormalities of T lymphocyte subsets in patients with progresive systemic sclerosis (PSS, scleroderma). J Lab Clin Med 1981;97:264.

25. Kahan A, Kahan A, Picard F, et al. Abnormalities of T lymphocyte subsets in systemic sclerosis demonstrated with anti-CD45RA and anti-CD29 monoclonal antibodies. Ann Rheum Dis 1991;50: 354.

26. Kantor T V, Whiteside TL, Friberg D, et al. Lymphokine-activated killer cell and natural killer cell activities in patients with systemic sclerosis. Arthritis Rheum 1992;35:694.

27. Keystone EC, Lau C, Gladman D, et al. Immunoregulatory T cell subpopulations in patients with scleroderma using monoclonal antibodies. Clin Exp Immunol 1982;48:443.

28. Gustaffson R, Totterman TH, Klareskog L, Hali-

cated in onset of chromosomal condensation. Proc Natl Acad Sci USA 1990;87:8617.

135. Wang JC. DNA topoisomerases. Annu Rev Biochem 1985;54:665.

136. Schulz MC, Brill SJ, Ju Q, et al. Topoisomerases and yeast rRNA transcription: Negative supercoiling stimulates initiation and topoisomerase activity is required for elongation. Genes Dev 1992;6:1332.

137. Hirakata M, Kanungo J, Pati U, et al. The autoantigenic domain of RNA polymerase III resides at the carboxyterminal domain. Arthritis Rheum 1992;35:S62.

138. Hwong CL, Chen CY, Shang HF, Hwang J. Increased synthesis and degradation of DNA topoisomerase I during the initial phase of human T lymphocyte proliferation. J Biol Chem 1993;268:18982.

139. Earnshaw WC, Machlin PS, Bordwell B, et al. Analysis of anti-centromere autoantibodies using cloned autoantigen CENP-B. Proc Natl Acad Sci USA 1987;84:4979.

140. Piccini G, Cardellini E, Reimer G, et al. An antigenic region of topoisomerase I in DNA polymerase chain reaction technique generated fragments recognized by autoantibodies of scleroderma patients. Mol Immunol 1991;28:333.

141. Eng WK, Pandit SD, Sternglanz R. Mapping of the active site tyrosine of eukaryotic DNA topoisomerase I. J Biol Chem 1989;264:13373.

142. Hardin JA. The lupus autoantigens and the pathogenesis of systemic lupus erythematosus. Arthritis Rheum 1986;29:457.

143. Tan EM. Antinuclear antibodies: Diagnostic markers for autoimmune diseases and probes for cell biology. Adv Immunol 1989;44:93.

144. Query CC, Keene JD. A human autoimmune protein associated with U1 RNA contains a region of homology that is crossreactive with retroviral p30gag antigen. Cell 1988;51:211

145. Adams TE, Alpert S, Hanahan D. Non-tolerance and autoantibodies to a transgenic self antigen expressed in pancreatic beta cells. Nature 1987;325:223.

146. Holt CM, Lindsey N, Moult J, et al. Antibody-dependent cellular cytotoxicity of vascular endothelium: Characterization and pathogenic associations in systemic sclerosis. Clin Exp Med 1989;78:359.

147. Marks RM, Czerniecki M, Andrews BS, Penny R. The effects of scleroderma serum on human microvascular endothelial cells. Induction of antibody-dependent cellular cytotoxicity. Arthritis Rheum 1988;31:1524.

148. Tan EM, Rodnan GP. Profile of antinuclear anti-

bodies in progressive systemic sclerosis (PSS). Arthritis Rheum 1975;18:430.

149. Townes AS. Complement levels in disease. Johns Hopkins Med J 1967;120:337.

150. Cunningham PH, Andrews BS, Davis JS. Immune complexes in progressive systemic sclerosis and mixed connective tissue disease. J Rheumatol 1980;7:301.

151. Seibold JR, Medsger TA Jr, Winkelstein A, et al. Immune complexes in progressive systemic sclerosis (scleroderma). Arthritis Rheum 1982;25:1167.

152. Siminovitch K, Klein M, Pruzanski W, et al. Circulating immune complexes in patients with progressive systemic sclerosis. Arthritis Rheum 1982;25:1174.

153. Furst DL, Davis JA, Clements PJ, et al. Abnormalities of pulmonary vascular dynamics and inflammation in early progressive systemic sclerosis. Arthritis Rheum 1981;24:1403.

154. Chen Z, Virella G, Tung HE, et al. Immune complexes and antinuclear, antinucleolar, and anti-centromenre antibodies in scleroderma. J Am Acad Dermatol 1984;11:461.

155. Pisko E, Gallup K, Turner R, et al. Cardiopulmonary manifestations of progressive systemic sclerosis: Association with circulating immune complexes and fluorescent antinuclear antibodies. Arthritis Rheum 1982;25:1167.

156. Hughes P, Cunningham J, Day M, et al. Immune complexes in systemic sclerosis: Detection by C1q binding. K cell inhibition and Raji cell immunoassays. J Clin Lab Immunol 1983;10:133.

157. Bernat RL, Borisy GG, Rothfield NF, Earnshaw WC. Injection of anticentromeric antibodies in interphase disrupts events required for chromosome movement in mitosis. J Cell Biol 1990;111:1519.

158. Jabs EW, Tuck-Muller CM, Anhalt GJ, et al. Cytogenetic survey in systemic sclerosis correlation of aneuploidy with the presence of anticentromere antibodies. Cytogenet Cell Genet 1993;63:169.

159. Boros P, Chen J, Bona C, Unkeless JC. Autoimmune mice make anti-Fc gamma receptor antibodies. J Exp Med 1990;11:1581.

160. Muryoi T, Andre-Schwartz J, Saitoh Y, et al. Self reactive repertoire of tight skin: Immunochemical and molecular characterization of anti-cytoplasmic antibodies. Cell Immunol 1992;144:43.

161. Muryoi T, Kasturi KN, Kafina MJ, et al. Self reactive repertoire of tight skin mouse: Immunochemical and molecular charcterization of anti-topoisomerase autoantibodies. Autoimmunity 1991;9:109.

162. Muryoi T, Kasturi KN, Kafina MJ, et al. Self reac-

tive repertoire of tight skin mouse: Immuno-chemical and molecular characterization of anti-topoisomerase I antibodies. Autoimmunity 1991; 9:109.

163. Shibata S, Muryoi T, Saitoh Y, et al. Immuno-chemical and molecular characterization of anti-RNA polymerase I autoantibodies produced by tight skin mice. J Clin Invest 1993;92:984.

164. Leff RL, Vazquez-Abad D, Everett ET, et al. Anti-topoisomerase-1 antibodies are not increased in the serum of tight-skin (TSK) mice. Arthritis Rheum 1993;6:S130.

165. Gruschwitz MS, Shoenfeld Y, Knupp M, et al. An-tinuclear antibody profile in UCD Line 200 chick-ens: A model for progressive systemic sclerosis. Int Arch Allergy Immunol 1993;100:307.

166. Irani AMA, Gruber BL, Kaufman LD, et al. Mast cell changes in scleroderma. Presence of MCT cells in the skin and evidence of mast cell activa-tion. Arthritis Rheum 1992;35:933.

167. Hawkins RA, Clamon HN, Clark RAF, Steiger-wald JC. Increased dermal mast cell population in progressive systemic sclerosis: A link to fibrosis? Ann Intern Med 1985;102:182.

168. Nishioka K, Kobayashi Y, Katayama I, Takijuri C. Mast cell numbers in diffuse scleroderma. Arch Dermatol 1987;123:205.

169. Seibold JR, Giomo RC, Clamon HN. Dermal mast cell degranulation in systemic sclerosis. Arthritis Rheum 1990;33:1702.

170. Fonseca E, Solis ZJ. Mast cells in the skin: Pro-gressive systemic sclerosis and the toxic oil syn-drome. Ann Intern Med 1985;102:864.

171. Gabrielli A, De Nictolis M, Campanati G, Cinti S. Eosinophilic fasciitis: A mast cell disorder? Clin Exp Rheumatol 1983;1:75.

172. Goto T, Befus D, Low R, Bienenstock LJ. Mast cell heterogenity and hyperplasia in bleomycin-in-duced pulmonary fibrosis in rats. Am Rev Respir Dis 1984;130:797.

173. Clamon HN, Giorno RC, Seibold JR. Endothelial and fibroblast activation in scleroderma: The myth of the "uninvolved skin." Arthritis Rheum 1991;34:1495.

174. Lee Cho K, Clamon HN. Mast cells, fibroblast, and fibrosis: New clues to the riddle of mast cells. Immunol Res 1987;6:145.

175. Lee Cho K, Giorno R, Claman HN. Cutaneous mast cell depletion and recovery in murine graft-vs-host disease. J Immunol 1987;138:4093.

176. Walker M, Harley R, Maize J, et al. Mast cells and their degranulation in the TSK mouse model of scleroderma. Proc Soc Exp Biol Med 1985;180: 323.

177. Tuveri MA, Passiu G, Mathieu A, Aloe L. Nerve growth factor and mast cell distribution in the skin of patients with systemic sclerosis. Clin Exp Rheumatol 1993;11:319.

178. Chanez P, Lacoste JY, Guillot B, et al. Mast cells' contribution to the fibrosing alveolitis of the scleroderma lung. Am Rev Respir Dis 1993;147: 1497.

179. Lightbroun AS, Sandhaus LM, Giorno RC, et al. Myocardial mast cells in systemic sclerosis: A re-port of three fatal cases. Am J Med 1990;89:372.

180. Grazia Cifone M, Giacomelli R, Famularo G, et al. Natural killer activity and antibody-dependent cellular cytotoxicity in progressive systemic scle-rosis. Clin Exp Immunol 1990;80:360.

181. Wright JZK, Hughes P, Powell NR. Spontaneous lymphocyte-mediated (NK cell) cytotoxicity in systemic sclerosis: A comparison with antibody-dependent lymphocyte (K cell) cytotoxicity. Ann Rheum Dis 1982;41:409.

182. Miller EB, Hiserodt JC, Hunt LE, et al. Reduced natural killer cell activity in patients with sys-temic sclerosis: Correlation with clinical disease type. Arthritis Rheum 1988;31:1515.

183. Silver R. Lymphokine activated killer (LAK) cell activity in the peripheral blood lymphocytes of systemic sclerosis (SSc) patients. Clin Exp Rheu-matol 1990;8:481.

184. Gustafsson R, Fredens K, Nettelbladt O, Haligren R. Eosinophil activation in systemic sclerosis. Arthritis Rheum 1991;34:414.

185. Varga J, Wright J, Earle L, et al. Eosinophil acti-vation in diffuse cutaneous systemic sclerosis. Arthritis Rheum 1993;36:S270.

186. Ishkawa O, Ishkawa H. Macrophage infiltration in the skin of patients with systemic sclerosis. J Rheumatol 1992;19:1202.

187. Koch AE, Litvak MA, Burrows JC, Polverini PJ. Decreased monocyte-mediated angiogenesis in scleroderma. Clin Immunol Immunopathol 1992; 64:153.

188. De Paulis A, Valentini G, Spadaro G, et al. Human basophil releasability. VIII. Increased basophil re-activity in patients with scleroderma. Arthritis Rheum 1991;34:1289.

189. Konig G, Luderschmidt C, Hammer C, et al. Lung involvement in scleroderma. Chest 1984;85:318.

190. Stevens TRJ, Hall ND, McHugh NJ, Maddison PJ. Spontaneous neutrophil activation in patients with primary Raynaud's phenomenon and sys-temic sclerosis. Br J Rheumatol 1992;31:856.

191. Cathcart MK, Krakauer RS. Immunologic en-hancement of collagen accumulation in progres-sive systemic sclerosis (PSS). Clin Immunol Im-munopath 1981;21:128.

192. Gonzalez-Amaro R, Alarcon-Segovia D, Alcocer-

Varela J, et al. Mononuclear cell-fibroblast interactions in scleroderma. Clin Immunol Immunopathol 1988;46:412.

193. Needleman BW, Ordonez JV, Taramelli D, et al. *In vitro* identification of a subpopulation of fibroblasts that produces high levels of procollagen in scleroderma. Arthritis Rheum 1990;33:842.

194. Worrall JG, Whiteside TL, Prince RK, et al. Persistence of scleroderma-like phenotype in normal fibroblasts after prolonged exposure to soluble mediators from mononuclear cells. Arthritis Rheum 1986;29:54.

195. Johnson RL, Ziff M. Lymphokine stimulation of collagen accumulation. J Clin Invest 1976;58:240.

196. Needleman BW, Wigley FM, Stair RW. Interleukin-1, interleukin-2, interleukin-4, interleukin-6, tumor necrosis factor α, and interferon-γ levels in sera from patients with scleroderma. Arthritis Rheum 1992;35:67.

197. Degiannis D, Seibold J, Czarnecki M, et al. Soluble and cellular markers of immune activation in patients with systemic sclerosis. Clin Immunol Immunopathol 1990;56:259.

198. Kahaleh MB. Soluble immunologic products in scleroderma sera. Clin Immunol Immunopathol 1991;58:139.

199. Southcott AM, Jones KP, Pantelidis P, et al. Interleukin-8 is associated with the presence of pulmonary fibrosis in systemic sclerosis. Arthritis Rheum 1993;36:S181.

200. Gabrielli A, DiLoret C, Taborro R, et al. Immunohistochemical localization of intracellular and extracellular associated TGFβ in the skin of patients with systemic sclerosis (scleroderma) and primary Raynaud's phenomenon. Clin Immunol Immunopathol 1993;68:340.

201. Gay S, Jones RE Jr, Huang GQ, et al. Immunohistologic demonstration of platelet-derived growth factor (PDGF) and sis-oncogene expression in scleroderma. J Invest Dermatol 1989;92:301.

202. Famularo G, Procopio A, Giacomelli R, et al. Soluble interleukin-2 receptor, interleukin-2 and interleukin-4 in sera and supernatants from patients with progressive systemic sclerosis. Clin Exp Immunol 1990;81:368.

203. Kulozik M, Hogg A, Lankat-Buttgereit B, et al. Colocalization of transforming growth factor β2 with α1(I) procollagen mRNA in tissue sections of patients with systemic sclerosis. J Clin Invest 1990;86:917.

204. Grushwitz M, Muller PU, Sepp N, et al. Transcription and expression of transforming growth factor type beta in the skin or progressive systemic sclerosis: A mediator of fibrosis? J Invest Dermatol 1990;94:197.

205. Deicher HRG, Denck F, Hoffman T. Identification of an LTB4 protein complex as evidence of endothelial cell cytotoxicity activity (ECA) in progressive systemic sclerosis (PSS), Z Rheumatol 1987;46:147.

206. Kahaleh MB. Endothelin, an endothelial-dependent vaoconstrictor in scleroderma: Enhanced production and profibrotic action. Arthritis Rheum 1991;34:978.

207. Roberts AB, Sporn MB, Assoian RK, et al. Transforming growth factor type β: Rapid induction of fibrosis and angiogenesis *in vivo* and stimulation of collagen formation *in vitro*. Proc Natl Acad Sci USA 1986;83:4167.

208. Snowden N, Herrick AL, Illingworth K, et al. Plasma transforming growth factor β1 in systemic sclerosis. Arthritis Rheum 1993;36:S272.

209. Peltonen J, Kahari L, Jaakkola S, et al. Evaluation of transforming growth factor beta and type I procollagen gene expression in fibrotic skin diseases by *in situ* hybridization. J Invest Dermatol 1990;94:365.

210. Spikakis PP, McCune BK, Tsokas M, et al. Immunohistological demonstration of transforming growth factor-β isoforms in the skin of patients with systemic sclerosis. Clin Immunol Immunopathol 1993;69:199.

211. Gabrielli A, Di Loreto C, Taborro R, et al. Immunohistochemical localization of intracellular and extracellular associated TGFβ in the skin of patients with systemic sclerosis (scleroderma) and primary Raynaud's phenomenon. Clin Immunol Immunopathol 1993;68:340.

212. Kulozik M, Hogg A, Lankat-Buttgereit B, Kreig T. Localization of transforming growth factor β2 with the α1(I) procollagen mRNA in tissue sections of patients with systemic sclerosis. J Clin Invest 1990;86:917.

213. Fava R, Olsen N, Keski-Oja J, et al. Active and latent forms of transforming growth factor beta activity in synovial effusions. J Exp Med 1989;169:291.

214. Nakamura T, Miller D, Ruoslahti E, Border WA. Production of extracellular matrix by glomerular epithelial cells is regulated by transforming growth factor-beta 1. Kidney Int 1992;41:1213.

215. Paralkar VM, Vukicevic S, Reddi AH. Transforming growth factor beta type 1 binds to collagen IV of basement membrane matrix: Implications for development. Dev Biol 1991;143:303.

216. Deguchi Y. Spontaneous increase of transforming growth factor β production by bronchoalveolar mononuclear cells of patients with systemic autoimmune diseases affecting the lung. Ann Rheum Dis 1992;51:362.

217. Moreland LW, Goldsmith K, Russell WJ, et al. Transforming growth factor β with fibrotic scleroderma lungs. Am J Med 1992;93:628.

218. Majewski S, Hunzelmann N, Schirren CG, et al. Increased adhesion of fibroblasts from patients with scleroderma to extracellular matrix components: *In vitro* modulation by IFN-γ but not by TGF-β. J Invest Dermatol 1992;98:86–91.

219. Yamakage A, Kikuchi K, Smith EA, et al. Selective upregulation of platelet-derived growth factor α receptors by transforming growth factor β in scleroderma fibroblasts. J Exp Med 1992;175:1227.

220. Klareskog L, Gustafsson R, Schneyiu A, Haligren R. Increased expression of platelet-derived growth factor type β receptors in the skin of patients with systemic sclerosis. Arthritis Rheum 1990;33: 1534.

221. Gay S, Jones RE Jr, Huang GQ, Gay RE. Immunohistologic demonstration of platelet-derived growth factor (PDGF) and sis-oncogene expression in scleroderma. J Invest Dermatol 1989;92: 301.

222. Needleman BW, Choi J, Burrows-Mezu A, Fontana JA. Secretion and binding of transforming growth factor-β by scleroderma and normal dermal fibroblasts. Arthritis Rheum 1990;33:650.

223. McWhirter A, Colosetti P, Rubin K, Black CM. Role of TGF-β in the acquisition of the scleroderma (SSc) phenotype. Arthritis Rheum 1993; 36:S162.

224. Aotsuka S, Nakamura K, Nakano T, et al. Production of intracellular and extracellular interleukin-1α and interleukin-1β by peripheral blood monocytes from patients with connective tissue diseases. Ann Rheum Dis 1991;50:27.

225. Umehara H, Kumagai S, Murakami M, et al. Enhanced production of interleukin-1 and tumor necrosis factor alpha by cultured peripheral blood monocytes from patients with scleroderma. Arthritis Rheum 1990;33:893.

226. Sandborg CI, Berman MA, Andrews BS, Friou G. Interleukin-1 production by mononuclear cells from patients with scleroderma. Clin Exp Immunol 1985;60:294.

227. Whicher JT, Gilbert AM, Westacott C, et al. Defective production of leucocytic endogenous mediator (interleukin-1) by peripheral blood leucocytes of patients with systemic sclerosis, systemic lupus erythematosus, rheumatoid arthritis and mixed connective tissue disease. Clin Exp Immunol 1986;65:80.

228. Bravo J, Sutej P, Lykens M. Pulmonary dysfunction in scleroderma: Role of cytokines. Arthritis Rheum 1993;36:S131.

229. Kawaguchi Y, Harigai M, Hara M, et al. Increased interleukin 1 receptor, type I, at messenger RNA and protein level in skin fibroblasts from patients with systemic sclerosis. Biochem Biophys Res Commun 1992;184:1504.

230. Kawaguchi Y, Harigai M, Suzuki K. Interleukin 1 receptor on fibroblasts from systemic sclerosis patients induces excessive functional responses to interleukin 1β. Biochem Biophys Res Commun 1993;190:154.

231. Feghali CA, Bost KL, Boulware DW, Levy LS. Mechanisms of pathogenesis in scleroderma: I. Overproduction of interleukin 6 by fibroblasts cultured from affected skin sites of patients with scleroderma. J Rheumatol 1992;19:1207.

232. Romero LI, Pincus SH. *In situ* localization of interleukin −6 in normal skin and atrophic cutaneous disease. Int Arch Allergy Immunol 1992;99:44.

233. Kahaleh MB, Yin T. Enhanced expression of high affinity interleukin-2 receptors in scleroderma: Possible role for IL-6. Clin Immunol Immunopathol 1992;62:97.

234. Palazzo E, Crestani B, Dehoux M, et al. Interleukin-6 production by monocytes and alveolar macrophages in scleroderma with lung involvement. Arthritis Rheum 1993;36:S182.

235. Kahaleh MB, LeRoy EC. Interleukin 2 in scleroderma: Correlation of serum level with extent of skin involvement and disease duration. Ann Intern Med 1989;110:446.

236. Alms WJ, Wigley FM, Wise R, et al. Immunologic analyses of broncho alveolar lavage (BAL) cells from scleroderma patients and controls. Arthritis Rheum 1992;35:S312.

237. Feghali CA, Bost KL, Boulware DW, Levy LS. Human recombinant interleukin-4 induces proliferation and interleukin-6 production by cultured human skin fibroblasts. Clin Immunol Immunopathol 1992;63:182.

238. Postlethwaite AE, Holness MA, Katai H, Raghow R. Human fibroblasts synthesize elevated levels of extracellular matrix proteins in response to interleukin-4. J Clin Invest 1992;90:1479.

239. Postlethwaite AE, Seyer JM. Fibroblast chemotaxis induction by human recombinant interleukin-4: Identification by synthetic peptide analysis of two chemotactic domains residing in amino acid sequences 70–88 and 89–122. J Clin Invest 1991;87:2147.

240. Prior C, Haslam PL. *In vivo* and *in vitro* production of interferon-gamma in fibrosing interstitial lung diseases. Clin Exp Immunol 1992;88:280.

241. Scheglovitova ON, Balabanova RM, Kulieva AM, et al. Interferon system in patients with rheumatoid arthritis and sclerodermia systematica. Acta Virol 1993;37:54.

242. Kahaleh B, Fan FS. Impaired gamma interferon production in scleroderma: Possible role for interleukin-10. Arthritis Rheum 1993;36:S50.

243. Southcott AM, Jones KP, Pantelidis P, et al. Interleukin-8 is associated with the presence of pulmonary fibrosis in systemic sclerosis. Arthritis Rheum 1993;36:S181.

244. Sollberg S, Peltonen J, Uitto J, Jimenez SA. Elevated expression of β1 and β2 integrins, intercellular adhesion molecule 1, and endothelial adhesion molecule 1 in the skin of patients with systemic sclerosis of recent onset. Arthritis Rheum 1992; 35:290.

245. Majewski S, Hunzelmann N, Johnson JP, et al. Expression of intercellular adhesion molecule-1 (ICAM-1) in the skin of patients with systemic scleroderma. J Invest Dermatol 1991;7:667.

246. Picker LJ, Kisimoto TK, Smith CW, et al. ELAM-1 is an adhesion molecule for skin-homing T cells. Nature 1991;349:796.

247. Carson CW, Beall LD, Hunder GG, et al. Serum ELAM-1 is increased in vasculitis, scleroderma, and systemic lupus erythematosus. J Rheumatol 1993;20:809.

248. Piela TH, Korn JH. ICAM-1-dependent fibroblast-lymphocyte adhesion: Discordance between surface expression and function of ICAM-1. Cell Immunol 1990;129:125.

249. Veale DJ, Kirk G, McLaren M, Belch JJF. Elevation of circulating soluble ICAM-1 in response to venous occulusion in patients with systemic sclerosis and their relatives. Arthritis Rheum 1993;36: S270.

250. Rudnicka L, Majewski S, Blasczczyk M, et al. Adhesion of peripheral blood mononuclear cells to vascular endothelium in patients with systemic sclerosis (scleroderma). Arthritis Rheum 1992;35:771.

251. Needleman BW. Increased expression of intercellular adhesion molecule 1 on the fibroblasts of scleroderma patients. Arthritis Rheum 1990;33: 1847.

252. Abraham D, Lupoli S, McWhirter A, et al. Expression and function of surface antigens on scleroderma fibroblasts. Arthritis Rheum 1991;34:1164.

SERGIO A. JIMENEZ
M. ERIC GERSHWIN

12

Animal Models of Systemic Sclerosis

ANIMAL MODELS of systemic connective tissue diseases have provided valuable insights into the intimate mechanisms and the pathogenesis of these diseases, and have provided the means to test potentially useful therapeutic interventions. Although animal models for systemic lupus erythematosus (SLE), rheumatoid arthritis (RA), ankylosing spondylitis, and other systemic rheumatic diseases have been extensively employed, studies with animal models for systemic sclerosis (SSc) are scarce. The principal reason for the scarcity of these studies is the lack of an animal model that exhibits all the aspects of SSc. However, a number of experimental systems that reproduce some of the pathologic alterations of this disorder have been described. This chapter reviews various animal models of SSc emphasizing their similarities and differences with the human disease. These animal models can be separated into two groups. In one group, the pathologic alterations are induced in normal animals by either administration of exogenous substances or by manipulation of their immune system. In the second group, the pathologic phenotype is the result of a genomic mutation that is transmitted genetically as a stable trait.

Induced Models of SSc

The following section describes several induced animal models that reproduce some of the pathologic alterations of the human disease.

HOMOLOGOUS DISEASE AND GRAFT-VERSUS-HOST DISEASE (GVHD)

The first animal model resembling SSc was the "homologous disease" in rats described by Statsny et al (1,2). These investigators injected donor lymphoid cells into neonatal Sprague-Dawley rats to induce immunologic tolerance. Challenge of the adult Sprague-Dawley neonates that matured with lymphoid cells from the original donor resulted in pathologic alterations in virtually all of the animals that were challenged. These alterations were caused by the immunological attack of the recipient's tissues by the donor's cells—a "graft-versus-host" response. Animals surviving the acute phase of the "homologous disease" evolved into a chronic stage characterized by severe dermatitis with dermal and subdermal fibrosis, prominent mononuclear cell infiltration, and atrophy of sebaceous glands and hair follicles. The mononuclear cell infiltration and the accumulation of connective tissue in the dermis and subcutaneous tissue in these animals resembled closely those characteristics present in affected skin from patients with SSc of recent onset, as pointed out by Jaffee and Claman (3) and Claman et al (4). Many aspects of GVHD, however, are not considered typical of SSc. These include the frequent occurrence of hemolytic anemia, thrombocytopenia, and inflammatory arthritis (1,2), and the development of lymphoid hyperplasia and malignant lymphomas (5,6). Furthermore, the vascular changes in SSc are characterized by luminal occlusion and subendothelial connective tissue deposition, whereas those in GVHD are vasculitic (1,2).

BLEOMYCIN-INDUCED FIBROSIS

Ichihashi et al (7) described the occurrence of fibrotic changes and thickening of the skin in mice receiving the antitumor antibiotic bleomycin, and Adamsom and Bowden reported changes in lung architecture in mice injected intraperitoneally with this antibiotic (8). The lungs of these animals showed a marked infiltration by mononuclear cells and accumulation of fibroblasts resulting in pulmonary fibrosis. Similar lesions in the lungs of rabbits given intratracheal bleomycin have been reported (9). In these rabbits, lung elastin and types I and III collagens were found to be increased. Severe chronic inflammatory and fibrotic changes in the lungs have also been observed following either systemic or intratracheal bleomycin administration to rats (10), hamsters (11), and baboons (12). The pathologic alterations observed in the lungs of these animals bear striking resemblance to the histopathologic changes present in the lungs of patients with SSc. The prominent infiltration of lung parenchyma with chronic inflammatory cells in this animal model suggested that the resulting fibrosis was mediated by cellular immune mechanisms. However, the occurrence of interstitial pulmonary fibrosis in nude athymic mice receiving bleomycin (13) indicates that participation of immunocompetent cells is not an essential requirement for the development of lung fibrosis, and may be the result of a direct effect of bleomycin on connective tissue-producing cells. This possibility has been supported by the studies of Clark et al (14), who showed that normal human dermal and lung fibroblasts cultured *in vitro* in the presence of bleomycin displayed an increase in their rate of type I procollagen synthesis. The cutaneous effects of administration of bleomycin were further studied by Mountz et al (15), who showed that rats injected repeatedly with sublethal doses of bleomycin developed skin hyperpigmentation and severe dermal fibrosis. Abnormalities in the structure of dermal collagen fibers were also documented in this study. These animals, therefore, appear to reproduce the cutaneous pathologic changes characteristic of the fibrotic phase of SSc. However, in contrast with human SSc, the cutaneous lesions induced by bleomycin display minimal skin inflammatory changes without lymphocytic infiltration. Furthermore, the animals do not develop an autoimmune response, as indicated by negative laboratory tests for antinuclear antibodies (ANA) in their sera.

FIBROSIS INDUCED BY INJECTIONS OF GLYCOSAMINOGLYCANS (GAGS) FROM THE URINE OF SSC PATIENTS INTO MICE

Another experimentally induced model of scleroderma is that of mice that were injected with GAGs isolated from the urine of SSc patients (16). In these studies, several GAG fractions were partially purified from the urine of normal individuals and SSc patients by ion-exchange chromatography. Slightly more than 50% of the animals injected with certain of the chromatographically separated GAG fractions obtained from urine of SSc patients developed fibrotic lesions in the skin and in internal organs including heart, lungs, and esophagus. The skin showed increased deposition of collagen, and the visceral changes included interstitial edema, mononuclear cell infiltration, and various degrees of fibrosis (17). However, studies by Fox et al (18), following an essentially identical protocol to that of the initial study by Ishikawa (16), failed to show any effects of the GAG fractions isolated from the urine of SSc patients on skin thickness of the injected animals nor any histologic evidence of fibrosis in the skin or internal organs. Further studies to determine whether certain macromolecules which are present in the urine of SSc patients are capable of inducing fibrotic changes are necessary to resolve these discrepancies. The identification and characterization of such molecules, if confirmed, could provide valuable insights into the pathogenesis of SSc.

FIBROSIS INDUCED BY EXPOSURE TO ORGANIC SOLVENTS

Occupational exposure of people to certain organic compounds has been associated with the occurrence of Raynaud's phenomenon (RP) and other clinical manifestations resembling SSc (19,20). Based on these observations, Yamakage and Ishikawa (21) exposed mice to several organic solvents, including vinyl chloride, and found that a significant number of the exposed animals developed skin changes similar to those found in patients with SSc. However, no biochemical studies of the connective tissue changes induced by these solvents nor immunologic studies in the affected animals were reported.

Genetically Transmitted Models of SSc

Although the experimentally-induced animal models discussed previously in this chapter reproduce some of the features of human SSc, none of them exhibit all of the three principal pathogenetic features observed in the human disease: cutaneous and visceral fibrosis, alterations of the microvasculature, and cellular and humoral immune abnormalities. However, there are several animal models that display some features of SSc as a result of a genetically transmitted trait. These genetically based models of SSc may be more enlightening with regard to the etiology and pathogenesis of this disease, because they should allow for the identification of gene defects that are responsible for their abnormal phenotypes. Identification of these mutated genes may provide valuable clues to enhance our understanding of the molecular mechanisms involved in the pathogenesis of SSc.

AVIAN SCLERODERMA

One of the most interesting genetically transmitted animal models of SSc is the University of California at Davis (UCD) line 200 (L200) chickens,

which were propagated from an original mutant discovered in 1942 by Bernier and first described by Gershwin et al (22) and van de Water and Gershwin (23). Adult L200 birds display a characteristic feature known as "self-dubbing," referring to the varying degrees of missing combs exhibited in greater than 90% of the birds of both sexes (Fig. 12.1). Initial involvement of the comb in L200 chickens is apparent by 1 to 2 weeks of age, and is followed by polyarthritis of peripheral joints and dermal lesions by 6 weeks of age (Fig. 12.2). In the original report, it was noted that birds with comb, skin, and joint involvement were generally dead by 10 weeks of age, and that the overall mortality of L200 chickens was 40% by 4 months. The cause of death in these chickens is usually secondary cutaneous infection. However, when the birds are housed indoors and in less crowded conditions than those found in

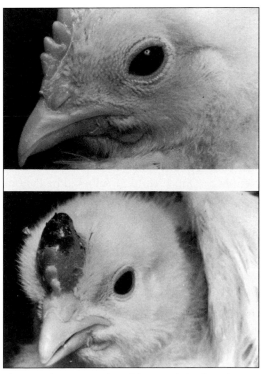

Figure 12.1. Seven-day-old control (*top*) and L200 (*bottom*) chickens. Note the severe swelling and early necrosis in the comb of the L200 chicken.

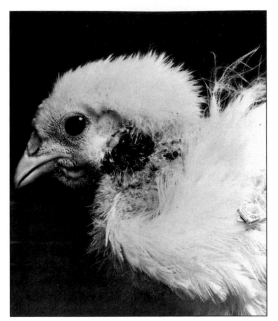

Figure 12.2. L200 chicken 8 weeks of age showing some comb loss and extensive neck involvement. Note the extremely thickened skin with necrosis.

conventional poultry establishments, infection is drastically reduced and the survival of the animals is substantially prolonged.

Pathologic Features

Early in the course of the disease there is an intense mononuclear cell (MNC) infiltration of the skin and comb (Fig. 12.3), followed by the proliferation of small blood vessels (Fig. 12.4), and increased deposition of collagen (Fig. 12.3). The lymphoid infiltration, which resolves later in the disease, is followed by the replacement of dermis, subcutaneous fat, and muscle with fibrous tissue. Involvement of internal organs is apparent in the esophagus, small intestine, lungs, heart, kidneys, and testicles. The connective tissue of the

esophagus and small intestine is thickened, with heavy collagen deposits extending into the muscle layers. By 1 week of age, 20% of the birds display interstitial fibrosis of the lungs (Fig. 12.5); involvement of this organ increases in incidence and severity until 6 weeks of age when 50% of the birds are affected. Pericardial effusions are observed in 40% of 6-month-old animals following early myocardial interstitial fibrosis and fiber degeneration. The kidneys are involved in nearly all animals, with swelling and thickening of the muscular layers of the renal arterioles (Fig. 12.6) and glomerulonephritis with deposition of IgG within the glomerulus.

MNC infiltration of the skin usually begins at 2 weeks of age with predominant infiltration by CD4+ T cells followed by CD8+ T cell infiltration (24–26). A portion of the T cells express surface B-L antigen, the chicken equivalent of Ia antigen, suggesting the presence of activated T cells. Distinct B cell clusters are also noted in progressing lesions. Further evidence suggests that L200 chickens have a major qualitative and quantitative T cell defect. L200 T cells respond poorly to a variety of diversely acting T cell mitogens, including Con A, PHA, and anti-chicken CD3. Indeed, they do not respond well even to phorbol myristate acetate in conjunction with ionomycin. Some of these abnormalities are similar to alterations in T cell function frequently observed in cells from patients with SSc.

Thymic Abnormalities

Mainstream thymocyte differentiation is initiated by the migration of blood-borne precursors into the thymic milieu, mediated by factors generally accepted as being released by thymic epithelial cells. The ensuing differentiation involves activation, T cell receptor (TCR) gene rearrangement and expression, generation and modulation

Figure 12.3. Light microscopy of skin sections from a L200 chicken stained with hematoxylin-eosin (*top*). The epidermis is atrophic. Notice the dense collagen bundles that have replaced the usual delicate collagen of the superficial dermis. The remaining dermis is infiltrated with chronic inflammatory cells, and adipose tissue has been replaced by fibroblasts and lymphocytes. Compare with sections of normal chicken skin (*bottom*). Notice the delicate superficial dermis; the subcutaneous tissue contains fat and striated muscle (magnification × 77).

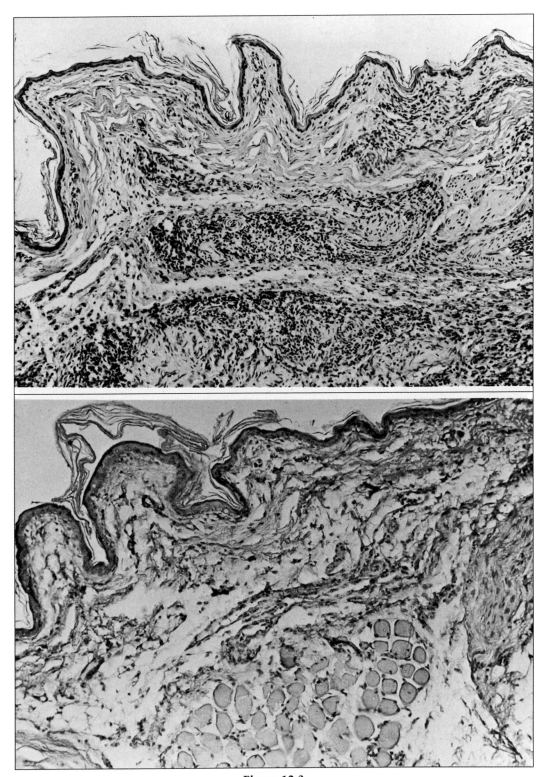

Figure 12.3.

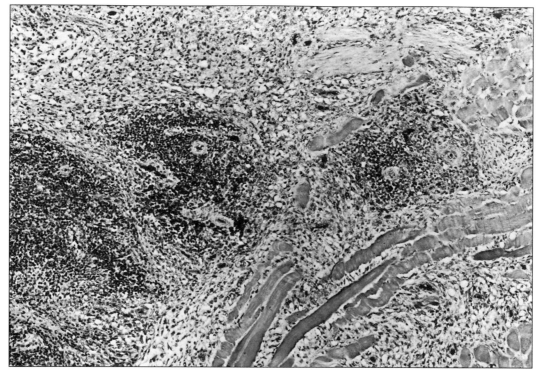

Figure 12.4. Light microscopy of a skin section from a L200 chicken 6 weeks of age stained with hematoxylin-eosin. Note the intense MNC infiltrate, particularly around blood vessels, as well as the swollen appearance of vessels (magnification × 77).

of accessory molecules, clonal expansion, and repertoire establishment. This complex differentiation process is accomplished through positive versus negative selection subsequent to emigration of cells to the periphery (27–30). Extensive phenotypic studies have delineated the major T cell maturation pathways, but the precise stromal compartments within which the discrete stages occur are not known. The emerging consensus is that positive selection is the domain of cortical epithelium, negative selection of macrophage/dendritic cells, and anergy, of medullary epithelium. This is clearly an oversimplified view that excludes intermediary, yet undoubtedly important, steps in the tightly regulated continuum of T cell differentiation. The genesis of the thymic stroma itself is also dependent on the T cells; thus, thymopoiesis involves a symbiotic maturation of multiple cell lineages.

Hence, a meaningful understanding of thymic contribution to pathology requires a detailed analysis of both T lymphocytic and stromal components.

Arguably, one of the most important roles of the thymus is to apply strict selection criteria to developing T cells. While recognition of foreign peptides bound to self major histo-compatibility complex (MHC) molecules is a fundamental feature of the TCR, potentially autoreactive T cells must be clonally deleted or functionally "silenced." Subsets of thymic stromal cells play key roles in these selection processes. Since negative selection occurs intrathymically and presumably at a distinct phase in T cell differentiation, inappropriate presentation of self peptides in the thymus, or disruption of the normal microenvironment encompassed within the stromal architecture, may instead lead to T cell dysfunction and perhaps predispose to the development of autoimmunity. Despite this, there have been very few detailed analyses of the status of the thymic microenvironment in autoimmune diseases. Recent studies have shown that L200 chickens have striking defects in the thymic subcapsular regions and in expression of MHC class II antigens in the cortex (31,32). Thus, it has been proposed that these unique defects may result in abnormal T cell maturation (31,32).

Extensive immunohistological studies employing a variety of specific antibodies were conducted by Gershwin et al to further delineate the thymic defect in L200 chickens (32,33). No differences were observed in chicken thymic stromal staining employing any of these antibodies in several normal control chicken lines at any ages tested. In contrast, however, striking differences were observed in restricted elements of the

thymic microenvironment of L200 chickens prior to onset of disease. The regions most affected were the subcapsule and the medulla. The monoclonal antibody MUI 70, which stains all type I epithelium (i.e., the entire subcapsular and perivascular epithelium) in a normal thymus, stained only perivascular epithelium, which is located predominantly in the medulla in the L200 thymus; the subcapsule was virtually negative. When the monoclonal antibodies MUI 51, MUI 53, and MUI 58, which identify sub-specificities within type I epithelium of normal chickens, were employed in L200 chickens, there was no significant staining of the subcapsule, and only isolated regions of perivascular epithelium were positive. Two additional striking abnormalities in L200 were identified with the monoclonal antibodies MUI 78 and MUI 36. There was an increase in isolated stellate MUI 78+

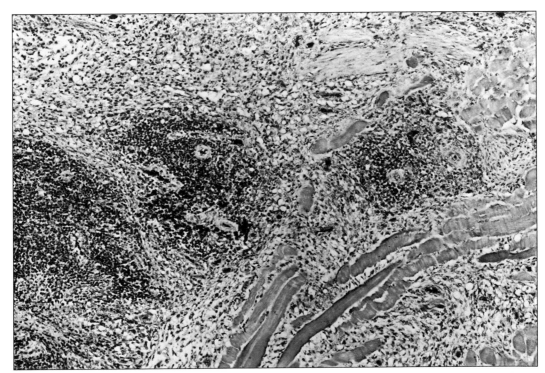

Figure 12.5. Light microscopy of a lung section from a 5-month-old L200 female chicken stained with hematoxylin-eosin. Note the infiltration of lymphoid cells and histiocytes. Severe interstitial fibrosis is seen predominantly around the bronchi (magnification × 77).

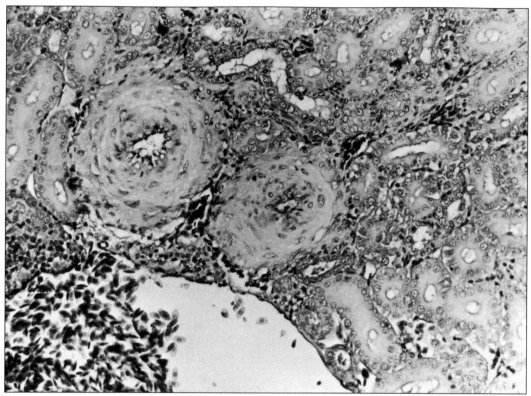

Figure 12.6. Light microscopy of a kidney section from a 3-month-old L200 chicken stained with hematoxylin-eosin. Note the severe occlusion due to medial and intimal hyperplasia. Also note the perivascular infiltrate (magnification × 400).

(monomorphic MHC class II) cells in the thymic cortex of L200; the medulla was essentially normal. A similar increase occurred in MUI 36 isolated positive cells in the L200 thymic cortex. In addition, a marked increase of staining occurred in the medulla, whereas this antibody stained only isolated B cells and a relatively rare subset of mature T cells and macrophages in the medulla of the normal chicken thymus. All alterations were unique for L200 chickens, were consistent for all ages (i.e., they did not undergo changes during the surveyed period), and have not been observed in any other strain studied to date (32,33). It should be emphasized that MUI 70 stains type I epithelium of every normal strain examined. Interestingly, when unaffected skin from L200 and L206 chickens were stained with MUI 70, markedly attenuated staining was observed,

whereas tissues from control, healthy chicken lines were strongly reactive (see Fig. 12.5).

T Cell Defects

The prominent cellular infiltrate in affected tissues of L200 chickens consists predominantly of lymphocytes with only a few esterase positive cells (monocyte/macrophages). Although initial studies indicated that no T cells were present (24), a subsequent study employing T cell-specific antibodies showed that the cellular infiltrates contained large numbers of T cells (25). Characterization of the infiltrating cells showed the presence of both T helper and T cytotoxic/suppressor cells with a T4:T8 ratio of 1.44 by 4 weeks of age. Furthermore, intense staining for the Ia antigen equivalent B-L antigen was found on all infiltrating cells as well as in fibroblasts.

Additional investigation of the phenotypic characteristics and function of peripheral blood lymphocytes (PBL), spleen cells, and thymocytes in comparison with skin infiltrating cells was carried out by Gruschwitz et al (26). These authors found by immunofluorescence and immunohistochemical analysis using monoclonal antibodies that the overwhelming majority of skin infiltrating MNCs in the deeper dermis and subcutaneous tissue were T cell receptor α/β (TcR2)+/CD3+/CD4+/class II+ cells, a small portion (5%–10%) of which were interleukin 2 (IL-2) receptor positive. In contrast, the inflammatory infiltrates in perivascular areas of the papillary dermis were mainly composed of TcR γ/β (TcR1)±class II-lymphocytes. Only a few B cells (T/B cell ratio >5) were detected. Functional *in vitro* studies showed a significantly decreased T cell mitogen-induced proliferation rate associated with a decreased capacity to produce IL-2 and to express IL-2 receptors. However, in contrast to the deficient *in vitro* IL-2 production, the sera of UCD L200 chickens contained significant levels of IL-2 bioactivity. These results indicate that the disease of UCD L200 chickens includes a numeric and/or a functional alteration of T cells similar to that observed in T cells from patients with SSc.

T cell activation is dependent upon calcium influx and protein kinase C activation, with subsequent lymphocyte proliferation-dependent interleukins such as IL-2. Since L200 chickens have both thymic defects and a diminished PBL response to IL-2, T cell function was further investigated (31). Interestingly, L200 T cells respond poorly *in vitro* to a variety of diversely acting T cell mitogens including Con A, PHA, and anti-chicken CD3 monoclonal antibody. Moreover, they do not respond well even to phorbol myristate acetate in conjunction with ionomycin. The addition of exogenous IL-2-containing supernatants concurrently with mitogenic stimulation also had no significant effect. Analysis of intracellular free calcium demonstrated that lymphocytes from L200 had a reduced influx of calcium (or release of intracellular stores) following stimulation. Analysis of chicken CD3, CD4, and CD8 expression revealed a 39% decrease in peripheral blood CD4+ cells in L200, although this decrease was not sufficient to explain the 80% to 90% decrease observed in proliferation assays and calcium influx. Thus, these extensive studies reveal the occurrence of a unique defect in T cell activation in these birds (31).

Autoantibodies in Sera of L200 Chickens

Serologic studies of autoantibody production showed that by 6 months of age, greater than 60% of L200 birds develop rheumatoid factor and a large spectrum of ANAs and anticytoplasmic antibodies (22,34). The ANAs display predominantly a finely speckled pattern by immunofluorescence. By enzyme-linked immunosorbent assay, 40% of L200 birds were found to have antibodies to single-stranded DNA (ssDNA). In contrast, antibodies to histones, RNA, poly A, or poly U were not detected. Precipitating antibodies to saline extracts from chicken liver were noted in 33% of L200 birds. The antigenicity of chicken liver extracts was shown by cell fractionation in conjunction with column chromatographic techniques, to be contained in several proteins, with apparent molecular weights in the range of 62,000 to 290,000 daltons, which were present in cytoplasm but not in isolated nuclei. L200 sera do not react against nuclear ribonucleoprotein, Sm, Scl-70, anticentromere, or SSB/La antigens. Thus, L200 chickens develop ANAs and anticytoplasmic antibodies that recognize a unique group of protein antigenic determinants found only in avian species, but do not develop those antibodies considered to be specific for human SSc, such as anticentromere or Scl-70 antibodies.

L200 chickens were found to have no detectable antibodies to native DNA (nDNA) or rabbit, rat, or mouse extractable nuclear antigen (ENA) however, 40% of L200 chickens were highly responsive to ssDNA versus 0% for a control line. In contrast, more than 50% of 1-month-old chickens expressed anticytoplasmic antibodies using an HEp-2 cell line, which is believed to be specific for cytoskeletal elements. Finally, by hemagglutination, 45 of 46 L200 chickens at 6 months of age were noted to have antibodies to type II collagen with a mean titer of 3.1 ± 1.4. In contrast, there were no detectable ANAs or anti-collagen antibodies present in control chickens.

Connective Tissue Alterations

To determine whether fibroblast activation is a factor that contributes to the development of fibrosis in L200 chickens, Duncan et al studied collagen, non-collagenous protein, and GAG production of 34 separate fibroblast lines derived from normal and fibrotic skin of L200 and from two control lines (35). The mean $\pm$SEM incorporation of ^{3}H-proline or ^{3}H-glucosamine into extracellular collagen, non-collagenous protein, or GAG by first passage fibroblast lines derived from fibrotic skin of diseased birds was three- to five-fold higher than that of fibroblast lines derived from the skin of controls. Similar differences were observed for cell-associated production, including collagen and non-collagenous protein production assessment using non-radioactive electrophoretic methods. The activated phenotype of fibroblast lines derived from the fibrotic skin of diseased birds persisted through at least 10 cell doublings in tissue culture. However, the ratio of type I:III collagen and the profile of GAG types produced were similar in all fibroblast lines, suggesting the occurrence of fibroblast biosynthetic activation rather than a change in the collagen phenotype (35). These observations are similar to those obtained with cultured human SSc fibroblasts.

To demonstrate a link between MNC infiltration and the development of skin fibrotic lesions in affected chickens, supernatants from cultures of skin pieces or from isolated MNC were obtained and assayed for their effect on collagen and GAG production of a chicken fibroblast cell line. Supernatants produced by skin from L200 fibrotic lesions stimulated fibroblast collagen and GAG production to a greater extent than supernatants generated from non-affected L200 skin or skin from normal control chickens. The enhanced fibroblast stimulatory activity produced by skin from fibrotic lesions was very likely produced by infiltrating MNC, because supernatants obtained from infiltrating MNC isolated from a skin lesion of an affected bird increased the synthesis of collagen and GAG by fibroblasts by approximately 100%. Moreover, lesion-derived MNC constitutively produced fibroblast-stimulatory activity after 24 to 72 hours of culture, indicating their prior *in vivo* activation. Interestingly, peripheral blood MNC from the same bird produced no fibroblast stimulatory activity, suggesting that only skin infiltrating MNC are activated *in vivo*.

Genetic Basis of Disease

The mode of inheritance of avian scleroderma has recently been investigated (36). Comb inflammation and lesions were used to determine the disease phenotype of 4-week-old chickens. All L200 males and 60% of L200 female chicks showed abnormalities. Crosses (F1) between L200 and eight partially inbred lines of chickens were all normal. Backcrosses of F1 cocks to L200 hens showed a higher incidence of cutaneous alterations in males than in females for all lines. It should be noted, however, that unlike mammals, female birds are heterozygotic for the sex chromosomes while male birds are homozygous for sex chromosomes. The incidence of affected birds varied among backcrosses from a low of 42% for backcross L217 males derived from a New Hampshire line, to a high of 88% for males of backcross L213 derived from a partially inbred Leghorn line, demonstrating the presence of genes that modify the penetrance of presumed major genes causing the disease. Backcross genotypes, segregating for haplotypes of the MHC derived from inbred lines, showed consistently lower penetrance of the scleroderma-like phenotype than homozygotes carrying the L200 haplotype (36).

Despite the remarkable similarities in immunologic and biochemical changes, there are important differences between the avian disease and human SSc. The onset of avian scleroderma is much more acute than human SSc and there is early mortality. Unlike the human disease where the female-to-male incidence ratio is 4:1, birds of either sex are equally affected. The vascular involvement in the avian disease is characterized both by proliferation of smooth muscle and subendothelial fibrosis, whereas in the human disease smooth muscle cell proliferation is not a prominent feature. Furthermore, as described in previous paragraphs, the nature of the autoantibodies detected is also different—anti-ssDNA antibodies, rheumatoid factor, and anti-type II collagen antibodies being more commonly present in the L200 chickens than in humans.

THE TIGHT SKIN (TSK) MOUSE

Another genetically based model of scleroderma is the tight skin mouse, a spontaneous dominant mutation that occurred in the inbred B10.D2 (58N)/Sn strain. Because a different mutation causing a tight skin phenotype has been recently described (see below), the original Tsk mutation will be referred here to as Tsk1. This mutation was identified at the Jackson Laboratories by Helen Bunker and reported in detail by Green et al (37). The most striking feature of heterozygous animals (Tsk1/ +) of this strain is the presence of thickened and tight skin that is firmly bound to the subcutaneous and deep muscular tissues. The Tsk1 mutation is lethal, and homozygous embryos degenerate *in utero* at 8 to 10 days of gestation. The Tsk1/+ mice display cutaneous and visceral changes that closely resemble those present in patients with SSc. Furthermore, the biochemical and molecular abnormalities that have been demonstrated in these animals (38,39) mimic the connective tissue alterations characteristic of SSc, particularly those related to the fibrotic stage of the disease.

Initial genetic studies mapped the Tsk1 mutation with respect to three visible mutations to mouse chromosome 2 (37). More recently, Siracusa et al (40) performed a more detailed analysis of the chromosomal location of the Tsk mutation, and were able to localize the Tsk gene to a 3.5 centiMorgan region closely linked to the β2 macroglobulin gene. More recent studies, however, showed that there was recombination between the β2 macroglobulin locus and the Tsk1 phenotype; these results localized the Tsk1 gene distal to the β2 macroglobulin gene (41).

Cutaneous Alterations

The tightness of the skin is readily detected at 7 days of age and is manifested by difficulty in gathering a fold of skin in the interscapular region (37–39). At 2 months of age, there is a hunched posture and prominent skin thickening with a pronounced hump in the interscapular region (Fig. 12.7). Studies by Menton and Hess (42) and Menton et al (43) confirmed the initial report of dermal thickening in Tsk1/ + mice, and demonstrated a decrease in pliability and an increase in stiffness of the skin. Electron microscopy (42) revealed changes in the connective tissue architecture of the dermis, including irregular spatial organization of collagen fibrils, which were of small diameter and were tightly packed. Furthermore, abundant deposition of fine microfibrillar material in the deep dermis was noted. Increased skin thickness was confirmed by Osborn et al (44) and Jimenez et al (38). Light microscopy studies of dorsal and tail skin from Tsk1/+ mice showed dermal thickening and replacement of adipose tissue by collagen deposits (Fig. 12.7). The thickened peritendinous fascia resulted in atrophy of tail and ankle tendons. Extensive replacement of the subcutaneous tissue by fibrosis was observed in the dorsal, lateral, and ventral thoracic regions, abdominal region, and in the fore and hind limbs. Prominent changes were also noted around the mammary glands, the brown fat of the scapular regions, and the ventral side of the sternum. Connective tissue surrounding the kidneys, adrenal glands, and pancreas was also affected (38,39).

Internal Organ Involvement

The most prominent visceral changes in Tsk1/+ mice occur in the lungs and heart. However,

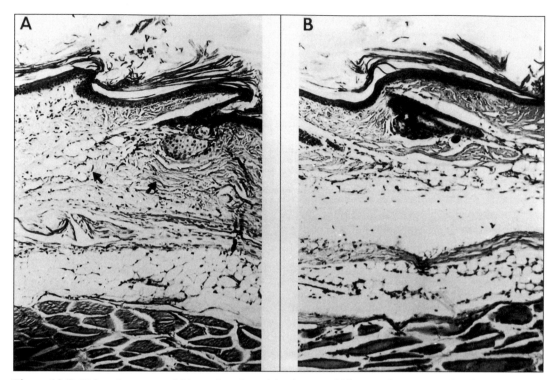

Figure 12.7. Light microscopy of skin sections from (*a*) Tsk1/+ and (*b*) normal mice stained with hematoxylin-eosin. Note the dermal thickening and the replacement of subcutaneous adipose tissue by homogeneously stained collagen (*arrows*) in the section from Tsk1/+ mouse skin (magnification × 100). (Reproduced with permission from Jimenez et al (38)).

vascular involvement has not been reported (37). The lung abnormalities are characterized by greatly distended lungs, which are present at birth. Histologically, the alterations in the lung resemble human emphysema, with little fibrosis. Szapiel et al (45) noted an accumulation of inflammatory cells in the interstitium and alveolar spaces. These alveolar spaces were markedly dilated with thin, disrupted walls and subpleural cysts and bullae. Rossi et al (46) found no evidence of infection in Tsk1/+ lungs, despite the presence of increased numbers of neutrophils in bronchoalveolar lavage fluids. The T and B cell levels were normal in the lungs of these mice. The cause of the pulmonary pathology is poorly understood and further studies will be necessary to clarify its pathogenesis and significance.

The cardiac enlargement reported by Green et al (37) was confirmed by Osborn and Bauer (47).

Myocardial hypertrophy in these mice is not caused by increased blood pressure nor valvular/arterial lesions. Osborn and Bauer (47) noted increased cardiac weight and electronmicroscopic evidence of moderately increased collagen deposits. No inflammatory cells were observed histologically. Osborn et al (48) carried out biochemical analysis of the collagen content of 1- and 12-month-old Tsk1/+ hearts compared to normal controls. They reported that type I collagen is markedly increased with a proportional decrease in types III and V collagen in Tsk1/+ myocardium.

Humoral Immune Abnormalities

Although MNC inflammatory infiltration of affected organs is not seen in the Tsk1/+ mouse, certain immunological abnormalities are present. ANAs, first observed by Osborn et al (personal communication), have been detected in approximately 50% of 8-month-old Tsk1/+ mice (49). Prior to this age, all animals tested were negative for ANA. These same serum samples were negative for anti-dsDNA antibody, as detected on *Crithidia luciliae*, and for SS-A/Ro, SS-B/La, Sm, RNP, and Scl-70 specificities when tested by immunodiffusion. However, antibodies that recognize the Scl-70 marker antigen (topoisomerase I) were demonstrated in supernatants from hybridomas established from Tsk1/+ mice splenocytes (49). These antibodies have been extensively characterized by Muryoi et al (50,51).

Cellular Immune Abnormalities

Several parameters of cellular immunity have been examined in Tsk1/+ mice (49). Responses to the T and B cell mitogens, concanavalin A, and lipopolysaccharide were found to be normal. The production of interleukin 2 was also found to be in the range of normal strains. However, a low autologous mixed lymphocyte response was observed, as is typical of autoimmune strains of mice (52) and of human SSc (53).

It has been suggested that mast cells may be important initiators of cutaneous fibrosis in SSc (54). Walker et al (55) examined this hypothesis in the Tsk1/+ model and found a two-fold increase in mast cell numbers compared to normal mouse skin up to 6 months of age. In these younger Tsk1/+ animals, the majority of mast cells were degranulated. By 15 months of age, the number of skin mast cells was comparable in the two groups and significantly reduced both in Tsk1/+ and normal controls compared to younger animals. These results suggest that mast cells may play an as yet undefined role in the progressive accumulation of connective tissue in the mutant. Similar increases in mast cells are seen in early stage human SSc, but these mast cell increases return to normal levels later (56). Walker et al (55) further studied the role of mast cells and fibrosis in Tsk1/+ mice by the administration of disodium cromoglycate, which inhibits mast cell degranulation, preventing mediator release. They observed that oral treatment of these mice significantly reduced both dermal mast cell degranulation and the width of the subcutaneous fibrous layer.

Abnormalities in Connective Tissue Metabolism

The histologic evidence suggesting an increase in collagen content and a possible alteration in its structure in the Tsk1/+ mouse has been confirmed by extensive biochemical studies (38,39, 57). The average total collagen content of skin from Tsk1/+ mice was 2.5-fold greater than that of control skin. Since there is evidence that shifts in collagen type are associated with certain pathological conditions, this possibility was examined in the Tsk1/+ mutant (Millan A and Jimenez SA, unpublished data). These studies failed to show qualitative differences in the collagens found in the skin of Tsk1/+ and normal mice. These results are similar to those reported in biochemical studies of affected skin from SSc patients showing increased collagen content but no alteration in the proportions of the various collagen types.

GAGs are the other major connective tissue component of skin. Ross et al (58,59) examined the GAG content of Tsk1/+ skin and found significant increases in total hexosamine and uronic acid for a given skin surface area, but not when expressed on a per milligram of wet weight basis. These findings are similar to the results of Rodnan et al (60) for SSc skin.

The role of collagen biosynthesis in the excessive accumulation of extracellular matrix in Tsk1/+ skin was further examined in an organ culture system (38). The results of these studies indicated that excessive biosynthesis was the primary mechanism of collagen accumulation in the Tsk/+ tissues. No qualitative differences in the products synthesized by Tsk/+ and normal skin organ cultures were found upon electrophoretic analysis (38,39). Studies by Uitto (61) and Jimenez et al (62) of collagen biosynthesis in organ cultures of SSc skin have shown similar findings.

Further *in vitro* studies of collagen biosynthesis and its regulation have been conducted with dermal fibroblast cultures established from

Tsk1/+ and normal littermate control mice (57). Collagen synthesis was examined by incorporation of ^{14}C-proline and production of ^{14}C-hydroxyproline by Tsk1/+ and control fibroblast cultures. Both parameters showed a greater than two-fold increase in the Tsk1/+ cultures. All of the increase was in the highly soluble fraction secreted into the culture medium. These findings are similar to results described in several studies of collagen and protein biosynthesis in cultures of SSc dermal fibroblasts (63–66). When the newly synthesized proteins from the Tsk/+ fibroblast and control cultures were analyzed by polyacrylamide slab-gel electrophoresis, quantitative but not qualitative differences were observed (57). This is similar to the findings of Uitto et al (67) with SSc and normal human fibroblasts. An increase in fibronectin synthesis is also seen in cultures of Tsk1/+ fibroblasts (63) similar to the increased fibronectin reported in SSc skin by Cooper et al (68).

At the molecular level, study of the expression of three collagen genes employing hybridizations with type-specific cDNAs for $\alpha 1(I)$, $\alpha 2(I)$, and $\alpha 1(III)$ procollagens showed a five-fold increase in steady-state mRNA levels for the corresponding transcripts in Tsk1/+ fibroblasts (57). In more recent studies, elevated type VI collagen mRNA levels were also found in cultured Tsk1/+ fibroblasts (69). These results are similar to the findings of a coordinate increase in types I and III procollagens and type VI collagen mRNAs in SSc fibroblasts (66,70).

The Molecular Defect in Tsk1/+ Mice

The observations that Tsk1/+ cells display an increased expression of multiple genes including those encoding for the $\alpha 1$ and $\alpha 2$ chains of type I procollagen, the $\alpha 1$ chain of type III procollagen, the three chains of type VI collagen, and the fibronectin gene, render it very unlikely that primary structural alterations in the regulatory regions of these multiple genes are responsible for their increased transcription in Tsk1/+ cells. If this were the case, it would have to be postulated that all the affected genes had undergone muta-

tions precisely in the same regulatory element that is responsible for their regulation under normal conditions. It is, therefore, more likely that the Tsk1 mutation affects a common regulatory mechanism that modulates the coordinate expression of several genes of the large family of extracellular matrix proteins. To evaluate this possibility, the cis acting elements responsible for increased transcription of the procollagen $\alpha 1(I)$ collagen gene in Tsk/+ fibroblasts were examined employing transient transfection of a series of human $\alpha 1(I)$ procollagen promoter—chloroamphenicol acetyl transferase (CAT) constructs into Tsk1/+ and normal fibroblast cultures (71). These transient transfection experiments allowed the mapping of the cis acting elements largely responsible for increased procollagen $\alpha 1(I)$ promoter activity in Tsk1/+ fibroblasts to sequences located between the initiation of transcription and -804 bp of the promoter. Subsequent studies examined DNA binding activity that recognized the mapped promoter region of the $\alpha 1(I)$ procollagen gene in nuclei from normal and Tsk1/+ cells (71). These studies indicated that abnormalities in regulatory DNA binding proteins may be responsible for the increased expression of collagen genes in Tsk1/+ cells. These results further suggest that the Tsk1 gene may be involved in the regulation of expression or activity of DNA-binding proteins that are capable of influencing the expression of genes encoding various collagens and other extracellular matrix proteins.

TSK/NZB MOUSE HYBRIDS

Despite the striking biochemical similarities to SSc, mice carrying the Tsk1 mutation do not develop the inflammatory and vascular changes nor the alterations in cellular immunity postulated to play a crucial role in SSc pathogenesis. Furthermore, the humoral immunologic dysregulation observed in Tsk1/+ mice occurs much later than the fibrotic process. An effort to breed a new murine model of SSc that might display more severe immunologic and inflammatory features, thus resembling more closely the human disease, was carried out by Bocchieri et al (72). The new murine model of SSc was developed by breeding the Tsk1/+ mice and the autoimmune disease-prone NZB mice to obtain an F1 hybrid displaying the connective tissue abnormalities of the Tsk1/+ parent and the autoimmune abnormalities of the NZB parent. The interscapular skin thickness in (Tsk1/NZB) F1 mice was significantly greater than in the (+/NZB) F1 littermates, and collagen biosynthesis in skin punch biopsies was more than 3.5 times greater in the (Tsk1/NZB) F1 mice than in controls. Hydroxyproline analyses confirmed that the increase in protein synthesis was primarily in collagen. These (Tsk1/NZB) F1 mice were tested for several cellular and humoral autoimmune manifestations. The results showed that autoantibodies, including ANAs, were present in their sera, and the proliferative response to autologous lymphocyte stimulation (AMLR) was decreased, as is commonly observed in murine and human autoimmune disorders. Thus, this new murine model for scleroderma combines and even exceeds the best features of the Tsk1 mutation. It displays several relevant immune system alterations comparable to the elements of autoimmunity reported in SSc. Additionally, the biochemical changes, including increased collagen synthesis, appear to be greater than the increased synthesis reported in Tsk1/+ mouse skin. Thus, the Tsk1/NZB mouse model more closely resembles the human disease condition than does its predecessor, the Tsk1/+ mouse. These results indicate that the (Tsk1/NZB) F1 mice may be of value for the study of the interactions between the immune system and connective tissue cells in the pathogenesis of SSc.

THE TSK2—A NOVEL MUTATION RESEMBLING SSC

A new mutation characterized by the occurrence of a tight skin phenotype in mice was first reported in 1986 (73). The mutation appeared in the offspring of a male from the 101/H mouse strain as a result of administration of the mutagenic agent, ethylnitrosourea. This novel mutation has been called Tsk2 and has been localized to mouse chromosome I (73). In similarity to the Tsk1 mutation, the Tsk2 mutation is inherited as an autosomal dominant trait and appears to be lethal *in utero*; therefore, only heterozygous Tsk2/+ animals survive. Preliminary studies to characterize the Tsk2/+ mice have shown that these animals indeed develop a "tight skin" phenotype, which becomes apparent at 3 to 4 weeks of age (74). Histologic examination of skin samples from affected animals showed marked thickening of the dermis and excessive deposition of thick collagen fibers extending into the subdermal adipose tissue (Fig. 12.8). In contrast to the histopathologic findings in Tsk1/+ mice, Tsk2/+ mice display the presence of a prominent infiltrate with mononuclear inflammatory cells in the lower dermis and in the adipose tissue septa (Fig. 12.9). Visceral fibrosis is not apparent at this age, although the adventitia of vessels in the lungs and heart appeared to be moderately increased in thickness and the lungs appeared slightly distorted with some dilatation and coalescence of alveolar spaces. No significant alterations in glycoproteins or GAGs were apparent in the sections stained with PAS and Alcian blue, respectively. Electronmicroscopic studies of Tsk2/+ skin showed that the collagen bundles appeared to be more abundant and more tightly packed than in skin from the normal control (Fig. 12.10). In biochemical studies, skin biopsies from four Tsk2 mice and matched controls were incubated with ^{14}C-proline. Incorporation of ^{14}C-proline into pepsin-resistant protein (largely representing collagen) was significantly higher in the Tsk2/+ mice than in the controls.

From these preliminary studies, it appears that the Tsk2 mutation mimics the Tsk1 mutation phenotypically, except that it is located on a different chromosome and must, therefore, involve a different gene. The occurrence of a novel and separate, chemically-induced mutation that results in the excessive accumulation of dermal collagen is of great relevance. This new

(*Text continues on p. 269.*)

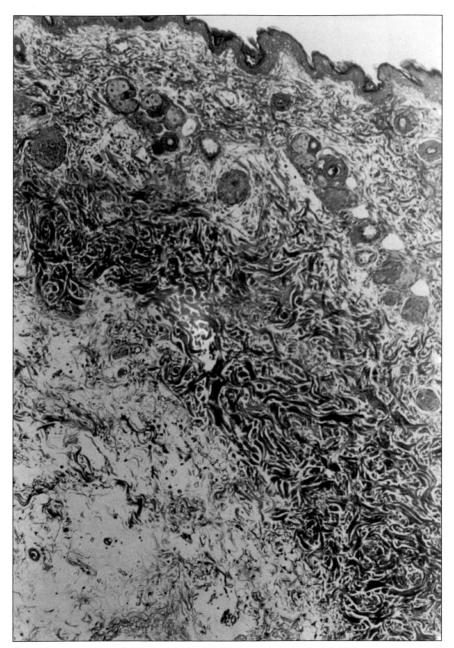

Figure 12.8. Light microscopy of skin section from a Tsk2 mouse stained with Masson trichrome. Note the dermal thickening and the infiltration of the subcutaneous adipose tissue by newly deposited connective tissue (magnification × 200).

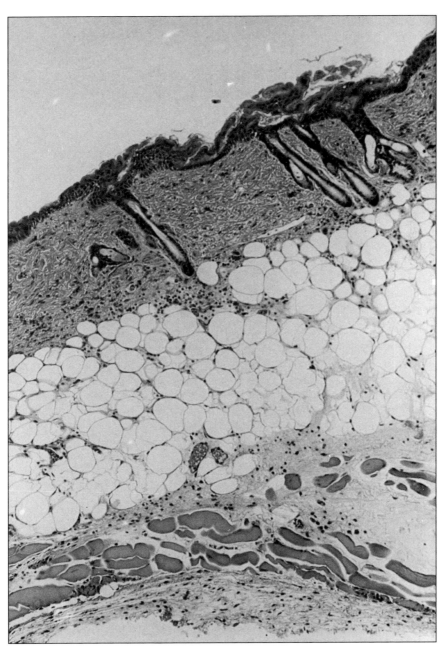

Figure 12.9. Light microscopy of skin section from a Tsk2 mouse stained with hematoxylin-eosin. Note the dermal thickening and the prominent presence of inflammatory cells in the lower dermis, adipose tissue septa, and in the tissue surrounding the panniculum carnosum below the adipose layer (magnification × 100).

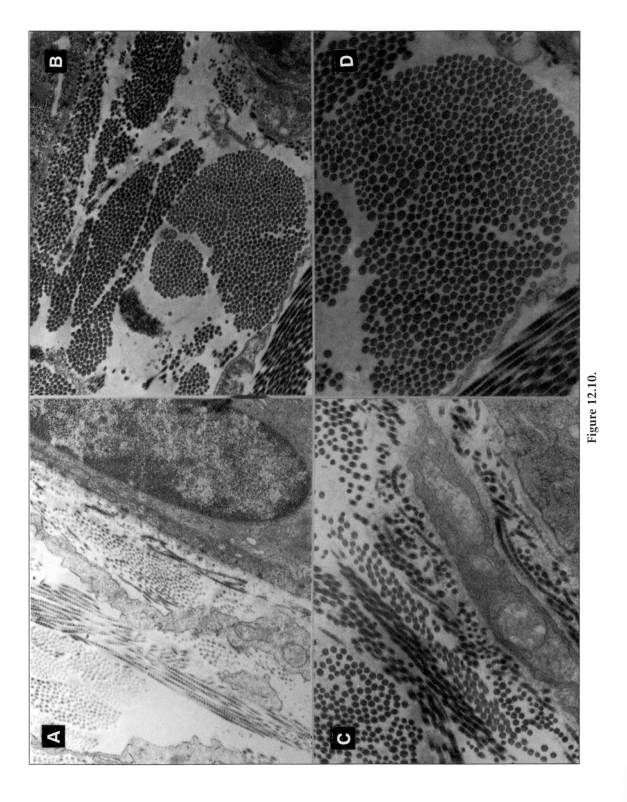

Figure 12.10.

268

mutation will allow the identification of a gene distinct from that affected by the Tsk1 mutation, which also controls the synthesis and accumulation of collagen in the mouse. The Tsk2 mutation that was originally caused by exposure to the toxic agent ethylnitrosourea is also particularly interesting, because of the recent realization that several human cutaneous fibrotic diseases resembling SSc appear to result from exposure to chemical substances, such as in the case of the Toxic Oil Syndrome and the L-tryptophan-induced Eosinophilia-Myalgia Syndrome. Studies to identify the mechanisms responsible for the connective tissue abnormalities in the Tsk2 mutation may, therefore, provide valuable information regarding the role of environmental exposures in the pathogenesis of SSc and other chemically-induced fibrotic diseases.

Summary

This review of the animal models for scleroderma described in the literature demonstrates that several induced and spontaneous systems are available in which to study various aspects of this complex disorder. Each model has its strengths in mimicking certain aspects of the disease—inflammatory, immunologic, or fibrotic—as well as important differences. It is apparent that each of these models can contribute to our knowledge of the mechanisms underlying this presently incurable disorder. The most extensively studied model from the histologic, immunologic, and biochemical viewpoint is the Tsk1 mutation. Its principal deficiencies are the absence of inflammatory, immunologic, vascular, gastrointestinal, and articular involvement, although more recent alterations in humoral immunity similar to those commonly observed in animal and human autoimmune diseases are present in these mice. Table 12.1 summarizes the available data on the most studied animal models of SSc, namely the UCD L200 chicken line, the Tsk1 mice, and the Tsk2 mice, in comparison to the features of human SSc. Further studies employing these models will undoubtedly extend our present knowledge and understanding of the cause and pathologic mechanisms of SSc. Furthermore, the existence of inherited animal models of SSc will allow the application of the techniques of genetics and molecular biology to address relevant questions related to the pathogenesis of SSc.

Table 12-1. Comparison of Animal Models and Human Scleroderma

Feature	UCD L200	TSK1/+	TSK2/+	HUMAN SSc
Clinical features				
Skin thickening	+	+	+	+
Visceral involvement				
Gastrointestinal	+	−	?	+
Vascular	+	−	?	+
Pulmonary	+	emphysema	?	fibrosis
Renal	−	?	?	+
Cardiac	+	+	?	+
Arthritis	+	−	−	+
Genetic transmission	+	+	+	rare

(*continued*)

Figure 12.10. Electron microscopic appearance of skin from normal mice (*a,c*) and Tsk2 mice (*b,d*). Note the abundance of tightly packed collagen fibers in samples from the Tsk2 mouse (magnification × 30,000 A,B: × 60,000 C,D). (Courtesy of Dr. Raul Fleishmajer).

Table 12.1—*continued*

Feature	UCD L200	TSK1/+	TSK2/+	HUMAN SSc
Immunological changes				
Mononuclear cell infiltrate	+(T cells)	−	+(? cells)	+(T cells)
Peripheral blood T cells	decreased	?	?	decreased
Mitogen proliferation	decreased	normal	?	decreased
IL-2 production	decreased	normal	?	increased
AMLR[a]	?	low	?	low
MLR[b]	?	normal	?	normal
ANA[c]	+	+	?	+
Sci-70	−	+	?	+
Anticentromere	−	−	?	+
anti-dsDNA	−	−	?	rare
Biochemical changes				
Increased tissue collagen	+	+	+	+
Collagen phenotype changes	−	−	−	−
Increased collagen biosynthesis	+	+	+	+
Increased post-translational enzymes	?	+	?	+
Collagenolytic activity	?	normal	?	normal
Abnormal collagen regulation	+	+	+	+
Increased procollagen gene expression	+	+	+	+
Increased procollagen gene transcription	?	+	?	+
Increased GAG[d]	+	+	?	+
Increased fibronectin	+	+	?	+

[a]AMLR: autologous mixed leukocyte reaction
[b]MLR: mixed leukocyte reaction.
[c]ANA: antinuclear antibodies.
[d]GAG: glycosaminoglycans.

References

1. Statsny P, Stembridge VA, Ziff M. Homologous disease in the adult rat, a model for autoimmune disease. J Exp Med 1963;118:635.
2. Statsny P, Ziff M. Immunologically induced experimental models of human connective tissue disease. Rheumatology 1967;1:198.
3. Jaffee BD, Claman HN. Chronic graft-versus-host disease (GVHD) as a model for scleroderma. I. Description of a model system. Cell Immunol 1983; 77:1.
4. Claman HN, Jaffee BD, Huff JC, Clark RAF. Chronic graft-versus-host disease as a model for scleroderma. II. Mast cell depletion with deposition of immunoglobulins in the skin and fibrosis. Cell Immunol 1985;94:73.
5. Gleichmann E, Gleichmann J. Pathogenesis of graft-versus-host reaction (GVHR) and GVH-like disease. J Invest Dermatol 1985;85(Suppl):115S.
6. Tateno M, Kondo N, Itoh T, Yoshiki T. Autoimmune and malignant lymphoma associated with host-versus-graft disease in mice. Clin Exp Immunol 1985;62:535.
7. Ichihashi H, Shinkai H, Takei M, Sano S. Analysis of the mechanism of bleomycin-induced cutaneous fibrosis in mice. J Antibiot (Tokyo) 1973;26: 238.
8. Adamson IYR, Bowden DH: The pathogenesis of bleomycin-induced pulmonary fibrosis in mice. Am J Pathol 1974;77:185.
9. Laurent GJ, McAnulty RJ, Corrin B, Cockerill P. Biochemical and histological changes in pulmonary fibrosis induced in rabbits with intratracheal bleomycin. Eur J Clin Invest 1981;11:441.
10. Kelley J, Newman RA, Evans JN. Bleomycin-induced pulmonary fibrosis in the rat. J Lab Clin Med 1980;96:954.
11. Clark JG, Overton JE, Marino BA, Uitto J, Starcher BC. Collagen biosynthesis in bleomycin-induced pulmonary fibrosis in hamsters. J Lab Clin Med 1980;96:943.
12. Collins IF, McCullough B, Coalson II, Johanson WG Jr. Bleomycin-induced diffuse interstitial pulmonary fibrosis in baboons. II. Further studies on connective tissue changes. Am Rev Respir Dis 1981;123:305.
13. Szapiel SV, Elson NA, Fulmer JD, Hunninghake

GW, Crystal RG. Bleomycin-induced interstitial pulmonary disease in the nude, athymic mouse. Am Rev Respir Dis 1979;120:893.

14. Clark JC, Starcher BC, Uitto J. Bleomycin-induced synthesis of type I procollagen by human lung and skin fibroblasts in culture. Biochim Biophys Acta 1980;631:359.

15. Mountz JD, Downs-Minor MB, Turner R, Thomas MB, Richards F, Pisko E. Bleomycin-induced cutaneous toxicity in the rat: Analysis of histopathology and ultrastructure compared with progressive systemic sclerosis (scleroderma). Br J Dermatol 1983;108:679.

16. Ishikawa H, Saito Y, Yamakage A, Kitabatake M. Scleroderma-inducing glycosaminoglycan in the urine of patients with systemic scleroderma. Dermatologica 1978;156:193.

17. Ishikawa H, Kitabatake M, Akiyama F. Biochemical characterization of scleroderma-inducing glycosaminoglycan. Acta Derm Venereol 1988;68:378.

18. Fox PK, White DD, Cavanagh M, Davies MG, Wusterman F. Failure to demonstrate fibrotic changes in the skin of mice injected with glycosaminoglycan fractions from the urine of scleroderma patients. Dermatologica 1982;164:80.

19. Yamakage A, Ishikawa H, Saito Y, Hattori A. Occupational scleroderma-like disorder occurring in men engaged in the polymerization of epoxy resins. Dermatologica 1980;161:44.

20. Black CM, Welsh KI, Walker AE, Bernstein RM, Catoggio LF, McGregor AR, Lloyd Jones JK. Genetic susceptibility to scleroderrna-like syndrome induced by vinyl chloride. Lancet 1983;11:53.

21. Yamakage A, Ishikawa H. Generalized morphea-like scleroderma occurring in people exposed to organic solvents. Dermatologica 1982;165:186.

22. Gershwin ME, Abplanalp HA, Castles Jl, Ikeda R, van der Water J, Eklund J, Haynes D. Characterization of a spontaneous disease of white leghorn chickens resembling progressive systemic sclerosis (scleroderma). J Exp Med 1981;153:1640.

23. van de Water J, Gershwin ME. Avian scleroderma: An inherited fibrotic disease of white leghorn chickens resembling progressive systemic sclerosis. Am J Pathol 1985;120:478.

24. van de Water J, Gershwin ME, Abplanalp H, Wick G, von der Mark K. Serial observations and definition of mononuclear cell infiltrates in avian scleroderma, an inherited disease of chickens. Arthritis Rheum 1984;27:807.

25. van de Water J, Haapanen L, Boyd R, Abplanalp H, Gershwin ME. Identification of T cells in early dermal lymphocytic infiltrates in avian scleroderma. Arthritis Rheum 1989;32:1031.

26. Gruschwitz MS, Moormann S, Kromer G, Sgonc R, Dietrich H, Boeck G, Gershwin ME, Boyd R, Wick G. Phenotypic analysis of skin infiltrates in comparison with peripheral blood lymphocytes, spleen cells and thymocytes in early avian scleroderma. J Autoimmun 1991;4:577–593.

27. Von Boehmer H, Kisielow P. Self-nonself discrimination by T cells. Science 1990;248:1369.

28. Lepesanti H, Reggio H, Pierres M, Nanquet P. Mouse thymic epithelial cells interact with and select a CD31owCD4+CD8+ thymocyte subset through an LFA-1-dependent adhesion-de-adhesion mechanism. Int Immunol 1990;2:1021.

29. Boyd RL, Hugo P. Towards an integrated view of thymopoiesis. Immunol Today 1991;12:71.

30. Blackman MA, Kappler JW, Marrack P. T cell specificity and repertoire. Immunol Rev 1988;101:5.

31. Wilson TJ, van de Water J, Mohr FC, Boyd RL, Ansari A, Wick G, Gershwin ME. Avian scleroderma: Evidence for qualitative and quantitative T cell defects. J Autoimmun 1992;5:261–276.

32. Boyd RL, Wilson TJ, van de Water J, Haapanen LA, Gershwin ME. Selective abnormalitites in the thymic microenvironment associated with avian scleroderma, an inherited fibrotic disease of L200 chickens. J Autoimmun 1991;4:369–380.

33. Boyd RL, Wilson TJ, Ward HA, Gershwin ME. Phenotypic characterization of chicken thymic stromal elements. Dev Immunol 1992;2:51.

34. Haynes DC, Gershwin ME. Diversity of autoantibodies in avian scleroderma: An inherited fibrotic disease of white leghorn chickens. J Clin Invest 1984;73:1557.

35. Duncan MR, Wilson TJ, van de Water J, Berman B, Boyd R, Wick G, Gershwin ME. Cultured fibroblasts in avian scleroderma, an autoimmune fibrotic disease, display an activated phenotype. J Autoimmun 1992;5:603–615.

36. Abplanalp H, Gershwin ME, Johnson E, Reed J. Genetic control of avian scleroderma. Immunogenetics 1990;31:291.

37. Green MC, Sweet HO, Bunker LE. Tight-skin, a new mutation of the mouse causing excessive growth of connective tissue and skeleton. Am J Pathol 1976;82:493.

38. Jimenez SA, Millan A, Bashey RI. Scleroderma-like alterations in collagen metabolism occurring in the TSK (tight skin) mouse. Arthritis Rheum 1984;27:180.

39. Jimenez SA, Bashey RI, Williams CJ, Millan AH. The tight skin (TSK) mouse as an experimental model of scleroderma. In: Greenwald RA, Diamond HS, eds. CRC handbook of animal models for rheumatic diseases. CRC Press, Inc. Boca Raton, FL, 1988:169–192.

40. Siracusa LD, Christner P, McGrath R Mowers SD, Nelson KK, Jimenez SA. The tight skin (TSK) mutation in the mouse, a model for human fibrotic diseases, is tightly linked to the β 2-microglobulin (B2m) gene on chromosome 2. Genomics 1993;17:748.

41. Everett ET, Pablos JL, Harns SE, LeRoy EC, Norris JS. The tight-skin (TSK) mutation is closely linked to β$_2$m on mouse chromosome 2. Mamm Genome 1944;5:55.

42. Menton DN, Hess RA. The ultrastructure of collagen in the dermis of tight-skin (TSK) mutant mice. J Invest Dermatol 1980;7:139.

43. Menton DN, Hess RA, Lichtenstein JR, Eisen AZ. The structure and tensile properties of the skin of tight-skin (TSK) mutant mice. J Invest Dermatol 1980;70:4.

44. Osborn TG, Bauer NE, Ross SC, Moore TL, Zuckner J. Tight-skin mouse: Physical and chemical properties of the skin. J Rheumatol 1983;10:793.

45. Szapiel SV, Fulmer JD, Hunninghake GW, Elson NA, Kawanami O, Ferrans VJ, Crystal RG. Hereditary emphysema in the tight-skin (TSK/+) mouse. Am Rev Respir Dis 1981;123:680.

46. Rossi GA, Hunninghake GW, Gadek JE, Szapiel SV, Kawanami O, Ferrans VJ, Crystal RG. Hereditary emphysema in the tight skin mouse. Am Rev Respir Dis 1984;129:850.

47. Osborn TG, Bauer NE. Physical and biochemical manifestations of cardiomyopathy in the tight-skin mouse. Arthritis Rheum 1984;27:S75A.

48. Osborn TG, Bashey RI, Moore TL, Fischer VW. Collagenous abnormalities in the heart of the tight-skinmouse. J Mol Cell Cardiol 1987;19:581.

49. Bocchieri MH, Henriksen PD, Kasturi KN, Muryoi T, Bona CA, Jimenez SA. Evidence for autoimmunity in the tight skin (TSK/+) mouse model of progressive systemic sclerosis. Arthritis Rheum 1991;34:599.

50. Muryoi T, Kasturi KN, Kafina MJ, Saitoh Y, Usuba O, Perlish JS, Fleischmajer R, et al. Self reactive repertoire of tight skin mouse: Immunochemical and molecular characterization of anti-topoisomerase I autoantibodies. Autoimmnun 1991;9:109.

51. Muryoi T, Andre-Schwartz J, Saitoh Y, Daian C, Hall B, Dimitriu-Bona A, Schwartz RS, et al. Self-reactive repertoire of tight skin (TSK/+) mouse: Immunochemical and molecular characterization of anti-cellular autoantibodies. Cell Immunol 1992;144:43.

52. Hom IT, Talal N. Decreased syngeneic mixed lymphocyte response (SMLR) in genetically susceptible autoimmune mice. Scand J Immunol 1982;15:195.

53. Morse JH, Budi BS. Autologous and allogeneic mixed lymphocyte reaction in progressive systemic sclerosis. Arthritis Rheum 1982;25:390.

54. Hawkins RA, Claman HN, Clark RAF, Steigerwald JC. Increased dermal mast cell population in progressive systemic sclerosis: A link in chronic fibrosis? Ann Intern Med 1985;102:182.

55. Walker M, Harley R, Maize J, DeLustro F, LeRoy EC. Mast cells and their degranulation in the TSK mouse model of scleroderma. Proc Soc Exp Biol Med 1985;180:323.

56. Pearson ME, Huff JC, Giorno RC, Panicheewa S, Claman HN, Steigerwald JC. Immunologic dysfunction in scleroderma: Evidence for increased mast cell releaseability and HLA-Dr positivity in the dermis. Arthritis Rheum 1988;31:672.

57. Jimenez SA, Williams CJ, Myers JC, Bashey RI. Increased collagen biosynthesis and increased expression of type I and type III procollagen gene in tight skin (TSK) mouse fibroblasts. J Biol Chem 1986;261:657.

58. Ross SC, Osborn TG, Dorner RW, Zucker J. Glycosaminoglycan content in skin of the tight-skin mouse. Arthritis Rheum 1983;26:653.

59. Dorner RW, Osborn TG, Ross SC. Glycosaminoglycan composition of tight skin and control mouse skins. J Rheumatol 1987;14:295.

60. Rodnan GP, Lipinski E, Luksick J. Skin thickness and collagen content in progressive systemic sclerosis and localized scleroderma. Arthritis Rheum 1979;22:130.

61. Uitto J. Collagen biosynthesis in human skin: A review with emphasis on scleroderma. Ann Clin Res 1971;3:250.

62. Jimenez SA, Yankowski R, Frontino PM. Biosynthetic heterogenetiy of sclerodermatous skin in organ cultures. J Mol Med 1977;2:423.

63. LeRoy EC. Increased collagen synthesis by scleroderma skin fibroblasts in vitro: A possible defect in the regulation or activation of the scleroderma fibroblasts. J Clin Invest 1074;54:880.

64. Buckingham RB, Prince PK, Rodnan GP, Taylor F. Increased collagen accumulation in dermal fibroblast cultures from patients with progressive systemic sclerosis (scleroderma). J Lab Clin Med 1978;92:5.

65. Jimenez SA, Bashey RI. Collagen synthesis by scleroderma fibroblasts in culture. Arthritis Rheum 1977;20:902.

66. Jimenez SA, Feldman G, Bashey RI, Bienkowski R, Rosenbloom J. Coordinate increase in the expression of type I and type III collagen genes in progressive systemic sclerosis fibroblasts. Biochem J 1986;237:837.

67. Uitto J, Bauer EA, Eisen AZ. Scleroderma: In-

creased biosynthesis of triple-helical type I and III procollagens associated with unaltered expression of collagenase by skin fibroblasts in culture. J Clin Invest 1979;64:921.

68. Cooper SM, Keyser J, Beaulieu AD, Ruoslahti E, Nimni ME, Quismorio FP Jr. Increase in fibronectin in the deep dermis of involved skin in progressive systemic sclerosis. Arthritis Rheum 1979;22:983.

69. Bashey RI, Philips N, Insigna F, Jimenez SA. Increased collagen synthesis and increased content of type VI collagen in myocardium of tight skin mice. Cardiovasc Res 1993:1061–1065.

70. Peltonen J, Kahari L, Uitto J, Jimenez SA. Increased expression of type VI collagen genes in progressive systemic sclerosis lesions *in situ*. Arthritis Rheum 1990;33:1829–1835.

71. Philips N, Bashey RI, Jimenez SA: Increased α1(I) procollagen gene expression in tight-skin (TSK) mice myocardial fibroblasts is due a reduced interaction of a negative regulatory sequence with AP-1 transcription factor. J Biol Chem 1995;270:9313.

72. Bocchieri MH, Christner PJ, Henricksen PD, Jimenez SA. Immunological characterization of (tight skin/NZB) F 1 hybrid mice with connective tissue and autoimmune features resembling human systemic sclerosis. J Autoimmun 1993;6:337.

73. Peters I, Ball ST. Tight skin-2 (TSK-2). Mouse News Lett 1986;74:91.

74. Christner PJ, Peters J, Hawkins D, Siracusa LD, Jimenez SA: The tight skin 2 (*Tsk2*) mouse: An animal model of scleroderma displaying cutaneous fibrosis and mononuclear cell infiltration. In Press, Arthritis Rheum 1995.

DANIEL E. FURST
PHILIP J. CLEMENTS

13

Pathogenesis, Fusion (Summary)

SCLERODERMA, or systemic sclerosis (SSc), is a multi-dimensional disease whose treatment is thus far unsuccessful, partly because its etiology and pathogenesis are unknown. While there are fibrosis-based, vascular-based, and immune-based hypotheses for the pathogenesis of systemic sclerosis, it has been difficult putting forward a unifying hypothesis. This review suggests the outlines of such a unitary hypothesis, realizing that it will need to be expanded and changed as more data become available.

The hypothesis (Fig. 13.1, Pathways I–X) postulates a genetic predisposition and an environmental stimulus, which result in immune activation and vascular injury. Immune activation induces immune-mediator release, vascular injury, fibroblast proliferation, collagen synthesis and deposition, and end-organ damage. Collagen, *per se*, incites further immune activation, thus closing the circle (Fig. 13.1, Pathway X). Mast cell activity feeds into that circle through the effects of serotonin and transforming growth factor-beta (TGF-β) on the vascular system, resulting in secondary vascular injury and fibroblast proliferation. Additionally, vascular injury induces Raynaud's phenomenon (RP), which itself results in further vascular damage.

Genetic Predisposition (Pathway I)

Genetic predisposition is supported by HLA data, familial data, and genetically predisposed animal models. There is an increase in HLA-DR8, HLA-DR11, and HLA-DR5 in some Caucasian SSc populations (1–3). There is also a significant increase in HLA-DR B1502 and HLA-DR B5-0102 or HLA-DR B1-0802 in Japanese SSc patients (4). Interestingly, a particular seven-amino acid sequence is shared among the DR11, DR5-0102, and DRB1-0802 patients. There is also some evidence derived from familial studies. For example, more than one family has been reported in which more than one member has had SSc (e.g., one family in which 6 of 45 members had connective tissue disease, two of whom had SSc (5); one family had identical twins, both of whom had SSc (6).

Genetically based animal models of SSc are described in detail by Jimenez and Gershwin in Chapter 12. The University of California at Davis (UCD) line 200 (L200) chicken develops a disease similar in many respects to human systemic sclerosis (7). These animals develop progressive inflammation and fibrosis of the esophagus, small intestine, lungs, heart, kidneys, skin, comb, and testicles. Furthermore, they manifest T cell infiltrates and develop rheumatoid factor and a number of antinuclear and anticytoplasmic antibodies (8). The incidence of disease among various back crosses using several chicken species was 42% to 88%, demonstrating that a number of genes modified the penetrance of the assumed causative genes (9). Despite the similarities, this model is not an exact copy of the human one, as it is more acute, and the vascular involvement

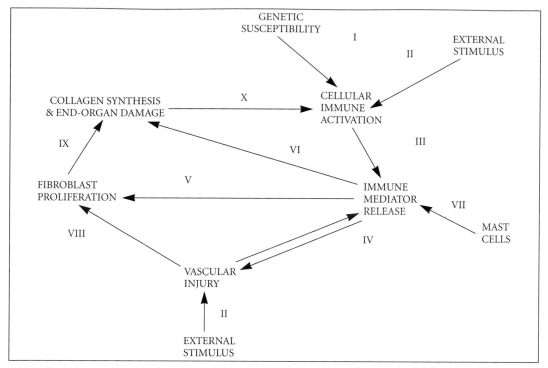

Figure 13.1. The proposed hypothesis for pathogenesis of systemic sclerosis is diagrammed. Each of the pathways (I–X) is explained in the text.

and autoantibodies are somewhat different than human SSc.

Another inherited scleroderma model is that of the tight skin mouse (Tsk-1) (10). Only the TSK1 heterozygote survives, and it manifests skin changes similar in many ways to SSc (10,11). On the other hand, the internal organ involvement appears somewhat different: lung changes are primarily emphysematous, with little fibrosis, while cardiac involvement includes increased collagen deposits (12). Antinuclear antibodies (ANAs) occur in approximately 50% of the animals, and some cross reactivity with topoisomerase I has been demonstrated (13).

A genetic pre-disposition, then, can be adduced from the evidence cited in the previous paragraphs, although it is probably multi-genetic and somewhat indirect.

Environmental Effects (Pathway II)

Over the last 75 years, several illnesses were reported that were apparently related to environmental materials and were similar to systemic sclerosis. Because these are reviewed in detail by Sternberg and Silver (Chapters 10 and 5), we will merely summarize some of the data here. Among the environmental factors associated with systemic sclerosis are silica and silicone, "toxic oil," and L-tryptophan.

An association between silica, silicosis, and scleroderma has been documented several times. German investigators estimated an odds ratio of 25 in coal miners (virtually all male) exposed to silica and 110 in miners with pulmonary silicosis (14). A possible association of augmentation mammoplasty (with silicone containing material) with scleroderma has been reported, although several recent large, case-controlled epidemiologic studies do not appear to support such an association (15).

Toxic oil syndrome (TOS) represents a foodborne disease with SSc-like features (16). Patients with this syndrome were part of an epidemic that affected approximately 20,000 individuals. The probable contaminants in this case were never completely identified but are thought to be aniline and anilide contaminants (17). During the chronic phase of this illness, scleroderma-like skin changes occurred in 22% of the patients and pulmonary hypertension occurred in 10% Some non-SSc-like involvement also occurred, including peripheral neuropathy and hepatomegaly (18).

Another environmentally-induced scleroderma-like illness is the eosinophilia-myalgia syndrome (EMS). This syndrome is in many ways similar to eosinophilic fasciitis and toxic oil syndrome (19,20). The putative agents for the syndrome appear to have resulted from a change in the manufacturing process of L-tryptophan (21).

Yet another example is the association of scleroderma-like skin changes with exposure to vinyl chloride and organic solvents (22). In these cases, the effects were principally to the skin and bones, although RP and abnormal serologies were also found. Evidence of toxic exposure, such as liver function abnormalities and bone marrow effects not typical of naturally occurring scleroderma, also occurred occasionally.

As with other rheumatic diseases, there is the possibility that systemic sclerosis may be triggered by viruses. Antitopoisomerase-I antibodies (Scl-70 antibodies), which are relatively specific for the diffuse form of systemic sclerosis, share a six-amino acid sequence with the P30[gag] protein of several retroviruses, including the simian sarcoma virus, the feline sarcoma virus, and the Maloney murine leukemia virus (23).

Another external stimulus that could initiate systemic sclerosis, according to our hypothesis, is

vascular injury, particularly associated with RP. LeRoy et al (Chapter 8) carefully review the evidence that vascular injury may induce systemic sclerosis. It is possible that early vascular injury aggravates or initiates RP. RP occurs in 90% to 95% of patients with systemic sclerosis (24). It may occur not only in the hands, feet, ears, nose, and other relatively cool extremities, but it has also been shown to occur in the kidneys, heart, and lungs (25–27). Thus RP seems to occur in several of the major end-organs which, like the skin and the fingers, can be damaged in SSc. Further, vascular abnormalities are clearly demonstrable by capillaroscopy even early in SSc (28). Whether the vascular injury precedes or follows RP is not clearly determined. In either event, RP may lead to further vascular injury by decreasing blood flow. Recurrent RP associated with SSc is characterized pathologically by concentric, intimal proliferation and adventitial fibrosis with consequent vascular narrowing and the clear potential for hypoxia and injury of the endothelial cells (29). This endothelial damage can result in release of endothelial adhesion molecules, intracellular adhesion molecules, TGF-β, IL-2, IL-6, and secondary products of platelet activation, all of which can induce the fibrosis so characteristic of systemic sclerosis (see Chapter 8). Damaged endothelial cells themselves can induce release of immune mediators capable of inducing collagen synthesis (30).

There is, therefore, ample support that environmental stimuli are associated with, and may trigger, SSc.

Cellular Immune Activation (Pathway III)

Our hypothesis posits that a combination of genetic background plus environmental stimuli activate the cellular immune system. The cellular immune aspects of scleroderma are fully reviewed by Varga and Jimenez (Chapter 7) and White (Chapter 11) and will only be outlined here. Monocyte/macrophages, T-helper lymphocytes, and other lymphoid cells are found in activated forms in the circulation and tissues of patients with systemic sclerosis (31,32). White (Chapter 11) reviews the evidence that T cells are activated within the tissues of SSc patients. Prescott et al observed very early migration of T cells (both CD4+ and CD8+ T cells, with a preponderance of CD4+ cells) into the skin of systemic sclerosis patients (33). Analysis of bronchoalveolar lavage (BAL) in SSc with alveolitis showed a contrasting increase in CD8+ with a reduced CD4+ prevalence, indicating that distinct T cell subpopulations may affect different organs in this disease (34).

There is also evidence of circulating T cell activation in SSc. HLA-DR molecule expression, IL-2 receptors, and soluble CD4 levels are increased in some but not all SSc patients (35–38), and serum adenine deaminase levels (another marker for T cell activation) are elevated in SSc patients (39).

Autoantibodies, as evidence of immune activation, are abundant in SSc. Antinuclear antibody, rheumatoid factor, and anti-single stranded DNA antibodies are found commonly (40). In addition, antitopoisomerase-1 (Scl-70), anti-RNA polymerase III, and anticentromere antibodies are relatively specific for SSc (41,42). Finally, IL-2, IL-4, and IL-6, and TNF-alpha levels are increased in systemic sclerosis sera (43).

Two examples of autoantibodies of potential importance are anti-centromere antibodies and antitopoisomerase antibodies. Anticentromere antibodies recognize centromeric proteins, which may down-regulate transcription, potentially altering later DNA-regulated events (44). Topoisomerase I ultimately relaxes super-coiled DNA and is necessary for RNA transcript production (45). Both auto-antibodies represent immune mediator release with potentially profound effects on later immune function through DNA regulation.

As was the case for genetic predisposition and environmental triggers, there are *some,* although not overwhelming, data supporting cellular immune activation in SSc.

IV–VI. Immune Mediator Release Resulting In: Vascular Injury (Pathway IV), Fibroblast Proliferation (Pathway V), and Collagen Synthesis (Pathway VI)

To remain within the logic of the present hypothesis (Fig. 13.1), one should identify cellular immune mediators that are released and which, in turn, affect either vascular integrity or cause increased fibrosis. Once again, Varga et al, White, and LeRoy et al (Chapters 7, 11, and 8, respectively) describe many aspects of immune mediator release in systemic sclerosis and how these mediators facilitate "communication" among vascular, immune, and fibroblastic cells.

VASCULAR DISEASE (PATHWAY IV)

In 1979, Kahaleh et al found that SSc sera kill human umbilical vein endothelial cells (46). Other authors confirmed this cytotoxicity *in vivo* in 40% of SSc patients (47). In addition, Evans et al demonstrated the deposition of IgM in the media and internal elastic lamina of small muscular arteries of SSc patients, suggesting that the vasculopathy found in SSc might be mediated by complement-fixing antibodies (48). The specific antigen responsible for this reactivity is unknown, although the viruses mentioned above have been suggested as possible etiologic agents.

While the mediator(s) of endothelial injury in SSc is/are not known, elevated levels of IL-1 and TNF have been found (43). As noted by LeRoy et al in Chapter 8, peripheral blood monocytes from SSc patients produce increased amounts of IL-1-beta, and IL-1 has been associated with pulmonary endothelial injury (37). Both TNF and IL-1 react with the endothelium through expression of endothelial cell adhesion molecule-1

(ECAM-1) and intercellular adhesion molecule-1 (ICAM-1) (49). These, in turn, can lead to adhesion of lymphocytes to endothelium and endothelial damage.

It is therefore easy to see that mediators released by lymphocytes can result in endothelial damage. The presence of such endothelial damage in SSc is documented by the increased serum levels of von Willebrand factor antigen found in SSc (50). Furthermore, in SSc, angiogenesis may be impaired, which could result in vascular abnormalities such as the capillaroscopic changes typically seen in SSc (see Chapters 17 and 8). Platelets are activated in SSc, as shown by increased levels of beta-thromboglobulin, platelet factor IV, and platelet circulating aggregates (51,52). Finally, coagulation and fibrinolysis are abnormal in SSc, as evidenced by increased plasminogen activator and variably decreased fibrinolytic activity (53–55).

FIBROBLAST PROLIFERATION (PATHWAY V)

Early studies showed that there was heterogeneity among fibroblast clones in SSc, and even in normals (56). For example, collagen production among six fibroblast clones varied by 17-fold in one study (57). SSc serum stimulated fibroblasts to proliferate: compared to normal serum, autologous or heterologous SSc serum increased fibroblast numbers by a factor of four to five (58).

Furthermore, IL-4, a protein produced by T cells and mast cells, is present in increased concentrations (as measured by IL-4 mRNA) in SSc blood and alveolar lavage fluid (59). Its potential importance lies in the fact that IL-4 promotes fibroblast proliferation and extracellular matrix production.

COLLAGEN SYNTHESIS (PATHWAY VI)

According to this hypothesis, mediator release, as well as vascular damage, can result in increased fibrosis. As will be noted, there is controversy surrounding the levels and activity of many of these cytokines in SSc. In this chapter, only selected cytokines (TGF-β, IFN-γ, IL-4) will be discussed as examples supporting the hypothesis of the pathogenesis of systemic sclerosis. The effects of TGF-β exemplify an instance of increased collagen production without, necessarily, fibroblast proliferation, while those of IL-4 demonstrate an example in which fibroblast proliferation occurs before increased collagen production.

Transforming growth factor-beta (TGF-β) increases fibrosis by several mechanisms. It stimulates extracellular matrix components, inhibits matrix degrading metalloproteineases, and *in vivo,* produces fibrosis in mice (60–62). Specifically, TGF-β increases collagen mRNA levels and can induce IL-6 production (63,64). TGF-β's role in SSc is supported by the finding that there is a tenfold increase in TGF-β mRNA levels in the alveolar lavage cells from SSc patients with lung involvement (65). *In vitro* patients with diffuse or limited SSc express increased amounts of TGF-β (66,67). Interestingly, TGF-β mRNA is detected in the cells infiltrating the dermis of patients with SSc in conjunction with fibroblasts expressing increased collagen mRNA (66–69). Despite some concern that some or all of these findings may be epiphenomena (70), it may well be that TGF-β, released from infiltrating mononuclear cells in early SSc as well as by skin fibroblasts, may be important in the production of fibrosis in this disease.

Interferon-gamma (IFN-γ) is another cytokine that may have a role in SSc. It counteracts the effects of TGF-β on collagen production and is a potent inhibitor of collagen production by T cells as well (72,72). Secretion of IFN-γ by peripheral blood mononuclear cells from SSc is lower than controls (73). Also, open studies of IFN-γ in SSc indicate some possible improvement in skin fibrosis (74).

There is ample evidence, then, that mediator release from immunologically activated cells can result in vascular damage, fibroblast proliferation, and increased collagen production.

Vascular Injury Induces: Immune Mediator Release (Pathway IV) and Fibroblast Proliferation (Pathway VIII)

The hypothesis, and existing data, requires some redundancy in the model, as vascular injury can induce immune mediator release, which secondarily results in fibroblast proliferation and increased collagen synthesis. Vascular injury can also result in fibroblast chemotaxis and fibroblast proliferation.

While data in scleroderma are sparse, there is support for the above position in other fibrotic models, such as the bleomycin-induced model for fibrosis. *In vitro* experiments, wherein supernatants from endothelial cells collected after exposure to bleomycin resulted in stimulation of collagen synthesis in control fibroblasts. The stimulation, it was found, was caused by TGF-β, an inducer of collagen synthesis (30).

Also, endothelial cell damage by activating platelets, can result in the release of substances that cause fibroblast proliferation. It has been found, for example, that the capillary endothelium in scleroderma tissue stains intensely for antibodies to platelet-derived growth factor (PDGF), thus evidencing an environment conducive to the release of platelet-derived factors causing fibroblast growth (66). In addition, *in situ* hybridization studies showed that fibroblasts in close proximity to blood vessels in early scleroderma indicated increased concentrations of collagen mRNA (67). Thus, endothelial damage activates platelets, which then release growth factors causing fibroblast chemotaxis and/or proliferation, as well as activation. This and other evidence amassed by Kahaleh in an article describing the role of the vascular endothelium in fibroblast activation and fibrosis (68), support the role of vascular injury in promoting fibroblast proliferation and collagen synthesis.

Mast Cells (Pathway VII)

The role of mast cells in systemic sclerosis has not been well established. Nevertheless, there is evidence supporting the possibility that they may be involved in fibrosis. For example, mast cell infiltration is often seen in SSc tissues (75). Furthermore, cutaneous fibrosis is often found in conditions characterized by eosinophilia, such as eosinophilic fasciitis and the eosinophilia myalgia syndrome, and evidence of eosinophil activation (elevated eosinophil granule proteins) is found in the skin of some SSc patients (76,77).

Interestingly, activated eosinophils secrete TGF-β and IL-4, which promote fibrosis, as outlined above (76–78). Furthermore, major basic protein, produced by eosinophils, induces platelet degranulation and, therefore, indirectly results in the release of cytokines, which may secondarily induce fibrosis (79).

Thus, while evidence is relatively sparse and somewhat indirect, eosinophils and mast cells may play a role in the pathogenesis of systemic sclerosis, feeding into the proposed hypothesis by secondarily inducing fibroblasts to produce collagen (see Fig. 13.1).

Increased Collagen Synthesis (Pathway IX)

Mediators capable of promoting collagen production have been described in previous paragraphs. Their presence implies either activation of fibroblasts, proliferation of fibroblasts, or both. Interleukin-1, which is produced by macrophages, may promote both fibroblast proliferation and fibrosis, perhaps through production of PDGF as well as of IL-1 (80). Additionally, TGF-β already discussed as an important mediator in the pathogenesis of SSc, has been shown to be capable of stimulating fibroblast collagen production (81).

T-Cell Activation by Collagen (Pathway X)

To complete the cycle resulting in SSc, one must postulate that collagen itself can result in immune activation. Otherwise, upon abrogation of the external stimuli, the disease can/will subside.

The evidence supporting this last step in the immune hypothesis is, today, relatively weak. Nevertheless, it has been shown that SSc lymphocytes respond to extracts of SSc skin collagen by migration inhibition, indicating a possible immune response to collagen. Furthermore, type I and type IV collagen, as well as purified collagen, activate T cells from SSc (82–84). Finally, SSc fibroblasts express ICAM-1, thus increasing their binding of T cells (85). Consequently, collagen and fibroblasts can induce immune activation, thus "closing the circle" and setting off a self-perpetuating cycle, which could explain the pathogenesis of SSc.

Significance of the Hypothesis

While our hypothesis has evidence supporting its existence, much work needs to be done to further define the existence (or need for change) of this construct. It is not likely that this is a final, complete, and unalterable pathogenetic conception; rather, its importance lies in the model it provides for potential treatment and for testing and learning more about the pathogenesis of systemic sclerosis.

References

1. Dunckley H, Jazwoinska EC, Gatenby PA, Serjentson W. DNA-DR typing shows HLA-DRwll RFLPs are increased in frequency in PSS and CREST variants in scleroderma. Tissue Antigens 1989;33:418–420.
2. Livingstone JZ, Scott TE, Wigley FM, Anhalt GJ, Bias WB, McLean RH, Hochberg MC. Systemic sclerosis (scleroderma), clinical, gentic, and serologic subsets. J Rheumatol 1987;14:512–518.
3. Gladman DD, Keystone EC, Baron M, Lee P, Cone D, Merrert H. Increased frequency of HLA-DR5 in scleroderma. Arthritis Rheum 1981;24:854–857.
4. Takeuchi F, Nakono K, Yamada H, Hong GH, Nabeta H, Yoshida A, Matsuta K, et al. Association of HLA-DR with PSS in Japanese. J. Rheumatol 1994; 21:857–863.
5. McGregor AR, Watson, A, Yunis E, Pandey JP, Takehara K, Tidwell JT, Ruggieri A, et al. Familial clustering of scleroderma spectrum disease. Am J Med 1988;84:1023–1032.
6. Cook NJ, Silman AJ, Propert J, Cawley MID. Features of systemic sclerosis (scleroderma) in an identical twin pain. Br J Rheumatol 1993;32:926–928.
7. Gershwin ME, Abplanalp HA, Castes JJ, Ikeda RM, Van der Water J, Eklund J, Haynes D. Characterization of a spontaneous disease of white leghorn chickens resembling progressive systemic scloersis (scleroderma). J Exp Med 1981;153:1640–1659.
8. Van de Water J, Gershwin ME. Avian scleroderma: An inherited fibrotic disease of white leghorn chickens resembling PSS. Am J Pathol 1985;120: 478–482.
9. Abplanalp H, Gershwin ME, Johnson E, Reed J. Genetic control of avian scleroderma. Immunogenetics 1990;31:291–296.
10. Green MC, Sweet HO, Bunker LE. Tight-skin, a new mutation of the mouse causing excessive growth of connective tissue and skeleton. Am J Pathol 1976;82:493–512.
11. Jimenez SA, Bashey RI, Williams CJ, Millan AH. The tight skin (TSK) mouse as an experimental model of scleroderma. In: Greenwald RA, Diamonds HS, eds. CRC handbook of animal models for rheumatic diseases. Boca Raton, CRC Press 1988;169–192.
12. Osborn TG, Bauer NE. Physical and biochemical manifestations of cardiomyopathy in the tight-skin mouse. Arthritis Rheum 1984;27:S75A.
13. Bocchieri MH, Henrikson PD, Kasturi KN, Muryvo T, Bona CA, Jimenez SA. Evidence for autoimmunity in the tight skin (TSK/+) mouse model of PSS. Arthritis Rheum 1991;34:559–565.
14. Haustein UF, Ziegler V. Environmentally induced systemic sclerosis-like disorders. Int J Dermatol 1985;24:147–151.
15. Wigley FM, Miller R, Hochberg MC, et al. Augmentation mammoplasty in patients with systemic sclerosis. Arthritis Rheum 1992;35:S46.

16. Toxic Epidemic Syndrome Study Group. Toxic epidemic syndrome, Spain, 1981. Lancet 1982;2:697–701.

17. Kilbourne EM, Bernert JR Jr, Posada de la Paz M, Hill RH, Abaitua-Borda I, Kilbourne BW, Zack MM. Chemical correlates of pathogenicity of oils related to the toxic oil syndrome in Spain. Am J Epidemiol 1988;127:1210–1227.

18. Abaitua Borda I, Posada de la Paz M. Current knowledge and future perspectives. WHO regional publications, European series #42. 1992;39–66.

19. Varga J, Griffin R, Newman JH, Jimenez SA. Eosinophilic fasciitis is clinically distinguishable from eosinophilia-myalgia syndrome and is not associated with L-tryptophan use. J Rheumatol 1991;18:259–263.

20. Hertzman PA, Borda IA. The toxic oil syndrome and the eosinophilia-myalgia syndrome: Pursuing clinical parallels. J Rheumatol 1993;20:1707–1710.

21. Belongia EA, Hedberg CW, Gleich GJ, White KE, Mayeno AN, Loegering DA, Dunnette Sl, et al. An investigation of the cause of the eosinophilia-myalgia syndrome associated with tryptophan use. N Engl J Med 1990;323:357–365.

22. Straniero NR, Furst DE. Environmentally-induced systemic sclerosis-like illness. Bailliere's Clin Rheumatol 1989;3:63–79.

23. Maul C, Jimenez S, Riggs E, Ziemnicka-Kotula D. Determination of an epitope of the diffuse systemic sclerosis marker DNA topoisomerase I. Proc Natl Acad Sci USA 1989;86:8492–8496.

24. Young EA, Steen VD, Medsger TA. Systemic sclerosis without Raynaud's phenomenon. Arthritis Rheum 1986;29(Suppl 4):S51.

25. Cannon PJ, Hassar M, Case OB, et al. The relationship of hypertension and renal failure in scleroderma to structural and functional abnormalities of the renal cortical circulation. Medicine 1974;53:1–46.

26. Furst DE, David JA, Clements PJ, Chopra SK, Theofilopoulos AN, Chia D. Abnormalities of pulmonary vascular dynamics and inflammation in early PSS. Arthritis Rheum 1981;24:1403–1408.

27. Alexander EL, Firestein GS, Weiss JL, Heuser RR, Leitl G. Wagner HN Jr, Brinker AJ, et al. Reversible cold-induced abnormalities in myocardial perfusion and function in systemic sclerosis. Ann Intern Med 1986;105:661–665.

28. Maricq HR, LeRoy EC, D'Angelo WA, Medsger Jr TA, Rodnan GP, Sharp GC. Diagnostic potential of *in vivo* capillary microscopy in scleroderma and related disorders. Arthritis Rheum 1980;23:183–189.

29. Rodnan GP, Myerowitz RL, Justh GO. Morphologic changes in the digital arteries of patients with

30. Phan SH, Gharee-Kermani M, Wolber F, Ryan US. Bleomycin stimulates production of TGF-beta by rat pulmonary artery endothelial cells. Chest 1991;99(Suppl 3):66S.

31. Roumm AD, Whiteside T, Medsger T, Jr. Lymphocytes in the skin of patients with progressive systemic sclerosis. Arthritis Rheum 1984;27:645–653.

32. Ferrarini M, Steen V, Medsger T Jr, Whiteside TL. Functional and phenotypic analysis of T-lymphocytes cloned from the skin of patients with systemic sclerosis. Clin Exp Immunol 1990;79:346–352.

33. Prescott RJ, Freemont PW, Jones CJ. Sequential dermal microvascular and perivascular changes in the development of scleroderma. J Pathol 1992;166:255–263.

34. White B, Wigley FM, Wise R, et al. Increased expression of CD8 and VG1 + γ/β T-cells in the lungs of systemic sclerosis patients. (submitted).

35. Fiocca U, Rosada M, Cozzi L, Ortolani C, DeSilv G, Estro G, Ruffatti A, et al. Early phenotypic activation of circulating helper memory T cells in scleroderma: Correlation with disease activity. Ann Rheum Dis 1993;52:272–277.

36. Clements P, Peter J, Agopian M, Telian NS, Furst DE. Elevated serum levels of soluble interleukin-2 receptor, interleukin-2 and neopterin in diffuse and limited scleroderma: Effect of chlorambucil. J Rheumatol 1990;17:908–910.

37. Kahaleh MB. Soluble immunologic products in scleroderma sera. Clin Immunol Immunopathol 1991;58:139–144.

38. Umehara H, Kumagai S, Ishida H, Suginoshita T, Maeda M, Imura H. Enhanced production of interleukin-2 in patients with progressive systemic sclerosis. Hyperactivity of CD-4 positive cells? Arthritis Rheum 1988;31:401–407.

39. Sasaki T, Nakajima H. Serum adenosine deaminase activity in systemic sclerosis (scleroderma) and related disorders. J Am Acad Dermatol 1992;27:411–414.

40. Furst DE, Clements PJ, Graze P, Gale R, Roberts N. A syndrome resembling PSS after bone marrow transplant. Arthritis Rheum 1979;22:904–911.

41. Tan EM, Rodnan GP, Garcia I, Moroi Y, Fritzler MJ, Peebles C. Diversity of antinuclear antibodies in PSS. Arthritis Rheum 1980;23:617–625.

42. Douvas AS, Achten M, Tan EM. Identification of a nuclear protein (Scl-70) as a unique target of human antinuclear antibodies in scleroderma. J Biol Chem 1979;254;3608–3616.

PSS (scleroderma) and Raynaud's phenomenon. Medicine 1980;59:393–408.

43. Needleman B, Wigley F, Stair R. Interleukin-1, interleukin-2, interleukin-4, interleukin-6, tumor necrosis factor alpha and interferon-gamma levels in sera from patients with scleroderma. Arthritis Rheum 1992;35:67–72.

44. Saunders WS, Chue C, Goebl M, Craig C, Clark RF, Powers JA, Eissenberg JC, et al. Molecular cloning of a human homologue of Drosophila heterochromatin protein HP1 using anti-centromere autoantibodies of antichromo specificity. J Cell Sci 1993; 104:573–582.

45. Wang JC. DNA topoisomerases. Ann Rev Biochem 1985;54:665–672.

46. Kahaleh MB, Sherer GK, LeRoy EC. Endothelial injury in scleroderma. J Exp Med 1979;149:1326–1335.

47. Cohen S, Johnson AR, Hurd E. Cytotoxicity of sera from patients with scleroderma. Arthritis Rheum 1983;26:170–177–178.

48. Evans DJ, Cushman SJ, Walport M. Progressive systemic sclerosis: Autoimmune arteriopathy. Lancet 1987;1:480–481.

49. Gruschwitz M, Von den Driesch P, Kellner P, et al. Expression of adhesion proteins in cell-cell and cell-matrix interactions in skin of patients with progressive systemic sclerosis. J Am Acad Dermatol 1992;27:169–177.

50. Mannucci PM, Lombardi R, Lattuada A, Perticucci E, Valsecchi R, Remuzzi G. Supranormal von Willebrand factor multimers in scleroderma. Blood 1987;73:1586–1591.

51. Kahaleh BM, Osborn I, LeRoy EC. Elevated levels of circulating platelet aggregates and beta-thromboglobulin in scleroderma. Ann Intern Med 1982; 96:610–613.

52. Lima J, Fonnolosa V, Fernandez-Cortijo J, Ordi J, Cuenca R, Khanashta MA, Vilardell M, et al. Platelet activation, endothelial cell dysfunction in the absence of anticardiolipin antibodies in systemic sclerosis. J Rheumatol 1991;18:1833–1836.

53. Godin-Ostro E, Mitrane M, Heller I, et al. Plasma plasminogen activator in systemic sclerosis. Arthritis Rheum 1985;28:80–87.

54. Cunliffe WJ, Menon IS. Blood fibrinolytic activity in disease of small blood vessels and the effect of low molecular weight dextran. Br J Dermatol 1969; 81:220–221.

55. Furey NL, Schmid FR, Kwan HC, et al. Arterial thrombosis in scleroderma. Br J Dermatol 1975;93: 683.

56. Botstein GR, Sherer GK, LeRoy EC. Fibroblast selection in scleroderma: An alternative model of fibrosis. Arthritis Rheum 1982;25:189–195.

57. Jimenez SA, MacArthur WM, Losher RJ, Rosen-bloom J. Selective inhibition of excessive scleroderma (PSS) fibroblast collagen synthesis by lymphokines from normal human mononuclear cells. Arthritis Rheum 1987;27(Suppl):S37.

58. Potter SR, Bienenstock J, Goldstein S, Buchan WW. Fibroblast growth factors in scleroderma. J Rheumatol 1985;12:1129–1135.

59. Alms WJ, Wigley FM, Wise R, et al. Increased expression of interleukin-4 mRNA in the bronchoalveolar lavage of systemic sclerosis patients with alveolitis. (Submitted)

60. Roberts A, Sporn M, Assovian RK, Smith JM, Roche NS, Wakefield LM, Heine UI, et al. Transforming growth factor type beta: Rapid induction of fibrosis and angiogenesis *in vitro* and collagen formation *in vitro*. Proc Natl Acad Sci USA 1986; 4167–4171.

61. Ignotz R, Massague J. Transforming growth factor-beta stimulates the expression of fibronectin and collagen and their incorporation into the extracellular matrix. J Biol Chem 1986;261:4337–4345.

62. Varga J, Rosenbloom J, Jimenez S. Transforming growth factor beta causes a persistent increase in steady state amounts of type I and III collagen and fibronectin mRNAs in normal human dermal fibroblasts. Biochem J 1987;247:597–604.

63. Reed M, Vernon R, Abrass I, Sage E. TGF-β1 induces the expression of Type I collagen and SPARC, and enhances contraction of collagen gels, by fibroblasts from young and aged doners. J Cell Physiol 1994;158:169–179.

64. Elias J, Lentz V, Cummings P. Transforming growth factor-beta regulations of IL-6 production by unstimulated and IL-1-stimulated human fibroblasts. J Immunol 1991;146:3437–3443.

65. Deguthi Y. Spontaneous increase of transforming growth factor beta production by bronchoalveolar mononuclear cells of patients with systemic autoimmune diseases affecting the lung. Ann Rheum Dis 1992;51:362–365.

66. Gay S, Jones R, Huang G, Gay R. Immunohistologic demonstration of platelet-derived growth factor (PDGF) and cis-oncogene expression in scleroderma. J Invest Dermatol 1989;92:301–303.

67. Scharffetter K, Lankat-Buttgereit G, Krieg T. Localization of collagen mRNA in normal and scleroderma skin by *in situ* hybridization. Eur J Clin Invest 1988;18:9–17.

68. Kahaleh MB. The role of vascular endothelium in fibroblast activation and tissue fibrosis, particularly in scleroderma (systemic sclerosis) and pachydermoperiotosis (primary pulmonary hypertension). Clin Exp Rheum 1992;10(Suppl 7):51–56.

69. LeRoy E, Smith E, Kahaleh M, Trojanowska M, Sil-

ver RM. A strategy for determining the pathogenesis of scleroderma: Is transforming growth factor-beta the answer? Arthritis Rheum 1989;32:817–825.

70. Paralkar VM, Vukicevic Reddi AH. Transforming growth factor beta type 1 binds to collagen IV of basement membrane matrix: Implications for development. Dev Biol 1991;143:303–308.

71. Duncan M, Berman B. Gamma interferon is the lymphokine and beta interferon the monokine responsible for inhibition of fibroblast collagen production and late but not early fibroblast proliferation. J Exp Med 1991;162:516–519.

72. Varga J, Olsen A, Herhal J, Constantine G, Rosenbloom J, Jimenez SA. Interferon-gamma reverses the stimulation of collagen but not fibronectin gene expression by transforming growth factor-beta in normal human fibroblasts. Eur J Clin Invest 1990;20:487–493.

73. Kahaleh B, Fan F-S. Impaired gamma interferon production in scleroderma: Possible role for interleukin-10. Arthritis Rheum 1993;36:S50.

74. Freundlich B, Jimenez S, Steen V, Medsger TA Jr, Szkolnicki M, Jaffe HS. Treatment of systemic sclerosis with recombinant interferon-gamma. Arthritis Rheum 1992;35:1134–1142.

75. Hawkins R, Claman H, Clark RA, Steigerwald JC. Increased dermal mast cell populations in systemic sclerosis: A link in chronic fibrosis? Ann Intern Med 1985;102:182–186.

76. Gleich G, Otteson E, Leiferman K, Ackerman S. Eosinophils and human disease. Int Arch Allergy Appl Immunol 1989;88:59–62.

77. Varga J, Wright J, Earle L, et al. Eosinophil activation in diffuse cutaneous systemic sclerosis. Arthritis Rheum 1993;36:S270.

78. Wong D, Elovi A, Matossian K, Nagura N, McBridge J, Chou MY, Garden JR, et al. Eosinophils from patients with blood eosinophilia express transforming growth factor-beta. Blood 1991;78:2702–2707.

79. Rohrbach M, Wheatley C, Slifman N, Gleich GJ. Activation of platelets by eosinophil granule proteins. J Exp Med 1990;172:1271–1274.

80. Kowaguchi Y, Harigi M, Hara M, et al. Increased interleukin-1 receptor, type I, at messenger mRNA and protein level in skin fibroblasts from patients with systemic sclerosis. Biochem Biophys Res Commun 1992;184:1504–1507.

81. Kahaleh MB, Smith EA, Soma Y, LeRoy EC. Effect of lymphotoxin and tumor necrosis factor on endothelial and connective cell tissue growth and function. Clin Immunol Immunopathol 1988;49:261–272.

82. Kondo H, Rabin BS, Rodnan GP. Stimulation of lymphocyte reactivity by a low molecular weight cutaneous antigen in patients with PSS (scleroderma). J Rheumatol 1979;6:30–37.

83. Alcocer-Varela J, Laffon A, Alarcon-Segovia D. Differences in the production of and/or the response to interleukin-2 by T-lymphocytes patients with various connective tissue diseases. Rheumatol Int 1984;4:39–44.

84. Hawrylko E, Spertus A, Mele CA, Oster N, Frieri M. Increased interleukin-2 production in response to human type 1 collagen stimulation in patients with systemic sclerosis. Arthritis Rheum 1991;34:580–587.

85. Stuart JM, Postlethwaite AE, Kang AH. Evidence for cell-mediated immunity to collagen in PSS. J Lab Clin Med 1976;88:601–607.

III
—

Organ Involvement

PIERRE YOUINOU
YVON-LOUIS PENNEC

14

Organ Involvement: Sjögren's Syndrome

SJÖGREN'S SYNDROME (SS) is presumably an autoimmune disease, in which exocrine glands are the site of intense immunologic activity (1–3). Lymphocytes and plasma cells infiltrate predominantly lacrimal and salivary glands, leading to keratoconjunctivitis sicca, xerostomia, and parotid gland enlargement (4–6). This may occur as sicca syndrome only (primary SS) or may be combined with connective tissue diseases (secondary SS), such as rheumatoid arthritis (RA), systemic lupus erythematosus (SLE), or systemic sclerosis (SSc). Several observations indicate that the pathogenesis of primary SS differs from that of the secondary condition (7–9); however, distinguishing between the two forms of the disease is difficult. Validation of proposed criteria (Table 14.1) for the classification of SS is currently underway (10).

The recognition of SSc as a separate disease is generally simple. SSc affects the skin, joints, muscle, and other selected organs, thus causing a wide variety of effects (11). Two types of patients with SSc have been observed: those with diffuse skin involvement and those with limited skin involvement. The term "diffuse scleroderma" is meant to describe patients who have cutaneous sclerosis in areas proximal to the elbows and knees and below the clavicles; the term "limited scleroderma" is meant to describe patients whose cutaneous sclerosis is limited to areas distal to the elbows, knees, and clavicles (12). The second group includes the CREST variant, which denotes the association of subcutaneous calcinosis, Raynaud's phenomenon, esophageal dysmotility, sclerodactily, and telangiectasia (13). In fact, many authors use the term CREST to connote patients who actually have limited cutaneous scleroderma. Consequently, the latter term will be used throughout this chapter. Interestingly, the best differentiated cases of SSc overlap with the various connective tissue diseases (14).

Although the association of SS with SSc is relatively common, the incidence of the former in subsets of the latter has not hitherto been unequivocally appreciated. The objective of this chapter is to describe the clinical, pathogenic, and serologic features of both disease components where SS and SSc develop together. Associated conditions are also explored.

Frequency of Association

HISTORICAL BACKGROUND

The coexistence of SS and SSc was first reported by Leriche (15) as the association of SS with pigmentation and scleroderma of the legs, as previously described by Sheldon (16); however, this association was subsequently not accepted as accurate by Weber (17). Since then, numerous case reports (18–25), including one by Sjögren himself (18) and three small studies (26–28), have been published. According to present criteria, however, the diagnosis of SS (10) or SSc (29) is unacceptable in some of these cases where lacrimal and salivary hyposecretion may be a result of SSc rather than SS (30), or may be caused

Table 14.1. European Preliminary Criteria for the Classification of Sjögren's Syndrome, As Established by Vitali et al[a]

1. Ocular symptoms
   Definition. A positive response to at least 1 of the following 3 questions:
   a. Have you had daily, persistent, troublesome dry eyes for more than 3 months?
   b. Do you have a recurrent sensation of sand or gravel in the eyes?
   c. Do you use tear substitutes more than 3 times a day?

2. Oral symptoms
   Definition. A positive response to at least 1 of the following 3 questions:
   a. Have you had a daily feeling of dry mouth for more than 3 months?
   b. Have you had recurrent or persistently swollen salivary glands as an adult?
   c. Do you frequently drink liquids to aid in swallowing dry foods?

3. Ocular signs
   Definition. Objective evidence of ocular involvement, determined on the basis of a positive result on at least 1 of the following 2 tests:
   a. Schirmer-I test ($\leq$ 5 mm in 5 minutes)
   b. Rose bengal score ($\geq$ 4, according to the van Bijsterveld scoring system)

4. Histopathologic features
   Definition. Focus score $\geq$ 1 on minor salivary gland biopsy (focus defined as an agglomeration of at least 50 mononuclear cells; focus score defined as the number of foci per 4 mm^2 of glandular tissue)

5. Salivary gland involvement
   Definition. Objective evidence of salivary gland involvement, determined on the basis of a positive result on at least 1 of the following 3 tests:
   a. Salivary scintigraphy
   b. Parotid sialography
   c. Unstimulated salivary flow ($\leq$ 1.5 ml in 15 minutes)

6. Autoantibodies
   Definition. Presence of at least 1 of the following serum autoantibodies:
   a. Antibodies to Ro/SS-A or La/SS-B antigens
   b. Antinuclear antibodies
   c. Rheumatoid factor

Exclusion criteria: preexisting lymphoma, acquired immuno-deficiency syndrome, sarcoidosis, or graft-versus-host disease.

[a] Vitali C, Bombardieri S, Moutsopoulos HM, et al. Preliminary criteria for the classification of Sjögren's syndrome. Results of a prospective concerted action supported by the European community. Arthritis Rheum 1993;36:340.

by primary SS with purpura of the lower extremities, which results in hyperpigmentation of the legs (i.e., an SSc-like syndrome) (16–20).

graph, a multicenter European study has recently defined diagnostic criteria for SS (10) that might be universally accepted (see Table 14.1).

PROGRESSIVE SYSTEMIC SCLEROSIS IN SJÖGREN'S SYNDROME

In seven reported series of patients with SS, a total of 452 cases (31–37), the proportion having SSc ranged from 1.4% in the first report to 7.8% in the seventh series. Variations can be accounted for by differences in the patient selection criteria. Nevertheless, the frequency of SSc in SS is lower than that of RA and SLE. In fact, several sets of criteria for the classification of SS have been proposed. As referred to in a previous para-

SJÖGREN'S SYNDROME IN PROGRESSIVE SYSTEMIC SCLEROSIS

No mention was made of concomitant SS in the early reviews on systemic sclerosis (38–40), whereas SS was noted in 1%, 3% and 5%, respectively, of the SSc patients in subsequent reports (41–43). Since sensitive methods to detect lacrimal and salivary gland dysfunction have become available, reports of large series of individuals with SSc have yielded a higher prevalence of associated SS (44–50). The proportion of patients with both disorders ranged from as low as 4% (46) to as high as 90% (44). In fact, two series had 26 patients in common (47–48) and, with regard to other studies, the criteria for diagnosing SS was markedly variable from one study to another. Alarcón-Segovia et al (44) employed a battery of nine tests, and their definition of SS relied on the positivity of any two of the tests. They concluded that SS was present in 23 out of 25 patients with SSc. Drosos et al (50) required the presence of a definite lymphocytic infiltration in the labial salivary gland biopsy to establish the diagnosis of SS. They detected disease in 10 out of 44 patients with SSc. If these figures are recalculated in accordance with the current criteria for SS, the average incidence of SS is 25% (see Table 14.1) (10).

It is not yet clear whether some of the patients described in the previous paragraphs presented with diffuse or limited forms of SSc. An important aspect of several studies is the finding that 46% of the patients with limited scleroderma suffer from SS (Table 14.2), suggesting that the prevalence in limited SSc is far higher than the 20% prevalence in diffuse SSc (47,48,50–53). Two instances of familial limited scleroderma and SS have also been reported (54,55). As a consequence, screening for SS should be routinely conducted in patients with limited scleroderma.

SSc often makes an overt appearance in the skin, although Raynaud's phenomenon (RP) commonly antedates this event. Seventy-three consecutive patients with isolated RP were followed-up for 15 years by Priollet et al (56). The diagnosis at the final visit was SS in only two of the patients.

An interesting finding that exemplifies the potentially close relationship between SSc and SS is the occurrence of these two conditions in the chronic phase of the graft-versus-host disease (GVHD) (57,58). The recipients of allogenic bone marrow develop a marked cutaneous sclerosis, symptoms of keratoconjunctivitis siccca, and xerostomia. The severity of sicca symptoms and lesions corresponds with that of GVHD. SS has occasionally been observed in cases of SSc following breast augmentation with silicone injection (59) and cases of bleomycin-induced scleroderma (60).

Clinical Characteristics

PROGRESSIVE SYSTEMIC SCLEROSIS WITH SJÖGREN'S SYNDROME

At first glance, the clinical presentation of SSc in SS patients is unremarkable, except for the frequent association of sicca features with limited forms of SSc (53). Sex ratio, age, disease duration, and specific features of CREST are identical in patients with and without SS (Table 14.3).

Despite the duration of the disease and the age of many of these patients, serious visceral complications are rare. Shearn (26) suggested that this was because the patients only had a mild

Table 14.2. Sjögren's Syndrome in Limited (CREST) and Diffuse Progressive Systemic Sclerosis

CREST	Diffuse	Reference
4/15 (27)[a]	2/20 (10)	47
12/32 (38)	6/23 (23)	48
8/12 (67)	13/50 (26)	50
3/29 (10)	5/32 (16)	52
20/22 (91)		53
14/23 (61)		54
61/133 (46)	26/128 (20)	

[a]Number of patients with Sjögren's syndrome (SS)/total number of patients with progressive systemic sclerosis (% of patients with SS).

biopsy (74). Lymphocytic infiltration of the salivary ducts can be regarded as a specific lesion for primary SS (75).

The histopathology of salivary glands from patients with SSc (Fig. 14.2) is characterized by moderate to extensive periglandular fibrosis (48–50,65). The sclerosis does not correlate with the extent or degree of cellular infiltration. The fibrotic event is specific to SSc and not associated with SS. It is found in SSc of recent onset (76) and also in healthy elderly volunteers (77). Major histocompatibility class II antigens are inappropriately expressed on ductal epithelial cells in patients with primary SS (78) and in those developing GVHD, which has a clinical picture of SSc and SS (79).

However, our study has indicated striking differences between SS secondary to limited scleroderma and primary SS (50). Parotid gland enlargement was rarely observed in the former, yet was commonly observed in the latter. This suggests that the pathogenesis of SS due to SSc is more related to collagen metabolism than to real inflammation, and, indeed, patients with systemic sclerosis do not respond to corticosteroids on a regular basis. However, the labial biopsies of our patients with limited scleroderma demonstrated predominantly inflammation and not fibrosis. It would be appropriate to compare their histopathological data on salivary gland biopsies to those of diffuse patients. Unexpectedly, patients with longer duration SSc and diffuse disease appeared not to have more gland fibrosis.

Serological Abnormalities

ANTINUCLEAR ANTIBODIES

Anticentromere antibodies and antibodies to Scl-70 are thought to be closely related to the limited (80) and diffuse (81) forms of SSc. The frequency of anticentromere antibodies is similar in SSc patients with and without SS (51,53).

Antibodies to Ro (SSA) and La (SSB) peptides have been reported in patients with primary SS (82). The most striking observation when SSc is complicated by SS is the decreased incidence of anti-Ro (SSA) and anti-La (SSB) antibodies (48,50,53). When the results obtained by Osial et

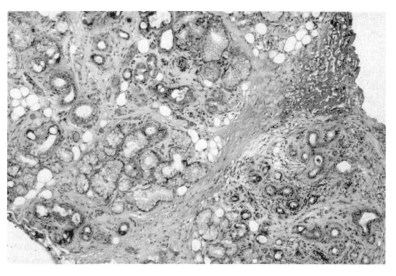

Figure 14.2. Labial salivary gland biopsy of a patient with progressive systemic sclerosis and Sjögren's syndrome showing periglandular and interlobular fibrosis.

al (48) and Drosos et al (50,53) are combined, the prevalence of anti-Ro (SSA) and anti-La (SSB) antibodies is 22% and 17% in SSc with SS, 5% and 3% in SSc only, and 79% and 38% in SS only. In normal controls, the prevalence is 1% and 0% (Table 14.4).

RHEUMATOID FACTORS

All three major classes of rheumatoid factors have been demonstrated in the sera and saliva of SS patients. Of note is the increased amount of serum IgA rheumatoid factor (83). These autoantibodies are more frequent in patients with primary SS than in patients with SS secondary to SSc (53), where the autoantibodies are more frequent than in patients with SSc only. They are correlated with a high lymphocytic infiltration in the labial salivary glands. Osial et al detected rheumatoid factor in 8 of 16 SS patients (50%) compared to 4 of 34 (12%) SS patients with normal biopsies (48).

MISCELLANEOUS

Consistent with the close relationship between SSc associated with SS and primary biliary cirrhosis is the frequent detection of anti-mitochodrial antibodies in SSc, even though only approximately 4% have evidence of liver disease (84). Various autoantibodies including anti-ery-throcyte, anti-smooth muscle, anti-thyroglobu-lin, and anti-salivary duct antibodies may occasionally be detected in patients with SSc and SS.

Treatment

To date, there is no ideal therapy for primary SS. Studies specifically devoted to treatment of SS complicating SSc are lacking, and a secondary SS is usually treated indirectly by treating the primary condition (85). The goals for therapy may be either the treatment of glandular and/or extraglandular disease. Currently, treatment for most patients is essentially symptomatic and often unsatisfactory.

Treatment includes substitution of the missing secretions and the prevention and treatment of the consequences of this lack of secretions. The mainstay of treatment for dry eyes is lubrication. This goal can be achieved through the use of a wide variety of commercially available tears, which differ primarily in their viscosity and the preservative used. The physician has to test several different preparations to determine which one is the best for each patient. Ointments that provide protection over a long period of time are also available, but they commonly produce blurring and are best used at night. The other steps taken to preserve tears include having the patient wear water-tight swimmer's goggles and

Table 14.4. Prevalence of Anti-Ro (SSA) and Anti-La (SSB) Antibodies in Progressive Systemic Sclerosis Patients with and without Sjögren's Syndrome (SS)[a]

Patient groups	No. positive/No. tested (% positive)	
	Anti-Ro (SSA) Antibody	Anti-La (SSB) Antibody
SSc + SS	9/41 (22)	7/41 (17)
SSc only	2/39 (5)	1/39 (3)
SS only	23/29 (79)	11/29 (38)
Normal controls	1/36 (3)	0/36 (0)

[a] From data reported in the following studies: (a Osial TA, Jr, Whiteside TL, Buckingham RB, et al. Clinical and serologic study of Sjögren's syndrome in patients with progressive systemic sclerosis. Arthritis Rheum 1983;26:500. b Drosos AA, Andonopoulos AP, Costopoulos JS, et al. Sjögren's syndrome in progressive systemic sclerosis. J Rheumatol 1988;15:965. c Drosos AA, Pennec YL, Elisaf M, et al. Sjögren's syndrome in patients with the CREST variant of progressive systemic scleroderma. J Rheumatol 1991;18:1685.

performing punctal occlusion using a variety of different types of stents, or even by performing a permanent punctal occlusion.

Treatment for dry mouth includes providing relief from its symptoms. The topical application of artificial salivary compounds (86) has been shown to increase parotid flow rates in SS patients, but the advantages of these compounds when compared to frequent ingesting of liquids are questionable. Stimulation of salivary flow using flavored lozenges and sugar-free chewing gums may also be of assistance. Mild increase of salivary flow rates may be obtained by potassium iodine or parasympathomimetic agents such as pilocarpine or neostigmine (87). The use of nandrolone decanoate, bromhexine or trithioparamethoxyphenylpropene has given equivocal results (88–91). In a small open study of ten patients lasting for 2 months, interferon-α (1×10^6 IU every week) was shown to be effective in increasing the saliva production of patients with primary SS (92). Finally, electrostimulation has been shown effective in stimulating increased production of saliva and in reducing the symptoms (93). Prevention of periodontal problems can be achieved by using toothpastes lacking detergents, by regular application of topical fluoride, and by careful dental supervision (1).

The presence of a chronic destructive inflammatory infiltrate in the exocrine tissue and the extensive serologic autoimmune reactivity suggest that patients with this disease might benefit from systemic treatment with anti-inflammatory agents. The results of such a general approach have been disappointing to date. Prednisone and piroxicam have failed to improve the histological and functional parameters of salivary and lacrimal glands in SS patients (94). Despite the promising results of an open study (95), hydroxychloroquine was not found to be of clinical benefit in a 2-year, double-blind crossover trial (96). Because minimal clinical improvement was observed and the side effects of cyclosporine-A could be serious, its use is not currently recommended (97). Cytotoxic drugs, such as cyclophosphamide, are contraindicated because they may increase the risk of the development of lymphoma in this disease (98).

Conclusions

The presence of SS modifies the clinical presentation of SSc, which is, usually, the limited variant. Conversely, the association of SSc alters the histopathological and serological pattern of SS. The GVHD is a fascinating model of the combination.

References

1. Talal N, Moutsopoulos HM, Kassan SS, eds. Sjögren's syndrome. Clinical and immunological aspects. Berlin: Springer-Verlag, 1987.
2. Talal N, ed. Sjögren's syndrome. A model for understanding autoimmunity. New York: Academic Press, 1989.
3. Alarcón-Segovia D. Primary Sjögren's syndrome. Six characters in search of an author. J Rheumatol 1989;16:1177.
4. Youinou P, Pennec YL. Immunopathological features of primary Sjögren's syndrome. Clin Exp Rheumatol 1987;5:173.
5. Youinou P, Moutsopoulos HM, Pennec YL. Clinical features of Sjögren's syndrome. Curr Opin Rheumatol 1990;2:687.
6. Moutsopoulos HM, Youinou P. New developments in Sjögren's syndrome. Curr Opin Rheumatol 1991;3:815.
7. Moutsopoulos HM, Mann D, Johnson A, et al. Genetic differences between primary and secondary sicca syndrome. N Engl J Med 1979;301:761.
8. Moutsopoulos HM, Webber BL, Vlagopoulos TP, et al. Differences in the clinical manifestations of sicca syndrome in the presence or absence of rheumatoid arthritis. Am J Med 1979;66:733.
9. Fox RI, Howell FV, Bone RC, et al. Primary Sjögren's syndrome. Clinical and immunopathologic features. Semin Arthritis Rheum 1984;14:77.
10. Vitali C, Bombardieri S, Moutsopoulos HM, et al. Preliminary criteria for the classification of Sjögren's syndrome. Results of a prospective concerted action supported by the European community. Arthritis Rheum. 1993;36:340.
11. Medsger TA Jr. Systemic sclerosis. In: McCarthy DJ

Jr, ed. Arthritis and allied conditions, 10th ed. Philadelphia: Lea & Febiger, 1985.

12. LeRoy EC, Black C, Fleischmajer R, et al. Scleroderma (systemic sclerosis). Classification, subsets and pathogenesis. J Rheumatol 1988;15:202.

13. Winterbauer RH. Multiple telangiectasia, Raynaud's phenomenon, sclerodactily and subcutaneous calcinosis. A syndrome mimicking hereditary hemorrhagic telangiectasia. Bull Johns Hopkins Hosp 1964;114:361.

14. Bennett RM. Scleroderma overlap syndromes. Rheum Dis Clin North Am 1990;16:185.

15. Leriche R. Traitement chirurgical du syndrome de Gougerot-Sj{im}ogren (oeil sec et bouche sèche). Résultat au bout de vingt-huit ans d'une double section du nerf vertébral. Presse Med 1947;55:77.

16. Sheldon JH. Sjögren's syndrome associated with pigmentation and scleroderma of the legs. Proc R Soc Med 1938;32:255.

17. Weber FP. Sjögren's syndrome, especially its nonocular features. Br J Ophtalmol 1945;29:299.

18. Sjögren H. Keratoconjunctivitis sicca and chronic polyarthritis. Acta Med Scand 1948;130:484.

l9. Holm S. Keratoconjunctivitis sicca and the sicca syndrome. Acta Ophtalmol 1949;33(Suppl):1.

20. Harrington AB, Dewar HA. A case of Sjögren's disease with scleroderma. Br Med J 1951;1:1302.

21. Ramage JH, Kinnear WF. Keratoconjunctivitis sicca and the collagen diseases. Br J Opthalmol 1956;40:41.

22. Piazzesi W. Su di un caso di sclerodermica con diplegia faciale e sindrome di Sjögren. Riv Pat Nerv Ment 1956;77:584.

23. Bertram U. Xerostomia. Clinical aspects, pathology and pathogenesis. Acta Odontol Scand 1967;1 (Suppl 49).

24. Appelboom T, Vandermoeten R, Vandenabeele G. Considérations pathogéniques à propos d'une association de syndrome CREST et de syndrome de Gougerot-Sjögren. Rev Rhum Mal Osteoarth 1975;42:127.

25. Trotta F, Potena A, Bertelli R, et al. Associazione sindrome di Reynolds-sindrome di Sjögren. Minerva Med 1980;71:1385.

26. Shearn MA. Sjögren's syndrome in association with scleroderma. Ann Intern Med 1960;52:1352.

27. Barrière H, Litoux P, Bureau B, et al. Deux observations de sclérodermie et syndrome de Gougerot-Sjögren. Bull Soc Fr Dermatol Syph 1973;80:122.

28. Youinou P, Le Goff P, Blain F, et al. Association d'une sclérodermie systémique, d'une hépatopathie et d'un syndrome de Gougerot-Sjögren. Nouv Presse Med 1976;5:1983.

29. Subcommittee for scleroderma criteria of the American Rheumatism Association diagnostic and therapeutic criteria committee. Preliminary criteria for the classification of systemic sclerosis (Scleroderma). Arthritis Rheum 1980;23:581.

30. Kerkham TH. Scleroderma and Sjögren's syndrome. Br J Ophtalmol 1969;2:131.

31. Stoltze CA, Hanbon DG, Pease GL. Keratoconjunctivitis sicca and Sjögren's syndrome. Systemic manifestations and hematologic and protein abnormalities. Arch Intern Med 1960;106:513.

32. Vanselow NA, Dodson VN, Angell DC, et al. A clinical study of Sjögren's syndrome. Ann Intern Med 1963;58:124.

33. Bloch KJ, Buchanan WW, Wohl MJ, et al. Sjögren's syndrome. A clinical, pathological and serological study of sixty-two cases. Medicine (Baltimore) 1965;44:87.

34. Denko CW. Antibodies in the sicca syndrome (Sjögren's syndrome). Arthritis Rheum 1965;8:970.

35. Shearn MA. Sjögren's syndrome. Philadelphia: Saunders, 1971.

36. Branson-Geokas B, Epstein MJ, Quismorio FP, et al. Sjögren's syndrome. Clinical and laboratory studies. Arthritis Rheum 1971;14:152.

37. Mason AMS, Gumpel JM, Golding PL. Sjögren's syndrome. A clinical review. Semin Arthritis Rheum 1973;2:301.

38. Beigelman PM, Goldman F Jr, Bayles TB. Progressive systemic sclerosis (scleroderma). N Engl J Med 1953;249:45.

39. Leinwand I, Duryee AW, Richter MN. Scleroderma based on a study of over 150 cases. Ann Intern Med 1954;41:1003.

40. Barnett AJ, Coventry DA. Scleroderma 1. Clinical features, course of illness and response to treatment in 61 cases. Med J Aust 1979;1:992.

41. Tuffanelli DL, Winkelmann RK. Scleroderma and its relationship to the "collagenoses," dermatomyositis, lupus erythematosus, rheumatoid arthritis and Sjögren's syndrome. Am J Med Sci 1962; 55:133.

42. Rodnan GP. The natural history of progressive systemic sclerosis (diffuse scleroderma). Bull Rheum Dis 1963;13:301.

43. Stava Z. Diffuse scleroderma. A clinical study of 65 cases. Dermatologica 1958;117:135.

44. Alarcón-Segovia D, Ibañez G, Hernandez-Ortiz J, et al. Sjögren's syndrome in progressive systemic sclerosis (Scleroderma). Am J Med 1974;57:78.

45. Fiessinger JN, Blanchet-Bardon C, Drouillat JP. Rapports entre la sclérodermie et le syndrome de Gougerot-Sjögren. Intérêt de la biopsie systémique des glandes salivaires labiales. Nouv Presse Med 1975;4:3177.

46. Grennan DM, Ferguson M, Ghobarey AE, et al. Sjögren's syndrome in SLE. Part 2. An examination

of the clinical significance of Sjögren's syndrome by comparison of its frequency in typical and atypical forms of SLE, overlap syndromes and scleroderma. N Z Med J 1977;85:376.

47. Cipoletti JF, Buckingham RB, Barnes L, et al. Sjögren's syndrome in progressive systemic sclerosis. Ann Intern Med 1977;87:535.

48. Osial TA Jr, Whiteside TL, Buckingham RB, et al. Clinical and serologic study of Sjögren's syndrome in patients with progressive systemic sclerosis. Arthritis Rheum 1983;26:500.

49. Coll J, Ferrando J, Vivancos J, et al. Incidence del sindrome de Sjögren in systemic scleroderma. Rev Clin Esp 1985;177:438.

50. Drosos AA, Andonopoulos AP, Costopoulos JS, et al. Sjögren's syndrome in progressive systemic sclerosis. J Rheumatol 1988;15:965.

51. Catoggio LJ, Bernstein RM, Black CM, et al. Serological markers in progressive systemic sclerosis. Clinical correlations. Ann Rheum Dis 1983;42:23.

52. Powell FC, Schroeter AL, Dickinson ER. Primary biliary cirrhosis and the CREST syndrome. A report of 22 cases. QJM 1987;62:75.

53. Drosos AA, Pennec YL, Elisaf M, et al. Sjögren's syndrome in patients with the CREST variant of progressive systemic scleroderma. J Rheumatol 1991;18:1685.

54. Camus JP, Emerit I, Reinert P, et al. Sclérodermie familiale avec syndrome de Sjögren et anomalies lymphocytaires et chromosomiques. Ann Med Int 1970;121:149.

55. Frayha RA, Tabbara KF, Geha RS. Familial CRST syndrome with sicca complex. J Rheumatol 1977; 4:53.

56. Priollet P, Vayssairat M, Housset E. How to classify Raynaud's phenomenon? Long-term follow-up study of 73 cases. Am J Med 1987;83:494.

57. Gratwhol AA, Moutsopoulos HM, Chused TM, et al. Sjögren-type syndrome after allogenic bone-marrow transplantation. Ann Intern Med 1977; 87:703.

58. Lawley TJ, Peck GL, Moutsopoulos HM, et al. Scleroderma, Sjögren-like syndrome and chronic graft-versus-host disease. Ann Intern Med 1977; 87:707.

59. Okano Y, Nishikai M, Sato A. Scleroderma, primary biliary cirrhosis and Sjögren's syndrome after cosmetic breast augmentation with silicone injection. A case report of possible human adjuvant disease. Ann Rheum Dis 1984;43:520.

60. Finch WR, Rodnan GP, Buckingham RB, et al. Bleomycin-induced scleroderma. J Rheumatol 1980;7:651.

61. Oddis CV, Eisenbeis CH Jr, Reidbord HE, et al. Vasculitis in systemic sclerosis. Association with Sjö-

gren's syndrome and the CREST syndrome variant. J Rheumatol 1987;14:942.

62. Youinou P, Pennec YL, Katsikis PD, et al. Raynaud's phenomenon in primary Sjögren's syndrome. Br J Rheumatol 1990;29:2052.

63. Skopouli FN, Talal A, Galanopoulou V, et al. Raynaud's phenomenon in primary Sjögren's syndrome. J Rheumatol 1990;17:618.

64. Kraus A, Caballero-Uribe C, Jakez J, et al. Raynaud's phenomenon in primary Sjögren's syndrome. Association with other extraglandular manifestations. J Rheumatol 1992;19:1572.

65. Rasker JJ, Jayson MI, Jones DE, et al. Sjögren's syndrome in systemic sclerosis. A clinical study of 26 patients. Scand J Rheumatol 1990;19:57.

66. Reynolds TB, Denison EK, Frakl HD, et al. Primary biliary cirrhosis with scleroderma, Raynaud's phenomenon and telangiectasia. Am J Med 1971; 50:302.

67. Vitali C, Tavoni A, Viegi G, et al. Lung involvement in Sjögren's syndrome. A comparison between patients with primary and with secondary syndrome. Ann Rheum Dis 1985;44:455.

68. Raminez-Mata M, Pena-Ancria F, Alarcón-Segovia D. Abnormal esophagal motility in primary Sjögren's. J Rheumatol 1976;3:6388.

69. Chisholm DM, Mason DK. Labial salivary gland biospy in Sjögren's syndrome. J Clin Pathol 1968; 21:656.

70. Greenspan JS, Daniels TE, Talal N, et al. The histopathology of Sjögren's syndrome in labial salivary gland biopsies. Oral Pathol 1974;37:217.

71. Tarpley TM Jr, Anderson LG, White CL. Minor salivary gland involvement in Sjögren's syndrome. Oral Surg 1974;37:64.

72. Daniels TE. Labial salivary gland biopsy in Sjögren's syndrome assessment as a diagnostic criterion in 362 suspected cases. Arthritis Rheum 1984; 27:147.

73. Pennec YL, Leroy JP, Jouquan J, et al. Comparison of labial and sublingual biopsies in the diagnosis of Sjögren's syndrome. Ann Rheum Dis 1990;49:37.

74. Leroy JP, Pennec YL, Soulier C, et al. Follow-up study of labial salivary gland lesions in primary Sjögren's syndrome. Ann Rheum Dis 1992;51:777.

75. Leroy JP, Pennec YL, Letoux G, et al. Lymphocytic infiltration of salivary ducts. A histopathologic lesion specific for primary Sjögren's syndrome? Arthritis Rheum 1992;35:481.

76. Jamin A, Gosselin B, Gosset D, et al. Histological criteria of Sjögren's syndrome in scleroderma. Clin Exp Rheumatol 1989;7:167.

77. Drosos AA, Andonopoulos AP, Costopoulos JS, et al. Prevalence of primary Sjögren's syndrome in an elderly population. Br J Rheumatol 1988;27:123.

78. Moutsopoulos HM, Hooks JJ, Chan CC, et al. HLA-DR expression by labial minor salivary gland tissues in Sjögren's syndrome. Ann Rheum Dis 1986;45:677.

79. Lindahl G, Lonnquist B, Hedfors E. Lymphocytic infiltration and HLA-DR expression of salivary glands in bone marrow transplant recipients. A prospective study. Clin Exp Immunol 1988;72:267.

80. Tan EM, Rodnan GP, Garcia I, et al. Diversity of antinuclear antibodies in progressive systemic sclerosis. Anti-centromere antibody and its relationship to CREST syndrome. Arthritis Rheum 1980; 23:617.

81. Shero JH, Bordwell B, Rothfield NF, et al. High titers of autoantibodies to topoisomerase I (Scl-70) in sera from scleroderma patients. Science 1986;231:737.

82. Moutsopulos HM, Zerva LV. Anti-Ro(SSA)/-La(SSB) antibodies in Sjögren's syndrome. Clin Rheumatol 1990;9:1.

83. Muller K, Oxholm P, Hoier-Madsen M, et al. Circulating IgA- and IgM-rheumatoid factors in patients with primary Sjögren's syndrome. Scand J Rheumatol 1989;18:29.

84. Barnett AJ. The systemic involvement in scleroderma. Med J Aust 1977;2:659.

85. Fox TI. Treatment of the patient with Sjögren's syndrome. Rheum Dis Clin North Am 1992;18:699.

86. Weisz A. The use of saliva substitute as treatment for xerostomia in Sjögren's syndrome. Oral Surg 1981;52:384–396.

87. Fox PC, van der Veen PF, Baum BJ, et al. Pilocarpine for treatment of xerostomia associated with salivary gland dysfunction. Oral Surg 1986;61:243.

88. Drosos AA, Vliet-Dascalopoulou E, Andonopoulos AP, et al. Nandrolone decanoate (decadurabolin) in primary Sjögren's syndrome: A double blind pilot study. Clin Exp Rheumatol 1988;6:53.

89. Prause JV, Frost-Larsen K, Hoj L, et al. Lacrimal and salivary secretion in Sjögren's syndrome. The effect of systemic treatment with bromhexine. Acta Ophtalmol 1984;62:489.

90. Manthortpe R, Frost-Larsen K, Hoj L, et al. Bromhexine treatment of Sjögren's syndrome. Effect on lacrimal and salivary secretion on proteins in tear fluid and saliva. Scand J Rheumatol 1981; 10:177–180.

91. Schiodt M, Oxholm P, Jacobsen A. Treatment of xerostomia in patients with primary Sjögren's syndrome with sulfarlem. Scand J Rheumatol 1986; 61(Suppl):250–252.

92. Shiozawa S, Morimoto I, Tanaka Y, Shozawa K. A preliminary study on the interferon-α treatment for xerostomia of Sjögren's syndrome. Br J Rheumatol 1993;32:52–54.

93. Talal N, Quinn JH, Daniels TE. The clinical effects of electrostimulation on salivary function of Sjögren's syndrome patients. A placebo controlled study. Rheumatol Int 1992;12:43–45.

94. Fox PC, Datiles M, Atkinson JC, et al. Prednisone and piroxican for treatment of primary Sjögren's syndrome. Clin Exp Rheumatol 1993;11:149.

95. Fox RI, Chan E, Benton L, et al. Treatment of primary Sjögren's syndrome with hydroxychloroquine. Am J Med 1988;85(Suppl 4A):62–67.

96. Kruize AA, Hené RJ, Kallenberg CGM, et al. Hydroxychloroquine treatment for primary Sjögren's syndrome: A two year double blind crossover trial. Ann Rheum Dis 1993;52:360–364.

97. Drosos AA, Skopouli FN, Costopoulos JS, et al. Cyclosporine-A (Cy-A) in primary Sjögren's syndrome: A double blind study. Ann Rheum Dis 1986;45:732.

98. Kassan S, Thomas TL, Moutsopoulos HM, et al. Increased risk of lymphoma in sicca syndrome. Ann Intern Med 1978;89:888–892.

CAROL M. BLACK
RON M. DU BOIS

15

Organ Involvement: Pulmonary

PULMONARY DISEASE is currently considered to be the major cause of death in patients with systemic sclerosis (SSc) (1). A recent study (2) found the median survival to be 78 months, with 60% dead at 5 years in patients who had diffuse skin disease and pulmonary involvement, but no cardiac or renal disease; early diagnosis enabling the institution of effective therapy to halt disease progression is a critical aim in the management of the patient with SSc.

The two major clinical manifestations of lung involvement are fibrosing alveolitis and pulmonary vascular disease. Aspiration pneumonia, pleural disease, spontaneous pneumothorax, drug-induced pneumonitis, associated pneumoconiosis, and neoplasm are infrequent complications. Pulmonary fibrosis occurs in more than 75% of the patients with SSc, and pulmonary vascular disease in approximately 50% (3). Post mortem reports have always yielded higher percentages than clinical studies. The lack of appropriate investigative procedures meant that, until recently, we were unable to diagnose lung involvement in its earliest stages. This is changing, particularly with respect to interstitial lung disease.

The first suggestion of lung involvement in scleroderma was made by Hippocrates in what was thought to be the first recorded description of the disease itself. More than 2000 years elapsed before Binz (1864) (4) noted pulmonary symptoms in recorded cases of scleroderma. He attributed these symptoms to an increased blood volume in the lungs caused by a marked distur-

bance of the cutaneous circulation. In 1877, Harley (5) suggested that there was fibrous degeneration of the lung tissue, and in 1891 Dinkler (6) commented that pressure on the vascular system and diminution of the surface area of the arterial circulation was involved in the etiology of the lung disease. However, it was not until after the careful work of von Notthaft in 1898 (7) and Matsui in 1924 (8) that both parenchymal interstitial change and vascular abnormalities were felt to be directly caused by scleroderma.

This chapter not only describes the clinical and histopathological aspects of pulmonary scleroderma, but also shows that modern investigative tools plus the growing body of information on the pathogenesis of the fibrotic lesion and vascular abnormalities make possible prediction of those at risk, early diagnosis, accurate staging, and sensitive prediction of progression. We hope that this will guide and change our therapeutic approach to pulmonary disease.

Pathogenesis

SSc produces two major patterns of abnormality within the lungs—a fibrosing alveolitis or a primary pulmonary vascular disease. Although both of these processes appear to be centered on the vessels, subsequent progression would suggest that the pathogenetic processes are quite different. Much has now been learned about the pathogenesis of fibrosing alveolitis through the use of bronchoalveolar lavage (BAL) and evaluation of lung biopsy samples: these approaches are not possible in pulmonary vascular disease.

FIBROSING ALVEOLITIS

Initiating Factors

Ultrastructural observation in human and animal models of lung fibrosis would support the concept that lung injury to the epithelium and endothelium is the first event in the pathogenesis of the fibrosing alveolitis that occurs in the context of SSc (FASSc), although the nature of the initiating factor is not known (9,10). It is likely that patients with SSc have a predisposition to develop pulmonary fibrosis. In support of this, a recent study has shown that fibrosing alveolitis occurring in SSc is associated with the presence of a class II major histocompatibility complex haplotype DR3/DR52a and/or the presence of the anti-DNA topoisomerase I antibody (Scl-70) in the serum (11). SSc patients with this class II haplotype or Scl-70 have a 16.7-fold excess risk of having pulmonary fibrosis as compared to SSc patients without these risk factors.

In predisposed individuals, the initial injurious process is followed by an influx of acute and chronic inflammatory cells that are responsible for initiating and maintaining the immunological and inflammatory responses, which results in further lung injury and, ultimately, fibrosis. The pathogenetic process is, therefore, a combination of inflammatory, destructive, and fibrotic changes and not just the deposition of connective tissue matrix proteins.

Immunological Mechanisms

Studies in cryptogenic fibrosing alveolitis (CFA) of lung biopsies, BAL cells, and epithelial lining fluid (sampled by BAL) have all demonstrated activation of immunological mechanisms, mirroring the substantial evidence for the involvement of immunological processes in the pathogenesis of SSc.

Histological examination of lung biopsies shows the presence of lymphoid follicles and abundant lymphocytes and plasma cells. Immunohistochemical studies have clarified the nature of the lymphoid aggregates, which have the morphological and immunohistochemical features of secondary follicles (with true germinal centers) as seen in reactive lymph nodes (12,13). Within the interstitium of the lung, macrophages express the phenotype of inflammatory cells, and lymphocytes are predominantly CD4+ helper/inducer subset cells with variable numbers of CD8+ suppressor/cytotoxic cells present. Many of the T cells express markers of activation, and the majority of T cells have the surface phenotype of antigen-primed, memory T cells (CD45RO+) (14). To investigate whether these antigen primed cells are clonally distributed, Southcott et al (15) analyzed the T cell antigen receptor repertoire using RNA extracted from open lung biopsies from patients with SSc and using specific primer pairs for 18 T cell antigen receptor alpha chain variable regions. These investigators showed that there is no difference between SSc patients, patients with cryptogenic fibrosing alveolitis, and lung tissue from normal individuals in terms of the numbers of families expressed and the range of families expressed. This does not completely exclude clonality, because homology at the antigen binding site can be present within variable regions of different family specificities. Further studies using detailed sequencing of large numbers of clones will be necessary to confirm or exclude this possibility.

The cells within the interstitium express a repertoire of cytokines, as confirmed by both polymerase chain reaction expansion of RNA from lung biopsy samples and *in situ* hybridization (Table 15.1). Scattered cells within the interstitium express mRNA for IL-4, IL-5, and γ-interferon (16,17). This range of cytokine production does not fall neatly within the TH1 and TH2 groups of T cells, indicating that it is not always possible to divide human T cell responses into inflammatory or delayed hypersensitivity types. In some studies, IgG and complement deposition have been observed within the alveolar wall and capillaries of patients with fibrosing

Table 15.1. Lymphocyte and Macrophage Secretory Products Expressed in Fibrosing Alveolitis in Systemic Sclerosis

	Product	Reference
Lymphocyte		
	IL–2	Southcott et al (16)
	—4	Hamid et al (17)
	—5	
	Rantes	Petrek et al[a]
	IFN-γ	Hamid et al (17)
Macrophage		
	IL–8	Southcott et al (25)
		Carre et al (24)
	TNF-α	Pantelidis et al (26)
	Fibronectin	Kinsella et al (29)
		Rossi et al (20)
	PDGF	Thornton et al (43)
	IGF-1	Rossi et al (20)
		Harrison et al (30)
	TGFβ	Deguchi (39)
		Moreland et al (40)
		Corrin et al (41)

[a]Unpublished data: Petrek et al.

alveolitis, but such deposition is not found in the majority of cases and is rarely identified under the electron microscope (9). The epithelial cells express HLA-DR class II major histocompatibility complex molecules (12).

In samples obtained by BAL, several studies have shown the presence of an excess of lymphocytes within the lower respiratory tract (18–22). Epithelial lining fluid contains high levels of immunoglobulin, particularly IgG and immune complexes (23).

Inflammatory Response

Macrophages. Mononuclear phagocytes are present in abundance within the lungs of patients with SSc and are capable of expressing a number of genes encoding cytokines and other mediators that can modulate inflammation (Table 15.1). Of particular relevance is interleukin-8 (IL-8), which may be the most potent neutrophil chemotactant found in humans and is a member of the recently described chemokine family of peptides. Macrophages from patients with SSc contain mRNA for IL-8, and IL-8 is also found in epithelial lining fluid from patients with

SSc (24,25). It is important to note that enhanced IL-8 expression is found mainly in patients with FASSc; much less is present in the lungs of patients that lack evidence of diffuse parenchymal disease, as identified by thin section computed tomography (CT).

Alveolar macrophages from patients with FASSc also spontaneously produce tumor necrosis factor-α (TNFα) in increased amounts by comparison with normal individuals or patients with sarcoidosis—a granulomatous condition with a much reduced tendency to fibrosis in comparison to SSc or fibrosing alveolitis (26). This cytokine may play an important role in inflammatory cell recruitment to the lung by increasing the expression on vascular endothelium of the adhesion molecules ICAM-1, E-selectin, and VCAM-1. The finding of soluble ICAM-1 and E-selectin in lung lavage samples from patients with SSc supports the concept of adhesion molecule upregulation within the lung (27).

Macrophages also release increased amounts of oxidant species in comparison to control cells, adding to the burden of injury of oxidant and granule proteases released by neutrophils (see below) (28).

Perhaps the best defined group of macrophage products believed to play important roles in the pathogenesis of fibrosing alveolitis in SSc is the growth factors. Fibroblasts require competence and progression growth factors in order to proceed from the resting G0 state through the G1, S, and G2 phases of growth to cell division. Spontaneous synthesis and secretion of fibronectin (competence) and insulin-like growth factor-1 (progression) by lower respiratory tract cells from patients with FASSc (20,29,30) are likely to contribute to the stimulation of resting fibroblasts to division *in vivo*.

Granulocytes. Neutrophil polymorphonuclear leukocytes are capable of producing host tissue damage through release of proteolytic enzymes, particularly neutrophil elastase and collagenase, and their capacity to generate potent oxygen radicals. There is evidence for their involvement in fibrosing alveolitis in SSc. They are present in increased numbers (up to 15-fold, particularly in smokers) in lung lavage samples, although they are less prominent in lung tissue (31). This suggests that there may be a chemotactic gradient that attracts neutrophils from the vascular compartment, through the interstitium, and into the air spaces. Studies of cells obtained by BAL from patients with cryptogenic fibrosing alveolitis have shown enhanced release of oxygen radicals by comparison with normal individuals (32–34). Epithelial lining fluid glutathione from these patients is predominantly oxidized, implying local oxidant production in the lower respiratory tract. The evidence would suggest that this is neutrophil-derived. There is some evidence that lung cells in SSc are also spontaneously releasing these injurious reactive oxygen species (35). The presence of neutrophil collagenase and myeloperoxidase in epithelial lining fluid confirms that neutrophil degranulation is likely to contribute to tissue injury (28,36).

The role of eosinophils and mast cells is less clear, but both are present in increased numbers in the lung interstitium (37). These cells, too, are capable of inducing lung injury through release of their secretory products, particularly eosinophil cationic protein and vasoactive amines.

Fibrogenesis

Excess collagen is present within the lungs of patients with FASSc. Precise control of fibroblast and other connective tissue matrix cells and their secretory products almost certainly involves finely tuned cellular interrelationships, including cell/cell contact, cell/extracellular matrix contact, and cytokine production in the local microenvironment. The mediator TGFβ is receiving increasing attention. This is a 25kD homodimer that exists in a number of isoforms; these isoforms are emerging as potent fibroblast chemotactants and stimulators of fibrogenesis. Macrophages, monocytes, neutrophils, and fibroblasts can all synthesize and secrete this potent cytokine (38).

A study by Deguchi, using a nuclear run-on assay, demonstrated increased TGFβ transcription in bronchoalveolar mononuclear cells in SSc by comparison with controls, and also showed increased spontaneous TGFβ synthesis by cultured mononuclear cells (39). However, in a second study, BAL cells from patients with SSc were shown to contain amounts of mRNA that were similar to those in cells from normal individuals, and epithelial lining fluid TGFβ concentrations were found to be lower in the disease population (40). The use of different methodologies may explain the varied results of these two studies: Deguchi was studying the dynamic situation, whereas the second study involved measurement of steady-state mRNA levels and concentrations of epithelial lining fluid protein. It is also possible that these discordant data were the result of patients being studied at different stages.

Immunohistochemical studies of open lung biopsy samples from patients with SSc (41) have shown marked TGF-β localization in alveolar type II pneumocytes and fibrous tissue underlying the type II cell hypertrophy as well as in alveolar macrophages, thus identifying a number of cell types in the production of TGF-β at disease sites. Pulmonary fibroblasts from patients with SSc respond to *in vitro* stimulation with TGF-β by enhanced procollagen production. Furthermore, TGF-β can inhibit protease secretion (serine, thio- and metalloproteases) and increase the secretion of the protease inhibitors α-1-antitrypsin, and tissue inhibitor of metalloproteases (TIMP) (42).

Other growth factors are implicated in the pathogenesis of fibrosis in SSc. BAL fluid from patients with SSc stimulates fibroblast proliferation. At least part of this activity has been shown to be due to insulin-like growth factor-1 (30). Interestingly, although platelet-derived growth factor (PDGF) has been shown to play an important role in the fibrogenesis of cryptogenic fibrosing alveolitis, there are fewer studies of this growth factor in FASSc. One group (43) has shown that alveolar mononuclear cells in SSc secrete increased amounts of PDGF in comparison to those of normal individuals, and Gay et al have shown high expression of PDGF in the endothelial cells of patients with scleroderma, although this was in the skin, not the lung (44,45). Cells that appear to be myofibroblasts may be cultured from lung lavage samples, and they show an increased proliferative response to stimulation with TGFβ and PDGF (46).

Other recent studies have focused on the vascular compartment as a source of fibroblast mitogens and stimulators of collagen synthesis. In this regard, endothelin 1 (a member of a family of four isopeptides that can be produced by endothelial and epithelial cells) is known to be a powerful chemoattractant for fibroblasts and can cause dermal fibroblasts to secrete increased collagen. Lung lavage fluid from patients with SSc contains increased levels of endothelin 1. *In vitro* fibroblast proliferation studies, with and without specific endothelin 1 inhibitors, have confirmed that endothelin 1 can exert a specific proliferative effect on fetal lung fibroblasts (47).

Fibrin and fibrinogen degradation products can stimulate fibroblasts. Studies by Gray et al have demonstrated that fibroblast replication is significantly enhanced by fibrinogen derived proteins (48).

Although injury and subsequent loss of lung tissue are irreversible, deposition of collagen is not an end stage process. There is clear evidence that collagen turnover takes place in both humans and animals: in animal models, approximately 10% of lung collagen is turned over every day (49). Therefore, it is relevant to concepts of therapy in humans to consider that the control of collagen synthesis could result in an overall diminution in total lung collagen content and improved lung function. The finely tuned controls of fibroblast proliferation and collagen deposition and the identification of a key component in these processes await further research. It is interesting to note that the studies by Jordana et al (50) have demonstrated the emergence of a specific phenotype of fibroblasts that proliferate more rapidly than other fibroblasts when passaged. These emerge from a population of fibroblasts obtained from disease sites, and this phenotype of fibroblasts then "breeds true." Jordana et al's findings are consistent with observations of fibroblast subpopulations, which can be identified after culturing dermal tissue from patients with SSc (51,52). It is, therefore, possible to speculate, that, once this subpopulation of fibroblasts has emerged, further fibroblast proliferation may not be responsive to the usual homeostatic controls.

PULMONARY VASCULAR DISEASE

The study of the pathogenesis of pulmonary vessel disease occurring either alone or in association with FASSc is significantly more difficult than that of FASSc alone. This is because there are no investigative tools capable of identifying early disease with the same degree of sensitivity as with FASSc. Local access to the vascular compartment does not have the advantage of a technique such as BAL, which samples the local inflammatory milieu.

Vasospasm in the pulmonary circulation may be important in the pathogenesis of pulmonary hypertension, but attempts to use the severity of attacks of "pulmonary vasospasm" as markers of subsequent pulmonary hypertension have not been successful. The occurrence of pulmonary Raynaud's in response to cold remains uncertain and there are conflicting reports in the literature (53). In patients with long-standing primary Raynaud's, the histopathological features of the digital arteries can resemble some of the changes seen in the vessels in scleroderma. A common mechanism is yet to be identified, but endothelial cell damage may be an early event (54).

The etiological factors involved in endothelial cell damage and subsequent microvascular obliteration have not been characterized. Proposed agents include granzymes, endothelial cell antibodies, activated adhesion molecules, and free radicals (55–58).

Consequences of endothelial cell perturbation may include loss of vasomotor control because of an excess production of endothelin or a diminished production and release of nitric oxide (NO), which is recognized as the endothelium-derived relaxing factor (59), and the release of other vasoactive mediators.

The potential for intervention in the course of pulmonary vessel pathology is demonstrated by a recent study which showed that, unlike patients with pulmonary hypertension occurring alone, there is significant improvement in pulmonary vascular resistance in response to increased inspired oxygen concentrations (798 ± 179 to 610 ± 152 dynes/s/cm^{-5} in SSc compared to 964 ± 80 to 852 ± 91 dynes/s/cm^{-5} in primary pulmonary hypertension) (60). The implication of this reversal of hypoxic vasoconstriction is that increased pulmonary vascular resistance is at least partly reversible and that further vessel insult may be avoided by appropriate therapy.

The most promising approach to pulmonary vessel disease is in the prediction of an "at-risk" group. Two studies have suggested that an HLA DR52 class II-linked haplotype may carry a poorer prognosis with regard to vessel disease, and that the association with DR52 (61,62) occurs in individuals with scleroderma and pulmonary hypertension. In addition, the observation of an increase in the prevalence of antinuclear antibodies (ANAs) (40% of 43 patients), particularly anti-Ku (23% of 33), in primary pulmonary hypertension in the absence of SSc would suggest an autoimmune (and possibly an immunogenetic) predisposition to this primary lung disorder. Pulmonary hypertension is found most frequently in patients with the limited form of SSc, 80% to 90% of whom carry anticentromere antibodies; although the presence of anticentromere antibody is associated with a decreased likelihood of fibrosing alveolitis, it is not predictive of the development of pulmonary hypertension (63,64).

Pathology

Most reports of lung pathology in SSc have been derived from post mortem studies that necessarily usually describe end-stage disease. Detailed description of ante mortem lung pathology has been restricted to a few patients and there is only one case report of lung ultrastructure (53,65).

The early descriptive post mortem work focused attention on two principal structures—the alveolar wall with the subsequent development of fibrosis and the pulmonary arterial tree with the establishment of the hypertensive lesion.

FIBROSIS

In established disease, the most common finding is bibasal interstitial fibrosis (66,67), which involves the acinar regions of the lung and the bronchioles. The fibrosing process envelopes local capillaries, producing an endarteritis in which the alveolar air spaces become distorted (68–70). Cysts are present predominantly in a subpleural location, and the overlying parietal pleura may be thickened and studded with inflammatory cells (71). Type II pneumocyte hyperplasia is seen and there is obliteration of the normal submucosal architecture. Inflammatory cells have also been observed in post mortem samples but were often thought to represent terminal pathological events, rather than the underlying primary condition (72). Alveolitis had been observed in earlier ante mortem studies, but it was uncertain as to whether the inflammatory cell infiltrate preceded, accompanied, or followed the fibrosis of the alveolar walls (20). More recent biopsy studies have confirmed that extensive inflammatory change is commonly seen (9). Pleural effusions missed in life are often present at autopsy.

The majority of studies of lung biopsies obtained from patients with SSc have focused on the fibrosing alveolitis variant at an advanced disease stage. It is now possible to detect early pulmonary change in SSc using high resolution CT. This provides an opportunity to examine lung biopsy changes at an earlier stage providing an insight into initiating and key events in pathogenesis. Our published paper described 49 open lung biopsies from 34 patients with interstitial lung disease, in many of whom the disease was at an early stage (Figs. 15.1, 15.2, and 15.3) (9). This study of the structural features of fibrosing alveolitis in SSc used high resolution CT scans to

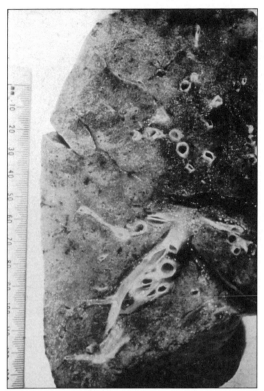

Figure 15.1. Autopsy lung from a patient with systemic sclerosis. Pale areas of sub-pleural interstitial fibrosis are seen especially in the posterior and diaphragmatic aspects of the lower lobe. (Courtesy of Professor B. Corrin, Royal Brompton Hospital.)

detect diffuse interstitial lung disease at an early stage. It included some patients with minimal or no chest radiographic and physiological abnormalities. What was striking about this subset of patients was the extent of pathological involvement in the lung even at this early stage (9,73).

In some samples there was minimal change. This allowed the examination of lung ultrastructure in SSc, with special reference to biopsies showing minimal change, anticipating that such changes might represent the earliest stages of the disease process. None of the patients in this study had clinically proven pulmonary hypertension. Biopsies were taken from the lower lobe in all patients; in 15 patients, a second biopsy was taken from the middle lobe. Examination of the lung

tissue by light microscopy showed the earliest changes to include an increase in macrophages together with occasional neutrophils, lymphocytes, and eosinophils in the intra alvcolar spaces, while lymphocytes and plasma cells were predominant in the interstitium and alveolar walls. However, fibroblasts and connective tissue matrix protein were also present, suggesting that these processes occur together from the earliest stages of the disease.

Alveolitis was not observed without fibrosis. Comparison of 22 biopsies from FASSc patients with biopsies from patients with CFA matched for age and sex, revealed no qualitative or quantitative differences other than a higher prevalence in the FASSc patients of focal lymphoid hyperplasia adjacent to bronchioles (23% and 5%, respectively). The pulmonary arteries of both groups showed fibrous thickening of the intima and medial hypertrophy. This was particularly evident in areas of marked fibrosis. No vascular abnormalities were seen where there was no parenchymal lung disease. Ultrastructural studies of 8 biopsies known to be abnormal on light microscopy showed evidence of endothelial injury together with interstitial edema and excess collagen deposition. Mast cells were occasionally in close contact with the interstitial fibroblasts. Of great interest was the fact that similar changes were seen in three biopsies that had appeared normal by light microscopy—the only observable ultrastructural difference was that these "normal" biopsies had less fibrosis and more edema than the abnormal ones. The lack of inflammatory cells in the biopsies does not favor alveolitis preceding structural damage, although it is possible that mediators released from inflammatory cells in adjacent parts of the lung could be responsible for the damage we observed. It was impossible, despite very careful observation, to determine whether endothelial or epithelial abnormalities predominated. Injury to capillary endothelial cells is likely to account for the interstitial edema and vascular leakage of proteins, including fibrinogen products. These mediators could act as potent fibroblast mitogens. The

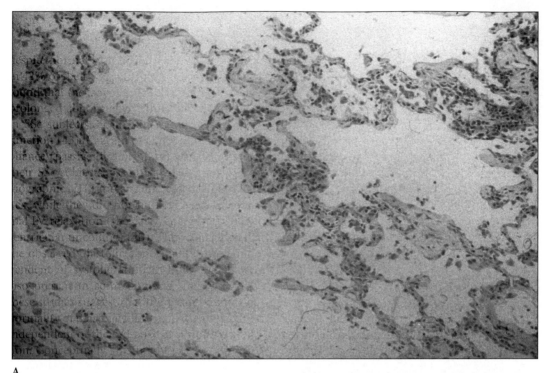

A

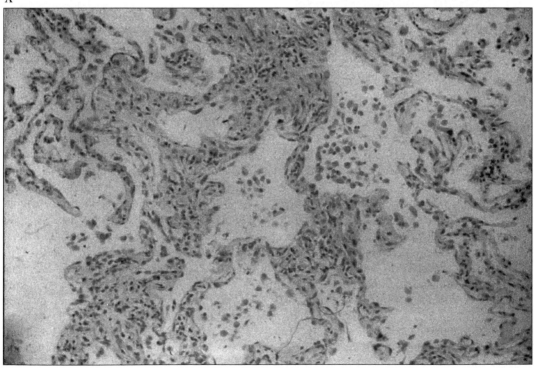

B

Figure 15.2. Varying degrees of fibrosing alveolitis in systemic sclerosis. Inflammatory activity persists throughout all stages of severity but is associated with increasing degrees of interstitial fibrosis: (*a*) mild disease,

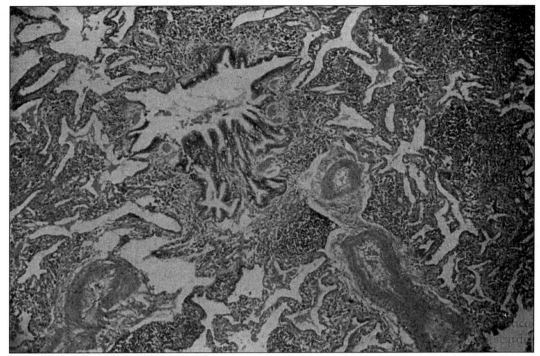

C

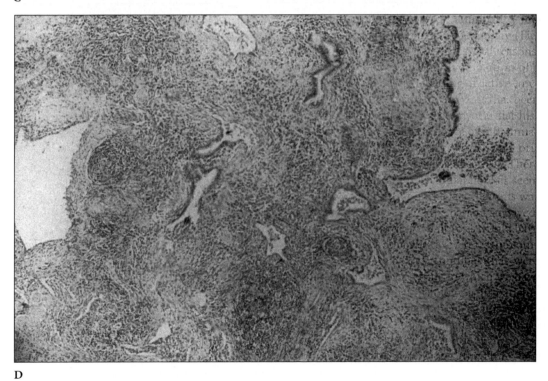

D

(*b*) moderate disease, (*c*) severe disease, (*d*) end stage disease in which there is complete loss of the alveolar architecture. (Courtesy of Professor B. Corrin, Royal Brompton Hospital.)

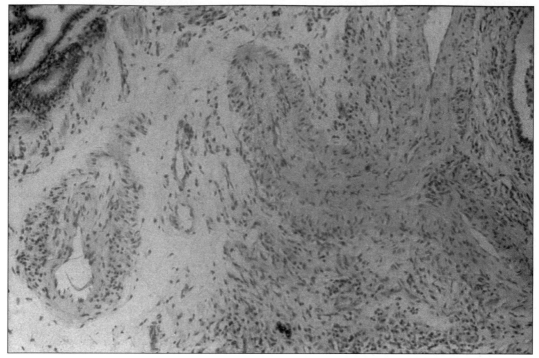

Figure 15.3. Pulmonary arterioles in fibrosing alveolitis. Note the marked medial hypertrophy and intimal fibrosis in the affected vessels (*arrows*). This change is limited to areas of the lung that show FA and does not necessarily indicate pulmonary hypertension. (Courtesy of Professor B. Corrin, Royal Brompton Hospital.)

occasional mast cells that were seen may also represent a further link between activated endothelial cells and fibroblasts: such a hypothesis has been suggested for the generation of skin fibrosis (74–76).

PULMONARY VASCULAR DISEASE

The vascular changes that lead to vessel obliteration consist of concentric intimal proliferation, medial hypertrophy, a variable degree of myxomatous degeneration, and marked perivascular fibrosis (66,77,78). The pulmonary arterioles bear the brunt of the disease, but vessels of all sizes can be involved (Fig. 15.4). Morphometric measurements performed on post mortem samples of pulmonary arteries from 58 patients with SSc and age, race, and sex-matched controls demonstrated that the area of the intima and percentage of luminal occlusion were greater in

SSc patients than in controls. As might be expected the greatest luminal occlusion was found in patients with limited cutaneous scleroderma, especially those who had clinical evidence of pulmonary arterial hypertension (79). Histological analysis of the pulmonary vascular tree in SSc reveals fibrinoid necrosis (present in primary pulmonary hypertension) and arteritis extremely rarely (69,80,81). As in other organs, the relationship between the fibrotic lesion and vascular pathology is unknown. Although it is possible to have severe vascular damage with little or no fibrosis, extensive fibrosis is almost always associated with vascular damage. The factors that determine the patient's pattern of pathological change are yet to be discovered. In view of the possibility of isolated vascular damage, the concept that fibrosis is always the initial event leading to vascular damage is hardly tenable. On the contrary, it is now known that immune (antibodies, T cells, adhesion molecules, granulocytes) or non-immune (toxins, chemicals, free radicals) factors influencing endothelial cell function and integrity may be the start of the process which leads to pulmonary fibrosis. Studies of the pathological appearances of lungs at an advanced stage of the disease process shed no light on the pathogenesis.

Clinical Features

The clinical symptoms and signs of pulmonary disease in scleroderma are summarized in Table 15.2. Symptoms are few and often undramatic, with a dissociation between the clinical features and evidence of the disease obtained by pathological and radiological investigation and pulmonary function tests. Some patients may have no symptoms of shortness of breath or cough, no radiological change, and normal lung function tests, and yet be found on high resolution CT scans or lung biopsy to have changes in the lung parenchyma. The reason for this is that the lungs have considerable reserve capacity: it is only when extensive disease is present that abnormalities on more routine investigations, such as chest radiography, become apparent. Symptoms occur at a very late stage of the natural history of the disease process and often as much as one third to one half of the lung may be involved before symptoms are present. The great advantage to the patient of presenting with disease outside the lung is that lung damage can be identified at an early stage because we are specifically looking for it, having been alerted to the possibility by the

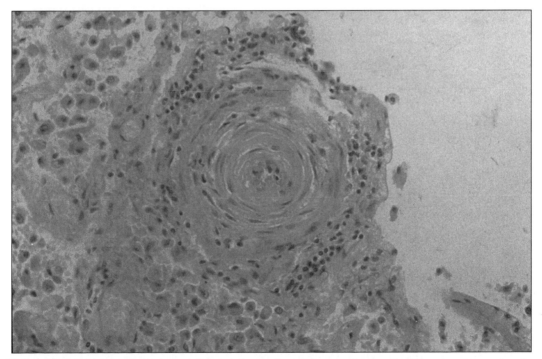

Figure 15.4. Primary pulmonary vessel disease in a patient with systemic sclerosis. Pulmonary artery showing marked lamellar intimal thickening ("onion skinning"). In primary pulmonary hypertension in SSc, these vascular changes occur in the absence of interstitium pulmonary inflammation or fibrosis. (Courtesy of Professor B. Corrin, Royal Brompton Hospital.)

Table 15.2. Pulmonary Disease in Systemic Sclerosis

Disorder	Symptoms	Signs	Specific Investigations	Therapeutic Possibilities
Pulmonary fibrosis	Dry cough Dyspnea	Reduced chest expansion Basal crackles	CXR, PFTs High resolution CT scan DTPA scan Bronchoalveolar lavage Lung biopsy	Steroids $+/-$ Cyclophosphamide Azathioprine D-penicillamine Cyclosporin α-interferon

Pulmonary vascular disease	Dyspnea	Loud P_2
		Right ventricular heave
		
		Right heart failure
			CXR
			Doppler
			
			Echocardiography
			  (cardiac catheter)
				Prostacyclin
				Nifedipine
				  (calcium channel-blocker)
				?ACE inhibitor
				?Warfarin
				Transplant

Rare Complications: Aspiration pneumonia: antibiotics
  Lung carcinoma: chemotherapy or radiotherapy
  Surgery: not usually an option

presence of extrapulmonary disease. Unfortunately, in many instances patients with scleroderma often have limited physical activity for reasons other than lung disease, which reduces the chances of symptomatic lung disease being identified early. However, the division of SSc into diffuse cutaneous (dcSSc) and limited cutaneous disease (lcSSc) permits rational monitoring and investigation of these subgroups. Diffuse cutaneous disease is often characterized by speedy internal organ involvement, early pulmonary fibrosis, and subsequent secondary pulmonary hypertension. Limited cutaneous disease often has a slowly progressive course with primary pulmonary hypertension appearing after 10 years of disease; pulmonary fibrosis, if present, often proceeds at an indolent rate.

FIBROSING ALVEOLITIS IN SSC (FASSC)

The most frequently noted respiratory symptom in this group of patients is dyspnea (65,82). It occurred in an average of 55% of 323 patients in 11 series (range 21%–80%) (53). It is usually first demonstrated on exertion, and only later evident at rest. Dyspnea is unfortunately not an early warning sign (83), as there are patients (particularly in the diffuse scleroderma group) who have no pulmonary symptoms but have objective evidence of established lung disease. Contrary to earlier reports (81,84), dyspnea does not necessarily predict a rapid downhill course in interstitial lung disease, and many patients are stable without significant deterioration in lung function (85). However, a small group of patients, as yet impossible to predict, progress to develop aggressive pulmonary fibrosis with dyspnea at rest, hypoxia, secondary pulmonary hypertension, right heart failure, and cardiorespiratory failure, which rapidly leads to death.

The cause of the dyspnea in fibrosing alveolitis is probably multi-factorial. Ventilation/perfusion mismatch is the major pulmonary physiological abnormality producing approximately 80% of the increase in alveolar-arterial (A-a) pO_2 gradient (86,87). A recent study has suggested that failure of the circulatory system is the limiting factor for exercise in SSc (88). Loss of compliance triggers stretch receptors, which results in reflex hyperpnea which adds to the sensation of breathlessness because of the thickened interstitium (89,90).

Pulmonary vascular change (78) is reflected in a reduced gas transfer measurement (carbon monoxide transfer factor or DLCO), particularly when corrected for alveolar volume (K_{co}), and contributes to dyspnea, as must the less common pleural disease, myocardial involvement, or chest wall thickening (91,92), which is a less common pleural disease. Although, when dyspnea is present, some form of pathology is expected and inevitably found if investigated with the appropriate tools, there is a poor correlation among symptoms, chest x-ray, and pulmonary function tests (93–95).

Cough is a less frequently reported symptom. It is usually non-productive (68,96) and, when persistent and refractory, is usually found in patients with severe pulmonary fibrosis. A productive and purulent cough reflects more advanced disease, when distortion of the alveolar and bronchiolar architecture gives rise to infection and pooling of secretions (97,98). Aspiration pneumonia should also be considered (see discussion later in this chapter). Hemoptysis is rare but raises four possibilities: an associated carcinoma, bronchial telangiectasia (99), hemoptysis and pulmonary hypertension in the setting of normotensive renal crises with micro-angiopathic hemolytic anemia and thrombocytopenia (100), or diffuse alveolar hemorrhage. Chest pain is uncommon but is usually the result of pleural or pericardial disease (66,72,80). Rarely, pneumothorax may be a complication of peripheral cystic changes.

The most commonly reported physical finding related to pulmonary interstitial involvement is bilateral basal fine inspiratory crackles (93). Other signs include pleural friction rubs (84), restrictive chest expansion, increased respiratory rate, and signs of pleural effusion. Digital clubbing is almost never observed, with a much lower frequency than when it is associated with either "lone" fibrosing alveolitis or other interstitial disease. The reasons suggested for this much lower frequency include poor peripheral microcirculation and almost universal sclerodactyly. It is also well documented that pulmonary disease may occur before or without the subsequent onset of skin changes, when it is known as scleroderma sine scleroderma. Unlike other forms of scleroderma, this occurs more frequently in males. The features that distinguish this group of patients from those with cryptogenic fibrosing alveolitis include the presence of Raynaud's phenomenon, scleroderma-related antibodies, abnormal nailfold capillary microscopy, esophageal dysmotility, and a time course which is usually slower than the more rapid decline of cryptogenic fibrosing alveolitis. The presence of any of these features in a patient who has hitherto been labeled as having cryptogenic fibrosing alveolitis should suggest a revision of that diagnosis. This is of particular importance because the prognosis is better if fibrosing alveolitis occurs in the presence of SSc, although patients who present with their lung disease before any other features of scleroderma have a worse prognosis than patients whose extra-pulmonary disease provide the presenting features.

Interestingly, when matched with patients suffering from cryptogenic fibrosing alveolitis for severity of gas transfer impairment, prognosis was better in SSc when total gas transfer was used as the index of comparison; however, prognosis was identical to cryptogenic fibrosing alveolitis when gas transfer corrected for alveolar volume (K_{co}) was the defining index (101).

PULMONARY ARTERIAL HYPERTENSION

Pulmonary hypertension (PHT) is a well recognized and often deadly complication of SSc. It occurs most frequently as an isolated event (89, 102,103) in limited cutaneous disease but also occurs secondary to pulmonary fibrosis in dcSSc. It is often a silent danger for many years, representing "on-going" arterial damage (104) (see below) only to present in the middle to late stages of lcSSc with a sudden onset of dyspnea. In the later stages of pulmonary fibrosis, PHT is associated with right heart failure (70,102). It may also occur secondary to pulmonary fibrosis. The frequency of pulmonary hypertension varies from study to study (11%–80%) (89,105,106) and depends on the methods used to delicate it. Noninvasion methods of estimating frequency are obviously not as sensitive as catheter studies. In three series of scleroderma patients undergoing cardiac catheterization (89,105,106), minimal

PHT was observed in many of them. As there was no follow-up, it is not known if all patients with PHT have progressive disease or if some remain stable (cf. the patients with stable pulmonary fibrosis and a relatively good prognosis). Although dyspnea is the most common symptom of scleroderma patients with PHT, up to one third may be asymptomatic. Physical findings may include a prominent a-wave in the jugular venous pulse, a loud pulmonary component of S2, and a right ventricular S4. These findings in isolation are unfortunately not very sensitive detectors (105). To date there are no predictors of PHT other than its association with lcSSc. The anticentromere antibody, which is closely associated with limited cutaneous scleroderma, is not an additional marker predicting the development of PHT within this group. This contrasts with the association of Scl-70 antibodies and the development of pulmonary fibrosis in diffuse disease (11).

OTHER PULMONARY COMPLICATIONS

Carcinoma of the Lung

Patients with scleroderma have an increased risk of lung cancer. Estimates of the number who will develop the complication vary but have been as high as 21% (98,107,108). All cell types have been reported. Cancer is associated with lung fibrosis. In a study of 680 scleroderma patients (109), 62% of the patients with pulmonary cancer had clinical evidence of parenchymal fibrosis. This association between excess cancers and fibrosis has also been shown in CFA and in asbestosis, where the excess risk of carcinoma occurs in relation to the presence of fibrosis (110–112). It was in 1956 that Spencer and Raeburn (113) pointed out the proliferation of cells of the terminal bronchiolar epithelium and showed that bronchiolar adenomatosis may occur as a reaction to fibrosis. Type II pneumocyte proliferation is a prominent feature of the alveolar walls in scleroderma lung. Taken together with an altered immune state and the presence of growth factors within the local microenvironment, this may predispose to the development of a malignancy. Lung cancer may also precede scleroderma or occur almost simultaneously in the absence of pulmonary fibrosis, giving rise to the suggestion of a pan-neoplastic event in a small number of individuals.

Aspiration Pneumonia

Scleroderma patients have abnormal esophageal function, which can result in aspiration of gastric contents and thus in aspiration pneumonia (98, 114,115). It has also been suggested that there is a distinct correlation between diffuse pulmonary disease and reflux, and that aggressive anti-reflux therapy may reduce the pulmonary damage owing to reflux in these patients (116).

Work-Related Scleroderma Lung Disease

There are many reports in the literature of scleroderma occurring in workers who are exposed to silica dust. The work of Erasmus, in 1957 (117), and Rodnan, in 1967 (118), showed that the prevalence of scleroderma in coal miners who were exposed to quartz exceeded that of the general population. Scleroderma was found in 17 of 100,000 hospital discharges in miners, compared to 6 in 100,000 discharges in nonminers. The presentation of and clinical and pathological features seen in these silica-exposed patients strikingly resembles the idiopathic disease. Other agents, such as vinyl chloride-related solvents, adulterated rapeseed oil, and L-tryptophan, can induce lung disease that resembles the changes seen in pulmonary scleroderma (119–122). (see Chapter 5 for a full discussion).

Respiratory Failure From Muscle Disease

This is rare, but there are several discrete cases related to chest wall involvement (91,92,123). It is difficult to establish whether this is the result of primary muscle disease, or is secondary to loss of respiratory drive. In at least one reported case (92), and in one of our own patients, response to steroids was notable. It may therefore be important to detect this type of respiratory failure early.

Rarely, respiratory failure may result from pronounced thoracic skin sclerosis. In one patient known to us, this resulted in type 2 respiratory failure with hypercapnia. In this individual, treatment with nocturnal nasal continuous positive airway pressure improved his resting carbon monoxide tensions and also his symptoms. One may speculate that this improvement was due to stretching of the cutaneous thickening, although such a change has not been demonstrated (personal observation).

Clues that extrapulmonary restriction are contributing to respiratory abnormalities on lung function are the presence of a high or inappropriately normal gas transfer measurement corrected for alveolar volume (K_{co}). Usually, in diffuse pulmonary disease and also pulmonary disease due to pulmonary vessel abnormalities, both the DLCO and the K_{co} are reduced. Pulmonary restriction caused by extrapulmonary factors, however, results in an increased K_{co} due to a disproportionately high blood flow for lungs that are being squeezed by extrathoracic abnormalities ("soggy sponge" effect).

Pulmonary Hemorrhage

Pulmonary hemorrhage has been reported to occur in scleroderma associated with renal disease (including Goodpasture syndrome) (53) and in scleroderma patients with normotensive renal crisis (84). As Goodpasture syndrome may be induced by D-penicillamine, a drug frequently used in scleroderma, a careful drug history must always be taken. Alveolar hemorrhage may also be present as part of the disease process.

CHILDHOOD SCLERODERMA AND PULMONARY DISEASE

Diffuse SSc is extremely rare in childhood. While the manifestations of lung disease in children are similar to those of affected adults, the disease often seems even more occult in childhood, with very few clinical manifestations but a high frequency of abnormal pulmonary function tests (124,125). Progression may be minimal or slow, but in a subgroup, as in the adult population, the

progress is rapid with early cardiopulmonary failure.

PROGNOSIS IN SYSTEMIC SCLEROSIS

It is difficult to give patients accurate information on the prognosis of scleroderma lung disease, with the exception of symptomatic isolated PHT. Sadly, in the latter case the prognosis is all too certain, with almost inevitable continued deterioration and death within 5 years. Our studies, and those of other investigators, have shown that patients who have a severely reduced K_{co} at presentation have a poor prognosis (101,126). Patients with PHT secondary to severe pulmonary fibrosis also have a decreased survival. For the remaining patients, the picture is less clear. Decline in diffusion capacity and/or progression of restrictive disease has been reported in several studies, with most authors considering the decline to be slow and gradual (78,96,126–128). More optimistically, some authors report that any changes seen occur at no greater rate than in a normal population (129,130). Colp et al considered that the pulmonary involvement occurs at a set point in time and then remains stable (131). Steen et al traced 48 patients over a 5-year period with little change in diffusion capacity or vital capacity (132). There is, however, a small group of patients in whom there is a rapid downhill course that is comparable to CFA (101,133), and some authors report that being male is an adverse prognostic feature (126,134). Added to these variables is the reported association by Peters-Golden (129) of severe Raynaud's portending a rapid deterioration, and the not unexpected finding by Steen et al (84) that smoking had an additional deleterious effect on lung function in scleroderma. A more recent study compared the prognosis of patients suffering from fibrosing alveolitis in SSc with patients in the same institution who suffer from cryptogenic fibrosing alveolitis (101). Sixty-eight patients with SSc were compared with 205 patients with cryptogenic fibrosing alveolitis. The outcome of patients presenting during the 10-year period from 1979 through 1989 was evaluated. During this period, 142 patients died from their cryptogenic fibrosing alveolitis, whereas only 11 had died from their fibrosing alveolitis in SSc. Survival from the time of presentation was lower in cryptogenic fibrosing alveolitis (odds ratio 3.3) even after adjustment for the age at presentation, smoking history, and the severity of lung function abnormalities at presentation. This indicates that even when corrections are made for the severity of the disease process at presentation, the natural history of scleroderma-associated fibrosing alveolitis is quite different from that of cryptogenic fibrosing alveolitis.

INVESTIGATIONS

Blood Tests

Routine blood tests are of little value in the assessment of fibrosing alveolitis in SSc. In severe cases, secondary polycythemia may be observed and a high neutrophil count may indicate superadded infection. Corticosteroid therapy may elevate total white count to 13 or $14 \times 10^9/1$, or even higher.

Raised levels of one or more classes of immunoglobulins, particularly IgG and IgM, may be seen. The presence of an anti-centromere antibody is found in 80% to 90% of patients with limited disease. This is more likely to be associated with primary pulmonary vascular disease. Scl-70 is more prevalent in diffuse disease (20%–40%) and is more likely to be present when pulmonary fibrosis exists (135–137).

Radiology

Chest Radiography. A typical chest radiograph of a patient with fibrosing alveolitis and SSc is characterized by small lung fields and reticulonodular shadowing. These occur particularly at the periphery of the lung and at the bases, obscuring the right and left heart borders and making the diaphragmatic surfaces irregular. Even in more subtle examples of fibrosing alveolitis, this distribution of radiographic abnormality should suggest the diagnosis. In more advanced cases, all lung zones are involved, at which point evidence of honeycomb shadowing may be present (138).

The chest radiograph may often be normal or present a diffuse "ground-glass" pattern. This pattern is highly suggestive of a more cellular pathological process and is the typical finding in the desquamative interstitial pneumonia form of diffuse lung disease (139); it is rarely seen in SSc. Lymphadenopathy is rarely observed with chest radiography but the presence of pleural disease may be noted. Cryptogenic organizing pneumonitis may be observed in SSc. The radiographic features are those of consolidation, which may be patchy and bilateral and are usually in a peripheral distribution (140–142). Cardiomegaly and prominent pulmonary arteries indicate secondary PHT.

High Resolution Computed Tomography. The use of high resolution computed tomography (CT) during the last 5 years has revolutionized the approach to diffuse lung disease (143–146). The pattern of abnormality may be characteristic in several diffuse lung diseases. For fibrosing alveolitis (either cryptogenic or FASSc), the pattern is virtually pathognomonic. The typical early change is of a peripheral rim of increased attenuation present posteriorly at the bases. As disease becomes more extensive, these changes are observed in the other lung zones and more centrally. A "ground-glass" pattern of opacification on CT is associated with a predominantly cellular biopsy, whereas a reticular pattern of abnormality is found in patients whose subsequent lung biopsy confirms a particularly fibrotic disease process (147,148) (Fig. 15.5). We have performed a semiquantitative comparison

Figure 15.5. (*a*) Computed tomography of a patient with cellular histology. Note the bilateral peripheral rim of "ground glass" attenuation in both lung fields. (*b*) Computed tomography of a patient with FASSc illustrating a more reticular pattern of abnormality in both peripheral lung fields associated with predominantly fibrotic change on lung biopsy.

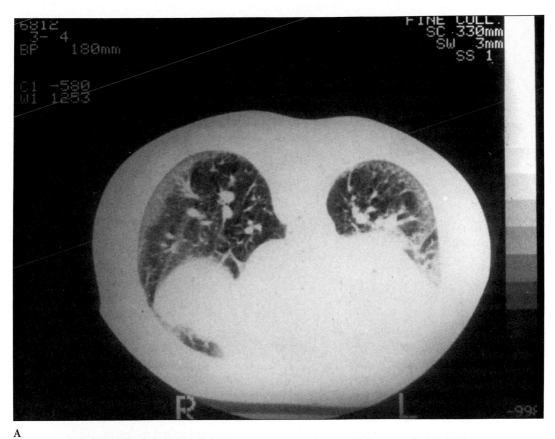

A

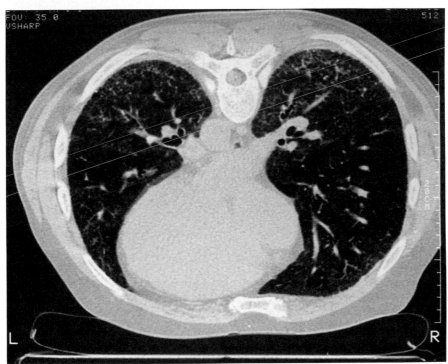

B

of the predictive value of these CT appearances. In 12 out of 13 instances, a reticular pattern was found to accurately predict predominantly fibrotic histology. A slightly lower accuracy (4 out of 7 correct predictions) was found when a "ground-glass" pattern predicted at least equivalent amounts of fibrosis and cellularity (147) (Table 15-3). This discrepancy may have occurred for two reasons. First, the presence of fine fibrosis beyond the resolution of the CT scanner would be missed. However, perhaps it is more likely that the overall scoring of relative degrees of cellularity and fibrosis was made on the basis of the whole CT, whereas the biopsy samples only a small peripheral part of the lung. This raises the question of which is the most appropriate "gold standard" investigation. Until this becomes clearer, patients who appear to have some cellularity on CT should still undergo a biopsy procedure for staging of the disease (see below) so that prognosis and better treatment strategies can be designed. CT confirms that pleural disease may be present. In contrast to the observation on plain chest radiography, mediastinal lymphadenopathy is commonly present. A dilated esophagus may also be seen.

Particularly in more subtle cases, it is important to perform both prone and supine scans to exclude the contribution of gravity to the radiographic appearances, resulting in vascular and interstitial pooling in the dependent areas.

Several studies have shown that high resolution CT scanning can identify disease before the chest radiograph has become abnormal (18, 149–152) (Fig. 15.6). In addition to identifying early disease, high resolution CT scanning can identify a disease pattern that predicts a better response to therapy and a better prognosis (151). Furthermore, the extent of disease present, defined by CT within the lavage lobe, correlates with the predominant type of inflammatory cell obtained by BAL of that same lobe—lymphocytes are present in excess before CT identifies disease, eosinophils appear as the lung becomes abnormal, and neutrophils are found in most abundance when at least 50% of the lavage lobe is involved in the disease process. That is, the predominant type of inflammatory cell traffic into the lungs depends upon disease extent. This would suggest that different inflammatory cells are involved in different stages of disease pathogenesis.

CT can also be used to exclude significant lung inflammation or fibrosis in patients with an isolated deficit in gas transfer. This situation would suggest a primary pulmonary vascular disease process rather than fibrosing alveolitis. Also, a pattern of consolidation seen on CT may suggest cryptogenic organizing pneumonitis.

Radionuclide Imaging

Ventilation/Perfusion Scans. Ventilation/perfusion scans show mismatching of perfusion to ventilation in fibrosing alveolitis. This probably reflects damage to the pulmonary vascular bed and means that ventilation/perfusion imaging is unreliable in excluding thromboembolic disease in both FA and FASSc. This is important because there is an increased incidence of pulmonary embolus in fibrosing alveolitis (although this has

Table 15.3. The Role of CT in Systemic Sclerosis

	Ground-Glass Opacification = Reticular Changes	Predominant Reticular Change
Prediction of biopsy appearances		
Predominant inflammation in lung biopsy	4/7	1/13
Predominant fibrosis in biopsy	3/7	12/13
Prediction of response to therapy		
Response to treatment	5/11	2/13
Decline in lung function or death within 1 year	0/11	3/13

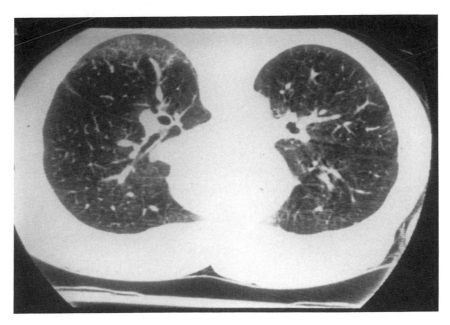

Figure 15.6. High resolution computed tomography of a patient with fibrosing alveolitis in systemic sclerosis (FASSc) but with a normal chest radiograph. Note that there is already a peripheral rim of increased attenuation in both lung fields (*arrows*) and that this is asymmetrical with the predominant abnormality being present in the left lung. This pattern of ground glass opacification is consistent with a more cellular biopsy appearance.

not been demonstrated in FASSc); the diagnosis of pulmonary embolus will therefore rely on the clinical features, identification of the venous source of emboli, and, in some instances, pulmonary angiography to identify proximal embolic lesions.

Gallium Scanning. Gallium scanning has been used to identify the presence of diffuse lung disease in many disorders, including SSc (20,21), and has been considered to be a marker of "activity." It is a highly sensitive test but is not specific, being positive in a wide range of diffuse processes that involve macrophage activation. In the presence of defined disease, however, gallium scanning adds nothing to the information obtained using other tests.

In attempts to measure degrees of activity, there have been reports of quantification of gallium uptake into the lungs in diffuse lung disease. These measurements are not universally reliable, and the test involves expensive isotope and requires the patient to visit the hospital on two oc-

casions—one visit for intravenous isotope administration and a second visit 2 to 3 days later to scan the lungs. Gallium scanning is not recommended for the evaluation of established fibrosing alveolitis in SSc (153,154).

^{99m}Tc-diethylinetriamine Pentacetate (DTPA). Other techniques of radionuclide imaging have been the subject of research (155,156). Of these, the clearance from the lung of inhaled ^{99m}Tc-diethylinetriamine pentacetate (DTPA) has been shown to be of value. The DTPA technique identifies early disease and also identifies a group of patients whose disease will run a more stable, non-progressive course, i.e., those with normal clearance (Fig. 15.7) (157,158). The speed of clearance of isotope depends upon the integrity of the epithelial barrier; therefore anything that disrupts this barrier, either inflammation or fibrosis, will increase the rate of clearance (159,160). DTPA clearance is highly sensitive: cigarette smoking produces increased clearance rates, thus the test is only of value in non-smok-

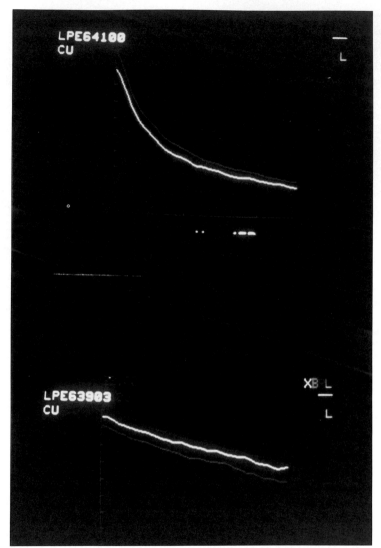

Figure 15.7. ^{99m}Tc-DTPA scans from a patient with FASSc (*left*) and a normal individual (*right*). Note that the rate of decline of isotope from both lungs of the patient with FASSc is biexponential in pattern with a more rapid initial phase. By contrast, the rate of decline of isotope from the lung of the normal individual is monoexponential and much slower than in the patient with lung fibrosis.

ers or those who have given up smoking for at least 1 month prior to assessment (160,161).

The role of DTPA in the management of SSc has been the subject of extensive study. Clearance of DTPA may be abnormal even when chest radiography and pulmonary function tests are normal (73). In established disease, clearance is en-

hanced in comparison with normal individuals (158). Furthermore, speed of clearance and change in clearance can predict subsequent pulmonary function test changes. Patients whose clearance is persistently abnormal are more likely to have a deterioration in pulmonary function tests at follow-up subsequent to the DTPA measurements. In contrast, persistently normal DTPA clearance predicts stable disease and therefore provides a good prognostic index. Significant improvement in pulmonary function tests occurred in six out of eight patients whose clearance returned to the normal range, whereas similar improvements were not seen in patients whose clearance remained normal or abnormally fast (158) (Table 15.4).

Lung Function Tests

Fibrosing alveolitis occurring alone or in the presence of SSc is characterized by a restrictive ventilatory defect of mechanical function resulting in reduced pulmonary compliance, vital capacity, and total lung capacity. Residual volume is usually decreased, unless there is coincident airflow obstruction caused by cigarette smoking, and lung recoil pressure is increased (87).

Carbon monoxide transfer factor (DLCO), which is a measure of diffusion capacity, is reduced and may be the only abnormality in early disease (162). In the majority of patients the gas transfer measurement adjusted for alveolar volume (K_{co}) is also reduced. This means that the total gas transfer depression is not purely attributable to a loss of lung volume, but rather that the capacity to exchange gas is impaired in the remaining lung.

Typical blood gas measurements will reveal a reduced PaO_2 value with a normal or low $PaCO_2$ measurement. In more advanced cases, the $PaCO_2$ will be reduced because of the increase in ventilatory drive in a patient with severe lung stiffening due to fibrosis. In terminal stages the $paCO_2$ may rise. The low PaO_2 is largely attributable to ventilation/perfusion mismatching. On exercise, hypoxemia is exacerbated and a widening of the A-a gradient is observed. Infrequently, abnormalities on exercise testing are the only physiological abnormalities; usually, by the time the patient seeks advice, there is already some abnormality in the gas transfer measurement at rest.

In a small percentage of patients, there is evidence of airflow obstruction on routine lung function assessment (94,124,127). Pulmonary function abnormalities thought to be representative of "silent" small airways disease have been seen in 15% to 42% of cases (94,127,163,164). However, the diagnosis of small airways abnormalities was based on flow rates at low lung volumes; these series lack normal control subjects and therefore the conclusions must be interpreted with caution. With the use in another series of more sophisticated lung function testing, isolated small airways abnormalities were not seen in SSc, except in smokers (165).

Similarly, abnormalities in gas transfer must be interpreted with caution. Any abnormality in "effective pulmonary blood flow" will affect the measurement of gas transfer. In SSc, in contrast to other diffuse lung diseases, there may exist a primary pulmonary vascular disease process either alone or in addition to the diffuse fibrosing process present in the lung interstitium. Thus, interpretation of isolated abnormalities in gas transfer could be due to either of these processes. It is particularly important that any follow-up studies should be done in the same laboratory

Table 15.4. ^{99m}Tc DTPA as a Predictor of Change in Pulmonary Function in Systemic Sclerosis

	n	Decline in Pulmonary Function
DTPA at presentation		
Rapid DTPA clearance at presentation	37	12
Normal DTPA clearance at presentation	16	0
Serial DTPA		
Persistently abnormal clearance	25	8
Persistently normal DTPA clearance	11	0
Abnormal DTPA clearance reverting to normal	5	0

with good quality control, because diffusion capacity is a measurement that may show a high coefficient of variation.

A severe depression in gas transfer measurement indicates an extremely poor prognosis. Patients whose gas transfer is less than approximately 50% at presentation are more likely to be dead within 5 years than those whose gas transfer is above this cut-off point (101). The same observation is true for gas transfer corrected for alveolar volume (K_{co}). Lung function measurements should be made sequentially to assess the progression of the disease process. Vital capacity and gas transfer measurements will usually suffice, and it is usually unnecessary to perform exercise tests as monitors of change in disease. Spirometry alone is inadequate for monitoring change. It is often sensible to plot out serial lung function studies in order to visualize more gradual change that may be missed if results are compared only with the previous set of measurements. In general, decline of pulmonary function to death is less sharp than in cryptogenic fibrosing alveolitis (101). However, severe lung disease may occur and rates of change should be monitored individually.

Bronchoalveolar Lavage

The use of bronchoalveolar lavage (BAL) to sample cells and non-cellular material from the lower respiratory tract has now been used for almost 20 years in the evaluation of diffuse lung disease. Initial hopes that this would provide an alternative to lung biopsy with high specificity for diagnosis have not been realized. There is still, however, a place for BAL in the evaluation of diffuse lung disease. The presence of abnormal numbers of granulocytes, particularly neutrophils and eosinophils (73,166,167), is typical for a patient with fibrosing alveolitis occurring alone or in the context of SSc. Excess lymphocytes are found in some individuals. In a typical patient with fibrosing alveolitis, BAL would show an increase in total cell returns of three- to six-fold (up to 6×10^5/ml of fluid return); of these, up to 20% may be neutrophils or eosinophils. Excess lym-

phocytes may be found (up to 20% of the total cells), and an increase in mast cells may be observed in a small percentage of patients (19,20, 31,168).

The predominant inflammatory cell provides a useful indication of the extent of the underlying disease process (see previous section on CT). Wells et al (169) have shown that the extent of lung disease in a single lobe, as defined by CT, correlates with the profile of inflammatory cells obtained from the same lobe. Miller et al (167) showed that an "active alveolitis," defined as the percent of total granulocytes (eosinophils and neutrophils) that is greater than the mean ± 2SD of the control population, in one lung site was accompanied in 15 of 17 instances by "active alveolitis" at a second site.

Lavage differential cell counts are also of value prognostically. The presence of excess granulocytes was associated with greater impairment of lung function in one study (166), but alveolitis may be present in individuals with normal chest radiography and pulmonary function tests (73,170). An excess of neutrophils is associated with an increased likelihood of disease progression if the alveolitis persists (166) and, in one retrospective (but uncontrolled) study, a decreased likelihood of response to treatment (171). Serial BAL is unhelpful as a monitor of disease and should be reserved for research purposes, although one study has shown that a persistent alveolitis was associated with lung function deterioration (166).

Lung Biopsy

The only lung biopsy technique that provides useful information is open lung biopsy, either through mini-thoracotomy or video-assisted thoracoscopic biopsy (172). Transbronchial biopsy is generally unhelpful: the samples are small, adequate samples being obtained in only approximately 35% of instances, and do not allow an assessment to be made of the relative degrees of cellularity and fibrosis (173). This comparison is important in assessing the likely response to treatment. A trephine drill biopsy technique has been used in the past in some units but it has now fallen into disuse (174). A "trucut" biopsy is hazardous, because it carries the risk of uncontrolled hemorrhage and air leak.

The more open approaches have the advantage of sampling lung that is clearly abnormal (175). The specificity of this approach can be improved further when CT images are used to guide the surgeon to the relevant sites (144,172,176). The surgeon may sample one or more sites, and the biopsy can be divided into parts that will be stored, if necessary, for immunohistochemical, molecular, and electron microscopical analysis, in addition to the more routine histological evaluation.

Not all patients need to undergo lung biopsy. Extensive disease, which is predominantly reticular on high resolution CT scanning, requires no biopsy confirmation especially in patients whose respiratory reserve is low. On the other hand, where there is "ground-glass" pattern, (suggesting a more cellular disease) biopsy is recommended to confirm the relative degrees of cellularity and fibrosis, because CT prediction is not as precise as it is with the predominantly reticular pattern. Furthermore, in a younger patient in whom prolonged potent therapy is being planned, it is very important to have all of the information available on which to make precise treatment judgments.

Pulmonary Vascular Investigations

All patients who attend our Units have an initial evaluation of their cardiovascular status using ECG, echocardiogram and, if necessary, right heart catheterization studies. A recent study from our Units has shown that echocardiography can accurately predict PHT, as subsequently confirmed by right heart catheterization (177). If a measurement of pressures can be estimated (i.e., in the presence of tricuspid regurgitation which allows a measurement of the gradient across the valve), there is excellent correlation with catheter values, and the need for invasive pressure measurements is now restricted to those patients whose echo measurements are borderline. However, in another study (105) utilizing right heart catheterization, only 67% of patients were correctly identified non-invasively using a range of techniques including echocardiography. In this study, a gas transfer below 43% predicted was the most sensitive predictor of PHT. In addition, the gas transfer measurement is a measurement of pulmonary vascular bed damage, especially if an abnormality occurs in the absence of any changes in lung volumes. In a study of 20 patients who were found at cardiac catheterization to have PHT, all had a reduction in DLCO (mean value 39% normal). Six of 20 had reduction in DLCO 1 to 6 years before clinical evidence of disease, and the 2-year survival in the group was 40% (103). Our studies have confirmed the severely worse prognosis in those patients with reduced gas transfer (101). A K_{co} of less than 50% of predicted was associated with a 2-year survival of approximately 40%, compared with a 95% survival if K_{co} is greater than 50% predicted. It is vital to be aware of early PHT, either occurring alone or in the presence of pulmonary fibrosis, because this predicts a worse prognosis and therefore indicates the need for a more aggressive treatment policy. Successful treatment strategies have still to be devised for pulmonary vessel disease and prospective controlled studies of treatment response and outcome measurements are needed.

Treatment

There is no sound evidence that any therapeutic agent used in pulmonary scleroderma has significantly altered its course: no controlled trials have been performed to date and these are urgently needed. This may be due either to the ineffectiveness of currently available drugs, or to the fact that scleroderma is a spectrum of disease. Pulmonary SSc has a variable rate of progression and pulmonary involvement has hitherto usually been identified at an established or late stage. Furthermore, the treatments used have been given for a variable length of time in an uncontrolled way to poorly stratified groups of patients. Most studies of treatment have been anecdotal, retrospective, or uncontrolled. Now that there is the potential (with the use of HRCT scans, DTPA imaging, and BAL) to recognize early inflammatory disease and predict outcome, prospective studies are urgently needed to analyze new agents and to establish the correct role for those already in use. The seeming lack of efficacy of our present therapies may be due to the timing of administration and the failure to use them in early disease. Once extensive lung damage and fibrosis are present, the best "response" to treatment that can be expected in many patients is a stabilization of disease progression; significant improvement in lung function indices will not be obtained at this advanced stage. However, stabilization must not be regarded as "failed treatment." Nowhere in scleroderma is early diagnosis and prevention more essential than in the lung.

The therapeutic strategies that have been used in the past include a bewildering array of agents. Para-aminobenzoic acid (82), colchicine (178), disodium EDTA (179), methysergide (72), and chlorambucil (86) have produced no improvement in pulmonary function. D-penicillamine (DP), a drug with immunosuppressive properties and an inhibitor of both collagen synthesis and cross-linking, has been used since 1961. There are at least five retrospective studies from three centers showing some benefit with this agent, some over a lengthy period of treatment (93,132, 180–182). The major improvement observed was an improvement or stabilization of DLCO. For example Steen et al (132) found that long-term therapy was associated with a significant increase in DLCO: predicted values rose from 76% to 87% among the treated group in comparison to controls (from 76% to 79%). This study and other studies showed no improvement in forced vital capacity (FVC). A D-penicillamine study monitoring response to treatment using changes in BAL as a response measure showed a decline in BAL lymphocyte content and an improvement in alveolitis (21). Clearly, the use of D-penicillamine

needs to be more completely defined, and controlled clinical trials are currently under way.

Probably the most widely used therapeutic agent in pulmonary SSc has been corticosteroids. A large volume of evidence would suggest a lack of success with the drug (20,67,72,183). However, an almost equally impressive literature indicates its therapeutic usefulness (96, 184,185). It is possible that it is best used in combination with cyclophosphamide (171,186,187). In one uncontrolled study, treatment of patients with FASSc with a regimen of daily oral cyclophosphamide and low-dose oral prednisolone was associated with sustained improvement in dyspnea and an increase in FVC in six of 14 patients: changes in DLCO were not significant, although minimal improvement was noted in five of 13 patients at 6 months (186).

Our observational study of a group of 30 patients with biopsy evidence of FASSc who were all treated subsequent to the biopsy procedure (performed to "stage" the relative degrees of cellularity and fibrosis) and followed for a minimum of 1 year in the same institution, have shown that 13 of 30 (43%) responded to therapy. Response was define as >15% improvement in either FVC or DLCO over pre-treatment values sustained over 1 year. The treatment regimens included high dose corticosteroids alone (60mg/day and then taper after 1 month) and low dose corticosteroid (20mg every other day) together with cyclophosphamide. It is interesting to note that, in common with CFA, high percentages of neutrophils in lavage returns predicted a poor response to therapy (171) (Table 15.5). The addition of plasmapheresis to an immunosuppressive regimen improved PFTs (188,189) in other uncontrolled observational studies.

The presence of alveolitis early in the disease, the ability to recognize it rapidly, plus the knowledge that the greatest decline in FVC occurs in the first 2 years of the disease (190), indicate that future studies must not only be controlled and prospective but also targeted at the early active stage.

Table 15.5. Treatment Response in Fibrosing Alveolitis in Systemic Sclerosis (FASSc)[a]

	n	Age	Lung function		BAL CELLS (%)		
			FVC	DLCO	Neutrophils	Eosinophils	Lymphocytes
Responders	13	48±11	65±18	48±18	5±4	7±7	11±14
Non responders	17	44±12	81±23[b]	60±15[b]	13±13[b]	4±4	12±9

[a]Results expressed as mean ± SD
[b]p<.05

PULMONARY VASCULAR DISEASE

Unfortunately, there are not yet available the means of detecting early PHT. Consequently we are called to treat this variety of scleroderma lung late in the natural history of the process. This inevitably has resulted in disappointing responses to therapy. Pulmonary vascular disease has two major components, a reversible pulmonary vasoconstrictive element and a fixed obliterative lesion. It is the latter component that probably leads to the almost universal failure of any vasodilator therapy to produce a sustained improvement, although short-term gain may be seen. Anecdotal short-term reports have advocated verapamil, hydralazine, ketanserin, and nifedipine (191–195), but evidence for long-term efficacy is still lacking, although sustained medium term efficacy has been shown for both nifedipine and captopril. Alpert et al (196) have reported six patients who showed an improvement in pulmonary vascular resistance following 3 to 6 months of oral treatment with nifedipine using the minimum dose required to achieve maximum response in a preliminary acute study. Using captopril, Alpert et al have shown more recently both short-term and medium-term benefit (6 months) (197). Mean pulmonary vascular resistance fell from 6.2 ±3.6 to 4.6 ±3.8 units in the short term study, and improvement was maintained after 3 to 5 months of oral therapy.

Intravenous therapy has been tried. Prostaglandin E, a vasodilator, failed to alter the pulmonary artery pressure (198,199) and caused an increase in pulmonary vascular resistance presumably by increasing stroke volume. The synthetic prostacyclin, iloprost, which is recognized as being able to reduce pulmonary vascular resistance (200), did not improve gas transfer in one study, suggesting that the pulmonary vascular bed in SSc is not amenable to dilatation (201).

Unpublished studies from our group, in which we infused prostacyclin directly into the pulmonary artery, have failed to produce significant falls in pulmonary vascular resistance as have infusions of 1-arginine, the substrate for nitric oxide which is the endothelial cell-derived relaxing factor, into the pulmonary vasculature (202).

For vasodilator therapy to be of any real value it must be effective over several years and this has yet to be established. Furthermore, a potential complication of vasodilator therapy that must be considered is the possibility of a precipitate fall in cardiac output due to decreased systemic vascular resistance. This can be life-threatening, particularly in the face of fixed increases in pulmonary vascular resistance.

In primary PHT, warfarin therapy increases survival (203) but this has not been tried in SSc. Oxygen therapy is a temporary help to patients with hypoxemia and PHT, and has been shown to improve pulmonary vascular resistance in one controlled prospective acute study (60). In view of the present failure to halt the disease by medical means, an increasing number of patients are being considered for transplantation. Single lung transplantation has been used to treat patients with CFA and primary PHT. To our knowledge, only four patients with SSc have received a lung transplant for either FASSc or PHT occurring alone, but the long-term outcome is not yet known. Clearly, the presence of significant extrapulmonary disease will preclude consideration for transplantation, particularly if there is renal disease. Also, the chances of recurrence in the transplanted organs are unknown.

References

1. Medsger TA. Systemic sclerosis, localized forms of scleroderma and calcinosis. In: McCarty DJ, Koopman WJ, eds. Arthritis and allied conditions: A textbook of rheumatology. Philadephia: Lea & Febiger, 1993:1253–1292.

2. Altman RD, Medsger TA Jr, Block DA, Michel BA. Predictors of survival in systemic sclerosis (scleroderma). Arthritis Rheum 1991;34:403–413.

3. Scully RE, Mark EJ, McNeely WF, McNeely BU. Case records of the Massachusetts General Hospital. N Engl J Med 1989;320:1333–1340.

4. Binz. Quoted in Wolters, M. Beitrag zur kenntniss der sklerodermie. Arch Dermatol U Syph 1892;24:695–738.

5. Harley J. A case of slowly advancing scleroderma attended by cardiac and gastric disorders. Br Med J 1877;1:107.

6. Dinkler M. Zur lehre von die sklerodermia. Dis Arch Klin Med 1891;48:514–577.

7. von Notthafft A. Neue arbeiten und anschihten uber sklerodermia. Zentralbl Allg Pathol Anat 1898;9:870–960.

8. Matsui S. Ober die pathologie und pathogenese von sklerodermia universalis. Mitteilungen Medizinischen Fakultat Universitat Tokyo 1924;31:55–116.

9. Harrison NK, Myers AR, Corrin B, Soosay G, Dewar A, Black CM, du Bois RM, et al. Structural features of interstitial lung disease in systemic sclerosis. Am Rev Respir Dis 1991;144:706–713.

10. Bocchieri MH, Jiminez SA. Animal models of fibrosis. In: LeRoy EC, ed. Rheumatic disease clinics of North America. Scleroderma. Philadelphia: WB Saunders, 1990;153–168.

11. Briggs DC, Vaughan RW, Welsh KI, Myers A, du Bois RM, Black CM. Immunogenetic prediction of pulmonary fibrosis in systemic sclerosis. Lancet 1991;338:661–662.

12. Haslam PL. Evaluation of alveolitis by studies of lung biopsies. Lung 1990;168(Suppl):984–992.

13. Campbell DA, Poulter LW, Janossy G, du Bois RM. Immunohistological analysis of lung tissue from patients with cryptogenic fibrosing alveolitis suggesting local expression of immune hypersensitivity. Thorax 1985;40:405–411.

14. Wells AU, Lorimer S, Jeffery PK, Majumdar S, Harrison NK, Sheppard MN, Corrin B, et al. Fibrosing alveolitis associated with systemic sclerosis is characterized by the presence of antigen-primed T cells in the lung interstitium. European Respiratory Journal, 1995;8:266–271.

15. Southcott AM, Gelder C, Barnes PJ, Morrison JFJ, du Bois RM. T cell receptor V alpha gene usage is not restricted in pulmonary fibrosis. Am Rev Respir Dis 1993;4:A11.

16. Southcott AM, Gelder CM, Morrison JFJ, Black CM, Barnes PJ, du Bois RM. Profiles of lymphokine gene expression in lung biopsies from patients with fibrosing alveolitis. Am Rev Respir Dis 1993;147:A756.

17. Hamid Q, Majumdar S, Sheppard M, Corrin B, Black CM, du Bois RM, Jeffery PK. Expression of IL-4, IL-5, INF gamma and IL-2 mRNA in fibrosing alveolitis associated with systemic sclerosis. Am Rev Respir Dis 1993;147:A479.

18. Harrison NK, Glanville AR, Strickland B, Haslam PL, Corrin B, Addis BJ, Lawrence R, et al. Pulmonary involvement in systemic sclerosis: The detection of early changes by thin section CT scan, bronchoalveolar lavage and 99m-Tc-DPTA clearance. Respir Med 1989;83:403–414.

19. Frigieri L, Mormile F, Grilli N, Mancini D, Ciappi G, Pagliari G, Magaro M, et al. Bilateral bronchoalveolar lavage in progressive systemic sclerosis: Interlobar variability, lymphocyte subpopulations, and functional correlations. Respiration 1991;58:132–140.

20. Rossi GA, Bitterman PB, Rennard SI. Evidence for chronic inflammation as a component of the interstitial lung disease associated with progressive systemic sclerosis. Am Rev Respir Dis 1985;131:612–617.

21. Edelson JD, Hyland RH, Ramsden M, Chamberlain DW, Kortan P, Meindok HO, Klein MH, et al. Lung inflammation in scleroderma: Clinical, radiographic, physiologic and cytopathological features. J Rheumatol 1985;12:957–963.

22. Pesci A, Bertorelli G, Manganelli P, Ambanelli U. Bronchoalveolar lavage analysis of interstitial lung disease in CREST syndrome. Clin Exp Rheumatol 1986;4:121–124.

23. Silver RM, Metcalf JF, LeRoy EC. Interstitial lung disease in scleroderma. Immune complexes in sera and broncoalveolar lavage fluid. Arthritis Rheum 1986;29:525–531.

24. Carré PC, Mortensen RL, King TEJ, Noble PW, Sable CL, Riches DWH. Increased expression of

the interleukin-8 gene by alveolar macrophages in idiopathic pulmonary fibrosis. J Clin Invest 1991;88:1802–1810.

25. Southcott AM, Jones KP, Pantelidis P, Black CM, Davies BH, du Bois RM. Interleukin-8 is associated with the presence of pulmonary fibrosis in systemic sclerosis. Am Rev Respir Dis 1993;147: A755.

26. Pantelidis P, Southcott AM, du Bois RM. Alveolar macrophages from fibrosing alveolitis patients secrete more TNF alpha than patients with sarcoidosis and normal individuals. Thorax 1994; 49:1146–1151.

27. du Bois RM, Hellewell PG, Hemingway I, Gearing AJ. Soluble cell adhesion molecules ICAM-1, ELAM-1, and VCAM-1 are present in epithelial lining fluid in patients with interstitial lung disease. Am Rev Respir Dis 1992;145:A190.

28. Wallaert B, Bart F, Aerts C, et al. Activated alveolar macrophages in subclinical pulmonary inflammation in collagen vascular diseases. Thorax 1988;43:24–30.

29. Kinsella MB, Smith EA, Miller KS, LeRoy EC, Silver RM. Spontaneous production of fibronectin by alveolar macrophages in patients with scleroderma. Arthritis Rheum 1989;32:577–583.

30. Harrison NK, Cambrey AD, Myers AR, Southcott AM, Black CM, du Bois, Laurent GJ, et al. Insulin-like growth factor-1 is partially responsible for fibroblast proliferation induced by bronchoalveolar lavage fluid from patients with systemic sclerosis. Clin Sci 1994;86:141–148.

31. Harrison NK, McAnulty RJ, Haslan PL, Black CM, Laurent GJ. Evidence for protein edema, neutrophil influx, and enhanced collagen production in lungs of patients with systemic sclerosis. Thorax 1990;45:606–610.

32. Cantin A, North SL, Fells GA, Hubbard RC, Crystal RG. Oxidant-mediated epithelial cell injury in idiopathic pulmonary fibrosis. J Clin Invest 1987; 79:1665–1673.

33. Cantin AM, Hubbard RC, Crystal RG. Glutathione deficiency in the epithelial lining fluid of the lower respiratory tract in idiopathic pulmonary fibrosis. Am Rev Respir Dis 1989;139: 370–372.

34. Borok Z, Buhl R, Grimes GJ, Bokser AD, Hubbard R, Holroyd KJ, Roum JH, et al. Effect of glutathione aerosol on oxidant-antioxidant imbalance in idiopathic pulmonary fibrosis. Lancet 1991;338:215–216.

35. Witt C, Neuhaus K, Winsel K, Brenke A, Hiepe F, Volk HD. Bronchoalveolar lavage in patients with systemic scleroderma and systemic lupus erythematosus: Characterization of cell activity by cytofluorometry, chemiluminescence and differential cell count. [German]. Z Erkrankungen Atmungsorgane 1991;176:21–29.

36. Sibille Y, Martinot JB, Polomski LL, et al. Phogocyte enzymes in bronchoalveolar lavage from patients with pulmonary sarcoidosis and collagen vascular disorders. Eur Respir J 1990;3:249–256.

37. Lorimer S, Wells AU, Walls S, Black CM, du Bois RM, Jeffery PK. Quantification of mast cells in fibrosing alveolitis associated with systemic sclerosis. Eur Respir J 1993;6:527S.

38. Gauldie J, Jordana M, Cox G. Cytokines and pulmonary fibrosis. Thorax 1993;48:931–935.

39. Deguchi Y. Spontaneous increase of transforming growth factor beta production by bronchoalveolar mononuclear cells of patients with systemic autoimmune diseases affecting the lung. Ann Rheum Dis 1992;51:362–365.

40. Moreland LW, Goldsmith KT, Russell WJ, Young KR Jr, Garver RI Jr. Transforming growth factor beta within fibrotic scleroderma lungs. Am J Med 1992;93:628–636.

41. Corrin B, Butcher D, McAnulty RJ, du Bois RM, Black CM, Laurent GJ, Harrison NK. Immunohistochemical localization of transforming growth factor beta 1 in the lungs of patients with systemic sclerosis, cryptogenic fibrosing alveolitis and other lung disorders. Histopathology 1994;24:145–150.

42. Sporn MB, Roberts AB, Wakefield LM, de Crombrugghe B. Some recent advances in the chemistry and biology of transforming growth factor beta. J Cell Biol 1987;105:1039–1045.

43. Thornton SC, Robbins JM, Penny R, Breit SN. Fibroblast growth factors in connective tissue disease associated interstitial lung disease. Clin Exp Immunol 1992;90:447–452.

44. Gay S, Jones RE, Huang GQ, Gay RE. Immunohistologic demonstration of platelet-derived growth factor (PDGF) and cis-oncogene expression in scleroderma. J Invest Dermatol 1989;92: 301–303.

45. Yamakage A, Kikuchi K, Smith EA, LeRoy EC, Trojanowska M. Selective upregulation of platelet-derived growth factor alpha receptors by transforming growth factor beta in scleroderma fibroblasts. J Exp Med 1992;175:1227–1234.

46. Ludwicka A, Trojanowska M, Smith EA, Baumann M, Strange C, Korn JH, Smith T, et al. Growth and characterization of fibroblasts obtained from bronchoalveolar lavage of patients with scleroderma. J Rheumatol 1992;19:1716–1723.

47. Cambrey AD, McAnulty RJ, Harrison NK, Dawes KE, Campa JS, du Bois RM, Black CM, et al. En-

dothelin is present in the lungs of patients with systemic sclerosis and stimulates lung fibroblast replication *in vitro*. Am Rev Respir Dis 1992;145: A15.

48. Gray AJ, Bishop JE, Laurent GJ. Partially degraded fibrin(ogen) stimulates the proliferation of human lung fibroblasts. Am Rev Respir Dis 1993; 147:A158.

49. Laurent GJ. Lung collagen: More than scaffolding. Thorax 1986;41:418–428.

50. Jordana M, Schulman J, McSharry C. Heterogeneous proliferative characteristics of human adult lung fibroblast lines and clonally derived fibroblasts from control and fibrotic tissue. Am Rev Respir Dis 1988;137:579–584.

51. Kahari VM, Sandberg M, Buorio T, Vuorio E. Identification of fibroblasts responsible for increased collagen production in localized scleroderma by in situ hybridization. J Invest Dermatol 1988;90:664–670.

52. Scharffeter K, Lankat-Buttgereit B, Krieg T. Localization of collagen mRNA in normal and scleroderma skin by *in situ* hybridization. J Clin Invest 1988;18:9–17.

53. Alton E, Turner-Warwick M. Lung involvement in scleroderma. In: Jayson MIV, Black CM, eds. Systemic sclerosis: Scleroderma. London: John Wiley & Sons, 1988:181–205.

54. Maricq HR. Raynaud's phenomenon and microvascular abnormalities in scleroderma (systemic sclerosis). In: Jayson MIV, Black CM, eds. Systemic sclerosis: Scleroderma. John Wiley & Sons, 1988:151.

55. Blann AD, Illingworth K, Jayson MIV. Mechanisms of endothelial cell damage in systemic sclerosis and Raynaud's phenomenon. J Rheumatol 1993;20:1325–1330.

56. Person JD. The endothelium: Its role in scleroderma. Ann Rheum Dis 1991;50:866–871.

57. Kahaleh MB, Sherer GK, LeRoy EC. Endothelial injury scleroderma. J Exp Med 1979;149:1326–1335.

58. Kahaleh MB. Vascular disease in systemic sclerosis: Endothelial cell-T lymphocyte-fibroblast interactions. Rheum Dis Clin North Am 1990;16: 53–73.

59. Palmer RMJ, Ferrige AG, Moncada S. Nitric oxide release accounts for the biological activity of endothelium-derived relaxing factor. Nature 1987; 327:524–526.

60. Morgan JM, Griffiths M, du Bois RM, Evans TW. Hypoxic pulmonary vasoconstriction in systemic sclerosis and primary pulmonary hypertension. Chest 1991;99(3):551–556.

61. Morse JH, Barst RJ, Whitman HH, Fotino M, Jacobs JC. Isolated pulmonary hypertension in the grandchild of a kindred with scleroderma (systemic sclerosis): "Neonatal scleroderma?" J Rheumatol 1989;16:1536–1541.

62. Lee P, Langevitz P, Alderdice CA, Aubrey M, Baer PA, Baron M, Buskila D, et al. Mortality in systemic sclerosis (scleroderma). QJM 1992;82:139–148.

63. Rich S, Kieras K, Hart K, Groves BM, Stobo JD, Brundage BH. Antinuclear antibodies in primary pulmonary hypertension. J Am Coll Cardiol 1986;8:1307–1311.

64. Isern RA, Yaneva M, Weiner E, Parke A, Rothfield N, Dantzker D, Rich S, et al. Autoantibodies in patients with primary pulmonary hypertension: Association with anti-Ku. Am J Med 1992;93:307–312.

65. Wilson RJ, Rodnan GP, Robin ED. An early pulmonary physiologic abnormality in progressive systemic sclerosis (diffuse scleroderma). Am J Med 1964;36:361–369.

66. D'Angelo WA, Fries JF, Masi AT, Shulman LE. Pathologic observations in systemic sclerosis (scleroderma). A study of fifty-eight autopsy cases and fifty-eight matched controls. Am J Med 1969;46:428–440.

67. Sullivan MA, Miller DK. Pulmonary manifestations in collagen disease. Arch Intern Med 1962; 110:769–781.

68. Oram S, Stokes W. The heart in scleroderma. Br Heart J 1961;23:243–259.

69. Twersky J, Twersky N, Lehr C. Scleroderma and carcinoma of the lung. Clin Radiol 1976;27:203–209.

70. Yousem SA. The pulmonary pathologic manifestations of the CREST syndrome. Hum Pathol 1990;21(5):467–474.

71. Church RE, Ellis ARP. Cystic pulmonary fibrosis in generalized scleroderma. Lancet 1950;1:392–394.

72. Ashba JK, Ghanem MH. The lungs in systemic sclerosis. Dis Chest 1965;47:52–64.

73. Harrison NK, Glanville AR, Strickland B, Haslam PL, Corrin B, Addis BJ, Lawrence R, et al. Pulmonary involvement in systemic sclerosis: The detection of early changes by thin section CT scan, bronchoalveolar lavage and 99m-Tc-DTPA clearance. Respir Med 1989;83:403–414.

74. Siebold JR, Giorno RC, Claman HN. Dermal mast cell degranulation in systemic sclerosis. Arthritis Rheum 1990;33:1702–1709.

75. Claman HN, Giorno RC, Seibold JR. Endothelial and fibroblastic activation in scleroderma. The myth of the "uninvolved skin." Arthritis Rheum 1991;34:1495–1501.

76. Gruber BL, Kaufman LD. Ketotifen-induced remission in progressive early diffuse scleroderma: Evidence for the role of mast cells in disease pathogenesis. Am J Med 1990;89:392–395.

77. Weaver AL, Divertie MB, Titus JL. Pulmonary scleroderma. Dis Chest 1968;54(6):490–498.

78. Young RH, Mark GJ. Pulmonary vascular changes in scleroderma. Am J Med 1978;64:998–1004.

79. Al-Sabbagh MR, Steen VD, Zee BC, Nalesnik M, Trostle DC, Bedetti CD, Medsger TA Jr. Pulmonary arterial histology and morphometry in systemic sclerosis: A case-control autopsy study. J Rheumatol 1989;16:1038–1042.

80. Sackner MA, Heinz ER, Steinberg AJ. The heart in scleroderma. Am J Cardiol 1966;17:542–559.

81. Weaver AL, Divertie MB, Titus JL. Scleroderma. Dis Chest 1968;54:490–498.

82. Sackner MA. Scleroderma, modern medical monographs. Vol. 26. New York: Grune & Stratton, 1966;76–115.

83. Leinwand I, Duryee AW, Richter MN. Scleroderma (based on a study of over 150 cases). Ann Intern Med 1954;41:1003–1041.

84. Steen VD. Systemic sclerosis. In: Caynon G, Zimmerman G, eds. The lung in rheumatic diseases. New York: Marcel Dekker, 1990;279–302.

85. Greenwald GI, Tashkin DP, Gong H, Simmons M, Duann S, Furst DE, Clements P. Longitudinal changes in lung function and respiratory symptoms in progressive systemic sclerosis. Am J Med 1987;83:83–92.

86. Agusti AGN, Roca J, Gea J, Wagner PD, Xaubert A, Rodriguez-Roison R. Mechanisms of gas-exchange impairment of idiopathic pulmonary fibrosis. Am Rev Respir Dis 1991;143:219–225.

87. Owens GR, Fino GJ, Herbert DL, Steen VD, Medsger TA, Pennock BE, Cottrell JJ, et al. Pulmonary function in progressive systemic sclerosis. Chest 1983;84:546–550.

88. Sudduth CD, Strange C, Cook WR, Miller KS, Baumann M, Collop NA, Silver RM. Failure of the circulatory system limits exercise performance in patients with systemic sclerosis. Am J Med 1993;95:413–418.

89. Sackner MA, Akgun N, Kimbel P, Lewis DH. The pathophysiology of scleroderma involving the heart and respiratory system. Ann Intern Med 1964;60:611–630.

90. Baldwin E, Cournand A, Richards DW Jr. Pulmonary insufficiency. I. Physiological classification, clinical methods of analysis, standard values in normal subjects. Medicine 1949;27:243–278.

91. Iliffe JD, Pettigrew NM. Hypoventilatory respiratory failure in generalized scleroderma. Br Med J 1983;286:337–338.

92. Chausow AM, Kane T, Levinson D, Szidon JP. Reversible hypercapnic respiratory insufficiency in scleroderma caused by respiratory muscle weakness. Am Rev Respir Dis 1984;130:142–144.

93. Steen VD, Owens GR, Fino JG, et al. Pulmonary involvement in systemic sclerosis (scleroderma). Arthritis Rheum 1985;28:759–767.

94. Guttadauria M, Ellman H, Emmanuel G, Kaplan D, Diamond H. Pulmonary function in scleroderma. Arthritis Rheum 1977;20:1071–1079.

95. de Muth GR, Furstenberg NA, Dabick L, Zarafonetis CJD. Pulmonary manifestations in scleroderma. Am J Med Sci 1968;255:94–104.

96. Hughes DTD, Lee FI. Lung function in patients with systemic sclerosis. Thorax 1963;18:16–20.

97. Guttadauria M, Ellman H, Kaplan D. Progressive systemic sclerosis; pulmonary involvement. Clin Rheum Dis 1979;5:151–166.

98. Weaver AL, Divertie MB, Titus JL. The lung in scleroderma. Mayo Clin Proc 1967;42:754–766.

99. Kim JH, Follett JV, Rice JR, Hampson NB. Endobronchial telangiectases and hemoptysis in scleroderma. Am J Med 1988;84:173–174.

100. Helfrich DJ, Banner B, Steen VD, Medsger TA Jr. Normotensive renal failure in systemic sclerosis (scleroderma). Arthritis Rheum 1989;32:1128–1134.

101. Wells AU, Cullinan P, Hansell DM, Rubens MB, Black CM, Newman-Taylor AJ, du Bois RM. Fibrosing alveolitis associated with systemic sclerosis has a better prognosis than lone cryptogenic fibrosing alveolitis. Am J Resp Clin Care Med 1994;149:1583–1590.

102. Salerni R, Rodnan GP, Leon DF, Shaver JA. Pulmonary hypertension in the CREST syndrome variant of progressive systemic sclerosis (scleroderma). Ann Intern Med 1977;86:394–399.

103. Stupi AM, Steen VD, Owens G, Barnes EL, Rodnan GP, Medsger TA Jr. Pulmonary hypertension in the CREST syndrome variant of systemic sclerosis. Arthritis Rheum 1986;29: 515–524.

104. Al-Sabbagh MR, Steen VD, Zee BC, Nalesnik M, Trostle DC, Bedetti CD, Medsger TA. Pulmonary arterial histology and morphometry in systemic sclerosis: A case-control autopsy study. J Rheumatol 1989;16(8):1038.

105. Ungerer RG, Tashkin DP, Furst D, et al. Prevalence and clinical correlates of pulmonary arterial hypertension in progressive systemic sclerosis. Am J Med 1983;75:65–74.

106. Germain BF, Howard TP, Soloman DA, et al. Cardiopulmonary function in the CREST syndrome. Clin Res 1981;29:164A.

107. Peters-Golden M, Wise RA, Hochberg M, Stevens

Wigley FM. Incidence of lung cancer in systemic sclerosis. J Rheumatol 1985;12(6):1136.

108. Talbott JH, Barrocas M. Carcinoma of the lung in progressive systemic sclerosis: A tabular review of the literature and a detailed report of the roentgenographic changes in two cases. Semin Arthritis Rheum 1980;9:191–217.

109. Roumm AD, Medsger TA Jr. Cancer and systemic sclerosis: An epidemiological study. Arthritis Rheum 1985;28:1336–1340.

110. Turner-Warwick M, Lebowitz M, Burrows B, Johnson A. Cryptogenic fibrosing alveolitis and lung cancer. Thorax 1980;35:469–499.

111. Browne K. Is asbestos or asbestosis the cause of the increased risk of lung cancer in asbestos workers? Br J Ind Med 1986;43:145–149.

112. Browne K. A threshold for asbestos related lung cancer. Br J Ind Med 1986;43:556–558.

113. Spencer H, Raeburn C. Pulmonary (bronchiolar) adenomatosis. J Pathol Bacteriol 1956;71:145–154.

114. Denis P, Ducrotte P, Pasquis P, Lefrancois R. Esophageal motility and pulmonary function in progressive systemic sclerosis. Respiration 1981;42:21–24.

115. Doll NJ, Salvaggio JE. Pulmonary manifestations of the collagen vascular disease. Semin Respir Med 1984;5:273–281.

116. Johnson DA, Drane WE, Curran J, Cattau EL, Ciarleglio C, Khan A, Cotelingam J, et al. Pulmonary disease in progressive systemic sclerosis: A complication of gastroesophageal reflux and occult aspiration? Arch Intern Med 1989;149:589–593.

117. Erasmus LD. Scleroderma in gold miners on the Witwatersrand with particular reference to pulmonary manifestations. South African J Lab Clin Med 1957;3:209–231.

118. Rodnan GP, Benedek TG, Medsger TA Jr, Cammarta RJ. The association of progressive systemic sclerosis (scleroderma) with coal miners' pneumoconiosis and other forms of silicosis. Ann Intern Med 1967;66:323–334.

119. Williams GH, Silman AJ. Review of the UK data on rheumatic diseases: 9. Scleroderma. Br J Rheumatol 1991;30:365–367.

120. Silman AJ. Epidemiology of scleroderma. Curr Opin Rheumatol 1991;3:967–972.

121. Silman AJ, Jones S. What is the contribution of occupational environmental factors to the occurence of scleroderma in men? Ann Rheum Dis 1992;51:1322–1324.

122. Welsh KI, Black CM. Environmental and genetic factors in scleroderma. In: Jayson MIV, Black CM, eds. Systemic sclerosis: scleroderma. John Wiley and Sons, 1988;33–34:33–47.

123. Russell DC, Maloney A, Muir AL. Progressive generalized scleroderma: Respiratory failure from primary chest wall involvement. Thorax 1981;39:219–220.

124. Garty B-Z, Althreya BH, Wilmott R, Scarpa N, Doughty R, Douglas SD. Pulmonary functions in children with progressive systemic sclerosis. Pediatrics 1991;88:1161–1167.

125. Falcini F, Pignone A, Matucci-Cerinic M, Camiciottoli G, Taccetti G, Trapani S, Zammarchi E, et al. Clinical utility of non invasive methods in the evaluation of scleroderma lung in pediatric age. Scand J Rheumatol 1992;21:82–84.

126. Peters-Golden M, Wise RA, Hochberg MC, Stevens MB, Wigley FM. Carbon monoxide diffusing capacity as predictor of outcome in systemic sclerosis. Am J Med 1984;77:1027–1034.

127. Bagg LR, Hughes DTD. Serial pulmonary function tests in progressive systemic sclerosis. Thorax 1979;34:224–228.

128. Schneider PD, Wise RA, Hochberg MC, Wigley FM. Serial pulmonary function in systemic sclerosis. Am J Med 1982;73:385–394.

129. Peters-Golden M, Wise RA, Schneider P, Hochberg M, Stevens MB, Wigley F. Clinical and demographic predictors of loss of pulmonary function in systemic sclerosis. Medicine 1984;63:221–231.

130. Schneider PD, Wise RA, Hochberg MC, Wigley FM. Serial pulmonary function in systemic sclerosis. Am J Med 1982;73:385.

131. Colp CR, Riker J, Williams MH Jr. Serial changes in scleroderma and idiopathic interstitial lung disease. Arch Intern Med 1973;132:506–515.

132. Steen VD, Owens GR, Redmond C, Rodnan GP, Medsger TA Jr. The effect of D-penicillamine on pulmonary findings in systemic sclerosis. Arthritis Rheum 1985;28:882–888.

133. Turner-Warwick M. Thoracic manifestations of multisystem diseases. In: Baum GL, Wolinskey E, eds. Textbook of pulmonary diseases. Boston: Little, Brown & Co, 1983;703–726.

134. Konig G, Luderscmidt C, Hammer C, Adelmann-Grill BC, Braun-Falco O, Fruhmann G. Lung involvement in scleroderma. Chest 1984;85:318–324.

135. Fritzler MJ, Kinsella TD, Garbutt E. A distinct serologic entity with anticentromere antibodies. Am J Med 1980;69:520–526.

136. Tan EM, Rodnan GP, Gardia I, Moroia Y, Fritzler MJ, Peebles C. Diversity of antinuclear antibodies in progressive systemic sclerosis. Arthritis Rheum 1980;23:617–625.

137. Catoggio LJ, Bernstein RM, Black CM, Hughes GRN, Maddison PJ. Serological markers in pro-

gressive systemic sclerosis: Clinical correlations. Ann Rheum Dis 1983;42:23–37.

138. Kerr IH. Radiology of interstitial lung disease. Semin Respir Med 1984;6:80–90.

139. Liebow AA, Steer A, Billinglsey JC. Desquamative interstitial pneumonia. Am J Med 1965;39:369–404.

140. Davidson AG, Heard BE, McAllister WAC, Turner-Warwick MEH. Cryptogenic organizing pneumonitis. QJM 1983;52:382–394.

141. Epler GR, Colby TV, McLoud TC, Carrington CB, Gaensler EA. Bronchiolitis obliterans organizing pneumonia. N Engl J Med 1985;312:152–158.

142. Cordier JF, Loire R, Brune J. Idiopathic bronchiolitis obliterans organizing pneumonia. Definition of characteristic clinical profiles in a series of 16 patients. Chest 1989;96:999–1004.

143. Mathieson JR, Mayo JR, Staples CA, Muller NL. Chronic diffuse infiltrative lung disease: Comparison of diagnostic accuracy of CT and chest radiography. Radiology 1989;171:111–116.

144. Hansell DM, Kerr IH. The role of high resolution computed tomography in the diagnosis of interstitial lung disease. Thorax 1991;46:77–84.

145. Muller NL, Miller RR. Computed tomography of chronic diffuse infiltrative lung disease: Part 1. Am Rev Respir Dis 1990;142:1206–1215.

146. Muller NL, Miller RR. Computed tomography of chronic diffuse infiltrative lung disease: Part 2. Am Rev Respir Dis 1990;142:1440–1448.

147. Wells AU, Hansell DM, Corrin B, Harrison NK, Goldstraw P, Black CM, du Bois RM. High resolution computed tomography as a predictor of lung histology in systemic sclerosis. Thorax 1992;47:738–742.

148. Muller NL, Miller RR, Webb WR, Evans KG, Ostrow DN. Fibrosing alveolitis: CT-pathologic correlation. Radiology 1986;160:585–588.

149. Warrick JH, Bhalla M, Schabel SI, Silver RM. High resolution computed tomography in early scleroderma lung disease. J Rheumatol 1991;18:1520–1528.

150. Schurawitzki H, Stiglbauer R, Graninger W, Herold C, Polzleitner D, Burghuber OC, Tscholakoff D. Interstitial lung disease in progressive systemic sclerosis: High-resolution CT versus radiography. Radiology 1990;176:755–759.

151. Wells AU, Hansell DM, Rubens MB, Cullinan P, Black CM, du Bois RM. The predictive value of appearances on thin section computed tomography in fibrosing alveolitis. Am Rev Respir Dis 1993;148:1076–1082.

152. Pignone A, Matucci-Cerinic M, Lombardi A, Fedi R, Fargnoli R, De Dominicis R, Cagnoni M. High resolution computed tomography in systemic sclerosis. Real diagnostic utilities in the assessment of pulmonary involvement and comparison with other modalities of lung investigation. Clin Rheumatol 1992;11:465–472.

153. Panos RJ, King TE Jr. Idiopathic pulmonary fibrosis. In: Lynch JP III, De Remee RA, eds. Immunologically mediated pulmonary diseases. Philadelphia: JB Lippincott, 1991;1–39.

154. Line BR, Hunninghake GW, Keogh BA, Jones AE, Jognston GS, Crystal RG. Gallium-67 scanning to stage the alveolitis of sarcoidosis: Correlation with clinical studies, pulmonary function studies, and bronchoalveolar lavage. Am Rev Respir Dis 1981;123:440–446.

155. Schmekel B, Wollmer P, Venge P, Linden M, Blom-Bulow B. Transfer of 99m-Tc DTPA and bronchoalveolar lavage findings in patients with asymptomatic extrinsic allergic alveolitis. Thorax 1990;45:525–529.

156. Chinet T, Dusser D, Labrune S, Collingnon MA, Chretien J, Huchon GJ. Lung function declines in patients with pulmonary sarcoidosis and increased respiratory epithelial permeability to 99mTc-DTPA. Am Rev Respir Dis 1990;141:445–449.

157. Harrison K, Glanville AR, Corrin B, Lawrence R, Woodcock A, Turner-Warwick M. Rapid 99m-Tc DTPA clearance from the lungs in idiopathic pulmonary haemosiderosis (IPH). Am Rev Respir Dis 1989;139:A472.

158. Wells AU, Hansell DM, Harrison NK, Lawrence R, Black CM, du Bois RM. Clearance of inhaled 99m-Tc DTPA predicts the clinical course of fibrosing alveolitis. Eur Respir J 1993;6:797–802.

159. Barrowcliffe MP, Jones LG. Solute permeability of the alveolar capillary barrier. Thorax 1987;42:1–10.

160. Jones JG, Minty BD, Lawler P, Hulands G, Crowley JCW, Veall N. Increased alveolar permeability in cigarette smokers. Lancet 1908;i:66–68.

161. Mason GR, Uszler JM, Effros RM, Reid E. Rapidly reversible alterations of pulmonary epithelial permeability induced by smoking. Chest 1983;83:6–11.

162. Steen VD, Graham G, Conte C, Owens G, Medsger TA Jr. Isolated diffusing capacity reduction in systemic sclerosis. Arthritis Rheum 1992;35:765–770.

163. Garty BZ, Athreya BH, Wilmott R, Scarpa N, Doughty R, Douglas SD. Pulmonary functions in children with progressive systemic sclerosis. Pediatrics 1991;88:1161–1167.

164. Manoussakis MN, Constantopoulos SH, Gharavi AE, Moutsopoulos HM. Pulmonary involvement in systemic sclerosis. Association with anti-Scl-70

antibody and digital pitting. Chest 1987;92:509–513.

165. Bjerke RD, Tashkin DP, Clements PJ, Chopra SK, Gong H, Bein M. Small airways in progressive systemic sclerosis (PSS). Am J Med 1979;66:201–209.

166. Silver RM, Miller KS, Kinsella MB, Smith EA, Schabel SI. Evaluation and management of scleroderma lung disease using bronchoalveolar lavage. Am J Med 1990;88(5):470–476.

167. Miller KS, Smith EA, Kinsella M, Schabel SI, Silver RM. Lung disease associated with progressive systemic sclerosis. Assessment of interlobar variation by bronchoalveolar lavage and comparison with noninvasive evaluation of disease activity. Am Rev Respir Dis 1990;141:301–306.

168. Haslam PL, Dewar A, Butchers P, Primett ZS, Newman-Taylor A, Turner-Warwick M. Mast cells, atypical lymphocytes and neutrophils in bronchoalveolar lavage in extrinsic allergic alveolitis. Am Rev Respir Dis 1987;135:35–47.

169. Wells AU, Hansell DM, Rubens MB, Cullinan P, Haslam PL, Black CM, du Bois RM. Fibrosing alveolitis in systemic sclerosis: Bronchoalveolar lavage findings in relation to computed tomographic appearances. Am J Resp Clin Care Med 1994;150:462–465.

170. Wallaert B, Hatron P-Y, Grosbois J-M, Tonnel A-B, Devulder B, Voisin C. Subclinical pulmonary involvement in collagen-vascular diseases assessed by bronchoalveolar lavage. Am Rev Respir Dis 1986;133:574–580.

171. Harrison NK, Wells AU, Hansell DM, Black CM, du Bois RM. Treatment of lung disease in systemic sclerosis: A clinical comparison of responders and non-responders. Am Rev Respir Dis 1992;145:A755.

172. Wong PS, Goldstraw P, Kaplan D. Early experience with video assisted thoracoscopic lung biopsy. Thorax 1993;48:440(A).

173. Wall CP, Gaensler EA, Carrington CB, Hayes JA. Comparison of transbronchial and open lung biopsies in chronic infiltrative lung disease. Am Rev Respir Dis 1981;123:280–285.

174. Wright PH, Heard BE, Steel SJ, Turner-Warwci M. Cryptogenic fibrosing alveolitis: Assessment by graded trephine lung biopsy histology compared with clinical radiographic and physiological features. Br J Dis Chest 1981;75:6170.

175. Heard B. Quantitative pathology of interstitial lung disease. Semin Respir Med 1984;6:20–30.

176. Carnochan FM, Walker WS, Cameron EWJ. Efficacy of video assisted thoracoscopic lung biopsy: An historical comparison with open lung biopsy. Thorax 1994;49:361–363.

177. Cailes JB, Phillips GD, Wells AU, Black CM, Evans TW, du Bois RM. Correlation of echocardiography and right heart catheter in systemic sclerosis. Am J Respir Crit Care Med 1994;149:A43.

178. Guttadauria M, Diamond H, Kaplan D. Colchicine in the treatment of scleroderma. J Rheumatol 1977;4:272–276.

179. Conner PK, Bashour PA. Cardiopulmonary changes in scleroderma—a physiological study. Am Heart J 1961;614:494–499.

180. Broll H, Tausch G, Eberl R. Zur behandlung der lungen fibrose mit D-penicillamin/Metalcaptase. Munch Med Wochenschr 1969;111:1580–1584.

181. DeClerk LS, Dequeker J, Francx L, et al. D-penicillamine therapy and interstitial lung disease in scleroderma: A long-term follow-up study. Arthritis Rheum 1987;30:643–650.

182. Dequekker J, Francx L, Mbuyl JM. Effect of longterm d-penicillamine, corticosteroid and no treatment on lung diffusing capacity in progressive systemic sclerosis. In: Maini R, ed. Modulation of autoimmunity and disease. New York: Praeger, 1981:283–290.

183. Dines DE. Pulmonary disease of vascular origin. Dis Chest 1968;54:3–12.

184. Kallenberg CGM, Janssen HM, Elema JD, The TH. Steroid-responsive interstitial pulmonary disease in systemic sclerosis. Chest 1984;86:489–492.

185. Nice CM, Menon ANK, Rigler LG. Pulmonary manifestations in collagen diseases. Am J Roentgenol 1959;81:264–279.

186. Silver RM, Warrick JH, Kinsella MB, Staudt LS, Baumann MH, Strange C. Cyclophosphamide and low-dose prednisone therapy in patients with systemic sclerosis (scleroderma) with interstitial lung disease. J Rheumatol 1993;20:838–844.

187. Johnson MA, Kwan S, Sneil NJ, Nunn AJ, Darbyshire JH, Turner-Warwick M. Randomized controlled trial comparing prednisolone alone with cyclophosphamide and low dose prednisolone in combination in cryptogenic fibrosing alveolitis. Thorax 1989;44:280–288.

188. Äkesson A, Wollheim FA, Thysell H, et al. Visceral improvement following combined plasmapheresis and immunosuppressive therapy in progressive systemic sclerosis. Scand J Rheumatol 1988;17:313–323.

189. Ferri C, Bernini L, Gremignai G, Latorraca A, Fazzi P, Tavon A, Solfanelli S, et al. Lung involvement in systemic sclerosis sine scleroderma treated by plasma exchange. Int J Artif Organs 1992;15:426–431.

190. Steen VD, Conte C, Owens G, Medsger TA Jr. Nat-

ural history of severe pulmonary fibrosis in systemic sclerosis (SSc). Arthritis Rheum 1990;33: S157.

191. Ohar J, Polatty C, Robichaud A, Fowler A, Vetrovec G, Glauser F. The role of vasodilators in patients with progressive systemic sclerosis. Interstitial lung disease and pulmonary hypertension. Chest 1985;88:263S–265S.

192. Fudman EJ, Kelling DG Jr. Transient effect of nifedipine on pulmonary hypertension of systemic sclerosis. J Rheumatol 1985;12:1191–1192.

193. Glikson M, Pollack A, Dresner-Feigin R, Galun E, Rubinow A. Nifedipine and prazosin in the management of pulmonary hypertension in CREST syndrome. Chest 1990;98:759–761.

194. Sfikakis PP, Kyriakidis MK, Vergos CG, Vyssoulis GP, Psarros TK, Kyriakidis CA, Mavrikakis ME, et al. Cardiopulmonary hemodynamics in systemic sclerosis and response to nifedipine and captopril. Am J Med 1991;90:541–546.

195. Seibold JR, Moloney RR, Turkevich D, Ruddy MC, Kostis JB. Acute hemodynamic effects of ketanserin in pulmonary hypertension secondary to systemic sclerosis. J Rhematol 1987;14:519–524.

196. Alpert MA, Pressly TA, Mukerji V, Lamber CR, Mukerji B, Panayiotou H, Sharp GC. Acute and long-term effects of nifedipine on pulmonary and systemic menodynamics in patients with pulmonary hypertension associated with diffuse systemic sclerosis, the CREST syndrome and mixed connective tissue disease. Am J Cardiol 1991;68: 1687–1691.

197. Alpert MA, Pressly TA, Mukerji V, Lambert CR, Mukerji B. Short- and long-term hemodynamic effects of captopril in patients with pulmonary hypertension and selected connective tissue disease. Chest 1992;102:1407–1412.

198. Baron M, Skrinskas G, Urowitz MB, Madras PN. Prostaglandin E therapy for digital ulcers in scleroderma. Can Med Assoc J 1982;126:42–45.

199. Baron M, Skrinskas G, Hyland R, Urowitz MB. Effects of prostaglandin E and other vasodilator agents in pulmonary hypertension of scleroderma. Br Heart J 1982;48:304–305.

200. Robin ED. Some basic and clinical challenges in the pulmonary circulation. Chest 1982;81:357–363.

201. Thurm CA, Wigley FM, Dole WP, Wist RA. Failure of vasodilator infusion to alter pulmonary diffusing capacity in systemic sclerosis. Am J Med 1991;90(5):547–552.

202. Baudouin SV, Bath P, Martin JF, du Bois RM, Evans TW. L-arginine infusion has no effect on systemic hemodynamics in normal volunteers, or systemic and pulmonary hemodynamics in patients with elevated pulmonary vascular resistance. Br J Clin Pharmacol 1993;36:45–49.

203. Rich S, Kaufmann E, Levy PS. The effect of high doses of calcium-channel blockers on survival in primary pulmonary hypertension. N Engl J Med 1992;327:76–81.

WILLIAM P. FOLLANSBEE

16

Organ Involvement: Cardiac

ALTHOUGH HEINE was the first to describe a patient with systemic sclerosis (SSc) who developed clinical cardiac involvement as a manifestation of their disease (1926) (1), Weiss and colleagues are credited with having first established that the heart is a target organ in the disease process (2). In their now classic 1943 description of nine cases (two of whom came to autopsy), Weiss et al noted symptoms of congestive heart failure which they attributed to the presence of myocardial fibrosis, and suggested that it represented a distinct clinical and pathologic entity. It is now recognized that cardiac involvement in SSc can be manifested as myocardial disease, pericardial disease, conduction system disease, or arrhythmias. While the cutaneous abnormalities typically antedate the development of myocardial disease, in rare cases cardiac disease can precede skin changes, presenting a difficult diagnostic challenge (3).

Symptoms

Symptoms of cardiac disease in SSc are diverse and frequently non-specific. Dyspnea and palpitations are among the most common symptoms. Typically dyspnea occurs with exertion. Orthopnea is less frequent, and may be occult because patients typically sleep with the head of their bed elevated in order to prevent esophageal reflux, thereby protecting them from experiencing orthopnea. Paroxysmal nocturnal dyspnea is usually a manifestation of advanced myocardial fibro-

sis. Symptoms of right ventricular failure, particularly peripheral edema and right upper quadrant discomfort due to hepatic congestion, occur in patients with advanced pulmonary disease, particularly pulmonary vascular disease.

Palpitations are a common symptom experienced by SSc patients, but may or may not be a manifestation of arrhythmia. In eliciting the history, it is helpful to determine whether palpitations are regular or irregular in cadence, whether they are transient or sustained, and under what circumstances they occur. Systemic sclerosis (SSc) patients with myocardial fibrosis, and particularly those who also have pulmonary fibrosis, may experience an awareness of a pounding of their heart beat even in the presence of a normal heart rhythm, particularly during exertion (sinus tachycardia). Alternatively, palpitations can be a manifestation of sinus bradycardia or bradycardia resulting from high grade heart block, especially in patients with conduction system disease or patients on beta blockers or calcium channel blockers, which inhibit sinus or AV node function. Palpitations can also be a manifestation of tachyarrhythmias, originating in either the atria or ventricles (4,5). Atrial premature beats and sustained atrial tachycardias are relatively common, and although usually benign, may be poorly tolerated hemodynamically in a patient with myocardial fibrosis. Ventricular ectopy, including sustained ventricular tachycardia, is also associated with SSc. It can present clinically as palpitations or as frank syncope. Syncope in a patient with severe pulmonary hypertension is a particularly ominous symptom, which can be a manifestation of ventricular tachycardia, high grade heart block, or acute right ventricular failure. Sudden cardiac death is a recognized complication of SSc.

Chest discomfort is another relatively common symptom in patients with SSc. While typical Heberden's angina can occur, the chest discomfort usually has a number of atypical features. Because of this, coexisting atherosclerotic coronary artery disease should always be considered in the SSc patient who experiences typical angina pectoris. Nevertheless, typical angina pectoris can also be a feature of SSc in the absence of epicardial coronary artery disease, and can result in myocardial infarction (6).

Prevalence and Prognostic Implication of Cardiac Involvement

Estimates of the prevalence of cardiac involvement in SSc have varied widely, primarily depending upon the method of assessment. Clinical symptoms associated with cardiac involvement are comparatively nonspecific, resulting in under-recognition of cardiac involvement even when it has reached a symptomatic stage. Dyspnea, for example, is a common symptom but is frequently attributed to pulmonary disease; coexisting left ventricular dysfunction may be overlooked. Chest pain is a common symptom in SSc, but because it is usually atypical in nature it may be attributed to musculoskeletal disease, lung and pleural disease, or esophageal disease. As a result, even potentially life-threatening underlying cardiac disease can go clinically undiagnosed (6). Early investigators stressed that significant clinical cardiac involvement in SSc is uncommon or even rare, and when present, it is a manifestation of disease in other organs, particularly the lungs or kidneys, which only secondarily involve the heart primarily through the presence of systemic or pulmonary hypertension (7–10). Other early investigators, however, emphasized the frequency of occult cardiac disease, particularly myocardial fibrosis, and suggested that it was associated with an unfavorable prognosis (11). More recent clinical studies have found evidence of myocardial disease in 20% to 25% of patients (12,13).

In contrast to clinical studies, autopsy studies have found the prevalence of cardiac abnormalities, particularly myocardial fibrosis and pericardial disease, to be quite high in SSc (Table 16.1) (14–17). Myocardial fibrosis has been noted in 30% to 81% of autopsied patients in these studies. The difference between the clinically

Table 16.1. Prevalence of Myocardial Fibrosis at Autopsy in Systemic Sclerosis

Author	Systemic Sclerosis		Controls		p
	n	Prevalence of Myocardial Fibrosis (%)	n	Prevalence of Myocardial Fibrosis (%)	
D'Angelo[a]	58	81	58	55	<0.01
McWhorter[b]	34	30			
Bulkley[c]	52	50			
Follansbee[d]	54	70	54	37	<0.005

[a] D'Angelo WA, Fries JF, Masi AT, et al. Pathologic observations in systemic sclerosis (scleroderma); a study of fifty-eight autopsy cases and fifty-eight matched controls. Am J Med 1969;46:428–440.
[b] McWhorter JE IV, LeRoy EC. Pericardial disease in scleroderma (systemic sclerosis). Am J Med 1974;57:566–575.
[c] Bulkley BH, Ridolfi RL, Salyer WR, et al. Myocardial lesions of progressive systemic sclerosis; a cause of cardiac dysfunction. Circulation 1976;53:483–490.
[d] Follansbee WP, Miller TR, Curtiss EI, et al. A controlled clinicopathologic study of myocardial fibrosis in systemic sclerosis (scleroderma). J Rheumatol 1990:17:656–662.

estimated prevalence of cardiac disease and the prevalence found at autopsy could be a manifestation of selection bias, with more advanced disease being represented in the autopsy population. Alternatively, however, the discrepancy could be a result of failure to recognize disease clinically when it is present pathologically. Support for this latter possibility is provided from clinical studies that used more sensitive diagnostic techniques, particularly thallium scintigraphy, to detect otherwise occult disease. The prevalence of cardiac abnormalities in SSc subjects in these studies has been very high, and similar to that reported in autopsy series (see Table 16.1) (18–25). Indeed, in four different studies using SPECT thallium scintigraphy, Kahan et al have reported thallium perfusion abnormalities in 100% of SSc patients tested (19, 20, 23, 25). The significance of these abnormalities using SPECT scintigraphy remains to be established in view of their apparently nearly universal presence in SSc patients. Some quantitative thresholds will have to be developed in order to define when perfusion abnormalities are clinically relevant. Nevertheless, studies using thallium scintigraphy clearly indicate that occult cardiac disease is common.

Similar findings have been reported from echocardiographic investigations of pericardial involvement. These investigations have found that clinically inapparent disease can be frequently demonstrated. Smith et al, for example, reported results of echocardiographic evaluations of 54 patients (26). While their sample had a high prevalence of abnormal electrocardiograms or cardiomegaly by chest roentgenography (35%), only seven (13%) had symptomatic evidence of pericardial effusion, but 22 (41%) had pericardial effusion by echocardiography. Overall, 37 (69%) had some abnormality on echocardiographic examination.

Studies using 24-hour ambulatory monitoring have also demonstrated frequent abnormalities that were otherwise clinically inapparent (4,5). While patients who experience palpitations commonly have atrial or ventricular ectopy with or without electrocardiographic abnormalities, ambulatory monitoring frequently detects arrhythmias or conduction system abnormalities in otherwise asymptomatic individuals.

The results of these studies, which utilized a variety of diagnostic techniques, indicate that the discrepancy between the frequency of clinically-apparent cardiac disease and that described in autopsy studies is a reflection of the presence of unrecognized, clinically-occult disease, rather than a manifestation of selection bias in the autopsy studies.

Clinically apparent cardiac involvement portends an unfavorable prognosis. Medsger and Masi found that, of organ system involvement, heart involvement is second only to kidney involvement in terms of its negative prognostic implication, with five-year mortality estimated to be 70% (27). Furst et al conducted a randomized, placebo-controlled prospective trial to examine the possible therapeutic benefit of immunosuppressive therapy with the alkylating agent chlorambucil (28). Ten "summary indices" were developed which combined clinical variables by organ systems, including a general cardiac index. Of the 10 indices tested, only the cardiac index score, which included cardiomegaly, symptomatic heart failure, symptomatic arrhythmias, and echo score, predicted survival. In a further analysis of the data from this trial, Clements et al proposed a cardiac scoring system to estimate prognosis (29). Two cardiopulmonary variables, left axis deviation and moderate or large pericardial effusion, were found to be independently predictive of mortality. Using a weighted scoring system based on these two factors, the authors identified four subgroups of their study sample with 6-year mortality rates that ranged from 21% to 100%. It should be noted, however, that approximately half of the subjects in this study had SSc with limited cutaneous involvement, a subgroup with a lower prevalence of cardiac disease in comparison to subjects exhibiting diffuse cutaneous involvement (30). Other cardiac factors, therefore, might be found to contribute independently to mortality in a diffuse scleroderma subset. In addition, the authors pointed out that

despite normal systolic left ventricular function in 42% of their SSc subjects (38). Montanes et al found that the isovolumic relaxation period was prolonged abnormally with isometric handgrip in SSc subjects, again suggesting diastolic dysfunction (43). Kazzam et al noted that LV compliance (passive distensibility) was decreased in their SSc subjects, as indicated by the apexcardiographic a/H ratio and increased left atrial index, while they did not find evidence of abnormal LV relaxation (the early, energy-dependent, ventricular uncoiling) (40). They concluded that the observed diastolic abnormalities were independent of systolic abnormalities, which were also present in some subjects. Taken together, these studies suggest that there can be some abnormality of diastolic filling in patients with SSc, independent of the presence of systolic dysfunction. Conceptually, this might not be surprising in view of the high prevalence of myocardial fibrosis. Clinically, diastolic dysfunction is typically manifested as dyspnea, particularly dyspnea on exertion.

Before completely accepting the concept of primary diastolic dysfunction in SSc, however, additional factors must be considered. First, it is important to exclude any confounding conditions that can also cause diastolic dysfunction, particularly systemic hypertension and coronary atherosclerosis. More importantly, none of the studies suggesting the presence of diastolic dysfunction have directly measured left ventricular filling pressure; all have depended upon indirect, non-invasive parameters. In the single hemodynamic study reported thus far, which examined a small number of SSc patients all of whom had demonstrable myocardial involvement, hemodynamic indices of diastolic function in the SSc patients were not significantly different from controls (46). Before any firm conclusions can be drawn about the prevalence or severity of diastolic myocardial dysfunction resulting from SSc, therefore, additional invasive hemodynamic investigations are necessary. From a diagnostic standpoint, it is important to note that left ventricular filling pressure can be perfectly normal at rest despite prominent diastolic dysfunction, particularly if the patient has been treated with diuretics. Therefore, if left ventricular filling pressure is normal at rest in a patient in whom diastolic dysfunction is a clinical concern, it is essential that the patient be exercised in the catheterization laboratory in order to define the pressure-volume relationships of the ventricle during exercise. Left ventricular end diastolic pressure can increase dramatically with comparatively small increases in cardiac output, thereby revealing the abnormal diastolic stiffness.

Myositis and Myocardial Disease

Skeletal muscle disease has been recognized as a potential manifestation of SSc since Westphal's original description of a single case in 1876 (47). A subgroup of patients with SSc can develop a clinical picture of polymyositis in overlap with SSc, manifested by persistent elevations of creatine phosphokinase and aldolase, proximal muscle weakness, and an abnormal electromyogram. Muscle biopsy typically reveals fibrosis with varying degrees of inflammation. Estimates of the frequency of skeletal muscle involvement in SSc have varied widely (48–50).

West et al reported findings from eight SSc patients with myositis. Three of the eight patients had evidence of coexisting myocardial disease, including conduction system abnormalities in two patients and left ventricular dysfunction in one patient (51). There have been 2 other case reports of single SSc patients with coexisting skeletal and myocardial muscle involvement (52,53). These reports have introduced the possibility that there could be an association between myocardial muscle disease ("myocarditis") and skeletal muscle disease ("myositis") in SSc.

In 1993, Follansbee et al reported findings from a study in which they examined the possible association of skeletal and myocardial muscle disease in 1,258 SSc patients between 1959 and 1988 (54). Of the 1,095 SSc patients who did not have renal involvement, 183 (17%) had evidence of skeletal myositis. Of these 183, 39 (21%) also had evidence of myocardial disease, compared to 90 of the remaining 912 (10%, p < 0.0001). Patients with skeletal myopathy had an increased risk of congestive heart failure (19 of 183 vs 38 of 912, p < 0.002) and cardiac death (15 of 183 vs 27 of 912, p < 0.002) compared to those without myopathy. An elevated creatine phosphokinase (CK) determination at any time in the course of the disease (206 of 1095 patients), typically an index of skeletal muscle disease in SSc, was also associated with an increased incidence of myocardial dysfunction (47 of 206 vs 82 of 889, p < 0.0001), congestive heart failure (21 of 206 vs 36 of 890, p < 0.001), and cardiac death (18 of 206 vs 24 of 889, p < 0.001) compared to patients with no documented elevation of CK.

Sufficient data were available on retrospective analysis for 25 patients in this subgroup to objectively confirm the presence of both skeletal muscle disease and myocardial muscle disease, while excluding confounding conditions such as coronary artery disease, hypertension, or valvular heart disease. These patients were characterized by a high prevalence of clinical congestive heart failure (68%), and a nearly universal presence of electrocardiographic abnormalities and rhythm disturbances. Of the 12 patients in whom objective measurements of LVEF were available, nine had ejection fractions below 35%, a striking degree of impairment compared to the general SSc population (18). Eighteen of the 25 patients died in follow-up, 12 of the 18 deaths (67%) were sudden deaths, and eight of the 12 who suffered sudden death had intractable congestive heart failure. These findings indicate that there is an association between skeletal muscle disease and myocardial disease in SSc, and that this subgroup of SSc patients is at high risk of congestive heart failure, arrhythmias and conduction system abnormalities, and sudden death.

The findings from one of the patients in this study are of particular interest since she died in the clinical context of active skeletal myositis, with accompanying relentless, progressive myocardial necrosis, and came to autopsy. She had severe congestive heart failure, persistent elevations of both total CK and the CK-MB subfraction, new right bundle branch block and left anterior fascicular block, intractable atrial flutter, an LVEF of 32%, and a cardiac index of 1.6 L/min/m². She subsequently developed progressive renal insufficiency. She did not respond to treatment with high dose ACE inhibition and nifedipine, and died of intractable heart failure. She was not treated with corticosteroids because of her active renal disease. At autopsy the myocardium was found to have widespread areas of myocardial myocytolysis (Fig. 16.2). Residual empty shells were left behind where the myocytes had once been (Fig. 16.2a). There were areas of contraction band necrosis, but there was no fibrosis evident and there was no evidence of inflammation, despite the absence of corticosteroid treatment (Fig. 16.2b). The epicardial coronary arteries were without significant obstruction. Most of the small arteries were anatomically normal (Fig. 16.2c), although a few small arteries showed medial hypertrophy (Fig. 16.2d). The case is of interest for several reasons. It is the first reported autopsy examination of a SSc patient who died in the setting of active "myocarditis." While the term "myocarditis" has been used for this clinical entity, the myocardial histology was notable for the absence of inflammation. Inflammation did not appear to be the primary mediator of the myocardial necrosis. There was also no significant myocardial fibrosis seen, which likely was a result of the fact that this was an early, acute process. Had the patient survived, it is assumed that myocardial fibrosis would have ensued. Of particular note, however, are the comparatively unique histologic findings that were present. The only other setting in which we have seen similar myocardial histology is in patients with recent heart transplantation. That is a situation in which the heart is made globally ischemic during explantation, and is then reperfused. The histologic findings, therefore, are consistent with the hypothesis that myocardial injury in SSc is at least in part mediated by intermittent myocardial ischemia due to vasospasm,

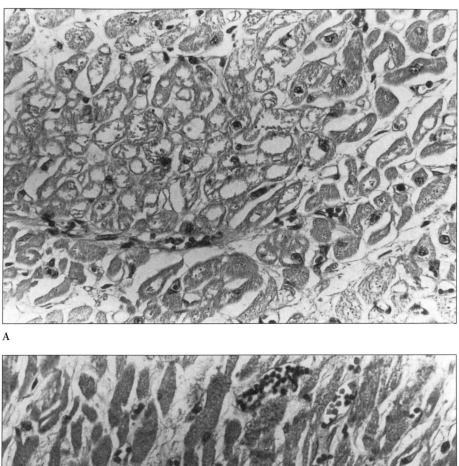

A

B

Figure 16.2. The autopsy findings from a patient who died in the clinical setting of fulminant "myocarditis" and "myositis" are illustrated. *A.* There are widespread areas of myocytolysis with myocyte necrosis and degeneration, leaving behind only empty shells where the myocytes had been. (Hematoxylin-eosin stain; × 500) *B.* There was a notable absence of inflammatory infiltrate or myocardial fibrosis. Contraction band necrosis was

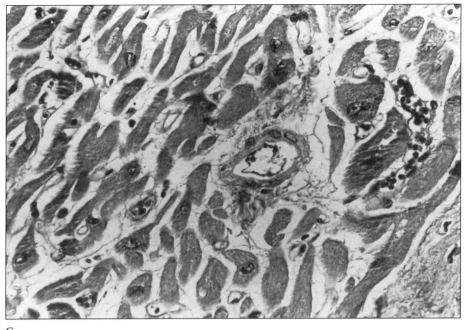

C

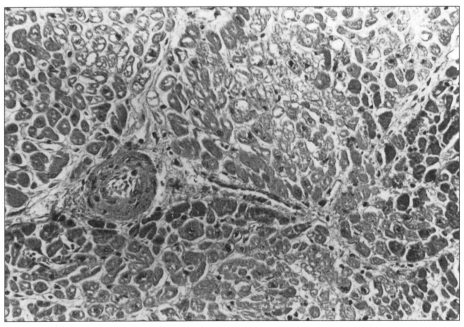

D

identified in the areas of myocytolysis. (Hematoxylin-eosin stain; × 500) *C.* Most of the small arteries were anatomically normal (Hematoxylin-eosin stain; × 500), although (*D.*) a rare artery showed prominent medial hypertrophy. (Hematoxylin-eosin stain; × 200) (Reproduced with permission from Follansbee WP, et al. Cardiac and skeletal muscle disease in SSc (scleroderma): A high risk association. Am Heart J 1993;125:194–203.)

followed by reperfusion, a "myocardial Raynauds phenomenon." In this particular case, if vasospasm was the mediator of injury, it was not responsive to aggressive vasodilator treatment, including both high dose ACE inhibition and calcium channel blockade.

The Coronary Vascular System

The arterial vascular system is an important target organ in SSc, and may be central to the pathogenesis of the disease (55,56). In the specific case of the myocardium, considerable supporting evidence has emerged to implicate the coronary vascular system in the pathogenesis of the myocardial fibrosis.

Chest pain is a not uncommon symptom in SSc, and while it usually has features atypical of angina, some patients experience typical Heberden's angina pectoris, suggesting the presence of myocardial ischemia (6). Because this is relative-

ly uncommon, however, when it occurs, consideration should be given to the presence of coexisting coronary artery atherosclerosis or possibly pulmonary hypertension with right ventricular angina. For example, of the nine SSc patients who suffered myocardial infarction in the absence of coronary atherosclerosis described by Bulkley et al, six had chest discomfort but only three had symptoms felt clinically to be angina pectoris (6). Nevertheless, the occurrence of typical angina in some SSc patients in the absence of other confounding conditions supports the hypothesis that compromise of myocardial blood flow is part of the disease process.

Thallium perfusion scintigraphy has provided stronger evidence than clinical symptomatology to support the hypothesis that the coronary arterial system is involved in the pathogenesis of myocardial scleroderma. As shown in Table 16.2, thallium perfusion defects are quite common in SSc patients—they may occur at rest, in response to exercise, or in response to cold pressor provo-

Table 16.2. Prevalence of Thallium Perfusion Abnormalities in SSc

Author	n	Condition	Method	Prevalence of ^{201}Tl Perfusion Defects (%)
Follansbee[a]	26	Exercise	Planar	77
Kahan[b]	20	Rest	SPECT	100
Kahan[c]	23	Rest	SPECT	100
Alexander[d]	13	Cold pressor	Planar	77
Follansbee[e]	29	Cold pressor	Planar	97
Kahan[f]	16	Rest	SPECT	100
Gustafsson[g]	21	Cold pressor	SPECT	71
Kahan[h]	12	Rest	SPECT	100

[a]Follansbee WP, Curtiss EI, Medsger TA Jr, et al. Physiologic abnormalities of cardiac function in progressive systemic sclerosis with diffuse scleroderma. N Engl J Med 1984;310:142–148.
[b]Kahan A, Devaux JY, Amor B, et al. Nifedipine and thallium-201 myocardial perfusion in progressive systemic sclerosis. N Engl J Med 1986;314:1397–1402.
[c]Kahan A, Devaux JY, Amor B, et al. Pharmacodynamic effect of dipyridamole on thallium-201 myocardial perfusion in progressive systemic sclerosis with diffuse scleroderma. Ann Rheum Dis 1986;45:718–725.
[d]Alexander EL, Firestein GS, Weiss JL, et al. Reversible cold-induced abnormalities in myocardial perfusion and function in systemic sclerosis. Ann Intern Med 1986;105:661–668.
[e]Follansbee WP, Kiernan JM, Curtiss EI, et al. Cold-induced thallium perfusion abnormalities in diffuse scleroderma and Raynaud's disease: Response to diltiazem therapy. Arthritis Rheum 1987;30(suppl 4):S117.
[f]Kahan A, Devaux J, Amor B, et al. Nicardipine improves myocardial perfusion in Systemic Sclerosis. J Rheumatol 1988;15:1395–1400.
[g]Gustafsson R, Mannting F, Kazzam E, et al. Cold-induced reversible myocardial ischaemia in systemic sclerosis. Lancet 1989;(Aug 26):475–479.
[h]Kahan A, Devaux JY, Amor B, et al. The effect of captopril on thallium 201 myocardial perfusion in systemic sclerosis. Clin Pharmacol Ther 1990;47:483–489.

cation. There is no evidence to suggest that there is any increased incidence of coronary atherosclerosis in this disease to account for the thallium perfusion defects that occur. While exercise-induced thallium perfusion defects are typically manifestations of coronary atherosclerotic disease, Follansbee et al reported angiographic findings from seven such SSc patients, and all were normal (18). Coronary arterial aneurysms have been described in a single case report, but they are not a recognized feature of the disease (57). Hence, the observed abnormalities in myocardial perfusion appear to result from abnormal resistance downstream at the level of the arterioles (the R2 vessels) or capillaries, or at the level of the myocardial interstitium (the R3 component of resistance reflecting wall tension), rather than being at the level of the epicardial or larger intramyocardial vessels (the R1 vessels) (58).

Thallium perfusion defects appear to reflect significant myocardial injury, at least in SSc patients with diffuse cutaneous involvement. In their study of 26 patients in this subgroup, Follansbee et al noted that patients with thallium defect size above the median had lower LVEF's than the remainder (18). This relationship was not seen in a similar study of patients with limited cutaneous involvement. In that subgroup, thallium defects were noted to be small, and were unrelated to left ventricular ejection fraction (30).

While there is no evidence that SSc patients are predisposed to coronary atherosclerosis, coronary artery disease is nevertheless widely prevalent in the general population, so the chance occurrence of both diseases is not rare. In that circumstance, the two disease processes may have an additive effect in impairing coronary blood flow. The hemodynamic effect of atherosclerosis in the proximal coronary vessels will be exacerbated by the increased resistance to perfusion downstream from small artery disease and/or interstitial myocardial fibrosis. Diastolic dysfunction will further compromise perfusion. Since left ventricular subendocardial perfusion, in particular, is virtually exclusively a diastolic phenomenon, increased diastolic wall tension

will further increase the resistance to subendocardial blood flow. Hence, the hemodynamic manifestations of the coronary athersclerostic plaque in the SSc patient may be disproportionate to the apparent severity of the obstruction seen on the angiogram. This potential interaction of disease in the proximal and distal coronary vascular tree also has at least theoretical implications on the suitability of these patients for coronary bypass surgery, since flow-through bypass grafts might be jeopardized by the high downstream resistance. There is insufficient clinical experience to know to what degree this is a clinically relevant concern.

Perhaps the most important early observation that stimulated interest in the role of the coronary vasculature in the pathogenesis of myocardial fibrosis in SSc came from the autopsy study of 52 patients performed by Bulkley et al (16). They noted that myocardial fibrosis in their subjects was associated with contraction band necrosis, a histologic lesion seen in the setting of myocardial ischemia followed by reperfusion (Figure 16.2b) (59–62). Contraction bands are dense hypereosinophilic transverse bands across the myofibril. They are distinct from coagulation necrosis, the typical lesion associated with ischemic myocardial infarction due to coronary atherosclerosis. Contraction bands are usually present in only very small numbers in the periphery of ischemic infarctions; in that context, they appear to result from reperfusion of the border zone of the infarction through collateral blood flow. They are also seen in patients with recent cardiopulmonary bypass surgery or heart transplantation, both situations in which the myocardium is ischemic and then reperfused. Bulkley et al noted that the severity of myocardial fibrosis found in their SSc subjects correlated with the presence of contraction band necrosis (16). From these findings, they hypothesized that myocardial fibrosis in SSc is a result of coronary artery vasospasm followed by reperfusion, a "myocardial Raynaud's phenomenon" (RP), thus accounting for the presence of contraction bands.

In a subsequent autopsy study of 54 subjects

and 54 controls, Follansbee et al found that contraction bands were not more frequent overall in their SSc subjects compared to controls (17). However, the subgroup of scleroderma subjects who had findings of primary myocardial involvement (i.e., myocardial fibrosis in the absence of systemic or pulmonary hypertension or other identifiable contributing cause) did have an increased prevalence of contraction bands. Furthermore, it was only in that subgroup that the combination of contraction band necrosis and severe myocardial fibrosis was noted to coexist. These observations suggest that it is this subset of patients with clinical evidence of myocardial involvement in the absence of systemic or pulmonary hypertension who are particularly predisposed to myocardial vasospastic injury.

If coronary artery vasospasm is present in SSc, it appears to be to some degree distinct from peripheral RP. There is a high prevalence of structural abnormalities in the small digital arteries in patients with SSc and RP. Rodnan et al noted that, of 25 digital arteries examined from 16 patients with SSc and RP who came to autopsy, 100% had intimal fibrosis and 79% had narrowing of the vessel lumen of at least 75% (63). Janevski noted that digital arteriograms revealed abnormal organic arterial stenoses and occlusions in all 12 SSc patients who were studied (64). According to the LaPlace relationship, the distending force holding a vessel open is proportional to its radius. As the radius of the vessel decreases, the vessel will be more predisposed to vascular collapse, because its wall tension is decreased. Hence, peripheral RP appears, at least in part, to be a manifestation of mechanical narrowing of the vessel lumen, upon which even normal variations in vascular tone can result in vessel occlusion. Abnormal platelet aggregation and/or abnormal serotonin metabolism may also contribute to the predisposition to vasospasm (65,66). In contrast to the periphery, however, the prevalence of small artery obstructive lesions in the heart appears to be much less. Bulkley et al observed that " . . . an occasional vessel . . . was narrowed by cellular intimal proliferation in

six . . . " of 52 patients (16). Post mortem microangiograms were performed in 12 of the subjects, and none showed significant abnormalities. Eight of nine patients with myocardial infarction and sudden death despite normal coronary arteries reported by this same group were found to have normal intramyocardial coronary arteries on multiple histological sections (6). Similarly, Follansbee et al noted small artery obstructive lesions in only three of their 54 SSc subjects, compared to none in 54 controls (p = ns) (17). Hence, if there is a "myocardial RP," it is at least somewhat distinct from peripheral RP in that there is a lesser prevalence of associated R2 vessel disease to account for the predisposition to vasospastic collapse of the lumen.

In an effort to confirm the presence of coronary vasospasm, a series of investigators have examined myocardial function and perfusion during cold pressor provocation in SSc patients, with somewhat equivocal results. Four studies have used cold pressor provocation in conjunction with thallium scintigraphy to assess myocardial perfusion (21,22,24,67), and 4 have examined the effects of cold on left ventricular function using either radionuclide ventriculography or echocardiography (21,39,68,69). Alexander et al noted that 10 of 13 (77%) SSc subjects without clinical cardiac disease had transient thallium perfusion defects induced by cold pressor challenge (21). Twelve of the 13 (92%) had cold-induced segmental wall motion abnormalities demonstrated by echocardiography, including all 10 with thallium perfusion defects. Long et al noted cold-provoked perfusion defects in four of their 10 (40%) subjects (67), and Gustafsson et al noted cold-provoked perfusion defects in 12 of 21 (57%) of their patients (24). Ellis and colleagues noted cold-induced wall motion abnormalities in eight of 15 (53%) SSc subjects studied by echocardiography (68). Five of eight who had inducible wall motion abnormalities did not have them when the examination was repeated after nifedipine therapy, but two subjects without abnormalities prior to nifedipine had them after nifedipine administration. In contrast to these reports, Siegel et al found that only two of nine (22%) SSc patients had an abnormal fall in LVEF induced by cold challenge, as assessed by radionuclide ventriculography; in both patients, the decline appeared to be attributable to a hypertensive blood pressure response (68). Moreover, normal subjects frequently have a decrease in ejection fraction and even segmental wall motion abnormalities produced early after cold pressor challenge (70).

Follansbee et al compared the response to cold pressor provocation of SSc patients to that of patients with Raynaud's Disease without scleroderma (22,69). If the abnormalities were of pathophysiologic consequence and not just the nonspecific manifestations of inducing peripheral Raynauds phenomenon, then they would be expected to be more frequent and/or more severe in SSc subjects, since patients with Raynaud's Disease are not known to develop cardiac abnormalities. Follansbee et al examined thallium perfusion during cold provocation in 29 SSc patients, and compared the findings to those from 17 patients with Raynaud's Disease without SSc (22). Cold-induced thallium perfusion defects were seen in both groups, although they were more common in the SSc patients (13% vs 9% of myocardial segments, $p < 0.05$). However, the defects were all mild in severity, and there was no significant change in their frequency or severity in either group when the examination was performed after diltiazem treatment. In a related study, these investigators examined the ejection fraction response to cold pressor challenge using radionuclide ventriculography for pre- and post-diltiazem therapy in 22 of the SSc patients and 13 of the Raynaud's Disease subjects, and compared them to the cold pressor response of 16 normal volunteers (69). All three groups had a decrease in LVEF with cold pressor, which was associated with an increase in arterial blood pressure; there was no significant difference in the response comparing the three groups, and no significant change in the response after diltiazem therapy.

Overall, the studies of cold-pressor challenge in SSc subjects have demonstrated a high prevalence of cold-induced thallium perfusion defects, and a variable prevalence of induced segmental wall motion abnormalities or a decreased LVEF; however, the pathophysiologic significance of these observations has not yet been demonstrated clearly. Further studies with adequate control groups, as well as clinical follow-up studies examining patient outcome, are necessary to determine whether the observed changes during cold provocation are of functional or clinical consequence. It is also significant to note that none of these studies using cold pressor provocation reported any incidence of electrocardiographic ST segment elevation during cold challenge. Hence, there was no evidence to suggest that these patients are subject to a Prinzmetals-like syndrome, with vasospasm of the epicardial or larger intramyocardial coronary vessels. If vasospasm is present, it appears to be at the level of the distal vasculature, not at the level of the large coronary arteries.

Additional studies have attempted to confirm the presence of coronary vasospasm/vasoconstriction by examining the effects on coronary perfusion of treatment with various vasodilators including nifedipine (19,71), diltiazem (22), nicardipine (23), captopril (25), and dipyridamole (20). Kahan and colleagues, in particular, have reported findings from an important series of studies in which they used resting SPECT thallium scintigraphy to examine SSc patients pre- and post-treatment with various vasodilators (19,20,23,25). The left ventricular myocardium in these studies was divided into nine segments, and the thallium uptake in each segment was visually quantitated on a scale from 0 (no uptake) to 2.0 (normal uptake). Hence, a completely normal study would have a global score of 18. A number of interesting observations can be made from the combined results of these studies, as shown in Table 16.3. First, thallium defects were not only universally present in every patient, they were widespread (average approximately 6 of the 9 segments), indicating a diffuse process. This is consistent with the observations from pathologic studies. Second, the defects were of only

Table 16.3. Effect of Vasodilator Therapy on Myocardial Thallium Uptake

Vasodilator	# pts	# pts abnormal	# abnormal segments pre Rx	# abnormal segments post Rx	Mean defect score pre Rx	Mean defect score post Rx
nifedipine[a]	20	20	5.3(2.0)	3.3(2.2)	.97(.24)	1.26(.44)
nicardipine[b]	16	16	6.0(2.0)	4.1(2.3)		
captopril[c]	12	12	6.5(1.9)	4.4(2.7)		
dipyridamole[d]	23	23	6.0(2.1)	4.1(2.5)	.92(.24)	1.13(.38)

( ) = standard deviation

[a]Kahan A, Devaux JY, Amor B, et al. Nifedipine and thallium-201 myocardial perfusion in progressive systemic sclerosis. N Engl J Med 1986;314:1397–1402.

[b]Kahan A, Devaux J, Amor B, et al. Nicardipine improves myocardial perfusion in Systemic Sclerosis. J Rheumatol 1988;15:1395–1400.

[c]Kahan A, Devaux JY, Amor B, et al. The effect of captopril on thallium 201 myocardial perfusion in systemic sclerosis. Clin Pharmacol Ther 1990;47:483–489.

[d]Kahan A, Devaux JY, Amor B, et al. Pharmacodynamic effect of dipyridamole on thallium-201 myocardial perfusion in progressive systemic sclerosis with diffuse scleroderma. Ann Rheum Dis 1986;45:718–725.

moderate intensity (mean defect score approximately 1.1, implying a reduction of thallium uptake of approximately 50%). This is consistent with a patchy process in the myocardium, rather than a process that causes transmural destruction, and, again, is consistent with pathologic observations. Third, the authors noted that thallium uptake improved with vasodilator treatment, a finding that they suggested supports the hypothesis that coronary vasospasm is present in SSc, and can be relieved by vasodilator treatment. They suggested that there may be a role for vasodilator therapy in preventing and/or treating myocardial damage in this population. However, some caution is warranted in interpreting these observations.

First, vasospasm is usually considered to be an episodic process. RP, for example, is not constantly present, at least at clinically detectable levels, but comes and goes depending upon conditions. In these thallium studies, however, every subject had reversible thallium perfusion defects present at rest, despite the fact that no provocative measures were used to stimulate coronary vasospasm. This would imply that there is chronic, pathologic coronary vasospasm constantly present, a heretofore unrecognized entity. Second, the vasodilator effect appeared to be nonselective. The response to the four different agents used was nearly identical with respect to the number of segments that improved, the magnitude of increase in thallium uptake in the defects, and the global defect score, despite the differences in the mechanism of action of the agents, the doses used, the duration of treatment, and the route of administration (Table 16.3). Third, if the response to vasodilator treatment does indicate the presence of vasospasm, the magnitude of the improvement in thallium uptake was still quite modest in degree (mean defect score increased from approximately 0.9 to 1.1, and the global defect score increased from approximately 10 to 12). The corollary is that the majority of the observed perfusion defects were not reversible with vasodilator treatment (post-treatment defect score of 1.1 and global perfusion score of 12), suggesting that they represented fibrosis, not vasospasm. It is still possible, of course, that the vasospastic component is more predominant earlier in the course of the disease, at which point perfusion abnormalities might be more completely reversible. Nevertheless, in view of the magnitude of the fixed perfusion defects that existed, the functional significance of the reversible component is not yet clear.

Finally, none of the studies demonstrating improvement in thallium perfusion defects with vasodilator therapy have examined the subsequent effect of that improvement on myocardial function. If these reversible perfusion defects do, in fact, represent resolution of ischemia, then one would expect that myocardial function would improve when the ischemia was alleviated. This has not been established and cannot be assumed.

While the improvement in thallium uptake with vasodilator treatment is consistent with the possible presence of coronary artery vasospasm, an alternative explanation should also be considered. Myocardial fibrosis in SSc is patchy and microscopic, as discussed previously. The spatial resolution of SPECT thallium perfusion imaging, however, is on the order of magnitude of 1 cm. It is possible, therefore, that the observed improvement in thallium uptake represents vasodilation with increased blood flow around islands of fibrosis that would tend to conceal them and make them appear to resolve, while the fibrotic areas are, in fact, unchanged. The findings of Duboc et al using positron emission tomography, however, argue against this interpretation (71). They examined myocardial blood flow using ^{38}K, and myocardial glucose metabolism using ^{18}FDG, in nine subjects with SSc pre- and post-treatment with nifedipine. They observed that ^{38}K uptake increased with nifedipine treatment, suggesting increased coronary blood flow, while ^{18}FDG activity decreased, suggesting a metabolic shift away from glucose as a primary energy source, implying improved tissue perfusion since glucose is not a preferred metabolic substrate in well perfused myocardium. The increased flow, therefore, appears to be metabolically significant rather than simply a reflection of increased flow around unaffected areas of fibrosis. If these findings are confirmed by subsequent studies in larger numbers of patients, they would provide strong evidence to support the vasospastic hypothesis.

If coronary vasospasm is present at rest and responds to vasodilator treatment, as the thallium studies imply, then one would expect coronary sinus flow measurements to show decreased coronary blood flow at rest with normal coronary vasodilator reserve in response to maximal coronary artery vasodilation. The single study of coronary flow and coronary vasodilator reserve in SSc subjects, however, found just the opposite (Fig. 16.3) (46). Mean coronary sinus blood flow at rest in seven SSc patients (89 $\pm$ 32 ml/minute/100 grams) was not significantly different from that observed in seven controls (100 $\pm$ 15 mls/minute/100 grams). There was a rather wide range in the resting levels found in the SSc subjects, so it is possible that there is a subgroup of patients who have decreased coronary blood flow at rest. Peak coronary blood flow in response to maximum vasodilation with intravenous dipyridamole, however, was markedly reduced in the SSc subjects (191 $\pm$ 45 mls/min/100 grams) compared to controls (399 $\pm$ 58 mls/min/100 grams, p < 0.01). This limitation in peak coronary blood flow and coronary vasodilator reserve could not be explained by vasospasm. It almost certainly represents the effects of interstitial myocardial fibrosis, plus or minus fixed small artery obstructive disease.

It has also been well demonstrated that the capillary bed can be damaged in SSc (72–76). Enlarged and deformed capillary loops surrounded by relatively avascular areas are readily apparent in the nailbeds, using nailfold capillary microscopy. The capillary bed is substantially destroyed, and the capillary loops that are left are dilated and distorted. Capillary destruction does not appear to be limited to the skin. Maricq et al demonstrated that skin capillary abnormalities are quantitatively related to internal organ involvement in the disease (77), a finding subsequently confirmed by other studies (78). Norton et al noted similar changes in the capillary bed of skeletal muscle of SSc patients (79). If the capillary bed of the coronary circulation is similarly damaged, it could contribute to the presence of fixed thallium perfusion defects, as well as to the observed reduction in peak coronary blood flow, and conceivably could account for some of the apparent improvement in thallium perfusion in response to vasodilator therapy. Preliminary data from our department, however, in which we have examined the myocardial capillary bed in autopsy specimens of SSc subjects compared to controls, have not indicated that the number or mor-

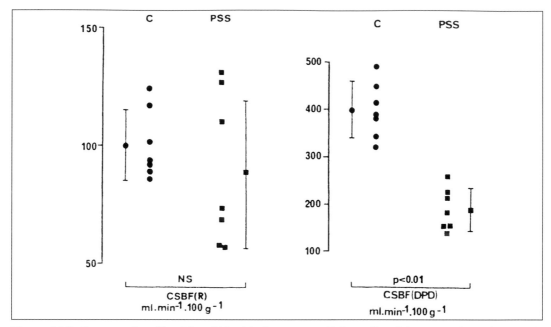

Figure 16.3. Coronary sinus blood flow (CSBF) is shown at rest (left panel) and during maximum hyperemia with intravenous dipyridamole (right panel) for seven patients with SSc and seven controls. The SSc patients all had diffuse cutaneous involvement and evidence of cardiac involvement. CSBF at rest was not significantly different comparing SSc to controls. However, peak CSBF was markedly decreased in the SSc group. (Reproduced with permission from Kahan A, et al. Decreased coronary reserve in primary scleroderma myocardial disease. Arthritis Rheum 1985;28:637–646.)

phology of capillaries is abnormal in the study subjects (Follansbee WP, unpublished data). Further investigation of the status of the capillary bed in SSc will be important.

In summary, the evidence accumulated to date suggests that there is a component of coronary artery vasospasm/vasoconstriction that occurs in SSc patients, and it appears to contribute to the development of myocardial fibrosis. However, the overall importance of this in the pathogenesis remains uncertain, and it is probably an over-simplification to assume that vasospasm is the sole or perhaps even the primary mediator of myocardial injury. There is substantial evidence, particularly the high prevalence of fixed thallium perfusion defects and the decrease in measured peak coronary arterial blood flow, to indicate that there are also fixed decreases in coronary

perfusion in many of these patients, unrelated to vasospasm. These latter findings likely result from interstitial myocardial fibrosis, with or without fixed small artery obstructive disease and/or destruction of the coronary capillary bed. It seems most reasonable to hypothesize that all of these factors interrelate in the pathophysiologic cascade. The potential efficacy of vasodilator therapy, while being theoretically attractive, remains unknown and untested. If vasospasm is central to the pathogenesis of myocardial fibrosis, treatment early in the course of the disease would likely have greater potential benefit than later treatment, since a limitation in peak coronary blood flow, once present, would be very unlikely to respond to vasodilator treatment. Prospective, randomized therapeutic trials will be essential to address these important issues.

Conduction System Disease and Arrhythmias

Conduction system disease, and atrial and ventricular tachyarrhythmias and bradyarrhythmias, are all well recognized manifestations of myocardial scleroderma. They may occur in patients with or without symptoms or clinically apparent myocardial involvement (4). In a study of 102 consecutive patients and a review of the literature, Follansbee et al examined the frequency of resting electrocardiographic abnormalities in patients with SSc (Table 16.4) (80). Based upon combined findings from 436 patients, they concluded that approximately 50% of SSc patients have a normal electrocardiogram (80). Not surprisingly, the prevalence of abnormalities detected is increased by 24-hour ambulatory monitoring, compared to a resting electrocardiogram (4,81).

Conduction system abnormalities can occur at any level. Approximately 5% of patients have first degree heart block, while 1% exhibit a higher grade—either second degree or third degree block (Table 16.4) (80). Right bundle branch block occurs in approximately 2% of patients, left bundle branch block in 1%, and left anterior

Table 16.4. Prevalence of Abnormalities on the Resting Electrocardiogram Based Upon Findings from 436 Patients[a]

Electrocardiographic Finding	Percent
Normal electrocardiogram	56
PR prolongation	5
Right bundle branch block	2
Left bundle branch block	1
Left anterior fascicular block	5
Intraventricular conduction defect	4
Second or third degree heart block	1
Left ventricular hypertrophy	7
Right ventricular hypertrophy	7
Low voltage QRS	5
Non-specific ST-T wave abnormality	7

[a] Follansbee WP, Curtiss EI, Rahko PS, et al. The electrocardiogram in systemic sclerosis (scleroderma). Study of 102 consecutive cases with functional correlations and review of the literature. Am J Medicine 1985;79:183–192.

fascicular block in 5%. An additional 4% have non-specific intraventricular conduction abnormalities. Conduction system abnormalities may result in symptomatic high degree heart block; death due to asystolic cardiac arrest has been documented, usually occurring in patients with advanced underlying conduction system disease (82,83). Estimates of the prevalence of conduction system abnormalities increase when 24-hour monitoring is employed. In a 24-hour ambulatory monitoring study of 53 patients, for example, Ferri et al detected conduction system abnormalities in 10 patients on the resting ECG, while 16 patients had them on ambulatory monitoring (5). Only 16 of 50 patients examined by Roberts et al had an abnormal ECG, but 62% had abnormal 24-hour ambulatory recordings (84). Similarly, 28 of 40 (70%) patients examined by Geirsson et al had a normal ECG at rest, while 65% had abnormal 24-hour ambulatory ECG recordings (81). In a report of 19 patients who underwent invasive electrophysiologic studies, Roberts and Cabeen noted that six had demonstrable intrinsic abnormalities in AV nodal function, while two had prolonged resting AH intervals (85). In a related report from the same group, only six of a total of 20 subjects who underwent invasive electrophysiologic studies had completely normal study (84). The patient sample was characterized by the presence of mild to moderate disease: 22% had clinically apparent cardiac involvement and 54% had renal involvement. However, the renal involvement was mild in all cases; none had renal crisis (personal communication).

Whether conduction system abnormalities result from direct intrinsic conduction system disease, or are instead a result of more diffuse myocardial disease, has been somewhat controversial. Loperfido et al reported findings from an electrophysiologic examination of a patient who had evolving conduction system disease on serial electrocardiograms (86). They noted the presence of a markedly prolonged H-V conduction interval, indicating advanced infranodal conduction system disease, despite the absence of detectable myocardial dysfunction by echocardiography and cardiac catheterization. Clements et al also emphasized that conduction system abnormalities and arrhythmias are frequently found in patients who lacked other evidence of myocardial disease, implying primary involvement of the conduction system (4). Supporting this hypothesis, Roberts and Cabeen noted that all seven subjects whom they examined at autopsy had an abnormal appearance of the proximal AV node, which they characterized as narrowing instead of the normal pear shaped appearance (85). There was only minimal evidence of fibrosis noted in the AV node, however, and only one of the subjects was judged to have scleroderma cardiomyopathy. Lev et al performed an extraordinarily detailed dissection of the conduction system of a SSc patient who died with complete heart block, and found marked replacement of the bundle branches by fibroelastic tissue (87). They concluded that collagenous proliferation is responsible for the damage. Their patient, however, also had significant myocardial fibrosis.

In contrast to these reports, Ridolfi et al examined the conduction systems of 35 SSc patients who came to autopsy (88). Thirteen of these patients had sinus node fibrosis, but it did not appear to be related to the presence or absence of myocardial fibrosis. The authors suggested that this could be related to pericardial disease, since the sinus node is directly contiguous to the pericardium. The AV node and main His bundles were histologically normal in all of the subjects. Fibrotic changes were seen in the proximal bundle branches of six patients, but did not clearly correlate with observed conduction abnormalities. The investigators concluded that, " ... although conduction abnormalities were more frequent in patients with myocardial disease, specific conduction system disease was not the cause in most patients." They postulated that the conduction disturbances are a result of a more diffuse myocardial process, rather than reflecting primary conduction system pathology. Follansbee et al noted that septal infarction pattern, an electrocardiographic abnormality which

they demonstrated to be associated with SSc, and ventricular conduction abnormalities are both associated with thallium perfusion defects in the septum or anteroseptal wall (80). Both septal infarction pattern and bifasicular block (either RBBB with left anterior fascicular block, or LBBB) were also associated with abnormalities in left ventricular function during exercise (Fig. 16.4). These findings suggest that the conduction abnormalities are a manifestation of a more diffuse myocardial process.

The truth, in all probability, includes both of these postulated mechanisms. Fibrosis is the hallmark of myocardial involvement with SSc, and is both a patchy and diffuse process. In most patients, ventricular conduction abnormalities are likely a manifestation of a diffuse fibrotic process involving both the ventricular conduction tissue as well as the myocardium itself. However, in some cases the fibrosis may more selectively involve the His purkinje system, with relative sparing of the myocardial muscle. In any given individual patient, electrocardiographic conduction abnormalities likely represent some variable contribution of primary conduction system disease and more diffuse myocardial fibrosis. Importantly, it should be understood that the absence of detectable abnormalities in myocardial function at rest by no means excludes the presence of myocardial fibrosis, which might only be functionally detectable with more sensitive exercise examinations.

It is perhaps to be expected that a patient population that is at risk of developing patchy myocardial fibrosis, as well as conduction system disease at any level, would also be at risk of developing atrial and ventricular arrhythmias, including sustained tachycardias. This has been clearly demonstrated to be part of the spectrum of the cardiac manifestations of SSc. Roberts et al, for example, noted that 32% of their 50 study subjects had supraventricular tachycardias on 24-hour ambulatory monitoring, 20% had coupled ventricular extrasystoles, and 10% had nonsustained ventricular tachycardia (84). In a subset of 20 patients who underwent invasive

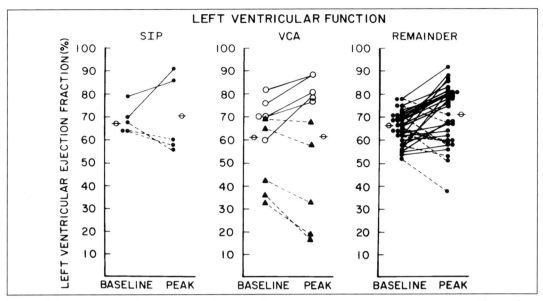

Figure 16.4. Baseline and peak exercise left ventricular ejection fractions are shown in patients with septal infarction pattern (SIP) or ventricular conduction abnormalities (VCA) compared to SSc patients without these findings. Patients with an abnormal ejection fraction response to exercise are shown by dashed lines, whereas those with a normal response are shown by solid lines. Of the patients with VCA, those with left bundle branch block or bifasicular block (right bundle branch block with left anterior fasicular block) are represented by solid triangles, whereas those without these abnormalities are shown by open circles. (Reproduced with permission from Follansbee WP, et al. The electrocardiogram in SSc (scleroderma). Study of 102 consecutive cases with functional correlations and review of the literature. Amer J Med 1985;79:183–192.)

electrophysiologic examination, seven had an abnormality of sinus node function, eight had an abnormality in the atrial refractory period, and seven had an abnormality in AV nodal function. The authors hypothesized that these abnormalities predisposed to the development of reentrant atrial tachyarrhythmias. Ferri et al recorded ventricular arrhythmias by ambulatory monitoring in 48 of 53 patients (91%), including 40% with multiform PVC's, 28% with ventricular couplets, and 13% with runs of ventricular tachycardia (5). Follansbee et al noted that 35% of their 48 patients had exercise-induced arrhythmias, including 4% with atrial ectopy alone, 21% with ventricular ectopy, and 10% with both atrial and ventricular ectopy (80). Ectopy was associated with an abnormal left ventricular ejection fraction response to exercise, and with the presence of thallium perfusion defects, supporting the hypothesis that arrhyth-

mias are a manifestation of a more diffuse myocardial process.

Kostis et al reported findings from a multicenter trial that performed 24-hour ambulatory recordings on 183 subjects (89). They detected ventricular ectopy in 67% of their patients, and, importantly, found that the ectopy was strongly correlated with both total mortality and with sudden cardiac death. Ventricular ectopy correlated with advancing age as well as with indices of cardiac and pulmonary involvement in the disease process. Other studies have also found that SSc patients are at risk of sudden death due to ventricular asystole or ventricular fibrillation (82). As discussed previously, the subset of SSc subjects who have skeletal and cardiac muscle disease have an extremely high prevalence of atrial and ventricular arrhythmias, including sustained tachycardias, and appear to be at particularly high risk of sudden cardiac death (54).

Marinato et al reported findings from a SSc patient who experienced recurrent syncope (90). An electrophysiologic evaluation revealed abnormalities of SA and AV nodal function, as well as a prolonged HV conduction time indicating infranodal conduction system disease. The patient subsequently suffered sudden death, and at autopsy had fibrosis of the SA and AV nodes, with atrophy of the left bundle branch. In addition, diffuse myocardial fibrosis with patchy myofibrillar degeneration was present. The authors speculated that the lesions in both the conduction system and the myocardium contributed to the development of the fatal tachyarrhythmia. Moser et al investigated the frequency of ventricular late potentials on signal averaged electrocardiography and their suitability as a marker of high risk of arrhythmias and sudden death (91). They noted that 26% of the 88 SSc subjects that were studied had some abnormality of the signal averaged electrocardiogram, but this was not different from a normal control group, 22% of whom also had some "abnormality" described. While 60% of SSc patients with ventricular late potentials had complex or frequent ventricular ectopy, 78% of patients with complex or frequent ventricular ectopy had normal signal averaged tracings. The authors concluded that the signal averaged electrocardiogram did not have sufficient diagnostic power to be useful as a screening tool for identifying high risk patients.

Gallagher et al described a single SSc patient with limited cutaneous involvement who had recurrent ventricular tachycardia, which was refractory to drug treatment (92). In this individual case, an open epicardial mapping procedure followed by cryoablation of the ventricular tachycardia pathway was successful in eliminating the clinical arrhythmia. Studies examining the potential role that electrophysiologic studies, ablative procedures, or implantable cardiac defibrillators might play in decreasing the incidence of sudden death in high risk SSc subjects have not been reported.

Pericardial Disease

Autopsy studies have demonstrated that pericardial abnormalities are common in SSc (Table 16.5). In a summary of autopsy findings from 31 reported subjects, Oram and Stokes noted that pericarditis, with or without pericardial effusion, was present in 22 (71%) (3). D'Angelo et al noted that pericardial abnormalities, including fibrinous pericarditis, fibrous pericarditis, and pericardial adhesions were present in 53% of their autopsy subjects, including 35% who had pericardial effusion (14). McWhorter and LeRoy found pericardial abnormalities in 62% of their autopsy subjects (15), and Bulkley et al in 33% of the subjects in their series (16). In this latter study, 10 of the 17 patients with pericardial abnormalities had uremia as a likely contributing etiologic factor.

In contrast to the reported autopsy experience, clinical pericardial disease is much less common (Table 16-5). Meltzer was the first to demonstrate significant pericardial effusions antemortem, as described in his 1956 report of two cases (93). While 53% of their autopsy subjects had pericardial disease at autopsy, D'Angelo et al noted that only 16% had clinically apparent pericardial involvement (14). Echocardiography improves the clinical detection of pericardial disease. In their study of 54 subjects, Smith et al noted that 41% had demonstrable pericardial effusions on echocardiography sometime in their disease course, while only seven of these 22 patients had clinically evident pericardial disease, all experiencing pericardial pain (26). None had hemodynamic embarrassment. The presence of a large pericardial effusion (> 200 mls) was associated with an unfavorable prognosis in this study, supporting earlier observations by McWhorter and LeRoy (15). Four of their 54 patients had large pericardial effusions; three of the four died within a short time, two with acute renal failure and one with congestive heart failure. The fourth developed malignant hypertension with acute renal failure, but survived. In a

Table 16.5. Prevalence of Pericardial Disease in SSc

Author	Prevalence of disease at autopsy	Prevalence of clinically symptomatic disease	Prevalence of disease echocardiographic study
Oram et al[a]	22/33 (71%)	"uncommon"	
Sackner et al[b]	18/25 (72%)	3/65 (5%)	
D'Angelo et al[c]	31/58 (53%)	9/58 (16%)	
McWhorter et al[d]	19/34 (56%)	15/210 (7%)	
Bulkley et al[e]	17/52 (33%)		
Smith et al[f]		7/54 (13%)	22/54 (41%)
Gottidiener et al[g]			2/11 (18%)
Gaffney et al[h]			3/16 (19%)
Follansbee et al[i]		1/26 (4%)	
Follansbee et al[j]		3/22 (14%)	

[a]Oram S, Stokes W. The heart in scleroderma. Br Heart J 1961;23:243–225.
[b]Sackner MA, Heinz ER and Steinberg AJ. The heart in scleroderma. Am J Cardiol 1966;17:542–559.
[c]D'Angelo WA, Fries JF, Masi AT, et al. Pathologic observations in systemic sclerosis (scleroderma); a study of fifty-eight autopsy cases and fifty-eight matched controls. Am J Med 1969;46:428–440.
[d]McWhorter JE IV, LeRoy EC. Pericardial disease in scleroderma (systemic sclerosis). Am J Med 1974;57:566–575.
[e]Bulkley BH, Ridolfi RL, Salyer WR, et al. Myocardial lesions of progressive systemic sclerosis; a cause of cardiac dysfunction. Circulation 1976;53:483–490.
[f]Smith JW, Clements PJ, Levisman J, et al. Echocardiographic features of progressive systemic sclerosis (PSS); correlation with hemodynamic and postmortem studies. Am J Med 1979;66:28–33.
[g]Gottdiener JS, Moutsopoulos HM, and Decker JL. Echocardiographic identification of cardiac abnormality in scleroderma and related disorders. Am J Med 1979;66:391–398.
[h]Gaffney FA, Anderson RJ, Nixon JV, and Blomqvist CG. Cardiovascular function in patients with progressive systemic sclerosis (scleroderma). Clin Cardiol 1982;5:569–576.
[i]Follansbee WP, Curtiss EI, Medsger TA Jr, et al. Physiologic abnormalities of cardiac function in progressive systemic sclerosis with diffuse scleroderma. N Engl J Med 1984;310:142–148.
[j]Follansbee WP, Curtiss EI, Medsger TA Jr, et al. Myocardial function and perfusion in the CREST syndrome variant of progressive systemic sclerosis. Exercise radionuclide evaluation and comparison with diffuse scleroderma. Am J Med 1984;77:489–496.

retrospective review of 210 patients, McWhorter and LeRoy noted clinical pericardial disease in 15 patients (7%) (15). Clinical disease occurred in two patterns. Four patients experienced symptoms of acute pericarditis with dyspnea, chest pain, fever, and a pericardial friction rub. Two of these patients suffered sudden death, presumed to be from an arrhythmia. In 11 patients, the clinical picture was that of chronic pericardial effusion with dyspnea, cardiomegaly, congestive heart failure, and pleural effusions, despite the absence of renal failure at the time of development of the pericardial effusion. Six of these 11 patients, however, died within 6 months of acute renal failure which developed at some time after the pericardial effusion; all had been treated with diuretics.

There are at least two potential explanations for the suggested association between pericardial effusion and subsequent acute renal failure. First,

the pericardial effusions appear to be a manifestation of activity of the underlying disease process, because they appeared prior to the onset of renal disease and in the absence of infection, heart failure, or other demonstrable contributing factors. It is possible that pericardial disease may simply be a marker of activity of the underlying SSc, thereby identifying patients at risk of also developing renal crisis unrelated to the pericardial effusion itself. Alternatively, however, it is possible that the presence of large pericardial effusion could compromise forward cardiac output, resulting in renal hypoperfusion, which, in turn, might trigger a cascade of events within the kidney leading to renal crisis. Both of these studies that found an association between pericardial effusion and renal failure were from the pre-ACE inhibitor era. It is not known whether ACE inhibitor therapy might modify this relationship. In addition, most if not all of these patients were treated with diuretics, presumably in an effort to treat their shortness of breath or perhaps, in some subjects, to treat hypertension, another potential marker of renal disease. Diuresis in the presence of pericardial effusion might further compromise renal blood flow, and thereby predispose to the development of acute renal failure.

While pericardial effusion in SSc typically is not hemodynamically significant, at least at clinically detectable levels, pericardial tamponade has been described in individual cases. Three of the subjects in McWhorter's chronic pericardial effusion group had evidence of hemodynamic embarrassment, including pulsus paradoxus and Kussmaul's sign, the latter suggesting the presence of a coexisting constrictive component (15). Uhl and Koppes described three patients who had well-documented evidence of pericardial tamponade that responded to pericardiocentesis (94). One of the three patients also had hemodynamics suggesting the presence of a coexisting constrictive component. Another came to autopsy and had marked pericardial fibrosis, again suggesting a possible constrictive component. The findings from this case are similar to a case described in the autopsy study of Bulkley et al (16).

In summary, occult pericardial disease is another common feature of SSc. Clinically apparent pericardial disease also occurs, but is less frequent. It can present as acute pericarditis, which may be associated with risk of arrhythmia and sudden cardiac death. Alternatively, it can present as chronic pericardial effusion. Chronic effusions are usually small and not hemodynamically significant, although they may be a marker of activity of the underlying disease. Large pericardial effusions can occur, however, and can lead to pericardial tamponade, possibly exacerbated by pericardial fibrosis contributing an additional component of constrictive physiology. Large pericardial effusions appear to be a marker of risk for development of subsequent renal crisis, and may directly contribute to its pathogenesis. Of interest, in developing a semiquantitative cardiac score to predict prognosis,

Clements et al noted that pericardial effusion and left axis deviation on the electrocardiogram were the two most important variables for defining risk (29).

Valvular Disease

There is no evidence to suggest that hemodynamically significant valvular abnormalities are part of the spectrum of cardiac involvement in SSc. There is evidence, however, to suggest that minor abnormalities do occur, particularly involving the mitral valve. D'Angelo et al noted that 38% of their autopsy subjects had areas of nodular thickening of the mitral valve, typically along its free edge (14). In 8% of the subjects, shortening of the mitral chordae tendinea was also described. Oram and Stokes noted that four of 32 patients in their collected autopsy series had vegetations consistent with non-bacterial verrucous endocarditis, two involving the mitral valve alone, and two involving both the mitral and tricuspid valves (3). In one, there was evidence of mitral chordal shortening. Sackner et al described similar findings in five of 25 patients in their autopsy series, four involving the mitral valve and one the tricuspid (95). Kinney et al described a SSc patient with the CRST syndrome who had a murmur of mitral regurgitation for approximately one year (96). An echocardiogram revealed irregular shaggy thickening of the anterior leaflet of the mitral valve. At subsequent autopsy, nodular thickening of the mitral valve was noted. Yunus et al described two SSc patients with isolated aortic regurgitation that was associated with evidence of nodular thickening of the aortic valve by echocardiography (97). Other isolated cases of valvular disease in SSc have been reported (98–100).

There is some evidence to suggest that there may be an increased incidence of mitral valve prolapse in SSc, a finding supported by this writer's personal observation. Comens et al noted that 32% of their 31 SSc patients had echocardiographic and auscultatory findings of mitral valve prolapse, compared to 10% of controls (101). Interestingly, the prevalence of mitral prolapse was also increased in patients with other connective tissue diseases studied by Comens et al, including those with systemic lupus erythematosus and mixed connective tissue disease. Two of 54 subjects undergoing echocardiography in the study by Smith et al (26), and two of 11 in the study by Gottdiener et al, had findings of mitral valve prolapse (38).

Cardiac Involvement in Systemic Sclerosis with Limited Cutaneous Involvement

Patients with SSc with limited cutaneous involvement (CREST syndrome) can also experience cardiac involvement. While there is some variability among studies, however, it appears that the frequency and severity of the cardiac involvement in CREST syndrome is significantly less than that seen in patients with diffuse cutaneous involvement.

Äkesson and Wollheim noted in their review of findings from 100 SSc patients that cardiomegaly was present in 24% of the patients with diffuse scleroderma, compared to only 3% of those with limited cutaneous involvement (102). An abnormal electrocardiogram was noted in 35% and 25% of the two groups, respectively. Geirsson et al suggested that the prevalence of cardiac involvement is the same in

CREST syndrome and diffuse scleroderma, although the findings from their series appear to be somewhat in contrast to this (81). In their study of 40 subjects, 21 of whom had limited cutaneous involvement, the CREST syndrome patients had a lower prevalence of lung involvement, cardiomegaly, cardiopulmonary symptoms, and an abnormal exercise electrocardiogram than did those with diffuse cutaneous involvement (Table 16.6).

Follansbee et al reported findings from an exercise radionuclide evaluation of 22 patients with CREST syndrome, and compared the findings to those obtained from a similar study of 26 patients with diffuse scleroderma (30). While the prevalence of thallium perfusion abnormalities was similar in the two groups (64% in CREST vs 77% in diffuse), the defects were significantly smaller in the CREST subjects. In addition, while 38% of the patients with diffuse scleroderma had exercise-induced thallium perfusion abnormalities in the absence of significant extramural coronary artery disease, this was not found in a single patient with CREST syndrome. In contrast to the patients with diffuse scleroderma, thallium perfusion defects in the CREST syndrome subjects were not associated with abnormalities in left ventricular function either at rest or during exercise. Importantly, unlike the diffuse scleroderma group, none of the CREST syndrome patients had an abnormal left ventricular ejection fraction at rest. Some CREST patients did have an abnormal left ventricular ejection fraction response to

Table 16.6. Prevalence of Cardiac Involvement Comparing CREST Syndrome and Diffuse Scleroderma in the Study by Geirsson et al[a]

	CREST Syndrome	Diffuse Scleroderma
Lung involvement	33%	68%
Cardiomegaly	10%	21%
Cardiopulmonary symptoms	43%	74%
Abnormal resting ECG	38%	37%
Abnormal exercise ECG	24%	37%
Abnormal 24 hour ECG	62%	68%

[a] Geirsson AJ, Blom-Bülow B, Pahlm O, et al. Cardiac involvement in systemic sclerosis. Sem Arthritis Rheum 1989;19:110–116.

exercise, but the abnormalities were all quantitatively mild; no patient had a peak exercise ejection fraction below 50%. Hence, while there was a similar frequency of thallium perfusion defects in the CREST syndrome patients, they did not appear to be functionally significant, unlike those seen in the diffuse scleroderma group.

Thirty-six per cent of the CREST syndrome patients in this study had an abnormal right ventricular ejection fraction. An abnormal right ventricular ejection fraction was not related to radiographic or pulmonary function testing indices of pulmonary fibrosis. However, it was associated with reduced lung diffusing capacity for carbon monoxide, an indicator of pulmonary vascular disease, suggesting that the abnormal right ventricular ejection fraction in the CREST syndrome patients was a manifestation of pulmonary hypertension. This relationship was not seen in the patients with diffuse scleroderma. While the incidence of pulmonary fibrosis is similar in patients with diffuse scleroderma compared to those with limited cutaneous involvement, patients with CREST syndrome are at risk of developing pulmonary vascular disease and severe pulmonary hypertension identical to that seen in patients with primary pulmonary hypertension, a complication which is rare in patients with diffuse disease (103).

Autopsy studies have also demonstrated that myocardial involvement in CREST syndrome patients can occur, although it appears to be less frequent and less severe than that seen in patients with diffuse cutaneous involvement. Bulkley et al noted that three of the 47 patients examined in their autopsy series had the CRST syndrome (16). None of these patients had histologic evidence of myocardial fibrosis. In contrast, Follansbee et al reported autopsy findings of 54 SSc subjects, 15 of whom had the CRST syndrome (17). The prevalence of myocardial fibrosis in their study was not significantly different in the CREST syndrome group (9 out of 15, or 60%) compared to those with diffuse scleroderma (24 out of 31, or 77%). However, compared to the diffuse scleroderma group, the fibrosis was mild

in degree in six of the nine CREST patients, and whereas 19% of the diffuse scleroderma patients had severe myocardial fibrosis, this was not found in any CREST syndrome patient. This suggests that there is a difference in the severity, if not the incidence, of myocardial fibrosis comparing the two groups. Furthermore, the CREST syndrome group in this autopsy study was heavily biased toward patients who had severe pulmonary hypertension, which likely contributed to the development of myocardial fibrosis, particularly in the right ventricle. To that degree, therefore, the study may have overestimated the actual prevalence of myocardial fibrosis in CREST syndrome. Nevertheless, it should be noted that, while none of the CREST syndrome patients in their prior clinical study had significant left ventricular dysfunction (30), there were three CREST syndrome patients in the autopsy series who did have left ventricular dysfunction with myocardial fibrosis in the absence of pulmonary hypertension (17). Hence, while this complication is uncommon in patients with limited cutaneous involvement, it can occur.

Patients with CREST syndrome may also be at risk of developing pericardial disease, but again it appears to be less severe than that experienced by patients with diffuse scleroderma. The echocardiographic study of Smith et al evaluated 54 patients, 13 of whom had CREST syndrome (26). In this study, CREST syndrome was defined by the presence of sclerodactyly alone without more proximal cutaneous involvement, as well as at least three of the cardinal features of CREST. Of the 11 patients in whom sufficiently detailed results were tabulated, five had pericardial effusions at some time in their course. However, these pericardial effusions were small in four of the five patients, and moderate in only one. None of the CREST syndrome patients had a large pericardial effusion, a complication seen in four diffuse scleroderma patients.

Valvular abnormalities may be seen in patients with CREST syndrome. Verrucous endocarditis with nodular thickening of the anterior leaflet of the mitral valve has been described in a patient with CREST syndrome (96), and the incidence of mitral valve prolapse appears to be similar in CREST syndrome and diffuse scleroderma (101). In both CREST syndrome and diffuse scleroderma, however, these valvular abnormalities are functionally mild and do not appear to be clinically significant.

Electrocardiographic abnormalities and arrhythmias may also occur in CREST syndrome patients, including even potentially life threatening arrhythmias (80,92). Geirsson et al noted a similar prevalence of abnormalities on the resting electrocardiogram comparing their patients with CREST syndrome (38%) to those with diffuse scleroderma (37%), but observed that an abnormal exercise electrocardiogram was more common in diffuse scleroderma (37%) than in CREST syndrome (24%) (84). Similarly, Follansbee et al noted that exercise-induced arrhythmia was significantly more frequent in diffuse scleroderma (12 of 26) than in CREST syndrome (3 of 22) (80). Geirsson et al (84) and Ferri et al (5) both observed that the frequency of arrhythmia on 24-hour ambulatory monitoring was not significantly different in CREST syndrome subjects compared to those with diffuse scleroderma. Reporting findings from a multicenter trial, Kostis et al observed that, using univariate analysis, patients with diffuse scleroderma were more likely to manifest supraventricular and ventricular tachycardias than were patients with CREST syndrome (89). However, using multivariate analysis, neither the extent of skin involvement nor the presence or absence of anticentromere antibody were independent predictors of arrhythmias or mortality. Cardiac arrhythmias in this study were strongly associated with mortality, and were related to indices of severity of cardiopulmonary and renal involvement.

In summary, SSc patients with limited cutaneous involvement are at risk of cardiac involvement in the disease process, which can in individual cases be severe or even life threatening. The overall frequency and severity of cardiac involvement, however, is significantly less in CREST syndrome patients than in those with diffuse cutaneous involvement, with the possible exception of arrhythmias which appear to have somewhat similar frequencies in the two groups.

Treatment: Theraputic Trials

There are no prospective or randomized trials available that have specifically investigated the efficacy of any therapy for the treatment of cardiac disease in SSc. No therapeutic agent, other than the use of ACE inhibition in patients with renal crisis, has yet been shown to consistently or predictably alter the course of the disease or, more specifically, its cardiac manifestations (104). As such, all therapies for cardiac involvement in SSc remain empiric and largely symptomatic at the present time. Nevertheless, some studies do provide some insight into possible treatments.

There is considerable evidence, as reviewed previously, to indicate that the vascular system is a target organ in SSc, and specifically that the coronary arterial system is integrally involved in the development of myocardial disease. Abnormal vascular reactivity to serotonin has been demonstrated in SSc patients, and treatment with ketanserin, a serotonin antagonist, has been investigated as a treatment of RP (66,105). Siebold and Jageneau found that ketanserin provided moderate to marked relief of symptoms of RP in 83% of SSc subjects, compared to 33% of patients with RP of other etiology (66). These investigators also noted some objective improvement demonstrated by digital plethysmography and healing of digital ulcerations. Coffman et al reported the findings from a multicenter, double-blind, placebo-controlled trial involving 222 patients (105). They noted a modest but significant reduction in the frequency, but no difference in the severity or duration, of RP episodes with ketanserin compared to placebo, and no difference in total finger blood flow. There was no difference in the response comparing patients with primary or secondary RP. There has been variable efficacy of ketanserin noted in other clinical studies (106,107). No trials have examined the effect of ketanserin on myocardial perfusion in SSc, but the results from the trials that examined its efficacy in treatment of peripheral vasospasm are not encouraging with regard to its potential cardiac benefits.

Multiple studies have demonstrated that SSc patients have thallium perfusion abnormalities which appear to improve with vasodilator therapy including nifedipine (19), nicardipine (23), captopril (25), and dipyridamole (20). However, while thallium perfusion defects have been shown to be important predictors of mortality (31), the therapeutic implication of the apparent benefit of vasodilator therapy is unknown and untested. One cannot assume that the improvement in thallium perfusion defects with vasodilator therapy will translate into an objective therapeutic benefit. There is evidence to suggest that vasodilator therapy has some, although limited, efficacy in the treatment of peripheral RP. Nifedipine has been shown in small studies to promote healing of digital ulcerations (108,109). However, while nifedipine has appeared to be the calcium channel blocker of preference for treatment of RP, it also has the effect of lowering lower esophageal sphincter tone, an adverse effect not found with diltiazem (110). Other vasodilators, for example the peripheral α1-receptor blocker prazosin, have also been suggested to be efficacious in the treatment of peripheral RP (111). Treatment with the ACE inhibitor captopril has well accepted efficacy in the treatment of renal crisis in SSc, a complication with a clear vasospastic component (112–114). Angiotensin is a powerful coronary artery vasoconstrictor, which adds at least theoretical support to a possible role of ACE inhibitor therapy in the treatment of myocardial scleroderma. Overall, the possible efficacy of vasodilator treatment in preventing or modifying the course of myocardial in SSc is an important area for future study. Prospective randomized trials will be essential to address this important question.

Elevated levels of platelets and beta-thromboglobulin have been demonstrated in SSc subjects, and they can be normalized by treatment with aspirin and dipyridamole (65). Whether these abnormalities are of pathophysiologic consequence, or are instead nonspecific markers of endothelial disease, is unknown, so the therapeutic advantage of antiplatelet therapy is at the present time conjectural. However, this is another promising area for further study.

Immunosuppressive therapy has been proposed to be a potentially useful treatment in SSc. Furst et al examined the therapeutic effect of immunosuppressive therapy with the alkylating agent, chlorambucil, in a randomized, placebo-controlled, prospective trial (28). Cardiac index score was the only organ system-based index of disease severity that predicted survival at the end of the trial. However, the results of the trial were disappointing in that there was no demonstrable benefit of chlorambucil therapy in this study group. There was some evidence with subgroup analysis that treadmill double product increased with chlorambucil therapy, but the authors correctly pointed out that this finding should be interpreted with caution, because there were a large number of results tested in subgroup analyses. The probability of finding a false-positive result is considerable. Furthermore, it is significant to note that 25 subjects who were initially enrolled in the trial withdrew within the first several months, some without ever taking the drug. Their entry data were analyzed but because there were no longitudinal data, they were not included in the final analysis. Six of these patients subsequently died of myocardial disease, raising the concern that the study population may have been biased toward less severe cardiac disease. This is further suggested by the fact that 24 of the 65 final study patients had limited cutaneous involvement. In one small trial, plasmapheresis in conjunction with cyclophosphamide and prednisone therapy appeared to be of therapeutic benefit in patients with moderate or severe scleroderma (115). Two patients in this trial had resolution of electrocardiographic abnormalities following treatment. Cyclosporin has also been proposed to have a possible role in the treatment of SSc, but there are no specific data available regarding its effects on the course of myocardial disease (116–118). Overall, the efficacy of immunosuppressive therapy in SSc is uncertain at the present time, and its potential effects on myocardial disease are completely unknown.

Isolated case reports have suggested possible beneficial effects of d-penicillamine treatment on cardiac involvement in SSc patients, including one patient who appeared to have dramatic improvement of advanced heart failure with this treatment (119,120). D-penicillamine appears to have some efficacy in the treatment of pulmonary disease, particularly in improving the diffusing capacity of carbon monoxide, which is of interest because it is a relatively specific marker of pulmonary vascular disease (121,122). In a retrospective analysis of d-penicillamine therapy, Steen et al found improved 5-year survival with d-penicillamine treatment, a finding supported by other studies (123,124). Of visceral involvement, there appeared to be particular benefit in decreasing kidney disease, although penicillamine is also associated with potential renal toxicity (125). There was no apparent benefit on cardiac involvement. The findings from this study must be interpreted with caution since it was a non-randomized study with retrospective analysis. Not all studies have shown benefit of penicillamine treatment (126). Furthermore, d-penicillamine has substantial, well-documented toxicities (127). Nevertheless, the role of d-penicillamine therapy in SSc deserves further study in prospective, randomized trials.

Treatment with colchicine does not appear to have significant benefit in the treatment of scleroderma, particularly with respect to any cardiac manifestations (128,129).

SSc patients are at risk of developing atrial or ventricular tachyarrhythmias, and ventricular ectopy in particular has been associated with long term mortality, including risk of sudden cardiac death (89). The approach to therapy of cardiac arrhythmias in this population, however, remains empiric. Specifically, the role of antiarrhythmic therapy has not been investigated. The potential risk of antiarrhythmic medications, particularly in patients with myocardial dysfunction, should not be underestimated because of their potential proarrhythmic effect and the increased risk of sudden death which might result (130). Cost and morbidity, particularly in terms of side effects, are also important issues to consider. Since patients at high risk of sudden cardiac death can now be identified, randomized therapeutic trials of efficacy of antiarrhythmic therapy are clearly warranted (54,89). Cryoablation of a ventricular tachycardia pathway has been successfully performed in a single patient, but this is obviously an invasive therapy that will not be appropriate in the majority of patients at risk (92). Implantation of cardiac defibrillators in high risk patients may be justified, and requires investigation.

References

1. Heine J. Über ein eigenartiges Krankheitsbild von diffuser Sklerosis der Haut und innerer Organe. Virchows Arch 1926;262:351–382.
2. Weiss S, Stead EA Jr, Warren JV, Bailey OT. Scleroderma heart disease, with a consideration of certain other visceral manifestations of scleroderma. Arch Intern Med 1943;71:749–776.
3. Oram S, Stokes W. The heart in scleroderma. Br Heart J 1961;23:243–225.
4. Clements PJ, Furst DE, Cabeen W, et al. The relationship of arrhythmias and conduction disturbances to other manifestations of cardiopulmonary disease in progressive systemic sclerosis (PSS). Am J Med 1981;71:38–46.
5. Ferri C, Bernini L, Bongiorni MG, et al. Noninvasive evaluation of cardiac dysrhythmias, and their relationship with multisystemic symptoms, in progressive systemic sclerosis. Arthritis Rheum 1985;28:1259–1266.
6. Bulkley BH, Klacsmann PG, and Hutchins GM. Angina pectoris, myocardial infarction and sudden cardiac death with normal coronary arteries: A clinicopathologic study of nine patients with progressive systemic sclerosis. Am Heart J 1978; 95:563–569.
7. Sackner MA, Akgun N, Kimbel P, et al. The pathophysiology of scleroderma involving the heart and respiratory system. Ann Intern Med 1964;60:611–630.

8. Oram S, Stokes W. The heart in scleroderma. Br Heart J 1961;23:243–259.

9. Tuffanelli DL, Winkelmann RK. Systemic scleroderma; a clinical study of 727 cases. Arch Dermatol 1961;84:359–371.

10. Sackner MA, Heinz ER, Steinberg AJ. The heart in scleroderma. Am J Cardiol 1966;17:542–559.

11. Leinwand I, Duryee AW, Richter MN. Scleroderma (based on a study of over 150 cases). Ann Int Med 1954;41:1003–1041.

12. Eason RJ, Tan PL, Gow PJ. Progressive systemic sclerosis in Auckland: A ten year review with emphasis on prognostic features. Aust NZ J Med 1981;11:657–662.

13. Lally EV, Jimenez SA, Kaplan SR. Progressive systemic sclerosis: Mode of presentation, rapidly progressive disease course, and mortality based on an analysis of 91 patients. Semin Arthritis Rheum 1988;18:1–13.

14. D'Angelo WA, Fries JF, Masi +AT, et al. Pathologic observations in systemic sclerosis (scleroderma); a study of fifty-eight autopsy cases and fifty-eight matched controls. Am J Med 1969;46:428–440.

15. McWhorter JE IV, LeRoy EC. Pericardial disease in scleroderma (systemic sclerosis). Am J Med 1974;57:566–575.

16. Bulkley BH, Ridolfi RL, Salyer WR, et al. Myocardial lesions of progressive systemic sclerosis; a cause of cardiac dysfunction. Circulation 1976; 53:483–490.

17. Follansbee WP, Miller TR, Curtiss EI, et al. A controlled clinicopathologic study of myocardial fibrosis in systemic sclerosis (scleroderma). J Rheumatol 1990:17:656–662.

18. Follansbee WP, Curtiss EI, Medsger TA Jr, et al. Physiologic abnormalities of cardiac function in progressive systemic sclerosis with diffuse scleroderma. N Engl J Med 1984;310:142–148.

19. Kahan A, Devaux JY, Amor B, et al. Nifedipine and thallium-201 myocardial perfusion in progressive systemic sclerosis. N Engl J Med 1986; 314:1397–1402.

20. Kahan A, Devaux JY, Amor B, et al. Pharmacodynamic effect of dipyridamole on thallium-201 myocardial perfusion in progressive systemic sclerosis with diffuse scleroderma. Ann Rheum Dis 1986;45:718–725.

21. Alexander EL, Firestein GS, Weiss JL, et al. Reversible cold-induced abnormalities in myocardial perfusion and function in systemic sclerosis. Ann Intern Med 1986;105:661–668.

22. Follansbee WP, Kiernan JM, Curtiss EI, et al. Cold-induced thallium perfusion abnormalities in diffuse scleroderma and Raynaud's disease: Response to diltiazem therapy. Arthritis Rheum 1987;30(suppl 4):S117.

23. Kahan A, Devaux J, Amor B, et al. Nicardipine improves myocardial perfusion in Systemic Sclerosis. J Rheumatol 1988;15:1395–1400.

24. Gustafsson R, Mannting F, Kazzam E, et al. Cold-induced reversible myocardial ischaemia in systemic sclerosis. Lancet 1989;(Aug 26):475–479.

25. Kahan A, Devaux JY, Amor B, et al. The effect of captopril on thallium 201 myocardial perfusion in systemic sclerosis. Clin Pharmacol Ther 1990; 47:483–489.

26. Smith JW, Clements PJ, Levisman J, et al. Echocardiographic features of progressive systemic sclerosis (PSS); correlation with hemodynamic and postmortem studies. Am J Med 1979; 66:28–33.

27. Medsger TA Jr, Masi AT. Survival with scleroderma— II: A life-table analysis of clinical and demographic factors in 358 male U.S. veteran patients. J Chron Dis 1973;26:647–660.

28. Furst DE, Clements PJ, Hillis S, et al. Immunosuppression with chlorambucil, versus placebo, for scleroderma. Results of a three-year, parallel, randomized, double-blind study. Arthritis Rheum 1989;32:584–593.

29. Clements PJ, Lachenbruch PA, Furst DE, et al. Cardiac score; a semiquantitative measure of cardiac involvement that improves prediction of prognosis in systemic sclerosis. Arthritis Rheum 1991;34:1371–1380.

30. Follansbee WP, Curtiss EI, Medsger TA Jr, et al. Myocardial function and perfusion in the CREST syndrome variant of progressive systemic sclerosis. Exercise radionuclide evaluation and comparison with diffuse scleroderma. Am J Med 1984;77:489–496.

31. Steen VD, Follansbee WF. Thallium perfusion abnormalities predict survival and cardiac dysfunction in patients with systemic sclerosis. Arthritis Rheum 1991;35:S37.

32. Follansbee WP. The cardiovascular manifestations of systemic sclerosis (scleroderma). Curr Probl Cardiol 1986;11:242–298.

33. Leinwand I, Duryee AW, Richter MN. Scleroderma (based upon a study of over 150 cases). Ann Intern Med 1954;41:1003–1041.

34. Sackner MA, Heinz ER, Steinberg AJ. The heart in scleroderma. Am J Cardiol 1966;17:542–559.

35. Nair CK, Goli-Bijanki R, Lyckholm L and Sketch MH. Inferior myocardial infarction complicated by mural thrombus and systemic embolization despite anticoagulation in progressive systemic sclerosis with normal coronary arteriograms. Am Heart J 1988;116:1357–1359.

36. Goetz RH. The heart in generalized scleroderma. Progressive systemic sclerosis. Angiology 1951;2: 555–578.

37. Eggebrecht RF, Kleiger RE. Echocardiographic patterns in scleroderma. Chest 1977;71:47–51.

38. Gottdiener JS, Moutsopoulos HM, and Decker JL. Echocardiographic identification of cardiac abnormality in scleroderma and related disorders. Am J Med 1979;66:391–398.

39. Siegel RJ, O"Connor B, Mena I, and Criley JM. Left ventricular function at rest and during Raynaud's phenomenon in patients with scleroderma. Amer Heart J 1984;108:1469–1476.

40. Kazzam E, Waldenström A, Landelius J, et al. Non-invasive assessment of left ventricular diastolic function in patients with systemic sclerosis. J Intern Med 1990;228:183–192.

41. Frayha R, Jubran F, Partamian L, Sawaya J. Hypertrophic nonobstructive cardiomyopathy in scleroderma. Arthritis Rheum 1978;21:609–611.

42. Gaffney FA, Anderson RJ, Nixon JV, and Blomqvist CG. Cardiovascular function in patients with progressive systemic sclerosis (scleroderma). Clin Cardiol 1982;5:569–576.

43. Montanes P, Lawless C, Black C, et al. The heart in scleroderma: A noninvasive assessment. Clin Cardiol 1982;5:383–387.

44. Kazzam E, Caidahl K, Hällgren R, et al. Noninvasive assessment of systolic left ventricular function in systemic sclerosis. Eur Heart J 1991; 12:151–156.

45. Butrous GS, Dowd PM, Milne J, et al. Non-invasive assessment of early cardiac involvement in systemic sclerosis. Postgrad Med J 1985;61:679–684.

46. Kahan A, Nitenberg A, Foult J, et al. Decreased coronary reserve in primary scleroderma myocardial disease. Arthritis Rheum 1985;28:637–646.

47. Westphal CFO. Zwei Falle von schlerodermie. Berlin: Charite-Annalen 1876;3:341–360.

48. Medsger TA, Rodnan GP, Moossy J, et al. Skeletal muscle involvement in progressive systemic sclerosis (scleroderma). Arthritis Rheum 1968;11: 554–568.

49. Thompson JM, Bluestone R, Bywaters EGL, et al. Skeletal muscle involvement in systemic sclerosis. Ann Rheum Dis 1969;28:281–288.

50. Clements PJ, Furst DE, Campion DS, et al. Muscle disease in progressive systemic sclerosis: diagnostic and therapeutic considerations. Arthritits Rheum 1978;21:62–71.

51. West SG, Killian PJ, Lawless OJ. Association of myositis and myocarditis in progressive systemic sclerosis. Arthritis Rheum 1981;24:662–667.

52. Yamaoki K, Yazaki Y, Matsunaga H, et al. An extensive primary myocardial fibrosis in progressive systemic sclerosis. A case report with autopsy findings. Jpn Circ J 1982;46:1159–1165.

53. Carette S, Turcotte J, Mathon G. Severe myositis and myocarditis in progressive systemic sclerosis. J Rheumatol 1985;12:997–999.

54. Follansbee WP, Zerbe TR, Medsger TA Jr. Cardiac and skeletal muscle disease in systemic sclerosis (scleroderma): A high risk association. Am Heart J 1993;125:194–203.

55. Norton WL, Nardo JM. Vascular disease in progressive systemic sclerosis (scleroderma). Ann Intern Med 1970;73:317–324.

56. Campbell PM, LeRoy EC. Pathogenesis of systemic sclerosis: A vascular hypothesis. Semin Arthritis Rheum 1975;4:351–368.

57. Chaithiraphan S, Goldberg E, O'Reilly M, Jootar P. Multiple aneurysms of coronary artery in sclerodermal heart disease. Angiology 1973:24: 86–93.

58. Follansbee WP. The heart in vasculitis. In: Leroy E, ed. Systemic vasculitis, the biologic basis. New York: Marcel Dekker, Inc, 1992;303–380.

59. Jennings RB, Sommers HM, Smyth GA, et al. Myocardial necrosis induced by temporary occlusion of a coronary artery in the dog. Arch Pathol 1960;70:68–78.

60. Sommers HM, Jennings RB. Experimental acute myocardial infarction. Histologic and histochemical studies of early myocardial infarcts induced by temporary or permanent occlusion of a coronary artery. Lab Invest 1964;13:1491–1503.

61. Herdson PB, Sommers HM, Jennings RB. A comparative study of the fine structure of normal and ischemic dog myocardium with special reference to early changes following temporary occlusion of a coronary artery. Am J Pathol 1965;46: 367–377.

62. Reichenbach DD, Benditt EP. Myofibrillar degeneration. A response of the myocardial cell to injury. Arch Path 1968;85:189–199.

63. Rodnan GP, Myerowitz RL, Justh GO. Morphologic changes in the digital arteries of patients with progressive systemic sclerosis (scleroderma) and Raynaud's phenomenon. Medicine (Baltimore) 1980;59:393–408.

64. Janevski B. Arteries of the hand in patients with scleroderma. Diagn Imag Clin Med 1986:55:262–265.

65. Kahaleh MB, Osborn I, LeRoy EC. Elevated levels of circulating platelet aggregates and beta-thromboglobulin in scleroderma. Ann Intern Med 1982;96:610–613.

66. Long A, Duffy G, Bresnihan B. Reversible my-

ocardial perfusion defects during cold challenge in scleroderma. Br J Rheum 1986;25:158–161.

67. Seibold JR, Jageneau AHM. Treatment of Raynaud's phenomenon with ketanserin, a selective antagonist of the serotonin[2] (5-HT$_2$) receptor. Arthritis Rheum 1984;27:139–146.

68. Ellis WW, Baer AN, Robertson RM, et al. Left ventricular dysfunction induced by cold exposure in patients with systemic sclerosis. Am J Med 1986; 80:385–392.

69. Follansbee WP, Kiernan JM, Curtiss EC, et al. Left ventricular function during cold pressor stimulation in diffuse scleroderma, Raynaud's disease, and normals. Arthritis Rheum 1987;30(suppl 4):S117.

70. Dymond DS, Caplin JL, Flatman W, et al. Temporal evolution of changes in left ventricular function induced by cold pressor stimulation. An assessment with radionuclide angiography and gold 195m. Br Heart J 1984;51:557–564.

71. Duboc D, Kahan A, Maziere B, et al. The effect of nifedipine on myocardial perfusion and metabolism in systemic sclerosis. A positron emission tomographic study. Arthritis Rheum 1991;34:198–203.

72. Brown GE, O'Leary PA. Skin capillaries in scleroderma. Arch Intern Med 1925;36:73–88.

73. Maricq HR, LeRoy EC, D'Angelo WA, et al. Diagnostic potential of in vivo capillary microscopy in scleroderma and related disorders. Arthritis Rheum 1980;23:183–189.

74. Lee P, Leung FY-K, Alderdice C, Armstrong SK. Nailfold capillary microscopy in the connective tissue diseases: A semiquantitative assessment. J Rheumatol 1983;10:930–938.

75. DeBure C, Fiessinger J, Priollet P, et al. Relationship between nailfold capillary microscopy and salivary capillary basement membrane width in Raynaud's disease and progressive systemic sclerosis. J Rheumatol 1985;12:279–282.

76. McGill NW, Gow PJ. Nailfold capillaroscopy: A blinded study of its discriminatory value in scleroderma, systemic lupus erythematosus, and rheumatoid arthritis. Aust NZ J Med 1986;16:457–460.

77. Maricq HR, Spencer-Green G, LeRoy EC. Skin capillary abnormalities as indicators of organ involvement in scleroderma (systemic sclerosis), Raynaud's syndrome and dermatomyositis. Am J Med 1976;61:862–870.

78. Joyal F, Choquette D, Roussin A, et al. Evaluation of the severity of systemic sclerosis by nailfold capillary microscopy in 112 patients. Angiology 1992;43:203–210.

79. Norton WL, Hurd ER, Lewis DC, Ziff M. Evi-

dence of microvascular injury in scleroderma and systemic lupus erythematosus: Quantitative study of the microvascular bed. J Lab Clin Med 1968;71:919–933.

80. Follansbee WP, Curtiss EI, Rahko PS, et al. The electrocardiogram in systemic sclerosis (scleroderma). Study of 102 consecutive cases with functional correlations and review of the literature. Am J Medicine 1985;79:183–192.

81. Geirsson AJ, Blom-Bülow B, Pahlm O, and Äkesson A. Cardiac involvement in systemic sclerosis. Sem Arthritis Rheum 1989;19:110–116.

82. Urai L, Veress G, Urai K. Scleroderma-Heart and conduction disturbances. Acta Medica Academiae Scientiarum Hungaricae, 1978;35:189–200.

83. Anuar M, Singham KT. Systemic scleroderma with complete heart block. Med J Malaysia 1983; 38:65–67.

84. Roberts NK, Cabeen WR, Moss J, et al. The prevalence of conduction defects and cardiac arrhythmias in progressive systemic sclerosis. Ann Intern Med 1981;94:38–40.

85. Roberts NK, Cabeen WR. Atrioventricular nodal function in progressive systemic sclerosis: Electrophysiological and morphological findings. Br Heart J 1980;44:529–533.

86. Loperfido F, Fiorilli R, Santarelli P, et al. Severe involvement of the conduction system in a patient with sclerodermal heart disease. An electrophysiological study. Acta Cardiol 1982;37:31–38.

87. Lev M, Landowne M, Matchar JC, Wagner JA. Systemic scleroderma with complete heart block. Report of a case with comprehensive study of the conduction system. Am Heart J 1966;72:13–24.

88. Ridolfi RL, Bulkley BH, Hutchins GM. The cardiac conduction system in progressive systemic sclerosis. Clinical and pathologic features of 35 patients. Am J Med 1976;61:361–366.

89. Kostis JB, Seibold JR, Turkevich D, et al. Prognsotic importance of cardiac arrhythmias in systemic sclerosis. Am J Med 1988;84:1007–1015.

90. Marinato PG, Thiene G, Menghetti L, et al. Clinicopathologic assessment of arrhythmias in a case of scleroderma heart disease with sudden death. Eur Heart J 1981;12:321–331.

91. Moser DK, Stevenson WG, Woo MA, et al. Frequency of late potentials in systemic sclerosis. Am J Cardiol 1991;67:541–543.

92. Gallagher JJ, Anderson RW, Kasell J, et al. Cryoablation of drug-resistant ventricular tachycardia in a patient with a variant of scleroderma. Circulation 1978;57:190–197.

93. Meltzer JI. Pericardial effusion in generalized scleroderma. Am J Med 1956;20:638–642.

94. Uhl GS, Koppes GM. Pericardial tamponade in

systemic sclerosis (scleroderma). Br Heart J 1979; 42:345–348.

95. Sackner MA, Heinz ER and Steinberg AJ. The heart in scleroderma. Am J Cardiol 1966;17:542–559.

96. Kinney E, Reeves W, Zelis R. The echocardiogram in scleroderma; endocarditis of the mitral valve. Arch Intern Med 1979;139:1179–1180.

97. Yunus MB, Radford CM, Masi AT, et al. Aortic regurgitation in scleroderma. J Rheumatol 1984;11: 384–386.

98. Jones EW. Valvular disease of the heart in systemic scleroderma. Br J Dermatol 1962;74:183–190.

99. Sabour MS, El Mahallauy MN. Mitral and aortic valve disease in a patient with scleroderma. Br J Dermatol 1966;78:15–23.

100. Roth LM, Kissane JM. Panaortitis and aortic valvulitis in progressive systemic sclerosis (scleroderma). Report of a case with perforation of an aortic cusp. Am J Clin Pathol 1964;41:287–296.

101. Comens SM, Alpert MA, Sharp GC, et al. Frequency of mitral valve prolapse in systemic lupus erythematosus, progressive systemic sclerosis and mixed connective tissue disease. Am J Cardiol 1989;63:369–370.

102. Åkesson A, Wollheim FA. Organ manifestations in 100 patients with progressive systemic sclerosis: A comparison between the CREST syndrome and diffuse scleroderma. Br J Rheumatol 1989; 28:281–286.

103. Salerni R, Rodnan GP, Leon DF, Shaver JA. Pulmonary hypertension in the CREST syndrome variant of progressive systemic sclerosis (scleroderma). Ann Int Med 1977;86:394–399.

104. McGee BA, Barnett MD, Small RE. Current options for the treatment of systemic sclerosis. Clin Pharmacy 1991;10:14–25.

105. Coffman JD, Clement DL, Creager MA, et al. International study of ketanserin in Raynaud's phenomenon. Am J Med 1989;87:264–268.

106. Engelhart M. Ketanserin in the treatment of Raynaud's phenomenon associated with generalized scleroderma. Br J Dermatol 1988;119:751–754.

107. Klimiuk PS, Kay EA, Taylor ML, et al. Ketanserin: An effective treatment regimen for digital ischaemia in systemic sclerosis. Scand J Rheumatol 1989;18:107–111.

108. Czirják L, Szegedi G. Nifedipine treatment for progressive systemic sclerosis. Arthritis Rheum 1986;29:1053–1054.

109. Woo TY, Wong RC, Campbell JP, et al. Nifedipine in scleroderma ulcerations. Int J Dermatol 1984; 23:678–680.

110. Jean F, Aubert A, Bloch F, et al. Effects of diltiazem versus nifedipine on lower esophageal sphincter pressure in patients with progressive systemic sclerosis. Arthritis Rheum 1986;29:1054–1055.

111. Surwit RS, Gilgor RS, Allen LM, Duvic M. A double-blind study of prazosin in the treatment of Raynaud's phenomenon in scleroderma. Arch Dermatol 1984;120:329–331.

112. Lopez-Ovejero JA, Saal SD, D'Angelo WA, et al. Reversal of vascular and renal crises of scleroderma by oral angiotensin-converting-enzyme inhibitor blockade. N Engl J Med 1979;300:1417–1419.

113. Zawada ET Jr, Clements PJ, Furst DA, et al. Clinical course of patients with scleroderma renal crisis treated with captopril. Nephron 1981;27: 74–78.

114. Chapman PJ, Pascoe MD, van Zyl-Smit R. Successful use of captopril in the treatment of "scleroderma renal crisis." Clin Nephrol 1986;26:106–108.

115. Dau PC, Kahaleh MB, Sagebiel RW. Plasmapheresis and immunosuppressive drug therapy in scleroderma. Arthritis Rheum 1981;24:1128–1136.

116. Knop J, Bonsmann G. Cyclosporin in the treatment of progressive systemic sclerosis. In: Schindler R, ed. First international symposium on cyclosporin in autoimmune disease. Basie, March 18–20, 1985;199–200.

117. Yocum DE, Wilder RL. Cyclosporin A in progressive systemic sclerosis. Am J Med 1987;83:369–370.

118. Amor B, Dougados M. Cyclosporine: Therapeutic effects in rheumatic diseases. Transpl Proc 1988;20(3 Suppl 4):218–223.

119. Muers M, Stokes W. Treatment of scleroderma heart by d-penicillamine. Br Heart J 1976;38: 864–867.

120. Kang B, Veres-Thorner C, Heredia R, et al. Successful treatment of far-advanced progressive systemic sclerosis by d-penicillamine. J Allergy Clin Immunol 1982;69:297–305.

121. Steen VD, Owens GR, Redmond C, et al. The effect of d-penicillamine on pulmonary findings in systemic sclerosis. Arthritis Rheum 1985;28:882–888.

122. De Clerck LS, Dequeker J, Francx L, Demedts M. D-penicillamine therapy and interstitial lung disease in scleroderma; a long-term followup study. Arthritis Rheum 1987;30:643–650.

123. Steen VD, Medsger TA Jr, Rodnan GP. D-penicillamine therapy in progressive systemic sclerosis (scleroderma); a retrospective analysis. Ann Int Med 1982;97:652–659.

124. Jimenez SA, Sigal SH. A 15-year prospective study

of treatment of rapidly progressive systemic sclerosis wit D-penicillamine. J Rheumatol 1991;18: 1496–1503.

125. Ntoso KA, Tomaszewski JE, Jimenez SA, Nielson EG. Penicillamine-induced rapidly progressive glomerulonephritis in patients with progressive systemic sclerosis: Successful treatment of two patients and a review of the literature. Am J Kidney Dis 1986;VIII:159–163.

126. Akesson A, Blom-Bülow B, Scheja A, et al. Long-term evaluation of penicillamine of cyclofenil in systemic sclerosis; results from a two-year randomized study. Scand J Rheumatol 1992;21:238–244.

127. Steen VD, Blair S, Medsger TA Jr. The toxicity of d-penicillamine in systemic sclerosis. Ann Int Med 1986;104:699–705.

128. Guttadauria M, Diamond H, Kaplan D. Colchicine in the treatment of scleroderma. J Rheumatol 1977;4:272–276.

129. Steigerwald JC. Colchicine vs. placebo in the treatment of progressive systemic sclerosis. In, Black CM, Myers AR, eds. Current topics in rheumatology; systemic sclerosis (scleroderma). New York: Gower Medical Publishing Limited, 1985;415–417.

130. Echt DS, Liebson RR, Mitchell LB, et al. Mortality and morbidity in patients receiving encainide, flecainide, or placebo. The cardiac arrhythmia suppression trial. N Engl J Med 1991;324:781–788.

HILDEGARD R. MARICQ
EDWIN A. SMITH

17

Organ Involvement: Peripheral Vascular

Systemic sclerosis (SSc), or scleroderma, is a disease of unknown origin with pathological changes of vascular and connective tissues in many organs, including muscle tissue and the skin. The earliest clinical signs and symptoms of SSc relate to disturbances in the peripheral vascular system, which is the subject of this chapter.

Pathogenesis

There is no reason to believe that the vascular and microvascular lesions occurring in the peripheral vascular system differ in their basic pathogenetic mechanisms from those of blood vessels in other organs. The detailed sequence of events, however, and the interaction of the various factors that play a role in the vascular and connective tissue changes leading to fibrosis may not be identical.

The participation of pathological mechanisms in immunological phenomena, connective tissue metabolism, coagulation and fibrinolysis, and in the endothelial cell function has been implicated in the pathogenesis of SSc. The activation of T cells and other lymphocytes, endothelial cell pathology, endothelial cell-blood leucocyte interactions, and the role of endothelial cells in the regulation of vascular tone and hemostasis have all received increased attention in recent years (1–12). The list of individual factors suspected to play a role in the pathogenesis of SSc has also increased rapidly and now includes a variety of cytokines, growth factors, vasoactive peptides such as endothelin, factors cytotoxic to endothelial cells, plasminogen activator and adhesion molecules (13–36). The mast cell is also suspected to play a role in the pathogenesis of SSc (37,38). The etiological agent is still unknown, although several candidates, including retroviruses, have been proposed (39–42).

All these factors act at the microvascular level and presumably injure the endothelial cells and trigger a cascade of events that leads to tissue injury and fibrosis; however, no conclusive evidence regarding the relative role and timing of these various factors in the pathogenesis of SSc has yet emerged from the numerous studies performed. None of the factors so far studied are specific to SSc, since they are also implicated in vascular injury in other diseases, such as atherosclerosis, diabetes, and hypertension.

Although endothelial injury has been observed in SSc (43–45), the exact sequence of the pathogenetic events is not clear, and there is yet no answer to the question of which factors play the primary role and which are epiphenomena.

Serum levels of substances presumably released by activated or injured endothelial cells in SSc have been measured to document endothelial cell injury (46–48). A difficulty in unraveling the pathogenesis of SSc derives from the fact that many studies use venous blood samples, which may not accurately reflect what is happening at the microvascular level. This could explain why a study by Blann et al (48) found no correlation between serum levels of suspected mediators of endothelial cell injury (tumor necrosis factor, circulating immune complexes, and oxidized lipoproteins) and indicators of endothelial injury (von Willebrand factor, angiotensin converting enzyme).

Pathology and Pathophysiology

The belief that vascular lesions precede fibrotic lesions is supported by data from studies of the peripheral vascular system. Raynaud's phenomenon (RP) generally precedes by months to years the diagnosis of SSc, which is based on a characteristic distribution of skin fibrosis. Microvascular lesions seen in uninvolved skin (49) also support this hypothesis.

Although the microvasculature is the main site of vascular pathology in SSc, large vessel disease can also occur. Furthermore, SSc can affect the digital artery, which is neither a large artery nor a microvessel. The closure of the digital artery in response to cold is believed to be the basis of RP, which is frequently the first symptom of SSc. This chapter, therefore, reviews the peripheral vascular system by arbitrarily dividing it into large vessels, the digital artery, and the microvasculature.

LARGE PERIPHERAL ARTERIES

The involvement of peripheral blood vessels other than the digital arteries is considered to occur so infrequently that it is rarely mentioned in textbooks. For this chapter, information was obtained from case reports and from arteriographic studies, as summarized below.

Furey et al (50) reported five cases of arterial thrombosis in SSc, with three of these cases involving larger arteries (and in one case also veins) of the extremities: (*a*) occlusion of both popliteal arteries; varying degree of intimal hyperplasia with marked narrowing of lumen in large and medium-sized arteries; (*b*) severe intimal fibrosis of major arteries of the foot with evidence of thrombosis and focal calcification; (*c*) arteries

and veins of the lower leg with mild to moderate intimal hyperplasia. Dorevitch (51) reported a lower limb amputation in a 34-year-old patient who had popliteal artery occlusion and marked intimal hyperplasia of the large vessels in the leg, as shown by histological examination. Shapiro (52) reported one case with thrombosis of both superficial femoral arteries and reviewed literature on large vessel thrombosis in SSc. He concluded that, in most cases, evidence of atherosclerotic origin of the reported lesions was minimal and that arterial occlusion could be related to the underlying SSc vascular disease, overlap with some other connective tissue disease (CTD), vasculitis, or to the antiphospholipid syndrome. Baril et al (53) reported another case of SSc with multiple thrombotic events in peripheral and visceral large vessels.

Youssef et al (54) reported four patients, three with the CREST syndrome and one with diffuse SSc, who had severe macrovascular disease with only minimal general vascular risk factors. All four showed involvement of the large arteries of the extremities: (*a*) severe narrowing of the left anterior tibial artery; (*b*) widespread arterial narrowing in the legs and severe right superficial femoral artery stenosis; (*c*) occlusion of left ulnar and radial arteries, arterial occlusion in multiple vessels bilaterally in the legs; (*d*) total occlusion of the two ulnar arteries.

Additional information comes from a study by Rodnan et al (55) of postmortem specimens obtained from the popliteal and posterior tibial arteries of one SSc patient. A photograph of a section of the posterior tibial artery shows an occlusive thrombus, intimal fibrosis, adventitial fibrosis, and telangiectasia of vasa vasorum.

Arteriographic studies of the hand have revealed defects in arteries proximal to the digital arteries in some patients with SSc. Dabich et al (56) found evidence of narrowing or occlusion of the ulnar artery in 16 of 31 patients with SSc, while the radial artery was involved in only two cases. The superficial palmar arch was affected in five patients. Jeune and Thivolet (57) also reported ulnar artery involvement in 13 of 22 SSc patients and radial artery abnormalities in two of 22 patients.

Jones et al reported five patients with progressive, severe, unilateral RP who were found by arteriography to have proximal occlusion of the radial and ulnar arteries (58). A transverse section through the distal ulnar artery (Fig. 17.1) shows marked intimal hyperplasia and virtual occlusion of the lumen. In another publication, Jones et al (59) described two patients who had undergone successful microsurgical revascularization. One of these patients had an occlusion of the radial artery at the level of the wrist, and an extensive occlusion of the distal ulnar artery and the superficial palmar arch, while the other patient had an occlusion of the distal ulnar artery and of the superficial palmar arch.

The conclusion that can be drawn from this review suggests that involvement of peripheral blood vessels of the lower extremities is indeed rare. The situation may be different regarding the upper extremities, in which over 50% of the pa-

tients have been shown by arteriography to have ulnar artery involvement.

DIGITAL ARTERIES

Digital artery abnormalities, both anatomical and functional, have long been the focus of studies trying to explain the frequent association of RP with SSc. RP is present in over 95% of these patients and usually precedes the diagnosis of SSc.

Although digital artery lesions were described earlier in a small number of patients with RP of varying severity, only one case of SSc was included (60). In that patient the ulnar, palmar, and digital arteries presented "conspicuous intimal thickening." Rodnan et al performed a thorough study of 16 unselected SSc patients from whom digital artery specimens were obtained during postmortem examinations (55). All patients but one suffered from diffuse SSc; the remaining patient had a typical CREST syndrome. All 25 specimens obtained from these patients showed structural abnormalities, of which severe intimal

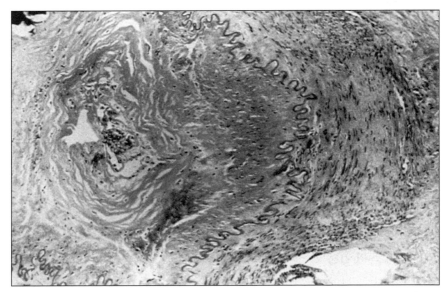

Figure 17.1. Transverse section through the distal ulnar artery showing marked intimal hyperplasia and virtual occlusion of the lumen. (Reproduced with permission from Jones NF, Imbriglia JE, Steen VD, Medsger TA. Surgery for scleroderma of the hand. J Hand Surg 1987;12A:391–400.)

fibrosis was the most prominent (Fig. 17.2). In many cases, the severe intimal fibrosis was associated with marked luminal narrowing and recent or old thrombosis.

These findings support the opinion already expressed by Lewis in 1933 (61) that structural narrowing is mainly responsible for RP associated with scleroderma, as opposed to the pathophysiological mechanisms in primary RP in which the digital arteries remain histologically normal. Therefore, it is generally believed that a normal vasoconstrictor response to cooling could trigger an RP attack in SSc patients. However, organic vascular changes in the wall of the digital arteries do not exclude the possibility that other factors, as discussed below, that are implicated in the pathogenesis of primary RP, may also operate in SSc. In recent years, the older hypothesis of hyperactivity of the sympathetic nervous system in RP has been replaced by that of a balance between α_1- and α_2-adrenergic receptor responses to cooling (62). In animal studies, cooling increases the α_2-adrenergic responsiveness while reducing the α_1-adrenergic responsiveness in cutaneous veins (63). Recently, it was found that vascular α_1- and α_2-adrenoreceptors, present in arteries and veins of the human skin, are modulated by cooling in a manner similar to that observed in animal models (64,65). Furthermore, α_2-adrenoreceptors are more prominently distributed in the distal than in the proximal vasculature and are also present in the digital vascular bed (66). Serotonergic receptors are also considered important, especially in vasoconstriction caused by body cooling (67,68).

It has been postulated, therefore, that an α_2-adrenergic mechanism may play a role in RP patients by producing RP attacks in response to cooling (62,64,69,70). Cold-induced potentiation of α_2-adrenergic vasoconstriction has indeed been reported in primary RP patients, but it is not known whether this is related to increased α_2-receptor sensitivity or to an increased number of receptors (70).

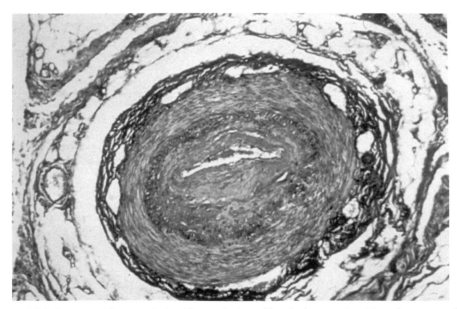

Figure 17.2. Digital artery with severe intimal hyperplasia and luminal narrowing. Note also severe adventitial fibrosis and marked telangiectasia of the vasa vasorum. (Reproduced with permission from Rodnan GP, Myerowitz RL, Justh GO. Morphologic changes in the digital arteries of patients with progressive systemic sclerosis (scleroderma) and Raynaud phenomenon. Medicine 1980;59:393–408.)

The possibility has also been considered that a decrease in the normal, cold-induced attenuation of the α_1-adrenergic response to cooling may increase the α_2-adrenergic vasoconstriction in RP patients, in whom a marked reduction of α_1-adrenergic reactivity compared to controls has been reported (62,64). Pharmacotherapy based on these hypotheses has been considered (64,71), but actual trials have not been proposed, as more research is needed to elucidate the mechanisms involved.

Most of these studies have been performed on normal volunteers and on patients with primary RP; only a few SSc patients have been included, making it impossible to draw conclusions regarding the relative importance of α_2-adrenergic and serotonergic receptors in SSc-related RP.

Recently, it has also been shown, in both primary and SSc related RP, that RP attacks can be produced by combined body and local cooling in fingers in which a digital nerve block has been performed (72). Pathophysiological explanations for such a response remain unknown, though humoral and local mechanisms are suggested.

The nature of a "local fault," proposed by Lewis (61) as the basis of RP, has remained elusive. It is interesting to note, however, that the patients described by Lewis, in whom he implied the local fault as a causal mechanism, all displayed nutritional changes in the skin of the fingers, such as chronic swelling, atrophy, and sclerodactyly. Some also showed limited flexion of the fingers or had tiny depressed scars left by "separation of a plug of tissue." Lewis concluded that the digital arteries are "almost certainly the seat of structural disease" in such patients. These reviewers believe that patients with such digital symptoms probably are in the early phase of SSc or represent the spectrum of SSc patients with the fewest clinically apparent changes.

There is little direct biopsy or autopsy information regarding the state of digital arteries in early SSc. Zweifler and Trinkaus (73) present plethysmographic data of RP patients and the results of their follow-up, suggesting that the RP in the early stages of SSc is due to organic changes rather than to a functional disorder, contrary to "the dominant view that Raynaud's phenomenon in early scleroderma is a functional disorder indistinguishable from Raynaud's disease."

Functional studies have shown a greater fall in digital systolic pressure in response to cooling in SSc patients than in those patients with primary RP (74,75), whose response is already abnormal when compared to controls (76). In addition, the critical closing pressure of the digital artery (77,78) is reached, in most patients, at higher cooling temperatures in SSc than in primary RP, and the digital artery remains closed for a short time, even when the occlusion cuff pressure is released. Already at average room temperature and without local cooling, the ratio of digital:brachial systolic blood pressure is lower than normal in SSc (79).

A variety of humoral and biorheological factors have also been implicated in RP, such as increased plasma levels of free serotonin (80) and endothelin-1 (25,32), increased platelet aggregation (81,82), and decreased red blood cell deformability (83,84). However, there have been few direct correlations with blood flow studies, making it difficult to evaluate the role of these factors in RP.

MICROVASCULATURE

The microvasculature, as usually defined (85), comprises blood vessels of less than 300μm in diameter and includes arterioles (sometimes classified into 1st through 4th order according to their successive branching from the feeding artery), a pre-capillary zone, capillaries, and venules. Some authors include the smallest arteries and small veins, as well. It is generally agreed that the primary site of vascular pathology in SSc is found at this level. This chapter focuses on the microvasculature of the hand and of the fingers, in particular, because the first evidence of SSc usually becomes apparent in the fingers: RP, edema, sclerodactyly, ulcerations, and pitting scars.

Histopathological studies of the muscle

microvasculature in SSc (43) have shown a striking loss of normal-sized capillaries and a shift of the distribution peak of microvessel diameter in SSc patients to 5.5 to 6.5 μm, as compared to 3.5 to 4.5 μm in normal subjects. The larger microvessels observed in increased numbers in SSc patients were venules. The major capillary abnormalities were an increase in thickness, reduplication of the capillary basement membrane, and endothelial swelling.

Numerous reports have described histopathological changes in the microvasculature of the skin in SSc. These include a reduction in the number of capillaries, swelling of endothelial cells, thickening and reduplication of the capillary basement membrane, increased capillary wall thickness and mucoid intimal hyperplasia in arterioles and small arteries, and perivascular cellular infiltrates (45–47). An increased turnover of skin endothelial cells to replace injured cells has been suggested as an explanation for the increased thymidine labeling of these cells (86). For additional information, the reader should refer to Chapter 18, Organ Involvement: Skin.

Superficial microvessels of the skin can also be studied by the *in vivo* microscopic methods first reported by Lombard in 1912 (87). With this technique, capillaries and venules, occasionally also arterioles, can be observed under a microscope after covering the observation site with oil and using reflected light for illumination. Although skin blood vessels have been observed by *in vivo* microscopic examination in many areas of the body, the preferred site is the nailfold.

Reports of nailfold capillary abnormalities seen by *in vivo* microscopy in the skin of patients with SSc date back to the 1920s (88,89). Sporadic publications appeared on this subject between 1950 and 1970 (90–97); these publications are reviewed by Jablonska (98). An increased interest in this area of research has occurred in the last two decades (99–118). Although, in many diseases, the relationship of nailfold capillary observations in clinically normal fingers to microvascular changes elsewhere in the body and to the systemic disease is questionable, the situation is different in SSc, where the fingers are the first location to show clinically observable symptoms, such as RP and sclerodactyly. In addition to the nailfold, the skin microvasculature of the rest of the hand is also easily accessible to *in vivo* microscopic examination.

Microvascular abnormalities observed in the nailfolds of SSc patients occur in a pattern that is characteristic of the scleroderma spectrum (SDS) disorders: SSc and closely related conditions such as the CREST variant of SSc, scleroderma sine scleroderma, dermatomyositis (DM), mixed connective tissue disease (MCTD), the overlap syndrome of SSc and systemic lupus erythematosus (SLE), and SSc-related RP preceding the diagnosis of SSc (103).

The most specific features of this scleroderma pattern of capillary changes (Fig. 17.3) are: (*a*) the presence of enlarged capillaries, especially at the edge of the nailfold, which show an increase in caliber of all three portions (arterial, apical and venous) of the capillary loop; and (*b*) a variable loss of nailfold capillaries, both along the edge and in the more proximal part of the nailfold, ranging from a "drop out" of a few capillaries (119) to avascular areas measuring from 0.4 to >4.0 mm^2 (120).

A less frequently observed feature is the "bushy" formation, which is the budding of small, thin capillaries apparently from a common "trunk" (not to be confused with capillary loops having two or three irregular branches instead of an average hairpin type loop). Bushy formations appear to represent angiogenesis and can be observed in association with avascular lesions; they are more frequently seen in DM and MCTD than in SSc.

Other microvascular abnormalities that are less specific and can be observed in SDS disorders and in other CTDs are: capillary hemorrhages, especially visible in the cuticle (during their slow elimination by "growing out" with the cuticle); enlarged and elongated capillaries, which have preserved relatively normal ratios of arterial vs. venous segments; thrombotic capillaries; and pericapillary hemorrhages. Some patients with

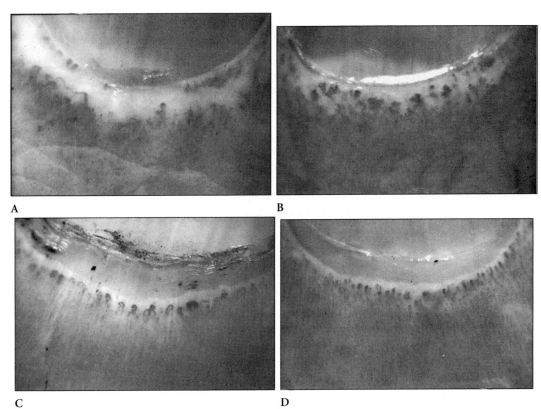

A   B

C   D

Figure 17.3. SD-type capillary patterns seen in patients with scleroderma spectrum (SDS) disorders. (*a*) "Active" pattern: extensive avascular area, destruction of capillaries with little increase in size of the remaining nailfold capillaries. (*b*) "Active" pattern: extensive relatively avascular area but also exhibiting evidence of capillary neo-formation—the presence of "bushy" capillaries. (*c*) "Slow" pattern: enormous capillaries with little capillary loss. (*d*) Numerous, moderately enlarged capillaries along the edge of the nailfold with little capillary loss—intermediate form, neither "active" nor "slow." In both 3*c* and 3*d* the capillary density along the edge of the nailfold is lower than normal, but there is not enough capillary loss to result in avascular areas.

SSc or DM exhibit yellow-orange staining of the cuticle, which probably is caused by the diffusion of plasma proteins into the cuticle from capillaries having an abnormal permeability or after capillary destruction. Comparisons of the data from *in vivo* and histological studies (121) have shown a good correlation with regard to capillary density, and demonstrate that the avascular zones observed *in vivo* cannot be ascribed to blanching from vasoconstriction.

The degree of avascularity shows a good correlation to the amount of periodic acid-Schiff positive material (121) containing immunoglobulins and found in the dermal papillae and cuti-

cle, as shown by immunofluorescence studies (122). The presence of extensive avascular areas is also related to an active disease and more internal organ involvement than the presence of extremely enlarged capillary loops associated with little capillary loss (106,123). Serial observations (Fig. 17.4) have revealed that, in the development of nailfold capillary abnormalities, the two aspects of the SDS pattern (enlargement of capillary loops and destruction of capillaries, resulting in avascular areas) do not necessarily proceed in a parallel fashion. In the active phase of the disease, extensive avascular areas can occur without appreciable increase in capillary size.

This is best illustrated in dermatomyositis (124), though it is also seen in SSc (Figs. 17-3 and 17-4b). The degree of avascularity discussed here ranges from 2 mm² to >4 mm² per nailfold. The loss of capillaries producing such extensive avascular areas is never preceded by the presence of enlarged loops (megacapillaries), as described for the loss of single capillaries in a few patients by Wong et al (125). On the other hand, extremely enlarged capillaries may be accompanied by a decreased density of capillaries at the edge of the nailfold but without any appreciable areas of complete avascularity (<0.4 mm² per nailfold).

The "white band" between the tips of the endrow capillaries and the cuticle is also considerably wider in many SSc patients (Fig. 17.5), but it is not clear whether this is related to a loss of capillaries or to the changed appearance of that part of the nailfold resulting from extravasation of plasma protein and/or other possible changes in the connective tissue.

The gradual enlargement of capillaries to enormous megacapillaries (sometimes clinically visible telangiectases) is a slow process (taking from several months to years) associated with a slowly progressing disease, while the development of avascular areas (Figs. 17.4a and 17.4b) can occur relatively quickly (in weeks to months)

(106,126,127). Regression of such lesions can also take place, but it is less frequent.

Clusters of enlarged capillaries can also be observed on the dorsal and palmar sides of the fingers and on the palm. Large clusters can be seen by the naked eye; they correspond to the punctate telangiectases associated with CREST. Ulcerations on the finger pads and on the dorsal skin of the joints are also surrounded by enlarged capillaries (103,106).

Because of the relationship between certain combinations of microvascular abnormalities and clinical disease activity, two patterns have been described that are at the opposite poles of the "activity range." The hallmark of the "active pattern" is a moderate to extensive capillary loss (as described above, covering 2 to more than 4 mm² per nailfold) often accompanied by marked permeability changes and capillary hemorrhages, but frequently shows little enlargement of the remaining capillary loops. On serial examination, changes in the size and distribution of capillary loops and avascular areas occur in a matter of weeks or months.

The "slow pattern" shows enormous capillary loops in the nailfold with little capillary loss (covering less than 2 mm² per nailfold) and/or CREST type capillary telangiectases. These le-

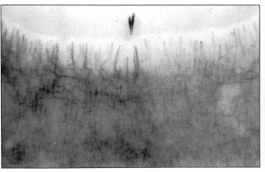
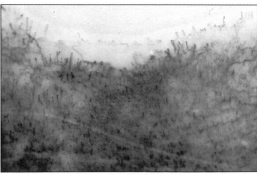

A   B

Figure 17.4. (*a*) A patient with recent onset SSc. Nailfold capillaries show no specific abnormalities. (*b*) The same nailfold 3 months later. Considerable loss of capillaries has occured during the interval: an active pattern. Clinically, the disease had progressed considerably. (Reproduced with permission from Maricq HR. Capillaroscopy in Raynaud's syndrome. Vasc Med Rev 1992;3:3–20.)

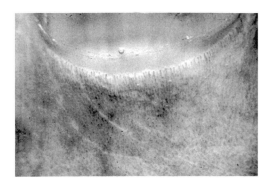 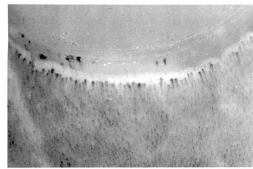

A   B

Figure 17.5. The "white band" often observed in SSc patients' nailfolds between the endrow capillaries and the cuticle. (*a*) Nailfold of a normal subject. (*b*) Nailfold of a SSc patient. Note not only the slight widening of the light zone along the edge of the nailfold but also its much brighter white coloration.

sions may remain stationary or evolve very slowly over the years. Change from one pattern to the other can occur in parallel with a change in disease activity.

The scleroderma-type (SD-type) nailfold capillary abnormalities have diagnostic value in the early stage of SSc and help to make a differential diagnosis between primary RP and RP in patients at risk for SDS disorders. These microvascular patterns have high specificity and sensitivity for such disorders and have increasingly been found to be the best predictors of the development of SDS in follow-up studies of RP patients (128–134).

The prognostic potential of capillary microscopy findings is related to their value in reflecting the disease activity. An "active pattern" has a bad prognosis because actively progressing SSc usually has a serious prognosis. Similarly, a "slow pattern" can indicate a favorable prognosis because a slowly progressing disease usually has a good prognosis. However, capillary patterns can change with a change in disease activity, and may not have a long-term prognostic value.

Capillary microscopy has also been used to differentiate between the localized and systemic forms of both scleroderma and lupus erythematosus (135). Furthermore, nailfold capillary abnormalities have been shown, by some investi-

gators, to correlate with indicators of internal organ involvement (102,136–139).

In vinyl chloride (VC) disease, a non-SDS disorder related to environmental exposure to vinyl chloride, nailfold capillary changes can be seen that are similar to those in the slow SDS pattern of SSc. VC disease can be distinguished from SSc by clinical features, and capillary changes in VC disease are much less numerous and often limited to isolated capillary enlargements (140). Capillary changes characteristic of SDS can also be helpful in the diagnosis of scleroderma sine scleroderma (141) and in differentiating SSc and eosinophilic fasciitis (142,143).

In addition to observations of morphological changes in the microvasculature, *in vivo* microscopic methods can be applied to functional studies. Capillaries in SSc patients display abnormal permeability characteristics, as shown by Na-fluorescein injections (144). Although this dye diffuses out of normal capillaries as well, the time course and distribution are quite different in SSc, where diffusion takes place in an irregular fashion, forming large "pools" next to some portions of the capillary, in contrast with the increased but uniform Na-fluorescein diffusion in diabetic patients (145). The Na-fluorescein injection method also helps to distinguish the isolated, large capillaries seen in hereditary hemorrhagic telangiectasia from those in CREST syndrome (146).

The skin blood flow in SSc has been shown to be abnormal by a variety of techniques, including direct microscopic observations of the capillary blood flow. Cooling decreases the blood flow in the skin of the finger, especially in the capillaries, more drastically in patients with SSc than in those with primary RP (147–150). Microscopic observations have demonstrated a complete standstill of the blood flow in the capillaries of SSc patients on exposure to cold, when the skin was still at relatively high temperature levels (151).

Clinical Signs and Symptoms

LARGE PERIPHERAL ARTERIES

Clinical signs and symptoms related to large artery involvement, a rare occurrence, depend on the degree of obstruction of the blood vessel and are similar to those produced by vascular obstructive lesions from any other cause; they need no special discussion here.

DIGITAL ARTERY

The main clinical symptoms and signs of digital artery involvement—whether by an organic lesion of the vessel wall, by a more subtle "local fault," or by a change in adrenergic receptors—are related to RP. The usual definition describes RP as an episodic, vasospastic attack, consisting of blanching and/or cyanosis of the fingers, followed by hyperemia, in response to cold or emotional stress and accompanied by feelings of numbness, tingling, and pain. This definition is both under- and overinclusive in its criteria. It does not specify that the vasospasm is not just an exaggerated (i.e., more intense than normal) vasoconstrictor response to environmental stimuli, but a qualitatively different response as well, i.e., an intense segmental response with demarcation. Furthermore, patients reporting all three phases of RP are a small minority (152), and even

the often stated requirement to have at least two of the three colors is not applicable to patients who have characteristic RP attacks of blanching but return to a normal digital color without passing through an appreciable hyperemic phase. The triggering stimulus, in the majority of cases, is an exposure to cold, while emotional stress is mentioned by some in addition to cold, with only a small proportion of subjects reporting the emotional stress alone.

Of the associated, subjective symptoms numbness is reported most often—approximately 80% to 90% of the attacks. Other symptoms occur much less frequently, with pain being the least frequent of all (Maricq HR, unpublished data). Compared with primary RP, patients with SSc more frequently experience both blanching and cyanosis and more often will have all 10 fingers involved (153,154). In addition, they may show a more or less permanent cyanosis of the fingers and of the whole hand, which presents a problem of terminology. By description, this condition corresponds to acrocyanosis. However, acrocyanosis is usually considered to be a benign vasomotor disturbance not associated with any systemic disease and not believed to have any associated blood vessel changes such as vessel wall lesions or "local fault." The pathology and pathogenesis of acrocyanosis have been studied rarely because of its benign nature. Lewis assumed that a heightened arteriolar tone combined with loss of tone in other minute vessels may be the basis of this disorder (155). As a result of this difficulty, SSc patients who show only a semipermanent cyanosis of hands usually still receive a diagnosis of RP.

MICROVASCULATURE

Of the microvascular lesions, those most prominent by clinical examinations are telangiectases, seen especially in the CREST variant of SSc. They appear as punctate telangiectases on fingers and palms and consist mostly of enlarged capillaries. When small, they may be confused with non-specific venular or other microvascular abnormalities. On the face, due to the different architecture of the vascular layers, the telangiectases are polygonal and show a network of venules.

In the nailfold, extremely large capillaries and large avascular areas can sometimes be seen with the naked eye as well. Most visible clinically in the nailfold are capillary hemorrhages in the cuticle.

Ulcerations on the fingertips and joints in SSc occur apparently as a result of local factors in combination with generally reduced digital skin blood flow and susceptibility to minor trauma. Such ulcerations are surrounded by a circle of enlarged capillaries, usually seen only in the early phase of normal wound healing (156). Splinter hemorrhages under the nail can also be observed.

Laboratory Examinations

Most laboratory procedures used in the evaluation of the peripheral vascular system in SSc are aimed to assist in the diagnosis of RP and to measure its severity and response to treatment by physiological testing. An exception is the method of capillary microscopy that is useful in making an early diagnosis of SDS disorders and in the differentiation of primary RP from RP associated with a connective tissue disease. Testing serum for antinuclear antibodies (ANA) is also helpful in this respect. This topic is addressed in Chapter 9.

There is no physiological test that can be used to diagnose RP in an individual patient, but some physiological tests can support the diagnosis of RP when this is already suspected on the basis of other information. They can also measure the degree of digital vascular response to cooling and the effect of treatment on RP severity.

COLOR CHARTS AS AN AID IN RP DIAGNOSIS

Usually, the clinical diagnosis of RP is made solely on the basis of the patient's history, because the RP is rarely observed by the physician. The diagnosis of RP can, however, be made more reliable by conducting a structured interview assisted by color charts that illustrate the color changes that occur during an attack of RP (157,158).

COLD PROVOCATION TESTS

Since it is very difficult to reproduce an RP attack in the laboratory, various cold provocation tests have been devised to estimate the degree of vasoconstriction in response to cold in RP patients compared to control subjects. Some of these tests also analyze the time necessary for the vascular parameter under study to return to baseline after the cold stimulus is removed.

The vascular parameters most often measured in such test procedures are skin blood flow, skin temperature, and digital arterial pressure. The cold challenge consists of local finger cooling, hand cooling, body cooling, or some combination thereof (147–149,159–164). Investigators have used a wide range of cooling temperatures, the most extreme of which reach 4°C for local cooling (immersion in ice water or in a cold box), 10°C with a cooling blanket for body cooling, and even 4°C in an environmental chamber (72).

In the simplest test, the hand is exposed to cold (by cold water immersion or in a cold air box) for a prescribed period of time, as the patient sits in a room maintained at average temperature. The return of skin blood flow is recorded by skin temperature measurements using a thermistor or thermocouple, or by laser Doppler flowmetry. There is a large overlap of responses to this test between patients with primary RP and SSc-related RP, and also between primary RP and normal subjects.

Another test is based on the principle of the critical closing phenomenon (77) of the digital artery on cooling. The finger is cooled by circulating cold water around its middle portion, and finger blood flow is arrested by an occlusion cuff placed on the proximal part of the finger (some models combine occlusion and cooling cuffs). After 5 minutes of occlusion the cooling is stopped, the cuff is deflated, and the finger systolic pressure is measured as the reopening pressure with an appropriate transducer on the fingertip (strain gauge, photoelectric transducer, or laser Doppler). The local cooling water temperature is decreased step-wise, usually from 30°C to 10°C in 5°C steps, while looking for abnormally low digital systolic pressure and/or failure to re-open after complete deflation of the occlusion cuff (159,160,162–164).

Observations of the nailfold capillary blood flow under the microscope can also be used with local and/or body cooling (151,165) to demonstrate a capillary flow standstill. This will be of distinctly longer duration in SSc than in primary RP, and will involve all of the nailfold capillaries (148,151).

Skin blood flow varies considerably in the fingers, depending on numerous factors such as room temperature, psychological stimuli, relationship to meals, drinking and smoking, diurnal variations, etc. Therefore, the tests based on digital skin blood flow are of questionable value for diagnosis, even under strictly controlled experimental conditions.

On the other hand, tests based on digital blood pressure measurements and on the critical closing phenomenon have shown better results when carried out under well-controlled experimental conditions. These tests have also shown good separation between primary RP and control subjects and between primary RP and SDS-related RP (75,78).

The results of such tests can, therefore, be of help in supporting the diagnosis of RP and may also be used to estimate the severity of RP and its response to treatment.

SKIN BLOOD FLOW MEASUREMENTS

Skin blood flow measurements can be used not so much for diagnostic purposes as to evaluate the adequacy of nutritional blood flow. These measurements have been performed at various local or environmental temperatures by means of several techniques such as venous occlusion plethysmography for total fingertip blood flow (147), isotope clearance methods for capillary

blood flow (147,166), laser Doppler flowmetry that measures skin blood flow but is likely to include not only capillary but also shunt flow in the skin (167,168), and video recordings of red cell velocity in the nailfold capillaries (150). Video microscopy can also be used to evaluate permeability changes in SSc capillaries, when combined with Na-fluorescein injection (144), and to detect capillary aneurysms, when combined with injections of cardiogreen (169,170). Blood flow measurements can also be performed to study the post-occlusive, reactive hyperemia response that is decreased in SSc patients (171).

The best estimate of nutritional blood flow is obtained by *in vivo* videomicroscopy of capillary blood flow, but this is technically more difficult than laser Doppler flowmetry. The results of the latter, however, are difficult to interpret in areas of the skin that contain many arterio-venous (A-V) shunts, which have a themoregulatory function. A-V shunts are numerous in the skin of the fingers, especially in the finger pad and in the nailbed, and are located in the lower dermis. It is, therefore, difficult to estimate the relative components of nutritive (i.e., capillary) vs. shunt flow, because the depth of the measurements in the skin by laser Doppler instruments varies as a function of the wave length of the laser and of the fibers separation used in different instruments.

IN VIVO MICROSCOPY TO DETECT MICROANGIOPATHIC PATTERNS

The examination of superficial blood vessels of the skin by *in vivo* microscopy has usually been performed on the nailfolds, but it is also desirable to look for microvascular abnormalities elsewhere on the hand (e.g., to document the presence of CREST-type telangiectases that may be too small for diagnosis by the naked eye).

Laboratories specializing in this technique have used low power objectives, giving a total magnification of 12X to 100X, with a variety of microscopes adapted for this application. The stereoscopes offer the best view, because they provide the observer with a three-dimensional view; however, stereoscopes usually do not have good photographic capability, and photographs are desirable to document and quantitate the microvascular abnormalities and to allow comparisons on follow-up.

To observe the overall pattern of the nailfold vascular bed, a range of 12× to 15× total magnification is best because it shows the entire nailfold area. A higher magnification can be used to evaluate details of some of the abnormalities seen at lower power. In order to visualize the microvessels of the skin under the microscope, the observed area must be covered by oil of good optical quality, such as immersion oil grade B (more viscous than that used in histology and thus less likely to run off). Because of finger-to-finger variations, especially in early disease, all 10 nailfolds should be examined to exclude any abnormalities. An adequate illumination source is needed for such examinations.

Among the clinical practitioners who have attempted to examine nailfold capillaries, the techniques vary greatly. In most cases, the instruments used range from hand held magnifiers (usually in the range of 10X) to ophthalmoscopes that give a view at approximately 40X and have a small field, not covering the whole nailfold. Some clinicians, however, use stereo microscopes and even take photographs.

The hand held instruments have severe limitations and, at best, can only serve to confirm gross abnormalities already suspected by naked eye examination or to support a diagnosis already made on some other basis. They cannot be considered adequate for a diagnostic examination in a patient with early suspected SSc, for differential diagnosis with other disorders that show capillary changes, or to classify patients with RP into primary RP and suspected SDS groups. Overrating and underrating of abnormalities are greatly increased by the use of hand held instruments. Also, although supposedly simpler, it is certainly more time consuming to examine properly the total nailfold areas of all fingers with an ophthalmoscope than with a stereomicroscope. The substitution of KY jelly

for immersion oil by some users of hand held instruments further lowers the quality of examination and limits its value.

Although capillary microscopy is technically a relatively easy procedure when photography is not included, the interpretation of observations requires experience. Only the "average normal" and the most extensive microvascular abnormalities can be reliably recognized by an inexperienced examiner. Since the examination of microvascular abnormalities in the fingers by *in vivo* microscopy has been proved to be useful as an early diagnostic test, the time has come to standardize the technique, the evaluation of results, and the terminology in order to make it a standard diagnostic test.

As an example of the present confusion in terminology, consider the use of the term "drop-out." "Drop-out" is sometimes defined as "drop-out of two contiguous" capillaries (119), which includes practically all patients with any SD-type capillary change, because of the well known decrease in the number of capillary loops along the edge of the nailfold in SSc. Others use "drop-out" to classify patients with limited and diffuse SSc, the latter reportedly associated with a "drop-out pattern," which refers to large avascular areas. This term, therefore, should no longer be used.

MISCELLANEOUS OTHER VASCULAR TESTS

Occasionally, additional examinations, such as Doppler studies and angiography, are required, especially when stenosis or occlusion of a blood vessel proximal to the digital artery is suspected (172).

TESTS USEFUL FOR THE CLASSIFICATION OF RAYNAUD'S PHENOMENON

Raynaud's phenomenon (RP) is usually classified into two main categories: primary RP (also called idiopathic RP or Raynaud disease) with no known disease association and a benign prognosis, and secondary RP associated with a variety of diseases, lists of which have been frequently published in articles and reviews on RP and need not be repeated here. The leading disorders associated with secondary RP are connective tissue diseases, especially SSc. The remainder consist of several diseases, each of which represents a small percent of the total secondary RP. Therefore, RP could be divided into three main groups: primary RP, CTD-associated secondary RP, and all other secondary RP. The diagnosis in the last group is the easiest, because the suspected, etiologically related disorder is usually already present at the time the patient seeks medical advice. The differential diagnosis between the two first groups presents difficulties because the diagnosis of primary RP can be made only by exclusion of all possible causes. However, since the RP associated with CTD, especially SSc, frequently precedes such CTD diagnosis, there is not enough evidence, or none at all, to make a diagnosis of secondary RP. Allen and Brown proposed criteria for differential diagnosis between primary and secondary RP that included a time factor, which was a waiting period of two years (173,174) for the diagnosis of primary RP. The other criteria were the presence of normal pulsations in the palpable arteries, no gangrene or minimal cutaneous gangrene, and absence of any causally related disease. These criteria, with slight modifications by some authors, are used to this date. The most serious problem with this classification has been the need for a waiting period; in addition, 2 years is not always an adequate length of time.

Thus, the largest group of patients with secondary RP that could not be differentiated from primary RP were those with not yet recognizable SSc; therefore, attempts have been made for years to find criteria to help make an early diagnosis of SSc. Since 1980, an increasing number of investigators have found that *in vivo* capillary microscopy of the fingers is useful in early diagnosis of SSc and other closely related SDS disorders, and thus could be used for early classification of RP (103,105,107–109,112,115–117). Follow-up studies (128–134) have supported this proposal.

Since these highly specific capillary abnormalities are present early (in patients with RP only or with minimal other symptoms suggesting SSc), the two-year waiting period of Allen and Brown loses its importance. Other signs of SSc not included among Allen and Brown's criteria, such as sclerodactyly and pitting scars (which when present alone cannot provide a basis for a formal diagnosis of SSc), are obviously also a basis to exclude the diagnosis of primary RP and have been used for this purpose in many studies. Testing for antinuclear antibodies (ANA) related to CTD, and especially for specific SSc-related ANA, has also been frequently used to improve the early diagnosis of SSc.

Some authors have suggested a short list of examinations to perform before a more thorough examination on initial contact with an RP patient in whom the cause of secondary RP is not readily evident for early classification into primary or CTD-related RP. These examinations include hand and chest roentgenographs and sedimentation rate, in addition to ANA tests and capillary microscopy (132,175). A thorough systemic examination of 138 RP patients with follow-up by Monin and Reggi (131) concluded that capillary microscopy gave the single best discrimination between the primary and secondary RP groups.

Treatment

The main goals in the treatment of vascular symptoms of SSc patients are the alleviation of RP and improvement of skin blood flow to prevent or treat ulcerations. These goals include treatments to produce vasodilation and those that are believed to ameliorate rheological factors in the blood, thereby improving blood flow in the microvasculature. Protective measures, based on current knowledge of the physiological mechanisms controlling the digital circulation, must be used regardless of whether additional treatment is needed. It is necessary, therefore, to inform patients that gloves are not sufficient for keeping hands warm, that mittens are a better choice for conserving heat and avoiding pressure, and that, preferably, the whole body should be kept warm.

The drug treatments that are briefly reviewed in this section, remain controversial and there is no generally accepted drug for the treatment of SSc's vascular problems. The evaluation of treatments is also made difficult by the lack of objective criteria to show improvement. Most studies have relied on the diary method, and laboratory studies have often been negative or have given results opposite to diary reports. The healing of chronic ulcerations is considered proof of drug efficacy in some patients, but healing can also occur spontaneously.

Consequently, many previously used drugs have been abandoned, as the early enthusiasm has not been supported by long term results and as new, more promising drugs have become available. The drawback of most drug treatments is the side effects that limit the drug's use. In addition, there is concern that a possible "steal phenomenon" may occur when the vasodilator drugs lower the blood pressure and thus further reduce the digital blood pressure in the hands of SSc patients, in whom it is already abnormally low.

The drugs that have been used during the last decade to treat RP in SSc patients include α_1-adrenergic receptor antagonists such as prazosin (176), direct acting vasodilators such as nitroglycerin (177), calcium channel blocking agents such as nifedipine, diltiazem and nicardipine (178–184), the prostacyclin analogues iloprost and cicaprost (185–192), the serotonin S_2 receptor antagonist ketanserin (193–200), the rheological agent pentoxiphylline (201) and, recently, the recombinant tissue plasminogen activator (202–204). The most controversial of these drugs has been ketanserin, with some studies reporting beneficial effects (194–197,200) and others finding no improvement compared to placebo (193, 198,199). Nifedipine seems to have become the favorite despite its side effects, which are reduced with new, delayed release formulations of the drug. Nifedipine has also been shown to have an-

tiplatelet properties (205). Other calcium channel blockers such as diltiazem and nicardipine have been reported as not effective (180,183). The stable prostacyclin analogue iloprost has shown favorable results in SSc patients, but the need for intravenous infusion excludes its use in outpatients.

However, another prostacyclin analogue that can be administered orally has now become available. The results of a study of this drug by Lou et al (189,192) are encouraging, as their patients reported a reduction in the severity of RP attacks, although the clinical and laboratory parameters of digital vasospasm did not show any statistically significant improvement. They believe that the lack of better results may be due to the low dosage and short treatment period of their preliminary study.

The most recent addition to the drug treatment possibilities is the recombinant tissue plasminogen activator (two case reports and a study of 10 patients) (202–204). Although one of the case reports described a prolonged improvement, the study by Klimiuk et al (203) reported only short lived improvement in skin blood flow. A summary of the drugs used in the treatment of RP in SSc patients is shown in Table 17.1.

Plasmapheresis has also been tried in the

Table 17.1. Pharmacologic Therapy for Raynaud's Phenomenon

Class	Drug Name	Trade Name
α_1-adrenergic blockers	Prazosin	Minipress
	Terazasin	Hytrin
Calcium channel blockers	Nifedipine	Procardia
		Procardia XL
		Adalat CC
	Diltiazem	Cardizem
		Cardizem SR
		Cardizem CD
	Nicardipine	Cardene
		Cardene SR
Direct vasodilator	Nitroglycerin	Nitrol Ointment
Prostglandin	PGE$_1$ Prostin VR	
Prostacyclin analogues	PGI$_2$ analogue (experimental)	Iloprost
Rheological agents	Pentoxiphylline	Trental

treatment of RP (including patients with SSc), and the authors claim prolonged improvement of RP and healing of ulcers (206,207).

Non-drug treatments, such as hand warming procedures, have been proposed, because drug treatments are often associated with side effects (208,209). Another non-drug therapy for RP, biofeedback treatment, is not believed to be effective in SSc even by those advocating it for primary RP (210).

In a few cases in which ulnar or radial occlusion was associated with RP, microsurgical repair was found beneficial (59). The standard sympathectomy is not advisable in SSc. Selective sympathectomy of digital arteries, first performed by Flatt in 1980 (211), has been advocated to treat RP. This surgical therapy has been applied to RP in scleroderma patients by Jones (58) and O'Brien (212). In the latter series, digital sympathectomy in 11 scleroderma patients relieved pain and ulceration. After a one year follow-up, mild recurrence of small ulcers was seen in four patients. More details regarding digital sympathectomy are given in Chapter 28.

References

1. Miller EH, Hiserodt JC, Hunt LE, et al. Reduced natural killer cell activity in patients with systemic sclerosis. Correlation with clinical disease type. Arthritis Rheum 1988;31:1515–1523.
2. Schleef RR, Bevilacqua MP, Sawdey M, et al. Cytokine activation of vascular endothelium. Effects on tissue-type plasminogen activator and type 1 plasminogen activator inhibitor. J Biol Chem 263: 5797–5803, 1988
3. Gustafsson R, Tötterman TH, Klareskog L, Hällgren R. Increase in activated T cells and reduction in suppressor inducer T cells in systemic sclerosis. Ann Rheum Dis 1990;49:40–45.
4. Matucci-Cerinic M, Lotti T, Lombardi A, et al. Cutaneous and plasma fibrinolytic activity in systemic sclerosis. Evidence of normal plasminogen activation. Int J Dermatol 1990;29:644–648.
5. Silver RM. Lymphokine activated killer (LAK) cell activity in the peripheral blood lymphocytes of systemic sclerosis (SSc) patients. Clin Exp Rheumatol 1990;8:481–486.
6. Claman HN, Giorno RC, Seibold JR. Endothelial and fibroblastic activation in scleroderma. The myth of the "uninvolved skin." Arthritis Rheum 1991;34:1495–1501.
7. Falanga V, Kruskal JB, Franks JJ. Fibrin and fibrinogen-related antigens in systemic sclerosis (scleroderma). J Am Acad Dermatol 1991;25: 771–775.
8. Kantor TV, Whiteside TL, Friberg D, et al. Lymphokine-activated killer cell and natural killer cell activities in patients with systemic sclerosis. Arthritis Rheum 1992;35:694–699.
9. Marasini B, Cugno M, Bassani C, et al. Tissue-type plasminogen activator and von Willebrand factor plasma levels as markers of endothelial involvement in patients with Raynaud's phenomenon. Int J Microcirc Clin Exp 1992;11:375–382.
10. Matucci-Cerinic M, Jaffa A, Kahaleh B. Angiotensin converting enzyme: An *in vivo* and *in vitro* marker of endothelial injury. J Lab Clin Med 1992; 120:428–433.
11. Rudnicka L, Majewski S, Blaszczyk M, et al. Adhesion of peripheral blood mononuclear cells to vascular endothelium in patients with systemic sclerosis (scleroderma). Arthritis Rheum 1992; 35:771–775.
12. Fiocco U, Rosada M, Cozzi L, et al. Early phenotypic activation of circulating helper memory T cells in scleroderma: Correlation with disease activity. Ann Rheum Dis 1993;52:272–277.
13. Drenk F, Deicher HRG. Pathophysiological effects of endothelial cytotoxic activity derived from sera of patients with progressive systemic sclerosis. J Rheumatol 1988;15:468–474.
14. Kahan A, Awada H, Sultan Y, et al. Tissue plasminogen activator (t-PA) activity and t-PA inhibition (PAI) in systemic sclerosis. Arthritis Rheum 1988;31:S112.
15. Umehara H, Kumagai S, Ishida H, et al. Enhanced production of interleukin-2 in patients with progressive systemic sclerosis. Hyperactivity of CD4-positive T cells? Arthritis Rheum 1988;31:401–407.
16. Gay S, Jones RE Jr, Huang G, Gay RE. Immunohistologic demonstration of platelet-derived growth factor (PDGF) and sis-oncogene expression in scleroderma. J Invest Dermatol 1989;92: 301–303.
17. Holt CM, Lindsey N, Moult J, et al. Antibody-dependent cellular cytotoxicity of vascular endothelium: Characterization and pathogenic associations in systemic sclerosis. Clin Exp Immunol 1989;78:359–365.
18. Kahaleh MB, LeRoy EC. Interleukin-2 in scleroderma: Correlation of serum level with extent of

skin involvement and disease duration. Ann Intern Med 1989;110:446–450.

19. Pandolfi A, Florita M, Altomare G, et al. Increased plasma levels of platelet-derived growth factor activity in patients with progressive systemic sclerosis. Proc Soc Exp Biol Med 1989;191:1–4.

20. Cifone MG, Giacomelli R, Famularo G, et al. Natural killer activity and antibody-dependent cellular cytotoxicity in progressive systemic sclerosis. Clin Exp Immunol 1990;80:360–365.

21. Degiannis D, Seibold JR, Czarnecki M, et al. Soluble interleukin-2 receptors in patients with systemic sclerosis. Clinical and laboratory correlations. Arthritis Rheum 1990;33:375–380.

22. Needleman BW. Increased expression of intercellular adhesion molecule 1 on the fibroblasts of scleroderma patients. Arthritis Rheum 1990;33:1847–1851.

23. Umehara H, Kumagai S, Murakami M, et al. Enhanced production of interleukin-1 and tumor necrosis factor α by cultured peripheral blood monocytes from patients with scleroderma. Arthritis Rheum 1990;33:893–897.

24. Kahaleh MB. Soluble immunologic products in scleroderma sera. Clin Immunol Immunopathol 1991;58:139–144.

25. Kahaleh MB. Endothelin, an endothelial-dependent vasoconstrictor in scleroderma. Enhanced production and profibrotic action. Arthritis Rheum 1991;34:978–987.

26. Majewski S, Hunzelmann N, Johnson JP, et al. Expression of intercellular adhesion molecule-1 (ICAM-1) in the skin of patients with systemic scleroderma. J Invest Dermatol 1991;97:667–671.

27. Gabrielli A, Danieli MG, Candela M, et al. The potential role of cytokines in the pathogenesis of systemic sclerosis (scleroderma). Int J Immunopathol Pharmacol 1992;5:135–140.

28. Gruschwitz M, von den Driesch P, Kellner I, et al. Expression of adhesion proteins involved in cell-cell and cell-matrix interactions in the skin of patients with progressive systemic sclerosis. J Am Acad Dermatol 1992;27:169–177.

29. Kantor TV, Friberg D, Medsger TA Jr, et al. Cytokine production and serum levels in systemic sclerosis. Clin Immunol Immunopathol 1992;65:278–285.

30. Needleman BW, Wigley FM, Stair RW. Interleukin-1, interleukin-2, interleukin-4, interleukin-6, tumor necrosis factor α, and interferon gamma levels in sera from patients with scleroderma. Arthritis Rheum 1992;35:67–72.

31. Sollberg S, Peltonen J, Uitto J, Jimenez SA. Elevated expression of β_1 and β_2 integrins, intercellular adhesion molecules 1, and endothelial leukocyte adhesion molecule 1 in the skin of patients with systemic sclerosis of recent onset. Arthritis Rheum 1992;35:290–298.

32. Yamane K, Miyauchi T, Suzuki N, et al. Significance of plasma endothelin-1 levels in patients with systemic sclerosis. J Rheumatol 1992;19:1566–1571.

33. Carson CW, Beall LD, Hunder GG, et al. Serum ELAM-1 is increased in vasculitis, scleroderma, and systemic lupus erythematosus. J Rheumatol 1993;20:809–814.

34. Gabrielli A, di Loreto C, Taborro R, et al. Immunohistochemical localization of intracellular and extracellular associated TGFβ in the skin of patients with systemic sclerosis (scleroderma) and primary Raynaud's phenomenon. Clin Immunol Immunopathol 1993;68:340–349.

35. Knock GA, Terenghi G, Bunker CB, et al. Characterization of endothelin-binding sites in human skin and their regulation in primary Raynaud's phenomenon and systemic sclerosis. J Invest Dermatol 1993;101:73–78.

36. Sfikakis PP, Tesar J, Baraf H, et al. Circulating intercellular adhesion molecule-1 in patients with systemic sclerosis. Clin Immunol Immunopathol 1993;68:88–92.

37. Claman HN. On scleroderma: Mast cells, endothelial cells, and fibroblasts. JAMA 1989;262:1206–1209.

38. Irani AA, Gruber BL, Kaufman LD, et al. Mast cell changes in scleroderma. Presence of MC_T cells in the skin and evidence of mast cell activation. Arthritis Rheum 1992;35:933–939.

39. Maul GG, Jimenez SA, Riggs E, Ziemnicka-Kotula D. Determination of an epitope of the diffuse systemic sclerosis marker antigen DNA topoisomerase I: Sequence similarity with retroviral p30^{gag} protein suggests a possible cause for autoimmunity in systemic sclerosis. Proc Natl Acad Sci USA 1989;86:8492–8496.

40. Abraham GN, Khan AS. Human endogenous retroviruses and immune disease. Clin Immunol Immunopathol 1990;56:1–8.

41. Dang H, Dauphinée MJ, Talal N, et al. Serum antibody to retroviral gag proteins in systemic sclerosis. Arthritis Rheum 1991;34:1336–1337.

42. Krieg AM, Gourley MF, Perl A. Endogenous retroviruses: Potential etiologic agents in autoimmunity. FASEB J 1992;6:2537–2544.

43. Norton WL, Hurd ER, Lewis DC, Ziff M. Evidence of microvascular injury in scleroderma and systemic lupus erythematosus: Quantitative study of the microvascular bed. J Lab Clin Med 1968;71:919–933.

44. Burch GE, Harb JM, Sun CS. Fine structure of

digital vascular lesions in Raynaud's phenomenon and disease. Angiology 1979;30:361–376.

45. Fleischmajer R, Perlish JS. Capillary alterations in scleroderma. J Am Acad Dermatol 1980;2:161–170.

46. Kahaleh MB, Osborn I, LeRoy EC. Increased factor VIII/von Willebrand factor antigen and von Willebrand factor activity in scleroderma and in Raynaud's phenomenon. Ann Intern Med 1981; 94:482–484.

47. Matucci-Cerinic M, Jaffa A, Kahaleh B. Angiotensin converting enzyme: An *in vivo* and *in vitro* marker of endothelial injury. J Lab Clin Med 1992;120:428–33.

48. Blann AD, Illingworth K, Jayson MIV. Mechanisms of endothelial cell damage in systemic sclerosis and Raynaud's phenomenon. J Rheumatol 1993;20:1325–1330.

49. Freemont AJ, Hoyland J, Fielding P, et al. Studies of the microvascular endothelium in uninvolved skin of patients with systemic sclerosis: Direct evidence for a generalized microangiopathy. Br J Dermatol 1992;126:561–568.

50. Furey NL, Schmid FR, Kwaan HC, Friederici HHR. Arterial thrombosis in scleroderma. Br J Dermatol 1975;93:683–693.

51. Dorevitch MI, Clemens LE, Webb JB. Lower limb amputation secondary to large vessel involvement in scleroderma. Br J Rheumatol 1988;27:403–406.

52. Shapiro LS. Large vessel arterial thrombosis in systemic sclerosis associated with antiphospholipid antibodies. J Rheumatol 1990;17:685–688.

53. Barile LA, Bravo G, Pizarro S. Large vessel arterial thrombosis in systemic sclerosis with antiphospholipid antibodies. J Rheumatol 1990;17:1721.

54. Youssef P, Englert H, Bertouch J. Large vessel occlusive disease associated with CREST syndrome and scleroderma. Ann Rheum Dis 1993;52:464–466.

55. Rodnan GP, Myerowitz RL, Justh GO. Morphologic changes in the digital arteries of patients with progressive systemic sclerosis (scleroderma) and Raynaud phenomenon. Medicine 1980;59:393–408.

56. Dabich L, Bookstein JJ, Zweifler A, Zarafonetis CJD. Digital arteries in patients with scleroderma. Arteriographic and plethysmographic study. Arch Intern Med 1972;130:708–714.

57. Jeune R, Thivolet J. Étude artériographique de la main au cours de 52 phénomènes de Raynaud d'étiologie diverse. Nouv Presse Méd 1978;7:2619–2623.

58. Jones NF, Imbriglia JE, Steen VD, Medsger TA.

Surgery for scleroderma of the hand. J Hand Surg 1987;12A:391–400.

59. Jones NF, Raynor SC, Medsger TA. Microsurgical revascularisation of the hand in scleroderma. Br J Plast Surg 1987;40:264–269.

60. Lewis T. The pathological changes in the arteries supplying the fingers in warm-handed people and in cases of so-called Raynaud's disease. Clin Sci 1937–38;3:287–319.

61. Lewis T, Pickering GW. Observations upon maladies in which the blood supply to digits ceases intermittently or permanently, and upon bilateral gangrene of digits; observations relevant to so-called "Raynaud's disease." Clin Sci 1933–34;1:327–366.

62. Lindblad LE, Ekenvall L, Etzell B-M. Bevegard S. Adrenoreceptors in Raynaud's disease. J Cardiovasc Pharmcol 1989;14:881–885.

63. Flavahan NA, Lindblad L-E, Verbeuren TJ, et al. Cooling and α1- and α2-adrenergic responses in cutaneous veins: Role of receptor reserve. Am J Physiol 1985;249:H950–952.

64. Flavahan NA. The role of vascular α2-adrenoceptors as cutaneous thermosensors. NIPS 1991;6:251–255.

65. Freedman RR, Sabharwal SC, Moten M, Migaly P. Local temperature modulates α1- and α2-adrenergic vasoconstriction in men. Am J Physiol 1992;263:H1197–1200.

66. Flavahan NA, Cooke JP, Shepherd JT, Vanhoutte PM. Human postjunctional alpha-1 and alpha-2 adrenoceptors: Differential distribution in arteries of the limbs. J Pharmacol Exp Ther 1987;241:361–365.

67. Coffman JD, Cohen RA. α-Adrenergic and serotonergic mechanisms in the human digit. J Cardiovasc Pharmacol 1988;11(suppl 1):S49–53.

68. Coffman JD, Cohen RA. Serotonergic vasoconstriction in human fingers during reflex sympathetic response to cooling. Am J Physiol 1988;254:H889–893.

69. Coffman JD. Raynaud's phenomenon. An update. Hypertension 1991;17:593–602.

70. Freedman RR, Moten M, Migaly P, Mayes M. Cold-induced potentiation of α_2-adrenergic vasoconstriction in primary Raynaud's disease. Arthritis Rheum 1993;36:685–690.

71. Brown MJ. Investigation of alpha 2-adrenoceptors in humans. Am J Med 1989;(suppl 3C):6S–9S.

72. Freedman RR, Mayes MD, Sabharwal SC. Induction of vasospastic attacks despite digital nerve block in Raynaud's disease and phenomenon. Circulation 1989;80:859–862.

73. Zweifler AJ, Trinkaus P. Occlusive digital artery

disease in patients with Raynaud's phenomenon. Am J Med 1984;77:995–1001.

74. Maricq HR. Microangiopathy in systemic scleroderma and related disorders. Int Angiol 1983;2: 119–128.

75. Maricq HR, Smith EA, Diat F, et al. Digital vascular responses to cooling in early scleroderma spectrum (SDS) disorders. Arthritis Rheum 1989; 32(suppl):R45.

76. Olsen N, Nielsen SL. Prevalence of primary Raynaud phenomena in young females. Scand J Clin Lab Invest 1978;38:761–764.

77. Krähenbühl B, Nielsen SL, Lassen NA. Closure of digital arteries in high vascular tone states as demonstrated by measurement of systolic blood pressure in the fingers. Scand J Clin Lab Invest 1977;37:71–76.

78. Maricq HR, Diat F, Weinrich MC, Maricq JG. Digital pressure responses to cooling in patients with suspected early vs definite scleroderma (systemic sclerosis) vs primary Raynaud's phenomenon. J Rheumatol (In press).

79. Henriksen O, Kristensen JK. Reduced systolic blood pressure in fingers of patients with generalized scleroderma (acrosclerosis). Acta Derm Venereol 1981;61:531–534.

80. Biondi ML, Marasini B, Bianchi E, Agostoni A. Plasma free and intraplatelet serotonin in patients with Raynaud's Phenomenon. Int J Cardiol 1988;19:335–339.

81. Kahaleh MB, Osborn I, LeRoy EC. Elevated levels of circulating platelet aggregates and beta-thromboglobulin in scleroderma. Ann Intern Med 1982;96:610–613.

82. Friedhoff LT, Seibold RJ, Kim HC, Simester KS. Serotonin induced platelet aggregation in systemic sclerosis. Clin Exp Rheumatol 1984;2:119–123.

83. Kovacs IB, Sowemimo-Coker SO, Kirby JDT, Turner P. Altered behaviour of erythrocytes in scleroderma. Clin Sci 1983;65:515–519.

84. Rustin MHA, Kovacs IB, Sowemimo-Coker SO, et al. Differences in red cell behaviour between patients with Raynaud's phenomenon and systemic sclerosis and patients with Raynaud's disease. Br J Dermatol 1985;113:265–272.

85. Rhodin JAG. Ultrastructure of the microvascular bed. In: The microcirculation in clinical medicine. Wells R, ed. New York: Academic Press, 1973.

86. Fleischmajer R, Perlish JS. [³H]Thymidine labeling of dermal endothelial cells in scleroderma. J Invest Dermatol 1977;69:379–382.

87. Lombard WP. The blood pressure in the arterioles, capillaries, and small veins of the human skin. Am J Physiol 1912;29:335–362.

88. Müller O. Die Kapillaren der menschlichen Körperoberfläche in gesunden und kranken Tagen. Stuttgart, Ferdinand Enke, 1922.

89. Brown GE, O'Leary PA. Skin capillaries in scleroderma. Arch Intern Med 1926;36:73–88.

90. Jablonska S, Bubnow B, Lukasiak B. Raynaud's syndrome; acrosclerosis; scleroderma. Br J Dermatol 1958;70:37–43.

91. Fukushiro R. Capillary microscopic examination in various skin diseases. Jpn J Dermatol 1965;75: 486–502.

92. Davis E, Landau J, eds. Clinical capillary microscopy. Springfield: CC Thomas, 1966.

93. Kawashima Y. Capillary microscopic examination in collagen disease. Jpn J Dermatol 1966;76: 24–31.

94. Ross JB. Nail fold capillaroscopy—a useful aid in the diagnosis of collagen vascular diseases. J Invest Dermatol 1966;47:282–285.

95. Buchanan IS, Humpston DJ. Nail-fold capillaries in connective-tissue disorders. Lancet 1968;1: 845–847.

96. Redisch W, Messina EJ, Hughes G, McEwan C. Capillaroscopic observations in rheumatic diseases. Ann Rheum Dis 1970;29:244–253.

97. Schmoranzer H. Vitalmikroskopische verlaufsbeobachtungen am nagelwall bei dermatomyositis und progressiver Sklerodermie. Z Haut-Geschl Kr 1970;45:663–673.

98. Jablonska S. Scleroderma and pseudoscleroderma, ed. 2. Warsaw: Polish Medical Publishers, 1975.

99. Maricq HR, Blume RS, LeRoy EC. Wide-field study of nailfold capillary bed in disorders of connective tissue. In: Ditzel J, ed. 6th European Conference on Microcirculation, Aalborg, 1970. Basel, Karger, 1971.

100. Rouen LR, Terry EN, Doft BH, et al. Classification and measurement of surface microvessels in man. Microvasc Res 1972;4:285–292.

101. Maricq HR, LeRoy EC. Patterns of finger capillary abnormalities in connective tissue disease by "wide-field" microscopy. Arthritis Rheum 1973; 16:619–628.

102. Maricq HR, Spencer-Green G, LeRoy EC. Skin capillary abnormalities as indicators of organ involvement in scleroderma (systemic sclerosis), Raynaud's syndrome and dermatomyositis. Am J Med 1976;61:862–870.

103. Maricq HR, LeRoy EC, D'Angelo WA, et al. Diagnostic potential of in vivo capillary microscopy in scleroderma and related disorders. Arthritis Rheum 1980;23:183–189.

104. Maricq HR. Widefield capillary microscopy. Technique and rating scale for abnormalities seen

in scleroderma and related disorders. Arthritis Rheum 1981;24:1159–1165.

105. Vayssairat M, Fiessinger JN, Housset E. Place de la capillaroscopie dans les acrosyndromes. Ann Med Interne 1980;131:41–41.

106. Maricq HR. The microcirculation in scleroderma and allied diseases. In: Davis E, ed. Advances in microcirculation. Basel, Karger, 1982.

107. Lee P, Leung FYK, Alderdice C, Armstrong SK. Nailfold capillary microscopy in the connective tissue diseases: A semiquantitative Assessment. J Rheumatol 1983;10:930–938.

108. Carpentier P, Franco A, Béani J-C, et al. Intérêt de la capillaroscopie périunguéale dans le diagnostic précoce de la sclérodermie systémique. Ann Dermatol Venereol 1983;110:11–20.

109. Spencer-Green G, Schlesinger M, Bove KE, et al. Nailfold capillary abnormalities in childhood rheumatic diseases. J Pediatr 1983;102:341–346.

110. Carpentier P, Franco A. Capillaroscopie et phénomène de Raynaud. J Mal Vasc 1984;9: 23–28.

111. Houtman PM, Kallenberg CGM, Wouda AA, The TH. Decreased nailfold capillary density in Raynaud's phenomenon: A reflection of immunologically mediated local and systemic vascular disease? Ann Rheum Dis 1985;44:603–609.

112. Chamot AM, Monti M. Indication à la capillaroscopie au lit unguéal dans le phénomène de Raynaud. Schweiz Med Wochenschr 1985;115:1852–1857.

113. DeBure C, Fiessinger J-N, Priollet P, et al. Relationship between nailfold capillary microscopy and salivary capillary basement membrane width in Raynaud's disease and progressive systemic sclerosis. J Rheumatol 1985;12:279–282.

114. Lee P, Sarkozi J, Bookman AA, et al. Digital blood flow and nailfold capillary microscopy in Raynaud's phenomenon. J Rheumatol 1986;13:564–569.

115. Houtman PM, Kallenberg CGM, Fidler V, Wouda AA. Diagnostic significance of nailfold capillary patterns in patients with Raynaud's phenomenon. An analysis of patterns discriminating patients with and without connective tissue disease. J Rheumatol 1986;13:556–563.

116. Wautrecht JC, Khouzam S, Bellens B, et al. Clinical interest of nail bed capillaroscopy. Microcirclulation 1987;2:487–488.

117. Joyal F, Choquette D, Roussin A, Senecal J-L. Nailfold capillary microscopy in Raynaud's phenomenon: A study of 454 patients. In: Boccalon H, ed. Angiologie. Paris: John Libbey Eurotext, 1988.

118. Duffy CM, Laxer RM, Lee P, et al. Raynaud's syndrome in childhood. J Pediatr 1989;114:73–78.

119. Campbell PM, LeRoy EC. Raynaud's phenomenon. Semin Arthritis Rheum 1986;16:92–103.

120. Maricq HR. Comparison of quantitative and semiquantitative estimates of nailfold capillary abnormalities in scleroderma spectrum disorders. Microvasc Res 1986;32:271–276.

121. Thompson RP, Harper FE, Maize JC, et al. Nailfold biopsy in scleroderma and related disorders. Correlation of histologic, capillaroscopic, and clinical data. Arthritis Rheum 1984;27:97–103.

122. Chen Z-Y, Dobson RL, Ainsworth SK, et al. Immunofluorescence in skin specimens from three different biopsy sites in patients with scleroderma. Clin Exp Rheumatol 1985;3:11–16.

123. Chen Z-Y, Silver RM, Ainsworth SK, et al. Association between fluorescent antinuclear antibodies, capillary patterns, and clinical features in scleroderma spectrum disorders. Am J Med 1984;77: 812–822.

124. Nussbaum AI, Silver RM, Maricq HR. Serial changes in nailfold capillary morphology in childhood dermatomyositis. Arthritis Rheum 1983;26: 1169–1172.

125. Wong ML, Highton J, Palmer DG. Sequential nailfold capillary microscopy in scleroderma and related disorders. Ann Rheum Dis 1988;47:53–61.

126. Carpentier PH, Maricq HR. Microvasculature in systemic sclerosis. In: LeRoy EC, ed. Rheumatic disease clinics of North America. Philadelphia: WB Saunders Co, 1990.

127. Maricq HR. Nailfold capillary abnormalities in patients with connective tissue diseases. In: Manabe H, Zweifach BW, Messmer K, eds. Microcirculation in circulatory disorders. Tokyo: Springer-Verlag, 1988.

128. Maricq HR, Weinberger AB, LeRoy EC. Early detection of scleroderma-spectrum disorders by in vivo capillary microscopy: A prospective study of patients with Raynaud's phenomenon. J Rheumatol 1982;9:289–291.

129. Harper FE, Maricq HR, Turner RE, et al. A prospective study of Raynaud's phenomenon and early connective tissue disease. A five-year report. Am J Med 1982;72:883–888.

130. Maricq HR, Harper FE, Khan MM, et al. Microvascular abnormalities as possible predictors of disease subsets in Raynaud's phenomenon and early connective tissue disease. Clin Exp Rheumatol 1983;1:195–205.

131. Monin A, Reggi M. Enquête étiologique d'un phénomenè de Raynaud. Étude prospecitve sur 138 cas. Arteres et Veines 1985;4:303–309.

132. Priollet P, Vayssairat M, Housset E. How to classify Raynaud's phenomenon. Long-term follow-up study of 73 cases. Am J Med 1987;83:494–498.

133. Fitzgerald O, Hess EV, O'Connor GT, Spencer-Green G. Prospective study of the evolution of Raynaud's phenomenon. Am J Med 1988;84:718–726.

134. Zufferey P, Depairon M, Chamot AM, Monti M. Prognostic significance of nailfold capillary microscopy in patients with Raynaud's phenomenon and scleroderma-pattern abnormalities: A 6 year follow-up study. Clin Rheumatol 1992;11:536–541.

135. Studer A, Hunziker T, Lütolf O, et al. Quantitative nailfold capillary microscopy in cutaneous and systemic lupus erythematosus and localized and systemic scleroderma. J Am Acad Dermatol 1991;24:941–945.

136. Cases A, Knobel H, Sobrino X, et al. Renal involvement in scleroderma: Relationship with capillary patterns. Kidney Int 1988;34:292.

137. Schmidt K-U, Mensing H. Are nailfold capillary changes indicators of organ involvement in progressive systemic sclerosis? Dermatologica 1988;176:18–21.

138. Groen H, Wichers G, ter Borg EJ, et al. Pulmonary diffusing capacity disturbances are related to nailfold capillary changes in patients with Raynaud's phenomenon with and without an underlying connective tissue disease. Am J Med 1990;89:34–41.

139. Joyal F, Choquette D, Roussin A, Levington C, Senécal J-L. Evaluation of the severity of systemic sclerosis by nailfold capillary microscopy in 112 patients. Angiology 1992;43:203–210.

140. Maricq HR. Vinyl chloride disease. In: Black CM, Myers AR, eds. Current topics in rheumatology. Systemic sclerosis (scleroderma). New York: Gower Med Publ Ltd, 1985.

141. Rosal EJ, Maricq HR. Nailfold capillary microscopy in 'systemic sclerosis sine scleroderma' (SSsS). Arthritis Rheum 1988;31(suppl):R47.

142. Rozboril MB, Maricq HR, Rodnan GP, et al. Capillary microscopy in eosinophilic fasciitis. A comparison with systemic sclerosis. Arthritis Rheum 1983;26:617–622.

143. Herson S, Brechignac S, Piette J-C, et al. Capillary microscopy during eosinophilic fasciitis in 15 patients: Distinction from systemic scleroderma. Am J Med 1990;88:598–600.

144. Bollinger A, Jäger K, Siegenthaler W. Microangiopathy of progressive systemic sclerosis. Evaluation by dynamic fluorescence videomicroscopy. Arch Intern Med 1986;146:1541–1545.

145. Bollinger A, Frey J, Jäger K, et al. Patterns of diffusion through skin capillaries in patients with long-term diabetes. N Engl J Med 1982;307:1305–1310.

146. Maire R, Schnewlin G, Bollinger A. Videomikroskopische untersuchungen von teleangiektasien bei morbus osler und sklerodermie. Schweiz Med Wochenschr 1986;116:335–338.

147. Coffman JD, Cohen AS. Total and capillary fingertip blood flow in Raynaud's phenomenon. N Engl J Med 1971;285:259–263.

148. Maricq HR, LeRoy EC. Capillary blood flow in scleroderma. Bibl Anat 1973;11:352–358.

149. LeRoy EC, Downey JA, Cannon PJ. Skin capillary blood flow in scleroderma. J Clin Invest 1971;50:930–939.

150. Jacobs MJHM, Breslau PJ, Slaaf DW, et al. Nomenclature of Raynaud's phenomenon: A capillary microscopic and hemorheologic study. Surgery 1987;101:136–145.

151. Maricq HR, Downey JA, LeRoy EC. Standstill of nailfold capillary blood flow during cooling in scleroderma and Raynaud's syndrome. In: Bevan JA, Comel M, Laszt L, eds. Blood Vessels. Basel, Karger, 1976.

152. Maricq HR, Weinrich MC, Keil JE, LeRoy EC. Prevalence of Raynaud's phenomenon in the general population. A preliminary study by questionnaire. J Chronic Dis 1986;39:423–427.

153. Carpentier P, Laperrousaz P, Magne JL, et al. Semiological analysis of Raynaud attacks. Int Angiol 1987;6:163–169.

154. Engelhart M, Kristensen JK. Colour changes during 'Raynaud's phenomenon' and finger blood supply during direct and indirect cooling procedures. Clin Exp Dermatol 1987;12:339–342.

155. Lewis T, Landis EM. Observations upon the vascular mechanism in acrocyanosis. Heart 1929–31;15:229–246.

156. Zimmer JG, Demis DJ. Burns and other skin lesions: Microcircular responses in man during healing. Science 1963;140:994–996.

157. Maricq HR, Weinrich MC. Diagnosis of Raynaud's phenomenon assisted by color charts. J Rheumatol 1988;15:454–459.

158. Maricq HR, Carpentier PH, Weinrich MC, et al. Geographic variation in the prevalence of Raynaud's phenomenon: Charleston, SC, USA, vs Tarentaise, Savoie, France. J Rheumatol 1993;20:70–76.

159. Nielsen SL, Lassen NA. Measurement of digital blood pressure after local cooling. J Appl Physiol 1977;43:907–910.

160. Nielsen SL. Raynaud phenomena and finger systolic pressure during cooling. Scand J Clin Lab Invest 1978;38:765–770.

161. Hirai M. Cold sensitivity of the hand in arterial occlusive disease. Surgery 1979;85:140–146.

162. Nilsson H, Jonason T, Leppert J, Ringqvist I. The effect of the calcium-entry blocker nifedipine on

cold-induced digital vasospasm. Acta Med Scand 1987;221:53–60.

163. Gates KH, Tyburczy JA, Zupan T, et al. The non-invasive quantification of digital vasospasm. Bruit 1984;8:34–37.

164. Engelhart M, Nielsen HV, Kristensen JK. The blood supply to fingers during Raynaud's attack: A comparison of laser-Doppler flowmetry with other techniques. Clin Physiol 1985;5:447–453.

165. Mahler F, Saner H, Boss C, Annaheim M. Local cold exposure test for capillaroscopic examination of patients with Raynaud's syndrome. Microvasc Res 1987;33:422–427.

166. Kristensen JK, Petersen LJ. Measurement of cutaneous blood flow by the ^{133}Xenon washout method. Clinical applications in dermatology. Acta Physiol Scand 1992;143:67–73.

167. Bonner RF, Nossal R. Principles of laser-Doppler flowmetry. In: Shepherd AP, Öberg PÄ, eds. Laser-Doppler Blood Flowmetry. Boston Dordrecht London: Kluwer Academic Publishers, 1990.

168. Johnson JM. The cutaneous circulation. In: Shepherd AP, Öberg PÄ, eds. Laser-Doppler Blood Flowmetry. Boston Dordrecht London: Kluwer Academic Publishers, 1990.

169. Bollinger A, Saesseli B, Hoffmann U, Franzeck UK. Intravital detection of skin capillary aneurysms by videomicroscopy with indocyanine green in patients with progressive systemic sclerosis and related disorders. Circulation 1991;83: 546–551.

170. Brülisauer M, Bollinger A. Measurement of different human microvascular dimensions by combination of videomicroscopy with Na-fluorescein (NaF) and indocyanine green (ICG) in normals and patients with systemic sclerosis. Int J Microcirc Clin Exp 1991;10:21–31.

171. Wigley FM, Wise RA, Mikdashi J, et al. The post-occlusive hyperemic response in patients with systemic sclerosis. Arthritis Rheum 1990;33:1620–1625.

172. Arneklo-Nobin B, Albrechtsson U, Eklöf B, Tylén U. Indications for angiography and its optimal performance in patients with Raynaud's phenomenon. Cardiovasc Intervent Radiol 1985;8: 174–179.

173. Allen EV, Brown GE. Raynaud's disease: A critical review of minimal requisites for diagnosis. Am J Med Sci 1932;183:187–200.

174. Allen EV, Brown GE. Raynaud's diseade affecting men. Ann Intern Med 1932;5:1384–1386.

175. LeRoy EC, Medsger TA. Raynaud's phenomenon: A proposal for classification. Clin Exp Rheumatol 1992;10:485–488.

176. Surwit RS, Gilgor RS, Allen LM, Duvic M. A dou-ble-blind study of prazosin in the treatment of Raynaud's phenomenon in scleroderma. Arch Dermatol 1984;120:329–331.

177. Fischer M, Reinhold B, Falck H, et al. Topical nitroglycerin ointment in Raynaud's phenomenon. Z Kardiol 1985;74:298–302.

178. Kahan A, Weber S, Amor B, et al. Étude controlée de la nifédipine dans le traitement du phénomène de Raynaud. Rev Rhum 1982;49:337–343.

179. Rodeheffer RJ, Rommer JA, Wigley F, Smith CR. Controlled double-blind trial of nifedipine in the treatment of Raynaud's phenomenon. N Engl J Med 1983;308:880–883.

180. Kahan A, Amor B, Menkes CJ. A randomised dou-ble-blind trial of diltiazem in the treatment of Raynaud's phenomenon. Ann Rheum Dis 1985; 44:30–33.

181. Kallenberg CGM, Wouda AA, Kuitert JJ, et al. Nifedipine in Raynaud's phenomenon: Relationship between immediate, short term and long term effects. J Rheumatol 1987;14:284–290.

182. Meyrick-Thomas RH, Rademaker M, Grimes SM, et al. Nifedipine in the treatment of Raynaud's phenomenon in patients with systemic sclerosis. Br J Dermatol 1987;117:237–241.

183. Rupp PAF, Mellinger S, Kohler J, et al. Nicardipine for the treatment of Raynaud's phenomena: A double blind crossover trial of a new calcium entry blocker. J Rheumatol 1987;14:745–750.

184. Wollersheim H, Thien T, van't Laar A. Nifedipine in primary Raynaud's phenomenon and in scleroderma: Oral versus sublingual hemodynamic effects. J Clin Pharmacol 1987;27:907–913.

185. Keller J, Kaltenecker A, Schricker KT, et al. Inhibition of platelet aggregation by a new stable prostacyclin introduced in therapy of patients with progressive scleroderma. Arch Dermatol Res 1985;277:323–325.

186. McHugh NJ, Csuka M, Watson H, et al. Infusion of Iloprost, a prostacyclin analogue, for treatment of Raynaud's phenomenon in systemic sclerosis. Ann Rheum Dis 1988;47:43–47.

187. Rademaker M, Cooke ED, Almond NE, et al. Comparison of intravenous infusions of iloprost and oral nifedipine in treatment of Raynaud's phenomenon in patients with systemic sclerosis: A double blind randomised study. Br Med J 1989; 298:561–564.

188. Constans T, Diot E, Lasfargues G. Iloprost for scleroderma. Ann Intern Med 1991;114:606.

189. Lau CS, McLaren M, Saniabadi A, et al. The pharmacological effects of cicaprost, an oral prostacyclin analogue, in patients with Raynaud's syndrome secondary to systemic sclerosis—a preliminary study. Clin Exp Rheumatol 1991;9:271–273.

190. Kyle MV, Belcher G, Hazleman BL. Placebo controlled study showing therapeutic benefit of ilopost in the treatment of Raynaud's phenomenon. J Rheumatol 1992;19:1403–1406.

191. Wigley FM, Seibold JR, Wise RA, et al. Intravenous iloprost treatment of Raynaud's phenomenon and ischemic ulcers secondary to systemic sclerosis. J Rheumatol 1992;19:1407–1414.

192. Lau CS, Belch JJF, Madhok R, et al. A randomised, double-blind study of Cicaprost, an oral prostacyclin analogue, in the treatment of Raynaud's phenomenon secondary to systemic sclerosis. Clin Exp Rheumatol 1993;11:35–40.

193. Bounameaux HM, Hellemans H, Verhaeghe R, Dequeker J. Ketanserin (5 HT$_2$-antagonist) in secondary Raynaud's phenomenon. J Cardiovasc Pharmacol 1984;6:975–976.

194. Roald OK, Seem E. Treatment of Raynaud's phenomenon with ketanserin in patients with connective tissue disorders. Br Med J 1984;289:577–579.

195. Seibold JR, Jageneau AHM. Treatment of Raynaud's phenomenon with ketanserin, a selective antagonist of the serotonin$_2$ (5-HT$_2$) receptor. Arthritis Rheum 1984;27:139–146.

196. Lukac J, Rovensky J, Tauchmannova H, Zitnan D. Effect of ketanserin on Raynaud's phenomenon in progressive systemic sclerosis: A double-blind trial. Drugs Exp Clin Res 1985;11:659–663.

197. van der Linden MMD, Hulsmans RFHJ, Jageneau AHM. The effect of ketanserin on Raynaud's phenomenon in scleroderma patients. A double-blind placebo-controlled study. Br J Dermatol 1986;115:583–594.

198. Kirch W, Linder HR, Hutt HJ, et al. Ketanserin versus nifedipine in secondary Raynaud's phenomenon. Vasa 1987;16:77–80.

199. Marasini B, Biondi ML, Bianchi E, et al. Ketanserin treatment and serotonin in patients with primary and secondary Raynaud's phenomenon. Eur J Clin Pharmacol 1988;35:419–421.

200. Lukac J, Rovensky J, Tauchmannova H, Zitnan D. Long-term ketanserin treatment in patients with systemic sclerosis and Raynaud's phenomenon. Curr Ther Res 1991;50:869–877.

201. Seibold JR, O'Byrne M, Harris JN. Open trial of pentoxiphylline in prophylaxis of digital ulceration in systemic sclerosis (abstract). Arthritis Rheum 1987;30(suppl 4):S120.

202. Fritzler MJ, Hart DA. Prolonged improvement of Raynaud's phenomenon and scleroderma after recombinant tissue plasminogen activator therapy. Arthritis Rheum 1990;33:274–276.

203. Klimiuk PS, Kay EA, Illingworth KJ, et al. A double blind placebo controlled trial of recombinant tissue plasminogen activator in the treatment of digital ischemia in systemic sclerosis. J Rheumatol 1992;19:716–720.

204. Bridges AJ, Spadone DP. Tissue plasminogen activator treatment of digital thrombosis in severe Raynaud's phenomenon. A case report. Angiology 1993;44:566–569.

205. Rademaker M, Meyrick Thomas RH, Kirby JD, Kovacs IB. The anti-platelet effect of nifedipine in patients with systemic sclerosis. Clin Exp Rheumatol 1992;10:57–62.

206. Dodds AJ, O'Reilly MJG, Yates CJP, et al. Haemorheological response to plasma exchange in Raynaud's syndrome. Br Med J 1979;2:1186–1187.

207. Jacobs MJHM, Jörning PJG, van Rhede van der Kloot EJH, et al. Plasmapheresis in Raynaud's phenomenon in systemic sclerosis: A microcirculatory study. Int J Microcirc Clin Exp 1991;10:1–11.

208. Jobe JB, Sampson JB, Roberts DE, Beetham WP. Induced vasodilation as treatment for Raynaud's disease. Ann Intern Med 1982;97:706–709.

209. Goodfield MJD, Rowell NR. Hand warming as a treatment for Raynaud's phenomenon in systemic sclerosis. Br J Dermatol 1988;119:643–646.

210. Freedman RR, Ianni P, Wenig P. Behavioral treatment of Raynaud's phenomenon in scleroderma. J Behav Med 1984;7:343–353.

211. Flatt AE. Digital artery sympathectomy. J Hand Surg 1980;5:550–556.

212. O'Brien BM, Kumar PAV, Mellow CG, Oliver TV. Radical microarteriolysis in the treatment of vasospastic disorders of the hand, especially scleroderma. J Hand Surg 1992;17B:447–452.

PHILIP J. CLEMENTS
THOMAS A. MEDSGER, JR.

18

Organ Involvement: Skin

Clinical and Pathologic Stages of Skin Involvement

CLINICAL PHASES OF SKIN THICKENING

There are three recognized phases of skin thickening in systemic sclerosis (SSc), which generally follow one another as the disease evolves: the edematous phase, the indurative phase, and the atrophic phase.

Edematous phase

Initially, the patient complains about "tight" or "puffy" fingers, especially on arising in the morning. This may be a sensation only, or there may be visible swelling, which subsides during the day only to recur in the evening or the next morning. In most instances, obvious swelling becomes constant, although it may vary in degree. Persistently enlarged digits are frequently referred to as "sausage fingers." Either pitting or non-pitting edema is present in the fingers, and similar changes may also affect the dorsum of the hands, forearms, legs, feet, and face (Fig. 18.1). Such edema may last indefinitely. Typically, such swelling is painless. The causes of edema are multiple and include increased extracellular connective tissue matrix deposition, inflammation, poor lymphatic return, and microvascular injury with fluid extravasation.

Indurative phase

Most often edema is gradually replaced by thickened, tight skin. In diffuse cutaneous SSc, this evolution is relatively rapid, occurring over the course of several months to years. Intense pruritus may precede, accompany, or follow the onset of skin thickening. In contrast, in patients with the limited cutaneous (CREST) form of SSc, the development of induration occurs very slowly over several years, to as many as 15 to 20 years.

In addition to obvious thickening, affected skin becomes increasingly shiny, taut, and tightly adherent to the underlying subcutis (Fig. 18.2). Transverse creases on the dorsum of the fingers disappear, and skin folds over joints become widened or "fat." During the indurative phase the dermis is markedly thickened, but the epidermis is thinned, leading to loss of skin creases and "choking out" of hair follicles, sweat glands, and sebaceous glands caused by collagenous deposition in the upper dermis. Hair loss in the extremities and decreased sweating result. Skin thickening indirectly impairs mobility of muscles, tendons, and joints. The indurative phase is the time at which a physician should be able to make the diagnosis of scleroderma on physical examination. The latter is quick, easy, and inexpensive to perform, as well as more reliable than a skin biopsy regarding diagnosis. The weight (and thickness) of a standard diameter, full-thickness, skin punch biopsy correlates closely with skin thickness at the same site estimated by physical examination (1) (Fig. 18.3). Erythema may occur, but the most frequent accompanying color change is hyperpigmentation, which may be impressive and always spares the mucous membranes. Increased pigmentation is promi-

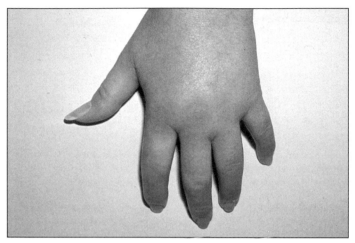

Figure 18.1. Hand of a woman with early scleroderma showing the "puffy" appearance typical of the "edematous" phase of early scleroderma.

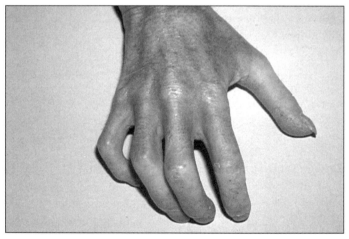

Figure 18.2. Hand of a man with scleroderma of several years duration, showing changes typical of the indurative phase: tight, thickened, shiny skin over the fingers, with little hair on the dorsum of the hand and fingers, loss of skin folds over the joints, and moderately severe flexion contractures of the fingers.

nent at the sites of hair follicles, with surrounding hypopigmentation resulting in a "salt-and-pepper" appearance (Fig. 18.4). Hyperpigmentation has been reported to be most striking along the course of superficial blood vessels (2) and tendons (3), as well as over the "belt line" on the anterior abdominal wall (4).

Facial changes result in a characteristic "pinched nose" or "mauskopf" appearance, some-times interpreted as an "expressionless" facies due to reduced mobility of eyelids, cheeks, nose, and mouth during ordinary conversation. Tightly pursed lips that lose their fullness, perioral subcutaneous fibrosis, and temporomandibular joint involvement all contribute to reduced oral aperture and radial furrowing around the mouth (Fig. 18.5). Lip retraction makes normal mouth closure impossible, accentuating the prominence

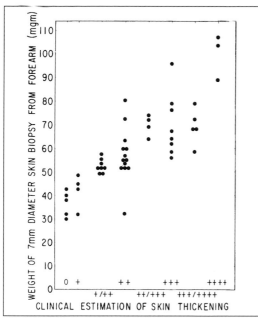

Figure 18.3. Correlation between weights of skin biopsy cores (7 mm surface diameter) obtained from the forearms of 50 consecutive patients with systemic sclerosis and diffuse cutaneous sleroderma and clinical estimation of skin thickness. 0=normal, $+$=slight but definite thickening, $++$=moderate thickening, $+++$=severe thickening, $++++$=extreme degree of thickening. All 5 patients judged to have normal, i.e., not thickened, forearm skin at the time of biopsy subsequently developed frank scleroderma in this area. (Reproduced with permission from Rodnan GP, et al. Skin thickness and collagen content in progressive systemic sclerosis (scleroderma) and localized scleroderma. Arthritis Rheum 1979;22:130–140.)

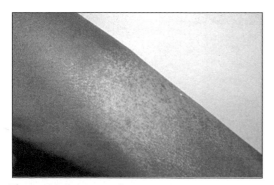

Figure 18.4. Increased pigmentation is prominent at the site of hair follicles, with surrounding hypopigmentation resulting in a "salt-and-pepper" appearance.

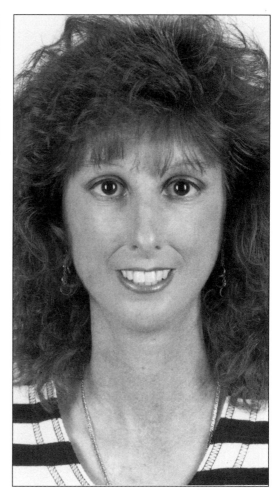

Figure 18.5. Face of a 37-year-old woman with systemic sclerosis and diffuse cutaneous thickening for 11 years. Note the "pinched" nose; shiny, taut skin with loss of normal skin folds; and retraction of the lips.

of the central incisor teeth. This microstomia interferes with eating and with proper prophylactic oral hygiene. Secondary Sjögren's (sicca) syndrome, if present, offers an additional threat to dentition.

In the limited cutaneous variant, skin thickening is less prominent than are mat-like telangiectasias, which represent clusters of dilated, tortuous capillary loops and venules (Figs. 18.6A and B). The latter increase over time, while skin thickening tends to recede. Thus, late-stage limit-

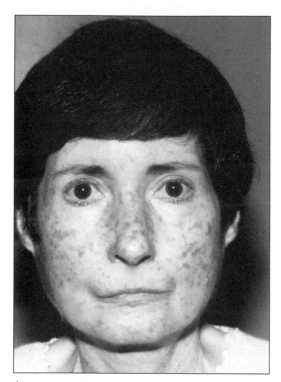

A

Figure 18.6. Telangiectasias affecting the face (*A*) and hands (*B*). These clusters of dilated and tortuous capillaries and venules are grossly visible and blanche on pressure with very slow refilling. They are more numerous later in the course of disease, especially in the atrophic phase.

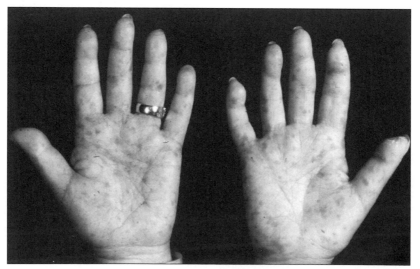

B

ed cutaneous SSc patients often have normal or near-normal digital and/or facial skin but myriad telangiectasias. In diffuse cutaneous SSc, this same sequence of events occurs, but skin thickening is a more prominent aspect of the physical examination during the first few years of disease, especially in areas such as the forearms and upper arms.

Atrophic phase

After several years, the thickened dermis softens and either reverts to normal thickness or actually becomes thinner than normal. The dermis often becomes more firmly adherent to underlying subcutaneous fat, leading to "binding down" or "tethering" that can be confused with dermal thickening. In this late stage, telangiectasias increase in number and tend to be the dominant visual feature (Figs. 18-6A and B). In many cases, the cutaneous examination alone cannot distinguish between limited SSc and late stage diffuse SSc. Consequently, it is hazardous to conclude that numerous telangiectasias alone define limited SSc; additional clinical, laboratory, and serologic data should all be used to form a conclusion about disease classification.

SPECIAL FEATURES OF SKIN INVOLVEMENT

Pathology

Biopsy specimens obtained during the active, indurative phase show loss of rete pegs and atrophy of epidermal skin appendages. Hair follicles and cutaneous glands are "choked out" by the excessive collagen deposition. There is a marked increase in compact collagen fibers in the reticular dermis. These fibers often extend into the uppermost portions of the subcutis. As seen by electron microscopy, there is an increase in thin collagen fibrils (similar to early wound healing) and in ground substance, representing new connective tissue matrix synthesis (5). The relative proportion of types I and III collagen is similar to the ratio in normal skin (6)—mRNA levels for both of these two collagen types are increased (7). Type

IV (basement membrane) collagen (8), fibronectin (9), and glycosaminoglycan (10) amounts also are increased in scleroderma skin, and type VI collagen is found in excess in perivascular regions. The overall excessive collagen deposition appears to be the result of greater production rather than diminished breakdown (11). Within the dermis, there is subintimal proliferation of connective tissue matrix proteins in small arteries and arterioles, leading to narrowed lumens and obliteration of some capillaries. The technique of wide field nailfold capillaroscopy (described more fully in Chapter 17 by Maricq) is a clinically useful method to visualize both the capillary "dropout" and tortuosity characteristic of scleroderma (12).

Inflammatory cell infiltration of vascular walls (true vasculitis) is absent. Variably large collections of mononuclear cells are encountered in perivascular and interstitial locations within the deep dermis and superficial subcutis, especially where induration is greatest and most recent. Nearly all of these are T-lymphocytes (Fig. 18.7) (13). The products of these cells (lymphokines) are believed to be responsible for the excessive stimulation of resident fibroblasts to overproduce procollagen. Degranulated mast cells, which have been linked to fibrosis, are detected in increased numbers and density in clinically involved sites (14). Direct immunofluorescence is negative for immunoglobulins and complement components both at the dermal-epidermal junction and in blood vessels (15).

Ulceration

The etiology of ulceration of skin affected by scleroderma is multifactorial. Digital tip ulcers are most commonly caused by ischemia (Fig. 18.8). In contrast, ulcers over the proximal interphalangeal (PIP) and melacarpophalangeal (MCP) joints, elbows, and tragus of the ear are probably attributable to contractures, tight stretching and thinning of skin, and extreme vulnerability to trauma. Large, deep, painful, punched out lateral malleolar ulcers are most often the result of vasculitis. The latter is not an

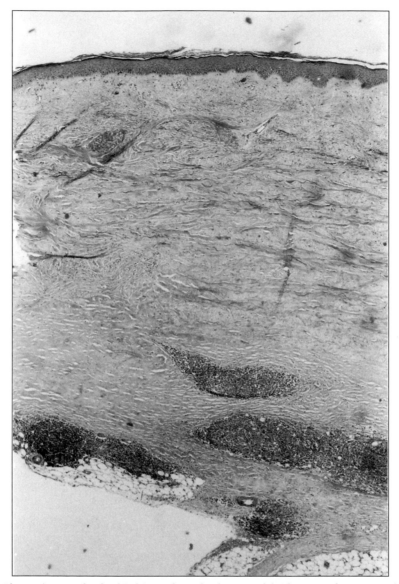

Figure 18.7. Photomicrograph of a skin biopsy from the dorsum of the forearm of a 44-year-old woman with systemic sclerosis and diffuse scleroderma. The epidermal appendages are atrophic. The dermis is thickened because of excessive deposition of collagenous connective tissue. The lower portion of the dermis contains large, dense collections of mononuclear cells, nearly all of which were identified as T-lymphocytes.

integral feature of systemic sclerosis but is instead related to secondary Sjögren's syndrome and often accompanied by palpable leg purpura, peripheral sensory (and occasionally motor) neuropathy, low serum complement levels, and serum anti-SSA/SSB antibody (16). All finger tip ulcers heal extremely slowly and frequently become secondarily infected. However, fear concerning inadequate wound healing after surgical debridement or elective surgical procedures (joint reconstruction, excision of calcinotic masses) appears to be unfounded (17).

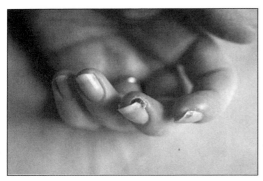

Figure 18.8. Ulcerations and areas of necrosis at the tips of the fingers (which involve the index and middle finger in this illustration) are felt to be secondary to ischemia which results from the obliterative vasculopathy and the vasospasm associated with systemic sclerosis and Raynaud's phenomenon.

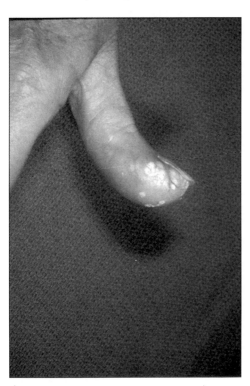

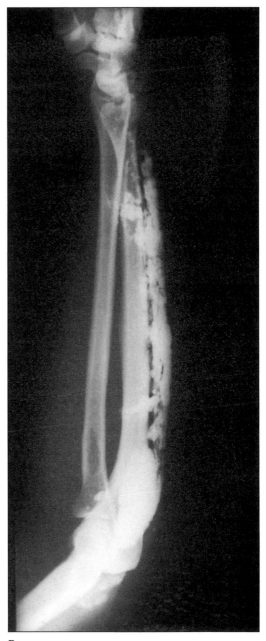

A   B

Figure 18.9. Patients with late-stage limited or diffuse cutaneous scleroderma frequently develop subcutaneous or intracutaneous calcinosis: (*A*) the tip of the thumb is swollen and white "calcific" material can be seen just under the surface of the skin of the distal digit; and (*B*) radiograph of the forearm of a 68 year-old woman with systemic sclerosis and limited cutaneous scleroderma showing extensive subcutaneous calcinosis. She subsequently died of septicemia from an abscess in an infected calcinotic mass. (Figure 18.9A kindly donated by Neil Jones, MD.)

Calcinosis

Patients with limited cutaneous involvement or late-stage diffuse SSc frequently develop subcutaneous and/or intracutaneous calcinosis. These deposits occur chiefly in the digital pads and periarticular tissues, but also occur in other sites of repeated pressure trauma such as the olecranon bursae, extensor surfaces of the forearms, prepatellar and infrapatellar bursal areas around the knees, and in the buttocks (Fig. 18.9). Calcinosis deposits vary in size from tiny punctate lesions of the fingers to large conglomerate masses. Calcinosis may be complicated by ulceration of overlying skin, spontaneous extrusion of calcareous material, and draining sinuses with difficult-to-eradicate secondary bacterial infection. The etiology of calcinosis in the connective tissue diseases, especially systemic sclerosis and dermatomyositis, is unknown, but prominent involvement of the microvasculature in these two disorders may be an important clue to the further investigation of the etiology and pathogenesis of calcinosis.

Natural History of Skin Involvement

CLINICAL METHODS FOR MEASURING SKIN INVOLVEMENT

Longitudinal studies over the past 20 years have provided us with a much clearer picture of the evolution of cutaneous involvement in systemic sclerosis (SSc) (18,19). Several measures have been employed to quantify and document changes in skin thickening over time (Table 18.1). Although some of these measures have shown promise of good reliability and reproducibility, most have not been useful in clinical settings (20–45).

There is mounting evidence that semiquantitative skin scoring by physical examination, a technique pioneered by Rodnan, is reliable, reproducible, readily available, and easy to use. He showed convincingly that affected forearm dermis of SSc patients was thickened (up to three times the thickness of controls) and that clinical

Table 18.1. Measurements of SSc Cutaneous Involvement

Modality	Measurement	References
Physical	Grip strength	20–23
	Maximum oral aperature	20, 22–26
	Finger flexion	20, 26
	Hand extension	22, 26
	Cutaneous temperature	27
	Palm prints (photocopy)	28
	Joint motion/contractures	21, 25, 27, 29
	Cutaneous hypoxia	30
	Percent skin area involved	24, 31
Skin elasticity	Suction cup	22, 23, 28
	Pierard tonometer	25
	Bachman skin mobility	32, 33
	Skin elastometer	34
Biopsy	Weight of uniform diameter	1
	Core	24
	Pathology	1, 35
	Amount of hydroxyproline	
Ultrasound/X-ray	High frequency ultrasound	36
	B-mode ultrasound	37
	Soft tissue radiographs	38–40
Semi-quantitative skin scoring	Original/modified Rodnan skin thickness score	41, 42
	UCLA skin score	43, 44
	Kahaleh modified skin score	45

assessment of cutaneous thickness (using a scale of 0–4, 0 being normal and 4 being extreme thickening) correlated well with the weight of 7 mm diameter skin punch biopsies from the same site (1) (Fig. 18.3). Shortly thereafter, Rodnan defined the total skin score (TSS) as the sum of skin thickness assessments (0–4) made by palpation of 26 separate cutaneous surface areas (maximum score of 104) (41). More recently, this "original" method has been modified (Figs. 18.10A and B) to eliminate areas that are difficult to grade and to employ a simpler (0–3) scale of 17 sites (maximum score of 51) (Fig. 18.11) (31,42). The modified Rodnan skin thickness score has recently been validated (46).

The inter-observer variability of the original Rodnan skin thickness score was documented by seven examiners who assessed (in a blinded fashion) skin thickness scores on 15 SSc patients (42): the mean ± within-patient standard deviation (SD) was 26.6 ± 5.4 units (Table 18.2). Similarly, the inter-observer variability of the *modified* Rodnan skin thickness score was documented in two independent studies in which multiple examiners from different institutions assessed many SSc patients in a blinded fashion (31,42): the mean ± within-patient SD was 18.3 ± 4.6 in one study and 17.7 ± 4.6 in the other (Table 18-2). Another study demonstrated that when the skin score was assessed by the same examin-

er on the same patient several times over a period of 2 to 8 weeks (blinded to previous score), the variability of the modified Rodnan technique was reduced by about half: the mean ± within-patient SD was 20.7 ± 2.45 (47).

Other semi-quantitative measurements for assessing skin thickness and/or tethering by clinical palpation have been described by Furst and Clements (43,44) (UCLA skin score = the sum of 10 separate body surface areas assessed on a 0–3 scale for tethering, maximum score of 30) and by Kahalen (45) (modified skin score = the sum of 22 body surface areas assessed on a 0–3 scale for thickness, maximum score of 66). The inter-observer coefficient of variation was 10% for the UCLA skin score and 6% for the Kahaleh technique. The intra-observer coefficient of variation for the UCLA technique was 8%. The fact that these were single institution studies where participating examiners worked closely together and were well versed in each other's technique may explain, in part, these low rates of variability.

Even so, the experience of Brennan et al and Clements et al suggests that the reliability of skin scoring, even among examiners from many different institutions, compares favorably to the ARA (American Rheumatism Association) and Ritchie joint tenderness counts regularly employed in studies of rheumatoid arthritis (RA) (Table 18.2) (31,42,48).

Table 18.2. Studies Which Document the Inter-Observer Variability of Semi-Quantitative Skin Scoring Techniques in SSc and of Joint Tenderness Counts in Rheumatoid Arthritis

Method of examination	# Pts	# Examiners	Mean	Within-Pt Std Devn	Coefficient Variation
1. Skin Scoring					
Original Rodnan (0–104)[42]	15	7	26.6	5.4	20%
Modified Rodnan (0–51)					
Brennan[31]	12	6	18.3	4.6	25%
D-pen[42]	22	33	17.7	4.6	25%
UCLA Skin Score					
(0–30)[43, 44]	12	2	—	—	10%
Kahaleh (0–66)[45]	20	3	27.8	1.6	6%
2. Joint Tenderness Counts					
ARA (0–68)[48]	66	3	18.2	7.8	43%
Ritchie (0–50)[48]	66	3	16.1	5.9	37%

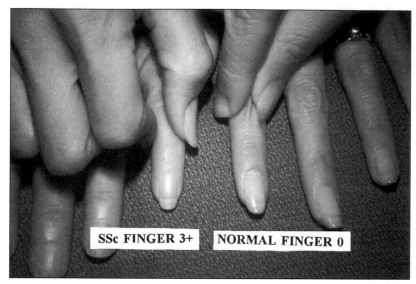

A

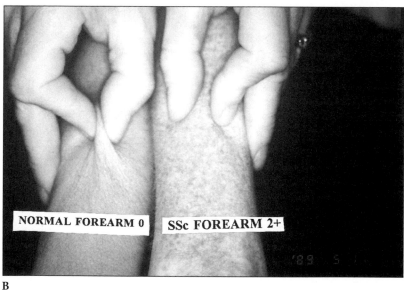

B

Figure 18.10. An estimate of skin thickness can accurately be made by palpating the skin as shown in these two illustrations: (*A*) The skin can be pinched into a skin fold over the middle phalanx of the normal finger (right side of illustration) while the skin of the indurated, sclerodermatous finger (left side of illustration) is less likely to do so. The picture actually illustrates "tethering" but the palpator can also appreciate and assess the skin's thickness during this maneuver. (*B*) The skin of the normal forearm can be pinched into a skin fold (leftt side of illustration) but is less likely to do so in the sclerodermatous forearm (right side). The inability to make a skin fold illustrates "tethering" but the skin's thickness can also be appreciated by the palpator. Note also the "salt-and-pepper" appearance (hypo- and hyperpigmentation) of the skin of the forearm. (Reproduced with permission from Clements PJ. J Muscolskel Med 1991;8:74–80.)

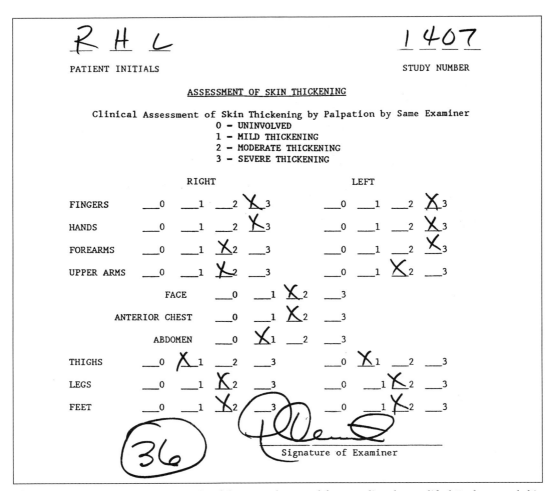

Figure 18.11. Illustrated is an example of the score sheet used for recording the modified-Rodnan total skin thickness score (the summated score from 17 body areas each assessed on a 0–3 scale for skin thickness). This patient has a score of 37 (which is quite high) and has skin thickening in a diffuse cutaneous pattern, both of which are indicators of increased risk for heart, lung, and/or kidney involvement and for decreased survival. The changes in skin score can be used to follow the patient's course as well as their response to treatment.

The percent of body surface area involved by thickening has also been proposed for assessing skin involvement, somewhat akin to assessing the percent of skin involved by burns or by psoriasis (24,31). Unfortunately, the site at which unaffected skin stops and affected skin begins is often very difficult to determine. Brennan et al recently demonstrated that the variability of this technique was twice that of the modified Rodnan skin thickness score (31).

METHODS FOR SUBGROUPING PATIENTS BASED ON THE DISTRIBUTION OF CUTANEOUS SSc

Numerous investigators have concluded that the extent and the degree of cutaneous involvement are predictive of survival and of certain visceral involvements in SSc. Currently, there are only two major proposals for subgrouping patients based on the distribution of cutaneous sclerosis: the three subset model (proposed by Barnett, Giordano, and Masi) (49–51) and the two subset model (proposed by Medsger, Leroy et al, and Steen and Medsger) (18,52,53). The groupings proposed for the three subset model are: *Type I,* sclerodactyly alone; *Type II* cutaneous sclerosis of the extremities; and *Type III,* cutaneous sclerosis of the trunk (central to axillae and/or inguinal regions). The groupings proposed for the two subset model are: *Limited,* skin thickness of the extremities distal to, but not proximal to, the elbows or knees and may affect the face but not the trunk; and *Diffuse,* skin thickness of the extremities, both distal and proximal to the elbows and/or knees, with or without facial involvement, may include the trunk. These models appear to predict outcome best when patients reach their maximum skin thickness (i.e., about 2–3 years after SSc onset).

In toto, the data suggest that the more central the cutaneous sclerosis (especially if the torso is involved), the greater the adverse impact on outcome. Studies evaluating the three subset model have usually shown that survival of patients with sclerodactyly alone (*Type I*) is significantly better than that of patients with truncal sclerosis (*Type III*) (49,50,51). Conversely, it is uncertain that survival of patients with sclerosis of the extremities (*Type II*) differs from that of patients with sclerodactyly alone or of patients with truncal sclerosis or is, in fact, intermediate between the two groups (49–51,54,55). Data evaluating the two subset model have usually suggested that patients with *diffuse* cutaneous scleroderma have a poorer prognosis for survival (18,52,53,55).

Two studies using semiquantitative skin scoring methodology have examined the issue of whether the degree of cutaneous thickening/tethering is predictive of outcome. Both found that patients with "high" initial skin scores (>15 using the UCLA skin score; >40 using the original Rodnan skin score) had significantly poorer survival (44,56). Six-year survival of patients with UCLA skin scores ≥15 was 40% and with skin scores of <15 was 73%; five-year survival of patients with original Rodnan skin scores ≥40 was 50% and with skin scores of <40 was 70%.

THE NATURAL HISTORY OF SSc SKIN INVOLVEMENT

Although this discussion will focus on the natural history of cutaneous scleroderma as documented for the two subset model, a similar scenario could be developed for the three subset model. In the course of *limited* cutaneous scleroderma, skin thickness tends to be insidious in onset, and to affect and be limited to the fingers, hands, and face (and to a lesser extent the distal forearms, and feet). Furthermore, the skin thickening tends to remain unchanged in distribution and severity over many years (see Fig. 3.2, Chapter 3). *Limited* SSc patients who have not developed *diffuse* cutaneous scleroderma within the first 3 years after SSc onset are unlikely to do so later (18,53).

Conversely, patients destined to develop *diffuse* cutaneous scleroderma typically have a rapid acceleration of cutaneous thickening within the first 2 years of disease, both in the degree of thickening and in the number of areas involved (Fig. 3.2, Chapter 3) (18,53). Skin swelling usually begins in the fingers and hands, and then progresses proximally to the forearms, upper arms and then frequently, but not always, to the torso (chest and abdomen). Similar central progression may occur in the lower extremities but is less common and less severe. In general, the peak extent and degree of skin thickening in *diffuse* SSc occurs within 1 to 3 years of SSc onset. Thereafter, cutaneous thickening plateaus and/or recedes, usually slowly, over many years. Such improvement begins centrally and then moves centrifugally down the extremities. Significant regression toward normal skin thickness may occur with time, even in diffuse SSc. However, rarely does all of the affected skin revert completely to normal. Skin atrophy (thinning) and tethering of this thin dermis to underlying subcutaneous tissue is a frequent finding in such late stages of scleroderma. Occasionally, a patient may have a recurrence of diffuse cutaneous SSc some time later in their disease.

Progression of skin thickening has been reported to be most rapid in the subset of patients destined to develop SSc renal crisis, especially in the months just prior to the onset of this complication (57). Similarly, skin thickness may rapidly decline once renal crisis has been brought under control (usually with the aid of angiotensin converting enzyme (ACE) inhibitors). These changes are most likely the result of changes in skin edema related to changes in aldosterone levels and sodium retention prior to and following renal crisis, rather than to disease modifying properties of these drugs.

PROGNOSTIC IMPORTANCE OF DIFFUSE VS LIMITED SSc

Although survival is significantly lower in patients with diffuse SSc (56% at 10 years from first diagnosis, vs 69% in patients with limited SSc) (18), there are other important clinical differences that help to differentiate between diffuse and limited SSc (see also Chapter 3). Diffuse cutaneous involvement is frequently associated with palpable tendon friction rubs, arthritis with joint contractures, serum antitopoisomerase and anti-RNA-polymerase III antibodies, and the frequent occurrence of early visceral disease (heart, lung, kidney, and gastrointestinal tract). Limited cutaneous involvement, conversely, is associated with subcutaneous calcinosis, multiple telangi-ectasias, autoimmune hypothyroidism, sicca/Sjögren's syndrome, serum anticentromere and anti-Th antibodies, and the occasional late development of pulmonary arterial hypertension (without interstitial fibrosis) and biliary cirrhosis.

Studies of Scleroderma Skin Fibroblasts in Tissue Culture

Dermal fibroblasts in scleroderma patients, especially those from the reticular portion of the dermis, synthesize increased amounts of collagen for several generations *in vitro* (58). Many factors influence these fibroblasts, including cytokines produced by activated immune cells and injured endothelium (Fig. 18.12) (59). Post-translational control of the connective tissue matrix composition does not explain the scleroderma fibroblast phenotype.

Several lines of evidence suggest that the overproduction of collagen by scleroderma fibroblasts is caused by a disorder at the transcriptional level. A subpopulation of fibroblasts may preferentially produce excessive procollagen (60), or the responsible fibroblasts may be normal and become expanded or activated by contact with certain substances, such as cytokines or growth factors (61). For example, in mice a specific regulatory element in the OC 2(I) procollagen gene

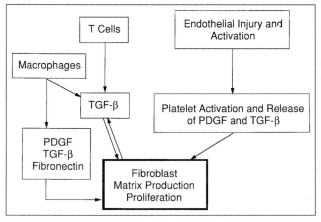

Figure 18.12. A hypothetical scheme of the pathogenesis of systemic sclerosis. (Reproduced with permission from LeRoy EC, et al. Rheumatology. In: Klippel JH, Dieppe TA, eds. London: Mosby Year Book Europe, 1994; 6(9):1–10.)

stimulates its mRNA via transforming growth factor β (TGF-β) (62). The secretion of collagen and fibronectin, a matrix protein recognized to be elevated at the transcriptional level in scleroderma fibroblasts and to enhance fibroblast proliferation, is stimulated by TGF-β (63). The latter cytokine itself activates fibroblasts, and its mRNA has been detected in affected dermis, especially around blood vessels, and colocalizes with procollagen I mRNA (64). TGF-β also stimulates mononuclear cell infiltration and angiogenesis *in vitro* and increases type IV collagenase (65–67). These functions are consistent with endothelial cell damage, telangiectasia production, and fibroblast activation. Platelet-derived growth factor (PDGF), which is found in platelets and several other cells, promotes fibroblast growth by paracrine or autocrine actions, and has been detected in the lower dermal lesions of systemic sclerosis (68). Scleroderma fibroblasts are unresponsive to added PDGF alone, but increase their collagen synthesis in response to PDGF when TGF-β is added first.

In summary, selected scleroderma skin fibroblasts are forced to proliferate and overproduce procollagen and other connective tissue matrix proteins. The stimulus for this pathologic response results from endothelial cell injury and immune cell activation resulting in cytokine production. When activated, skin and other connective tissue fribroblasts are also capable of producing cytokines and of responding to them in a paracrine fashion, resulting in a positive feedback loop.

Treatment

Despite the knowledge that extensive cutaneous thickening is a poor prognostic sign in SSc, there are as yet no controlled studies which show conclusively that the natural history of diffuse disease can be altered or that associated visceral involvement can be ameliorated or prevented. Nevertheless, since skin is the largest and most accessible of affected organs, and its involvement

alone may cause considerable morbidity, its course during treatment has been documented in the majority of the controlled therapeutic trials reported in the past 20 years (Table 18.3).

Numerous therapies have been suggested to reduce skin thickness (reviewed in Chapters 26 and 27). In Table 18.3 we list some trial characteristics and the methods used to document changes in skin involvement in 22 reported controlled trials (of 16 treatments) in which the course of skin involvement was documented (21–27,29,32,35,41,43,69–79). Claims favoring active over control therapies have been reported in these trials (and, at that, not unanimously) only for apheresis, colchicine, cyclofenil, cyclosporin A, D-penicillamine, photopheresis, and potassium paraaminobenzoic acid (POTABA) (22,24,71,72,74,78). More recent randomized, placebo-controlled trials failed to substantiate efficacy for colchicine and potaba on skin involvement (32,73), while other studies of cyclofenil were inconclusive (23). A photopheresis versus D-penicillamine trial did not result in a distinct benefit of either treatment on skin disease, but could be interpreted as showing a small and equal amount of skin softening with both therapies (24). Randomized, placebo/sham-controlled trials have not been reported for apheresis, cyclosporin, photopheresis, and D-penicillamine. Only a few abstracts have appeared to date about the use of methotrexate. Multicenter randomized, double-blind controlled trials of D-penicillamine (USA), photopheresis (USA), alpha-interferon (UK), and methotrexate (Canada) are currently underway, and all have change in skin thickening as a major outcome variable.

There are several methodologic problems inherent in the above-reported studies that cloud their interpretation: (*a*) The natural history of skin involvement (particularly diffuse skin involvement) is one of initial worsening and later improvement, even without specific treatment. The improvement reported for some of these therapies, especially when compared to historical controls, may actually reflect the natural history of cutaneous SSc. (*b*) Until a treatment is shown

Table 18.3. Controlled Therapeutic Trials in Which the Course of Skin Involvement was Studied and the Methods Used to Document Skin Involvement (Adapted from Pope[69].)

	Trial Design	Quantitative Skin Score	Bx	Skin Mobility Elasticity	Other	Efficacious for Skin	Authors (references)
					Measures of Skin Involvement		
Antihypertensive	DB-PL				Skin map	No	Fries[70]
Anti-platelet	DB-PL				Skin induration (+ or - in 8 sites)	No	Beckett[29]
Apheresis	SB-no RX	Rodnan				Yes	Weiner[71]
Chlorambucil	DB-PL	UCLA				No	Furst[43]
Colchicine	DB-PL			Elasticity		Yes	Alarcon-Segovia[72]
Colchicine	DB-PL		+	Elasticity		No	Steigerwald[73]
Cyclofenil	DB-PL			Suction cup	Visual analogue	Yes	Gibson[22]
Cyclofenil	DB-PL			Suction cup		?	Blom-Bulow[23]
Cyclosporin	Open-PL*	UCLA			Mini skin score (3 areas, 0–3 score)	Yes	Clements[74]
DMSO	Open-OE					No	Binnick[27]
DMSO	SB-OE		+		Mini skin score (dorsum hand, 0–5 score)	No	Tuffanelli[73]
DMSO	Open OE					No	Scherbel[21]
D-penicillamine	Open-HX	Rodnan				Yes	Steen[41]
Factor XIII	DB-PL			Pierard		?	Guillevin[25]
5-FU	DB-PL	Rodnan	+			No	Casas[26]
Ketanserin	DB-PL			Pinchability		No	Ortonne[76]
Ketotifen	DB-PL	Kahaleh	+		Hydroxyproline content (skin bx)	No	Gruber[35]
Photopheresis	SB-DPEN	Rodnan	+		% surface area		Rook[24]
Potaba	DB-PL		+	Mobility		No	Bushnell[77]
Potaba	Open-HX				Chart review for changes in skin	Yes	Zarafonetis[78]
Potaba	DB-PL	Rodnan			Bachman skin mobility	No	Clegg[32]
Total nodal irridiation	SB-no RX	Rodnan			Visual analogue	No	O'Dell[79]

Binding: DB = Double blind. SB = Single blind. Open = Open study (not blinded). Control: PL = Placebo. PL* = Matched placebo controls with another trial. No Rx = Control was 'No Therapy'. HX = Historical control. OE = Other extremity as the control. DPen = D-penicillamine as an active control.

clearly to be effective or "active," trials using "active" controls rather than placebos are unwise, because they run the risk that the new therapy will have a course parallel to the "active" control, leaving the unanswerable question, "Were both therapies equally effective, or equally ineffective?" (c) Therapy-induced improvement in skin may be limited to the skin and unrelated to other organ system outcome. (d) Trials that have included large numbers of limited cutaneous SSc patients (and thus patients having little opportunity to show improvement in skin thickening) have probably prejudiced the trials against showing efficacy for the treatment of skin thickening.

REFERENCES

1. Rodnan GP, Lipinski E, Luksick J. Skin thickness and collagen content in progressive systemic (scleroderma) and localized scleroderma. Arthritis Rheum 1979;22:130–140.
2. Jawitz JC, Albert MK, Nigra TP, Bunning RD. A new skin manifestation of progressive systemic sclerosis. J Am Acad Dermatol 1984;2:265–268.
3. Sukenik S, Kleiner-Baumgarten A, Horowitz J. Hyperpigmentation along tendons in progressive systemic sclerosis. J Rheumatol 1986;13:474–475.
4. Fam AG, Lee P. The belt sign in scleroderma. J Rheumatol 1990;17:725–726.
5. Hayes RL, Rodnan GP. The ultrastructure of skin in progressive systemic sclerosis (scleroderma). I. Dermal collagen fibers. Am J Pathol 1971;63:433–442.
6. Krieg T, Perlish JS, Mauch C, Fleischmajer R. Collagen synthesis by scleroderma fibroblasts. Ann NY Acad Sci 1985;460:375–386.
7. Jiminez SA, Feldman G, Bashey RI, Bienkowski R, Rosenbloom J. Coordinate increase in the expression of type I and type III collagen genes in progressive systemic sclerosis. Biochem J 1986;237:837–843.
8. Gay RE, Buckingham RB, Prince RK, Gay S, Rodnan GP, Miller EJ. Collagen types synthesized in dermal fibroblast cultures from patients with early progressive systemic sclerosis. Arthritis Rheum 1980;23:190–196.
9. Fleischmajer R, Perlish JS, Krieg T, Timpl RP. Variability in collagen and fibronectin synthesis by scleroderma fibroblasts in primary culture. J Invest Dermatol 1981;76:400–403.
10. Buckingham RB, Prince RK, Rodnan GP. Progressive systemic sclerosis (PSS, scleroderma) dermal fibroblasts synthesize increased amounts of glycosaminoglycans. J Lab Clin Med 1983;101:659–669.
11. Uitto J, Halme J, Hannuksela M, Peltokallio P, Kivirikko KI. Protocollagen proline hydroxylase activity in the skin of normal human subjects and of patients with scleroderma. Scand J Clin Lab Invest 1969;23:241–247.
12. Maricq HR, Weinberger AB, LeRoy EC. Early detection of scleroderma-spectrum disorders by in vivo capillary microscopy. J Rheumatol 1982;9:289–291.
13. Roumm AD, Whiteside TL, Medsger TA Jr, Rodnan GP. Lymphocytes in the skin of patients with progressive systemic sclerosis: Quantitation, subtyping and clinical correlations. Arthritis Rheum 1984;27:645–653.
14. Hawkins RA, Claman HN, Clark RAG, Steigerwald JC. Increased dermal mast cell populations in progressive systemic sclerosis: A link in chronic fibrosis? Ann Intern Med 1985;102:182–186.
15. Connolly SM, Winkelmann RK. Direct immunofluorescent findings in scleroderma syndromes. Acta Derm Venereol 1981;61:29–36.
16. Oddis CV, Eisenbeis CH Jr, Reidbord HE, Steen VD, Medsger TA Jr. Vasculitis in systemic sclerosis: A subset of patients with the CREST variant, Sjögren's syndrome and neurologic complications. J Rheumatol 1987;14:942–948.
17. Jones NF, Raynor SC, Medsger TA Jr. Microsurgical revascularization of the hand in scleroderma. Br J Plast Surg 1987;40:264–269.
18. Medsger TA Jr. Systemic sclerosis (scleroderma), localized forms of scleroderma, and calcinosis. In: McCarty DJ, Koopman WJ, eds. Arthritis and allied conditions. Philadelphia: Lea & Febiger 1993;1253–1292.
19. Clements PJ, Lachenbruch P, Furst D, Paulus H. The course of skin involvement in systemic sclerosis (SSc) over 3 years in a trial of chlorambucil versus placebo. Arthritis Rheum 1993;36:1575–1579.
20. Furst DE, Clements PJ, Harris R, Ross M, Levy J, Paulus HE. Measurement of clinical change in progressive systemic sclerosis: A one-year double-blind placebo-controlled trial of N-acetylcysteine. Ann Rheum Dis 1979;38:356–361.
21. Scherbel AL. The effect of percuatneous dimethyl sulfoxide on cutaneous manifestations of systemic sclerosis. Ann NY Acad Sci 1983;411;120–130.
22. Gibson T, Grahame R. Cyclofenil treatment of scleroderma—A controlled study. Br J Rheumatol 1983;22:218–223.
23. Blom-Bülow B, Oberg K, Wollheim FA, Persson B,

Jonson B, Malmberg P, Bostrom H, et al. Cyclofenil versus placebo in progressive systemic sclerosis. A one-year double-blind crossover study of 27 patients. Acta Med Scan 1981;210:419–428.

24. Rook AH, Freundlich B, Jegasothy BV, Perez MI, Barr WG, Jimenez SA, Rietschel RL, et al. Treatment of systemic sclerosis with extracorporeal photochemotherapy. Results of a multicenter trial. Arch Dermatol 1992;128:337–346.

25. Guillevin L, Chouvet B, Mery C, De Gery A, Thivolet J, Godeau P, Delbarre F. Treatment of progressive systemic sclerosis using factor XIII. Pharmatherapeutica 1985;4:76–80.

26. Casas JA, Saway PA, Villarreal I, Nolte C, Menajovsky BL, Escudero EE, Blackburn WD, et al. 5-fluorouracil in the treatment of scleroderma: A randomized, double blind, placebo controlled international collaborative study. Ann Rheum Dis 1990;49:926–928.

27. Binnick SA, Shore SS, Corman A, Fleischmajer R. Failure of dimethyl sulfoxide in the treatment of scleroderma. Arch Dermatol 1977;113:1398–1402.

28. Bluestone R, Graham R, Holloway V, Holt PJL. Treatment of systemic sclerosis with D-penicillamine: A new method of observing the effects of treatment. Ann Rheum Dis 1970;29:153–159.

29. Beckett VL, Conn DL, Fuster V, Osmundson PJ, Strong CG, Chao EYS, Chesebro JH, et al. Trial of platelet-inhibiting drug in scleroderma. Double-blind study with dipyridamole and aspirin. Arthritis Rheum 1984;27:1137–1143.

30. Silverstein JL, Steen VD, Medsger TA Jr, Falanga V. Cutaneous hypoxia in patients with systemic sclerosis (scleroderma). Arch Dermatol 1988;124:1379–1382.

31. Brennan P, Silman A, Black C, Bernstein R, Coppock J, Maddison P, Sheeran T, et al. Reliability of skin involvement measures in scleroderma. Br J Rheumatol 1992;31:457–460.

32. Clegg CI, Reading JC, Mayes MD, Seibold JR, Harris C, Wigley FM, Ward JR, et al. Comparison of aminobenzoate potassium and placebo in the treatment of scleroderma. J Rheumatol 1994;21:105–110.

33. Bachman DM. Quantifying skin mobility in scleroderma. Arch Dermatol 1961;83:598–605.

34. Ballou SP, Mackiewicz A, Lysikiewicz A, Neuman MR. Direct quantitation of skin elasticity in systemic sclerosis. J Rheumatol 1990;17:790–794.

35. Gruber BL, Haufman LD. A double-blind randomized controlled trial of ketotifen versus placebo in early diffuse scleroderma. Arthritis Rheum 1992;34:362–366.

36. Äkesson A, Forsberg L, Hederstrom E, Wollheim F. Ultrasound examination of skin thickness in patients with progressive systemic sclerosis (scleroderma). Acta Radiol Diagnosis 1986;27:472–477.

37. Myers SL, Cohen JS, Sheets PW, Bies JR. B-mode ultrasound evaluation of skin thickness in progressive systemic sclerosis. J Rheumatol 1986;13:577–580.

38. Dykes PJ, Marks R. Measurement of skin thickness: A comparison of two *in vivo* techniques with a conventional histometric method. J Invest Dermatol 1977;69:275–278.

39. Black CM. A modified radiographic method for measuring skin thickness. Br J Dermatol 1969;81:661–666.

40. Bliznak J, Staple TW. Roengenographic measurement of skin thickness in normal individuals. Radiology 1975;116:55–60.

41. Steen VD, Medsger TA Jr, Rodnan GP. D-penicillamine therapy in progressive systemic sclerosis (scleroderma). Ann Intern Med 1982;97:652–658.

42. Clements PJ, Lachenbruch PA, Seibold JR, Zee B, Brennan P, Silman A, Allegar A, et al. Skin thickness score in systemic sclerosis (SSc): An assessment of inter-observer variability in three independent studies. J Rheumatol 1993;20:1892–1896.

43. Furst DE, Clements PJ, Hillis S, Lachenbruch PA, Miller BL, Sterz MG, Paulus HE. Immunosuppression with chlorambucil, versus placebo, for scleroderma: Results of a three-year, parallel, randomized, double-blind study. Arthritis Rheum 1989;32:584–593.

44. Clements PJ, Lachenbruch PA, Ng SW, Simmons M, Sterz M, Furst DE. Skin score. A semiquantitative measure of cutaneous involvement that improves prediction of prognosis in systemic sclerosis. Arthritis Rheum 1990;33:1256–1263.

45. Kahaleh MB, Suttany GL, Smith EA, Huffstutter JE, Loadholt CB, LeRoy EC. A modified scleroderma skin scoring method. Clin Exp Rheumatol 1986;4:367–369.

46. Ramsden MF, Goldsmith CH, Lee P, Sebaldt R, Baer P. Clinical assessment of scleroderma: Observer variation in five methods. Arthritis Rheum 1986;29:S61.

47. Clements PJ, Lachenbruch PA, Seibold JR, White B, Weiner S, Martin R, Weinstein A, et al. Inter- and intraobserver variability of total skin thickness score (modified-Rodnan) in systemic sclerosis (SSc) J Rheumatol (in press).

48. Eberl DR, Fasching B, Rahfls V, Schleyer I, Wolf R. Repeatability and objectivity of various measurements in rheumatoid arthritis. Arthritis Rheum 1976;19:1278–1286.

49. Barnett AJ, Miller MH, Littlejohn GO. A survival study of the patients diagnosed over 30 years (1953–1983): The value of a simple cutaneous

classification in the early stages of the disease. J Rheumtol 1988;15:276–283.

50. Giordano M, Valentini G, Migliaresi S, Picillo V, Vatti M. Different antibody patterns and different prognoses in patients with scleroderma with various extent of skin sclerosis. J Rheumatol 1986;13: 911–916.

51. Masi AT. Classification of systemic sclerosis (scleroderma): Relationship of cutaneous subgroups in early disease to outcome and serologic reactivity. J Rheumatol 1988;15:894–898.

52. LeRoy EC, Black C, Fleischmajer R, Jabłońska S, Krieg T, Medsger TA Jr, Rowell N, et al. Scleroderma (systemic sclerosis): Classification, subsets, and pathogenesis. J Rheumatol 1988;15:202–205.

53. Steen VD, Medsger TA Jr. Epidemiology and natural history of systemic sclerosis. Rheum Dis Clin North Am 1990;16:1–10.

54. Ferri C, Bernini L, Cecchetti R, Latorraca A, Marotta G, Pasero G, Neri R, et al. Cutaneous and serologic subsets of systemic sclerosis. J Rheumatol 1991;18:1826–1832.

55. Vayssairat M, Baudot N, Abuaf N, Johanet C. Long-term follow-up study of 164 patients with definite systemic sclerosis: Classification considerations. Clin Rheumatol 1992;11:356–363.

56. Medsger TA Jr, Steen VD, Ziegler G, Rodnan G. The natural history of skin involvement in progressive systemic sclerosis. Arthritis Rheum 1980;22:720–721.

57. Steen VD, Medsger TA Jr, Osial TA, Ziegler GL, Shapiro AP, Rodnan GP. Factors predicting development of renal involvement in progressive systemic sclerosis. Am J Med 1984;76:779–786.

58. Uitto J, Bauer EA, Eisen AZ. Scleroderma: Increased biosynthesis of triple-helical type I and type III procollagens associated with unaltered expression of collagenase by skin fibroblasts in culture. J Clin Invest 1979;64:921–930.

59. LeRoy EC, Smith EA. Systemic sclerosis: Etiology and pathogensis. In: Klippel JH, Dieppe TA, eds. Rheumatology London: Mosby Year Book Europe, 1994;6(9):1–10.

60. Botstein GT, Sherer GK, LeRoy EC. Fibroblast selection in scleroderma: An alternative model of fibrosis. Arthritis Rheum 1982;25:189–195.

61. LeRoy EC. Increased collagen synthesis by scleroderma skin fibroblasts *in vitro*. J Clin Invest 1974;54:880–889.

62. Ramirez F, DiLiberto M. Complex and diversified regulatory programs control the expression of vertebrate collagen genes. FASEB J 1990;4:1616–1623.

63. Zu WD, LeRoy ED, Smith EA. Fibronection release

by systemic sclerosis and noraml dermal fibroblasts in response to TGF-β. J Rheumatol 1991;18: 241–246.

64. Kulozik M, Hogg A, Lankat-Buttgereit B, Krieg T. Localization of transforming growth factor β2 with α1(I) procollagen mRNA in tissue sections of patients with systemic sclerosis. J Clin Invest 1990; 86:917–920.

65. Roberts AB, Sporn MB, Assoian RK, Smith JM, Roche NS, Wakefield LM, Heine UI, et al. Transforming growth factor β: Rapid induction of fibrosis and angiogenesis *in vivo* and stimulation of collagen formation *in vitro*. Proc Natl Acad Sci USA 1986;83:4167–4171.

66. Takehara K, LeRoy EC, Grotendorst GR. TGF-β inhibition of endothelial cell proliferation: Alteration of EGF binding and EGF-induced growth regulatory (competence) gene expression. Cell 1987;49:415–422.

67. Brown PD, Levy AT, Margulies IMK, Liotta LA, Stetler-Stevenson WG. Independent expression and cellular processing of M,72,000 type IV collagenase and interstitial collagenase in human tumorigenic cell lines. Cancer Res 1990;50:6184–6191.

68. Gay S, Jones RE Jr, Huang G-Q, Gay RE. Immunohistologic demonstration of platelet-derived growth factor (PDGF) and sis-oncogene expression in scleroderma. J Invest Dermatol 1989;92: 301–303.

69. Pope J, Bellamy N. Outcome measurement in scleroderma clinical trials. Sem in Arthritis Rheum 1993;23:22–33.

70. Fries JF, Wasner C, Brown J, Feigenbaum P. A controlled trial of antihypertensive therapy in systemic sclerosis (scleroderma). Ann Rheum Dis 1094;43: 407–210.

71. Weiner SR, Kono KH, Osterman HA, Levy J, Paulus HE, Pitts WH. Preliminary report on a controlled trial of apheresis in the treatment of scleroderma. Arthritis Rheum 1987;30:S27.

72. Alarcon-Segovia D, Ramos-Niembro F, Kershenobich D, Rojkind M. Treatment of scleroderma by modification of collagen metabolism. A double-blind trial with colchicine vs placebo. J Rheumatol 1974;(Suppl)1–97.

73. Steigerwald JC. Colchicine vs placebo in the treatment of progressive systemic sclerosis. In: Black CM, Myers AR, eds. Systemic sclerosis (scleroderma). New York: Gower Medical, 1985;415–417.

74. Clements PJ, Sterz M, Danovitch G, Hawkins R, Lachenbruch PA, Ippoliti A, Paulus HE. Cyclosporin (CsA) in systemic sclerosis (SSc): Results of

a 48-week open safety study in 10 SSc patients. Arthritis Rheum 1993;36:75–83.

75. Tuffanelli DL. A clinical trial with dimethylsulfoxide in scleroderma. Arch Dermatol 1966;93:724–725.

76. Ortonne JP, Torzouli C, Dujardin P, Fraitag B. Ketanserin in the treatment of systemic sclerosis: A double-blind controlled trial. Br J Dermatol 1989; 120:261–266.

77. Bushnell WJ, Galens GJ, Bartholonew LE, Thompson G, Duff IF. The treatment of progressive systemic sclerosis: A comparison of para-amino-benzoate and placebo in a double blind study. Arthritis Rheum 1966;9:495.

78. Zarafonetis CJD, Dabich L, Skovronski JJ, DeVol EB, Negri D, Yuan W, Wolfe R. Retrospective studies in scleroderma: Skin response to potassium para-aminobenzoate therapy. Clin Exp Rheum 1988;6;261–268.

79. O'dell JR, Steigerwald JC, Kennaugh RC, Hawkins R, Holers VM, Kotzin BL. Lack of clinical benefit after treatment of systemic sclerosis with total lymphoid irradiation. J Rheumatol 1989;16:1050–1054.

KEN BLOCKA

19

Organ Involvement: Musculoskeletal

WHILE TETHERING of the skin is the clinical hallmark of systemic sclerosis (SSc), many patients may develop musculoskeletal symptoms during the course of their illness. Manifestations may include varying degrees of muscle weakness and rheumatic complaints ranging from simple arthralgias to frank arthritis. The articulations, if involved, may be associated with distinctive radiographic abnormalities.

The objective of this chapter is to provide an overview of the spectrum of musculoskeletal involvement in SSc and allied disorders and, as such, to further underscore the multi-system nature of this condition. Many of the musculoskeletal features to be described will apply equally well to limited cutaneous scleroderma, the preferred designation for the condition formerly known as the CREST syndrome (see *CREST Syndrome* section later in this chapter). The localized forms of scleroderma are not associated with musculoskeletal problems and thus will not be considered in this discussion. Finally, the shortened term "scleroderma" will be used interchangeably with SSc throughout this review.

Historical Background

The potential for musculoskeletal involvement was recognized in the earliest descriptions of scleroderma, with Rodnan and his associates providing many of the initial comprehensive reviews on the subject (1,2).

Forget published the first account of joint disease in scleroderma in 1847. He described a 33-year-old woman "whose wrists bore all the traces of leeches and cupping glasses" (3). While joint symptoms were readily identified, it remained unclear whether the rheumatic complaints were truly arthritic or merely a consequence of the skin tightening itself.

In 1896, Dercum (4) observed narrowing of the proximal interphalangeal (PIP) and distal interphalangeal (DIP) joints on hand roentgenograms of a patient with scleroderma, which supported the belief in scleroderma's potential to affect tissues other than the skin. This finding was confirmed in a subsequent series of 8 patients reported by Osler in 1898 (5).

Joint involvement was affirmed to be an integral feature of scleroderma following a review of the subject in 1920 by Adrian and Roederer (6). The authors suggested, perceptively, that there existed a primary inflammation of the synovial membrane, which could lead secondarily to atrophy of bone and cartilage. The association of SSc and joint involvement has since been well established and the subject of numerous reviews and reports (7–11).

In 1876, Westphal (12) first reported skeletal muscle involvement in SSc in a woman with marked shoulder girdle atrophy. The existence of a primary myopathy was subsequently confirmed by several investigators over the years and has been nicely reviewed by Medsger (13). Of interest, an early explanation for the myopathy was that of direct muscle invasion from overlying

409

cutaneous and subcutaneous fibrosis leading to compression atrophy.

A recurring problem in the interpretation of much of the earlier clinical data, according to Medsger, pertained to the diagnostic classification of the primary underlying process. A myopathic component is known to occur in many connective tissue disorders, but this would appear to be especially true of scleroderma. Tuffanelli and Winkelmann (14) coined the term "sclerodermatomyositis" to describe those individuals in whom the features of scleroderma and polymyositis seemed to be equally represented. It is now recognized that many of these patients would fulfill the clinical and serologic criteria for mixed connective tissue disease (MCTD) or overlap syndrome.

Clinical Presentation

RHEUMATOLOGIC

Articular involvement has been described as an initial manifestation in 12% to 65% of patients with scleroderma and as an eventual manifestation in up to 46% to 97% of patients (7,11). Generalized arthralgias and stiffness are the usual presentations; however, true joint inflammation may occur and be the source of initial diagnostic confusion. The onset may be acute or insidious, oligoarticular, or polyarticular in pattern. Virtually all joints may be affected with the fingers, wrists, and ankles predominating. A minority of patients may report the coincidental onset of a "creaking" or a palpable rubbing sensation on joint movement. As the cutaneous involvement progresses, there is an inexorable tethering and contracture of the underlying joints with impairment of movement and function.

Clinical findings are often minimal at the onset, aside from features which may betray the presence of early scleroderma such as subtle sclerodactyly or diffuse soft tissue swelling. Some patients may exhibit localized joint tenderness, redness, or swelling, and joint effusions may be detectable although these are usually small. Early flexion contractures are not uncommon especially in the fingers, wrists, and elbows. Bowing of the fingers has been suggested as a useful early diagnostic sign (15).

Tendon and tendon sheath involvement is also common especially in the knees, fingers, wrists, and ankles and may lead to a distinctive "leathery" crepitus, which may be both audible and palpable. The bursae may be similarly affected especially in the olecranon, trochanteric, and subscapular regions. Subscapular bursal involvement may mimic pleural friction rubs, and bursal involvement around the hip may be confused with primary hip disease (16).

Bursitis (primarily of the olecranon region) was identified in 10 out of 40 patients in a report by Lagana (17). It was suggested that the bursitis could consist of three forms: dry (with friction rub), effusive, or septic. In this series, the bursitis tended to be bilateral, and fistulae with recurrent infection were common.

Involvement of the periarticular structures in scleroderma has been attributed to the formation of fibrinous deposits within the tendon sheaths, bursae, and fascial planes (18). Calcification may also occur and, while generally asymptomatic, may give rise to acute calcific periarthritis (19). Additional reported sequelae have included nerve entrapment, especially of the median nerve (2), and rare instances of tendon rupture (20,21).

MUSCULAR

While the majority of SSc patients have no symptoms related to skeletal muscle, physical examination will often disclose unsuspected weakness and/or muscle atrophy. In two large studies limited to typical SSc patients without overlap, muscle weakness, often occurring independent of atrophy, was found in more than 80% of patients (22,23). While disuse atrophy and impaired nutrition represent the most important causes of weakness, especially in the more advanced stage of the disease, up to 10% of patients will also have clinical, biochemical, or histologic evidence of a true inflammatory myopathy (22,23).

Clements et al (23) have suggested two principal patterns of muscle involvement. The first is a simple and relatively non-progressive myopathy that is likely to occur in the majority of patients and is characterized by minor proximal weakness and normal or slight elevations of the CPK. The EMG may show increased polyphasic potentials of normal or decreased amplitude and duration, but without the insertional irritability and fibrillation that characterizes classic polymyositis. Muscle atrophy may or may not be apparent. The second pattern is a more aggressive form of limb girdle muscle weakness with significant CPK elevation, which is pathologically and electromyographically indistinguishable from classic polymyositis. This form is most likely to occur in the context of an overlap disorder such as MCTD or sclerodermatomyositis.

Excluding obvious examples of overlap with polymyositis, biopsies may be abnormal in up to 50% of individuals with SSc (22,24). The most prominent abnormality is the presence of increased collagen and fat in the interstitial, perivascular, and rarely the perineural areas (22). Focal mononuclear cellular infiltrates may be present along with infrequent changes of the myofibril ranging from atrophy, loss of striation, and variability in diameter, to degeneration and necrosis. Studies using electron microscopes have shown decreased numbers of mitochondria, vacuolization, granular degeneration, and vascular changes such as capillary wall thickening and lumen obliteration (25).

Patients with common simple myopathy will often show a waxing and waning course and are typically refractory to corticosteroids. These patients are distinguished from the smaller subset of patients with the more typical features of polymyositis whose symptoms are much more readily responsive to steroid therapy.

Clements et al (23), in their series of 23 patients, also described a single patient with proximal muscle weakness, significantly elevated muscle enzymes, and a muscle biopsy showing only

fibrosis and muscle fiber atrophy. The EMG showed generalized denervation of distal musculature with normal nerve conduction studies. This patient improved on corticosteroids, and it was suggested that the weakness could have been caused by an unusual neuropathic process relating to the underlying disease.

Laboratory Signs

Mild to moderate elevation of the erythrocyte sedimentation rate (ESR), low titer antinuclear antibody (ANA) elevation, and rheumatoid factor positivity may occur in many patients (26, 27). These tests are non-specific, however, and do not serve to distinguish SSc patients with musculoskeletal manifestations from those not so affected. A minority of patients in whom the presence of symmetrical polyarthritis antecedes the appearance of diagnostic skin changes may be initially misdiagnosed as having rheumatoid arthritis (RA), especially if they are found to be rheumatoid factor positive (28). The presence of rheumatoid factor does not seem to correlate with the clinical or radiographic pattern of arthritis including the comparatively rare subset of patients with joint erosions on x-ray (10). No other useful laboratory markers have been demonstrated.

Frank polymyositis is more frequently identified in scleroderma patients with anti-RNP antibodies pointing to the likelihood of underlying MCTD or an overlap syndrome. Moreover, the PM-Scl antibody may identify a subset of patients with myositis and/or more limited scleroderma that is more prone to inflammatory myopathy and arthritis (29).

Joint effusions have occasionally been reported, with analysis generally revealing normal or modestly increased leukocyte concentrations of less than 2000 cells/mm^3 and a predominantly mononuclear infiltrate (26,30). Rarely, frankly inflamed synovial fluid with inclusion-containing cells indistinguishable from the ragocytes of RA have been reported (31). Immunocytologic studies have revealed that these inclusion bodies contain large amounts of fibrin and/or fibrin breakdown products as well as the immunoglobulins IgG and IgM (32).

In addition to soft tissue and periarticular calcification, intra-articular (free or intrasynovial) calcification can occur in scleroderma (33,34). Radiographs reveal cloud-like radio-dense regions conforming to a portion of the joint or the entire articulation (Fig. 19.1). Aspiration of joint contents may reveal a chalky joint effusion containing hydroxyapatite crystals (35). The pathogenesis is not known, but the association of inflammatory changes with this phenomenon suggests that dystrophic calcification of diseased synovium may have taken place (33).

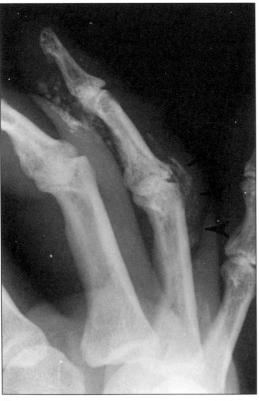

Figure 19.1. Conglomerate soft tissue calcification as well as calcification of the extensor tendon in a 62-year-old female with long-standing scleroderma.

Radiographic Features

Many distinctive radiographic abnormalities have been recognized in patients with SSc and have been the subject of several major reviews (1,2,11,36–38). These findings have been definitively characterized and detailed by Resnick (39), and his work has served as the principal reference for the following discussion.

It should be emphasized that perhaps the most common radiographic abnormality in SSc patients is that of generalized osteopenia irrespective of menopausal status (40). Seldom a source of symptoms, this finding likely relates to impaired intestinal absorption of calcium, disuse, or diminished osseous perfusion (16).

For ease of discussion, the radiographic abnormalities that are most commonly recognized in the hands of SSc patients may be classified as either non-articular or articular (Table 19.1).

NON-ARTICULAR

Non-articular abnormalities, whether singly or in combination, are among the most distinctive radiographic findings in SSc. They appear in up to two-thirds of scleroderma patients and are much less common (less than 5%) in the other connective tissue disorders. These changes are not diagnostic for SSc, however, having been reported to occur in nearly 40% of patients with primary Raynaud's (41).

Digital cutaneous atrophy is, by definition, almost universal in patients with scleroderma. While various measurements have been devised to detect this finding (41,42), the presence of skin

Table 19.1. Radiographic Findings in the Hands of Patients with SSc

Non-articular	Articular
Skin atrophy	Juxta-articular demineralization
Subcutaneous calcinosis	Joint space narrowing
Digital tuft resorption	Erosions

atrophy is much more readily appreciated clinically than radiographically.

Subcutaneous calcification is commonly seen in patients with scleroderma, an association first reported by Thibierge and Weissenbach in 1911 (43). Calcinosis is also one of the hallmark findings in the more limited form of scleroderma identified by the acronym CREST (see *CREST Syndrome* later in this chapter).

The hand is most commonly affected, with deposits at this location identified in greater than 85% of all patients with calcinosis. Subcutaneous calcification, however, may occur in other articular and non-articular locations throughout the body including strategically troublesome sites such as the ischial tuberosities, lateral malleoli, and at the thoracic outlet. Radiographs limited to the hands, therefore, may significantly underestimate the prevalence of this particular complication with the feet, knees, and legs representing other commonly affected locations (44).

The calcification may occur in linear, punctate, or conglomerate patterns and, at times, may show a remarkable predilection for tendon sheaths (Fig. 19.1) or the synovium and joint capsules (Fig. 19.2). The prevalence of this finding is thought to correlate with the severity and duration of the scleroderma, but seems unrelated to vascular factors such as the severity of the Raynaud's or the presence or absence of digital vasculitis. In contrast to that associated with dermatomyositis, resorption and/or disappearance of subcutaneous calcification has only been rarely reported (10).

Clinically, the presence of soft tissue calcification may be first detected by the appearance of subcutaneous nodularity or thickening in the soft tissues of the hands and fingers. These lesions, especially when arising over pressure points, may become subject to inflammation, ulceration, secondary infection, and, occasionally, the extrusion of whitish calcific material.

The extruded material is almost always calcium hydroxyapatite, although a single patient has been described where aspiration of a subcutaneous nodule yielded cholesterol crystals (45).

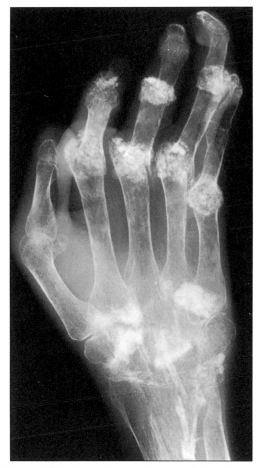

Figure 19.2. Dramatic capsular, synovial, and intra-articular calcification in a 68-year-old female with scleroderma. Note also the severe destructive arthropathy and subluxations occurring at the MCP and PIP joints.

On microscopic examination of the skin, the precipitates of calcium are revealed as pleomorphic crystals in the shape of needles and plates appearing to arise in the elastic fibers of connective tissue (46). These crystals have been identified as hydroxyapatite following both x-ray diffraction and electron microscopy (47).

The pathogenesis of subcutaneous calcinosis in scleroderma or other connective tissue disorders, such as dermatomyositis, is not understood. There would seem to be no evidence of an underlying derangement of calcium or phosphorous metabolism, and parathyroidectomy has not been associated with any improvement (48). Calcium binding studies have yielded contradictory results (49,50). The apparent predilection of calcification for sites of repetitive stress or pressure suggests a possible role for soft tissue trauma (2). Protein rich in gamma carboxyglutamic acid is increased locally in the calcinosis of both SSc and dermatomyositis (51). Urinary excretion of this vitamin K-dependent calcium binding protein has also been found to be increased in these disorders, but the putative role of this substance remains unclear. (52). Nishikai has suggested a correlation between anticentromere antibodies and the presence of subcutaneous calcification; however, the significance of this observation is uncertain (44).

Osseous resorption of the digital tuft represents the most distinctive and dramatic radiographic abnormality in scleroderma patients. Occurring in 40% to 80% of patients (41,42,53), this process may lead to a penciling, sharpening, or even complete loss of the distal phalanx (Fig. 19.3). In rare instances, resorption of the middle phalanx may also occur. Severe bony osteolysis is suggested to occur more frequently in children with scleroderma (54).

ARTICULAR

Radiographic abnormalities of the articulations themselves are known to occur, but with less frequency than the extra-articular abnormalities described in previous paragraphs. Rabinowitz et al (28), in their series of scleroderma patients, were struck by the similarity of some of their findings, such as joint space narrowing and erosions, to that found in RA. Caution is necessary, however, in the attribution of these findings to scleroderma because of the possibility for true overlap with RA, such as is now recognized to occur in MCTD. Nonetheless, in SSc patients vigorously screened to exclude possible RA overlap (10), rheumatoid-like articular findings were observed in a significant minority of patients. This would support the existence of a primary

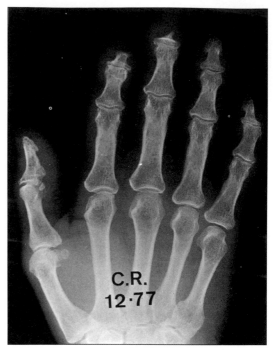

Figure 19.3. Severe resorptive changes of the distal 2nd and 3rd phalanges in a 54-year-old female with scleroderma.

arthropathy in SSc that is unexplained by overlap with RA.

A spectrum of articular changes, ranging from juxta-articular osteoporosis and joint space narrowing to frank erosions, has been reported throughout the distal interphalangeal (DIP), proximal interphalangeal (PIP), and metacarpophalangeal (MCP) joints as well as the wrist (11,38,55). Patterns have ranged from that resembling erosive osteoarthritis or psoriatic arthritis with relative sparing of the MCP joints (56–58) to changes reminiscent of rheumatoid arthritis (Fig. 19.4). The pathogenesis of these lesions is unclear, although it would seem likely, based on the limited number of synovial biopsies, that true synovial inflammation may be operative in at least some cases.

A seemingly distinctive erosion or focal resorptive change, localized to the dosal aspect of the MCP and PIP heads, has also been reported (10) (Figs. 19.5 and 19.6). These lesions, which

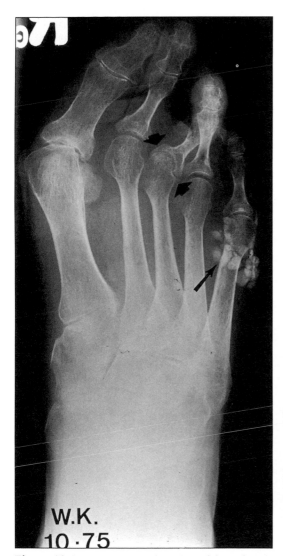

Figure 19.4. Large excavated erosion of the 3rd MTP joint along with soft tissue calcification in a 55-year-old female with chronic scleroderma.

feature in some patients with SSc (60). The described abnormalities include bilateral resorption of the trapezium and adjacent metacarpal bone along with intra-articular calcification and erosions. Resnick postulates that the frequently associated muscle atrophy and skin tightening may give rise to a chronic muscle tendon imbalance with secondary osseous resorptive changes.

With the exception of an increased active joint count in patients with erosions, computer-assisted analysis of multiple clinical and laboratory variables has failed to show correlation with any radiographic abnormality (10,11).

LESS COMMON SKELETAL FINDINGS

In addition to soft tissue and periarticular calcification, intra-articular calcification has also been occasionally reported in SSc (33,34). While

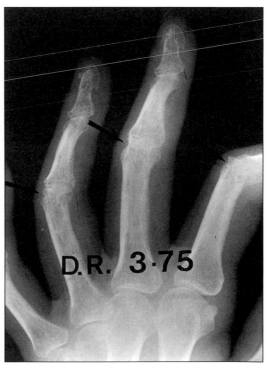

Figure 19.5. Unusual erosions localized to the dorsal aspect of the proximal phalanges in a 47-year-old female with scleroderma.

are best detected on oblique radiographic projections of the digits, have also been rarely reported in RA. Their etiology is unclear, but may relate to capsular or ligamentous traction rather than true synovial inflammation (59).

Resnick has suggested that selected involvement of the carpometacarpal phalangeal joint is an under-appreciated and relatively distinctive

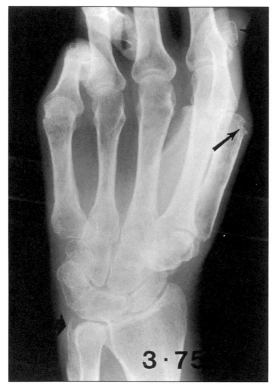

Figure 19.6. Well-demarcated isolated erosion of the dorsal aspect of proximal phalanx of the thumb in a 60-year-old female with deforming contractures of the fingers.

any articulation may be affected, this phenomenon has been identified most frequently in the elbow, radial ulnar joint, first carpometacarpal phalangeal joint, MCP joints, metatarsal phalangeal joints, knees, and hips (Fig. 19.7). Intra-articular calcification may also be associated with osseous resorption. The combination of these abnormalities in the carpometacarpal joint of the thumb is felt by some authors to constitute a distinctive arthropathy for SSc (60). Hydroxyapatite crystals have been identified on aspiration of these joints although their cause and pathogenetic role remains unclear. Intra-articular calcification and other less-common skeletal findings, described in the following paragraphs, are summarized in Table 19.2.

Perhaps one of the most characteristic radiographic abnormalities in SSc relates to the extraordinary propensity for osseous resorption. In addition to the well recognized resorptive tendency of terminal digital tufts, osteolysis has been reported in a number of other skeletal sites, most notably the ribs (38,61), the mandible (62), the distal clavicle (63), the humerus (64), and the cervical spine (65,66).

Rib involvement is characterized by superior surface resorptive changes especially of the posterior portions of the third to sixth ribs (Fig. 19.8) (38,61). Identical changes have been reported in conditions involving muscle atrophy resulting from chest wall restriction, such as

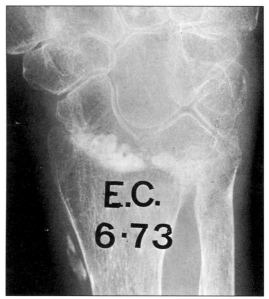

Figure 19.7. Intra-articular calcification of the radioulnar joint.

Table 19.2. Less Common Skeletal Findings in SSc

Intra-articular calcification
Osseous resorption at non-articular sites
Thickening of periodontal membrane
Ankylosis
Periostitis

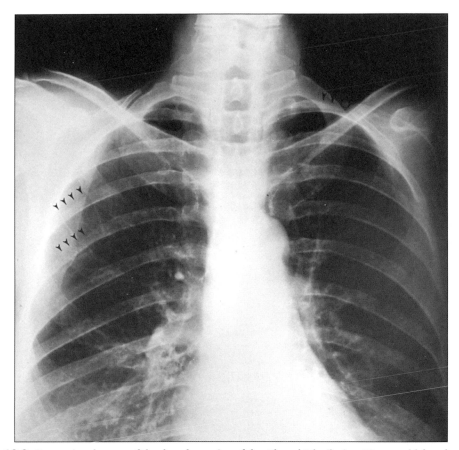

Figure 19.8. Resorptive changes of the dorsal margins of the 4th and 5th ribs in a 70-year-old female with advanced scleroderma.

in chronic obstructive pulmonary disease or in denervation such as polio. This has led to speculation that the rib changes in scleroderma may relate to intercostal muscle atrophy with loss of mechanical stress to costal surfaces, leading secondarily to osseous resorption (67).

Extensive mandibular resorption may also occur (68). This finding appears to relate to tightness of the facial skin, decreased oral aperture, and atrophy of the masticatory muscles, and may reflect ischemia and/or an external pressure affect. A relatively characteristic dental finding in scleroderma is thickening of the periodontal membrane. This abnormality, which was identified in 20% of patients in one series (69), may

lead to the loss of the lamina dura and eventual loosening of dentition.

Additional rarely observed findings include hip ankylosis (70), synostosis of the carpal bones with periostitis (71), and an increased association with osteonecrosis of the femoral head (72–74) (Fig. 19.9). Concurrent acute gout has been described in four patients with scleroderma, but this is generally felt to be quite rare (75).

Finally, while localized forms of scleroderma, such as cutaneous morphea, are not associated with visceral or articular abnormalities, linear forms of the condition may result in severe skeletal deformities, especially in children (en coupe de sabre deformity) (76).

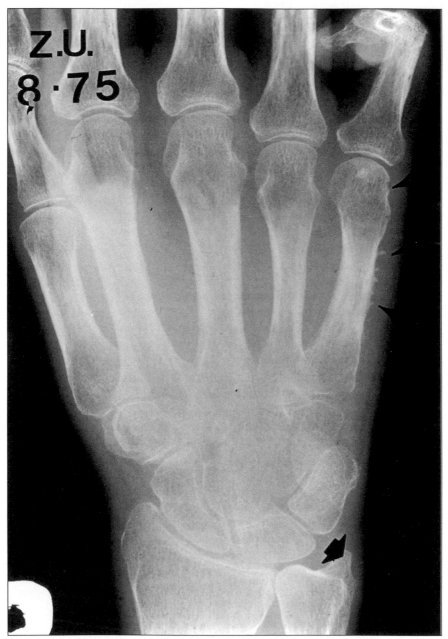

Figure 19.9. Fluffy periostitis of the shaft of the 5th metacarpal in a 48-year-old female with scleroderma. Note also tiny erosion of the metacarpal head and a shallow erosion of the ulnar styloid.

DIFFERENTIAL DIAGNOSIS

The differential diagnosis of the radiographic abnormalities of scleroderma has been extensively reviewed by Resnick (39). While highly suggestive of scleroderma, the resorption of the terminal phalanges of the hands (and less commonly the feet) may occur in several other disorders including: Raynaud's disease without scleroderma; frostbite; electrical or burn injuries; neuropathic disease (especially diabetes mellitus, leprosy, and meningomyelocele); psoriasis; hyperparathyroidism; and Lesch-Nyhan syndrome. These conditions are generally readily excluded on clinical grounds and by other identifying radiographic features.

Resorption of the ribs may not only be seen in scleroderma, but also in other collagen disease including poliomyelitis, restrictive lung disease, neurofibromatosis, and hyperparathyroidism. A useful differentiating feature is that the latter conditions tend to result in resorption of the inferior rib surfaces in contrast to scleroderma, which is typically associated with resorption of superior rib surfaces.

The differential diagnosis for soft tissue calcification is very extensive and may include other collagen vascular diseases such as dermatomyositis and renal osteodystrophy, various parathyroid disorders, fat necrosis, myositis ossificans, hypervitaminosis D, milk alkali syndrome, and sarcoidosis. Intra-articular calcification should be differentiated from calcium pyrophosphate deposition disease (and its various metabolic and endocrine associations), idiopathic hydroxyapatite disease, intra-articular osseous bodies, and synovial osteochondromatosis.

Pathogenesis

While the pathogenesis of scleroderma remains poorly understood, investigators (10) have drawn attention to the rheumatoid-like changes in the joint x-rays of a substantial minority of SSc patients, even in those patients specifically screened to exclude disease overlap with RA. These changes, which include juxta-articular demineralization, joint space narrowing, and occasional frank erosions, raise the possibility that a rheumatoid-like synovitis might contribute to the joint pathology in some patients.

There is some support for the existence of a true synovitis in the literature, although the number of case reports is rather limited. Rodnan described sub-synovial and perivascular infiltrates of lymphocytes and occasional plasma cells similar to that of early RA in the synovial biopsies of 14 out of 29 patients (2). Clark reported similar findings in his series of synovial biopsies, with the additional observation that the degree of inflammatory infiltrate appeared to correlate with rheumatoid factor positivity (26).

Despite these early changes, the synovial biopsies of SSc patients with more advanced disease consistently fail to show the expected progression to synovial hyperplasia and pannus formation typical of RA. A process of superficial fibrin accumulation and atrophy of the synovial lining cells occurs, which leads to a fibrosis similar to that observed in the overlying dermis (30,56). Of interest, increased mast cells have been found in the synovial fluid and synovial tissues of SSc patients (77). Mast cells are found in many fibrotic conditions and may significantly influence the proliferation and function of endothelial cells and fibroblasts, either directly or through mediator generation.

Several other mechanisms have been raised as potential explanations for the articular abnormalities of SSc. These include the possible role of ischemic necrosis (72) and neuropathic arthropathy (63,78). These conditions are supported by the finding of an obliterative microvascular angiopathy in the synovial biopsy of some SSc patients similar to that in other affected tissues (30). The effect of sustained tendon traction and/or the tethering effect of the skin on underlying demineralized bone is a likely explanation for focal resorptive changes on the dorsal surfaces of selected interphalangeal joints. This mechanism, along with chronic tissue ischemia and muscle atrophy, may account for the extensive osteolysis observed at non-articular skeletal sites. Finally, it is recognized that chondral atrophy and joint space narrowing can arise as a consequence of long-standing deformity in chronic disease (79).

Clinical Course and Management

While greater than 90% of patients will report rheumatic symptoms during the course of their illness, arthritis is rarely a dominant clinical complaint. The principal musculoskeletal symptoms pertain to the stiffness, contractures, and deformities of the joints secondary to the progressive hardening and tethering of the overlying skin. As there is no effective treatment for scleroderma, the management is essentially supportive and symptomatic.

Corticosteroids may have short-term value, especially in the early "edematous phase" of the disease or where there is evidence of significant primary joint or muscle inflammation. There is no evidence, however, that corticosteroids will, in any way, positively influence the disease process itself. Moreover, one or two reports have suggested that high dose corticosteroids may in fact precipitate a decline in renal function (80).

For the most part, the minor rheumatic symptoms of scleroderma will respond to simple non-steroidal anti-inflammatory drug treatment. Caution should be exercised, however, with this class of drugs because of the enhanced risk of gastroesophageal abnormalities and impaired renal function in this group of patients.

The early institution of physiotherapy may attenuate, but not prevent, the development of contractures. Dynamic splinting has not been shown to be of any value (81). Surgical intervention is generally not advisable, although PIP arthroplasties have been successfully undertaken in isolated patients (82). Finally, because of the propensity of SSc patients to ischemic vasculitis and/or ulceration, patients must be followed closely for signs of secondary infection and the risk of septic arthritis or osteomyelitis.

There is no reliable treatment for the management of subcutaneous calcinosis. Surgical excisions, especially of large cumbersome deposits or sites prone to repeated skin breakdown or ulceration, may represent an option in some patients. Soft tissue calcific deposits contain increased amounts of carboxyglutamic acid (51) and may respond to low dose anti-coagulant therapy (52). Colchicine has also been advocated to suppress reactive inflammation at sites of calcification (83).

Patients with significant muscle weakness should be investigated for the possibility of a myositic component to their disease with CPKs, EMGs, and, if need be, muscle biopsy. The few patients with evidence of a significant inflammatory myopathy generally respond to corticosteroid therapy. Steroid resistant cases may also be offered trials with azathioprine or methotrexate, although clinical experience is limited with these agents. None of these agents have been shown to influence the course of the scleroderma itself.

The clinical course of the musculoskeletal component of scleroderma generally parallels the course of the underlying disorder, although the rheumatic symptoms may be more prominent at the onset of the illness, tending to recede as the disease progresses. With the possible exception of an enhanced association of the risk of calcinosis with the presence of anti-centromere antibodies (44), laboratory values have not been shown to correlate with the course or prognosis of the musculoskeletal symptoms. Multivariate analysis (84) has shown that proximal muscle weakness, joint swelling, and deformity are more likely to be present at entry in patients with decreased survivorship. These abnormalities were not nearly as powerful predictors, however, as the presence of cardiac, pulmonary, or renal involvement.

Musculoskeletal Involvement and Allied Disorders

CREST SYNDROME

CREST is an acronym for a more limited form of systemic sclerosis characterized by the presence of calcinosis, Raynaud's phenomenon, esophageal dismotility, sclerodactyly, and telangiectasia (85). The musculoskeletal manifestations of CREST syndrome are for the most part indistinguishable from that of SSc. A comparison of 55 patients with SSc and 10 patients with CREST syndrome (skin involvement limited to sclerodactyly) showed a virtually identical array and frequency of radiographic abnormalities (10). There was, however, less tendency for radiographic progression over a similar follow-up period, supporting the contention that CREST may be a more benign variant of scleroderma (86).

It should be noted that the term "CREST syndrome" is generally regarded to be outmoded primarily because most patients with diffuse SSc will also fulfill the diagnostic criteria requirement for the diagnosis of CREST. The preferred convention is to divide SSc into "diffuse" and "limited" forms. Diffuse cutaneous scleroderma is defined as skin thickening proximal to elbows and/or knees with or without facial involvement. Limited cutaneous scleroderma is defined as skin involvement distal to elbows and/or knees with or without facial involvement (87).

MIXED CONNECTIVE TISSUE DISEASE

Occasionally, patients may exhibit scleroderma with overlapping features of one or more connective tissue diseases, such as RA, systemic lupus erythematosus (SLE), or polymyositis. A particular form of overlap syndrome, mixed connective tissue disease (MCTD), may be associated with an increased prevalence of antibodies to ribonucleoprotein (88,89).

Patients with MCTD may exhibit overlapping clinical and radiographic features, although not necessarily concurrently. Radiographic features typical for RA occurring in association with typical SSc changes, such as subcutaneous calcinosis and tuft resorption, are now well described in MCTD (90–92).

The recognition of MCTD and the possibility for disease overlap has raised into question the validity of some of the "rheumatoid-like features" reported in an earlier series of ostensibly pure SSc patients (28). Subsequent series (10), which were rigorously screened to exclude MCTD and RA, have nonetheless reconfirmed the existence of an apparently distinctive arthropathy in SSc with the potential for articular erosions and joint space narrowing. Furthermore, the erosions of SSc tend to be infrequent, non-progressive, and unassociated with rheumatoid factor positivity, whereas the opposite tends to apply with regard to the erosions of MCTD (93).

EOSINOPHILIC FASCIITIS

Also known as Schulman's syndrome, eosinophilic fasciitis is characterized by the subacute onset of diffuse inflammation and/or induration of the skin of the extremities, often apparently following a period of excessive exertion (94). Polyarthralgias, polyarthritis, muscle atrophy, and carpal tunnel syndrome have been observed (95).

Radiographic abnormalities are generally confined to osteopenia, although erosions of hands and wrists (96) and periostitis of the long bones (97) have been reported.

References

1. Rodnan GP. The nature of joint involvement in progressive systemic sclerosis (diffuse scleroderma). Clinical study and pathologic examination of synovium in 29 patients. Ann Intern Med 1962; 56:422–438.
2. Rodnan GP, Medsger TA Jr. The rheumatic mani-

in progressive systemic sclerosis. Arthritis Rheum 1982;25:1497–1500.

71. Bjorsand AJ. New bone formation and carpal synostosis in scleroderma. A case report. Am J Roentgenol 1968;103:616–619.

72. Wilde AH, Mankin HJ, Rodnan GP. Avascular necrosis of the femoral head in scleroderma. Arthritis Rheum 1970;13:445–447.

73. Taccari E, et al. Avascular necrosis of the femoral head in long term follow-up of systemic sclerosis: Report of 2 cases. Clin Rheumatol 1989;3:386–392.

74. Martinez-Cordero E. Avascular necrosis of bone in systemic sclerosis. Clin Rheumatol 1992;11:443–444.

75. Durback MA, Schumacher HR. Acute gouty arthritis in 4 patients with systemic sclerosis. J Rheumatol 1988;15:1503–1505.

76. Hoggins GS, Hamilton MC. Dentofacial defects associated with scleroderma. Oral Surg 1969;27:734–736.

77. Mican JM, Metcalfe DD. Arthritis and mast cell activation. J Allergy Clin Immunol 1990;4(2):677–683.

78. Khrten I. CRST syndrome and "neuropathic" arthropathy. Arthritis Rheum 1969;12:636–638.

79. Salter RB, McNeill OR, Carbin R. Pathologic changes in articular cartilage associated with persistent joint deformity: An experimental investigation. In: Studies of rheumatoid disease: Proceedings of the third Canadian conference on research in the rheumatic disease. Toronto, 1965:33–47.

80. Helfrich DJ, Medsger TA. Normotensive renal failure in systemic sclerosis (scleroderma). Arthritis Rheum 1989;32:1128–1134.

81. Seeger MW, Furst DE. Effects of splinting in the treatment of hand contractures in progressive systemic sclerosis. Am J Occup Ther 1987;41:118–121.

82. Norris RW, Brown HG. The proximal interphalangeal joint in systemic sclerosis and its surgical management. Br J Plast Surg 1985;38:526–531.

83. Fuchs D, et al. Colchicine suppression of local inflammation due to calcinosis in dermatomyositis and progressive systemic sclerosis. Clin Rheumatol 1986;5:527–530.

84. Altman RD, Medsger TA, Bloch DA, Michel BA. Predictors of survival in systemic sclerosis (scleroderma). Arthritis Rheum 1991;34:403–413.

85. Rodnan GP, Medsger TA, Buckingham RB. Progressive systemic sclerosis—CREST syndrome: Observations on natural history and late complication in 90 patients. Arthritis Rheum 1975;18:423.

86. Carr RD, Heisel EB, Stevenson TD. CRST syndrome: A benign variant of scleroderma. Arch Dermatol 1965;92:519–525.

87. LeRoy EC, Black C, Fleishmajer R. Scleroderma (systemic sclerosis): Classification, subsets and pathogenesis. J Rheumatol 1988;15:202–205.

88. Sharp GC, et al. Mixed connective tissue disease. An apparently distinct rheumatic disease syndrome associated with a specific antibody to an extractable nuclear antigen (ENA). Am J Med 1972;52:149–159.

89. Sharp GC, et al. Association of antibodies to ribonucleic protein and Sm antigens with mixed connective tissue disease, systemic lupus erythematosus, and other rheumatic diseases. N Engl J Med 1976;295:1149–1154.

90. Udoff EJ, Genant HI, Kozin F, Ginsberg M. Mixed connective tissue disease: The spectrum of radiologic manifestations. Radiology 1977;124:613–618.

91. Halla JT, Hardin JG. Clinical features of the arthritis of mixed connective tissue disease. Arthritis Rheum 1978;21:497–503.

92. Bennett RM, O'Cornnell DJ. The arthritis of mixed connective tissue disease. Ann Rheum Dis 1978;37:397–403.

93. Catoggio LJ, Evison G, Harkness JA, Maddison PJ. The arthropathy of systemic sclerosis (scleroderma): Comparison with mixed connective tissue disease. Clin Exp Rheumatol 1983;1(2):101–112.

94. Velayos EE, Masi AT, Stevens MB, Shulman LE. The "CREST" syndrome. Comparison with systemic sclerosis (scleroderma). Arch Intern Med 1979;139:1240–1244.

95. Lee P. Eosinophilic fasciitis—new associations and current perspectives. J Rheumatol 1981;8:6–8.

96. Fernandez-Herlihy L. Eosinophilic fasciitis: Report of a 22-year follow-up study. Arthritis Rheum 1981;24:97–98.

97. Giordano M, Ara M, Cicala C, Valentin G, Chianese U, Vatti M. Eosinophilic fasciitis. Ann Intern Med 1980;93:645.

20

Organ Involvement: Renal

KIDNEY INVOLVEMENT in systemic sclerosis (SSc) may be manifested by scleroderma renal crisis (SRC). Until recently, it was the most severe complication and the most frequent cause of death in patients with this disease. Fortunately, over the last 10 to 15 years, the outcome of SRC has improved dramatically with the use of angiotensin converting enzyme (ACE) inhibitors. Diagnosing the onset of renal crisis as soon as possible is extremely important so prompt therapeutic intervention can achieve the best possible outcome. Renal abnormalities independent of renal crisis have been noted, but usually they can be attributed to other problems. Further understanding of the pathogenesis of renal disease in scleroderma may lead to additional improvement in the therapy of renal crisis and perhaps the disease in general. This chapter reviews the pathogenesis, clinical setting, and appropriate therapy of this serious complication of SSc.

Pathogenesis of Renal Involvement

The pathogenesis of renal events in SSc remains incompletely understood, but the damage seems to evolve from a series of insults to the kidney (Fig. 20.1). The primary process, as seen in vessels in other organs, is injury of the endothelial cells, which results in intimal thickening and intimal proliferation of renal intralobular and arcuate arteries. Inflammatory cells, including lymphocytes and other mononuclear cells, are conspicuously absent in the pathologic examination of these arteries. The thickened abnormal vessel wall allows platelet aggregation and adhesion to occur. Release of platelet factors increases vascular permeability and may participate in the production of increased collagen and fibrin deposition contributing to the lumenal narrowing (1).

The narrowed arterial vessels are the primary cause of decreased renal perfusion, particularly cortical blood flow. However, episodic vasospasm, or what has been called "renal Raynaud's" phenomenon, has been carefully demonstrated in early classic studies by Cannon (2). He showed that three of four patients had a significant reduction in cortical blood flow following cold water hand immersion. Additionally, Cannon found that patients with progressive renal failure had severely reduced cortical blood flow, whereas those with normal or minimal clinical renal abnormalities had normal or only slightly diminished blood flow. A variety of techniques, including xenon-133 washout, I^{131} hippurate, and static 99mTc DTPA scans, have been used to assess blood flow and renal dysfunction, but these techniques have not been successful in the early identification or prediction of renal crisis (2–5).

Decreased blood flow leads to decreased perfusion of the juxtaglomerular apparatus, which causes release of renin as well as hyperplasia of the juxtaglomerular apparatus (6). The hypertension associated with SRC is renin-mediated, as demonstrated by the presence of markedly elevated peripheral plasma renin levels and the

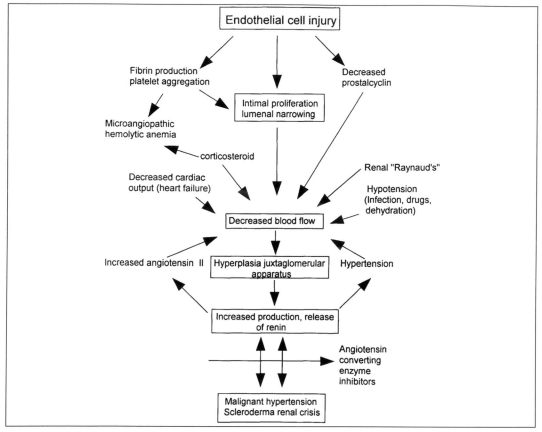

Figure 20.1. A potential pathogenetic mechanism for scleroderma renal crisis with multiple factors contributing to a "viscious" cycle resulting in malignant hypertension and renal failure.

dramatic improvement in hypertension following nephrectomy (2).

Kovalchik demonstrated hyperreninemia and an exaggerated renin response to a cold pressor test in patients without clinical evidence of SRC who had marked vascular changes on renal biopsy (7). However, prior to the actual onset of renal crisis, hyperreninemia is not consistently present (8,9), and when detected is not predictive of SRC (8–10). Although renin-angiotensin system abnormalities play a role in the pathogenesis of SRC, something else must occur to trigger the acute onset and rapid progression of renal failure, which is then fueled by the hyperreninemia.

These vascular changes are present in patients without renal crisis and, like plasma renin activity, do not predict development of SRC (7,11). Renal biopsies from diffuse scleroderma patients without renal abnormalities had vessels that showed the typical intimal proliferation and thickening (7). An autopsy series showed that even limited cutaneous scleroderma patients, who very rarely get renal crisis, had thickened vessels compared to normals (11) (Fig. 20.2). Thickening of the vessels or the degree of lumenal occlusion was not correlated with age, disease duration, or last serum creatinine. Vascular changes are frequently present in scleroderma patients, but additional factors beyond the vascular changes and hyperreninemia must be present to trigger the acute crisis event.

The precipitation of SRC may result from situations in which renal blood flow is further compromised. Some authors have reported an increased frequency of SRC onset during cold months, suggesting the possibility of "renal Raynaud's" phenomenon (2,12), although our more recent data do not confirm this association (13). Cardiac dysfunction that decreases renal perfusion, i.e., large pericardial effusions, arrhythmias, or congestive heart failure, have preceded SRC in some patients (8,14). Pregnancy, with its alterations in blood volume and flow, has been reported to precipitate renal crisis (15), but our extensive experience has not supported this theory (16).

Sepsis and dehydration causing hypotension could contribute to the problem. Several drugs are capable of causing decreased renal perfusion. Calcium channel blockers used in the management of Raynaud's phenomenon (RP) and ACE inhibitors may produce hypotension. Nonsteroidal anti-inflammatory agents may deplete vasodilating prostaglandins, thus compromising renal blood flow. There is no convincing evidence that any of these drugs precipitate SRC, but cautious use of them is prudent in SSc patients at high risk for SRC.

Corticosteroids have long been implicated in the development of SRC (17,18). Patients most likely to receive steroids are those with early inflammatory disease, and the same patients are at greatest risk for SRC. A significant association of antecedent *high* dose (>40mg prednisone) with corticosteroid administration with patients who had normotensive SRC has been noted (19). Since these compounds are capable of inhibiting prostacyclin production and increasing ACE activity, they could contribute to the pathogenesis of SRC.

Narrowed arteries/arterioles and decreased blood flow from a variety of sources are likely to cause ischemia of the juxtaglomerular apparatus, which results in increased renin. The increased renin causes increased angiotensin II, further vasoconstriction, elevated blood pressure, and renal ischemia. The end result is a vicious cycle as demonstrated in Figure 20-1.

Renal Pathology

Pathologic changes of "scleroderma kidney" are very similar to those observed in other forms of

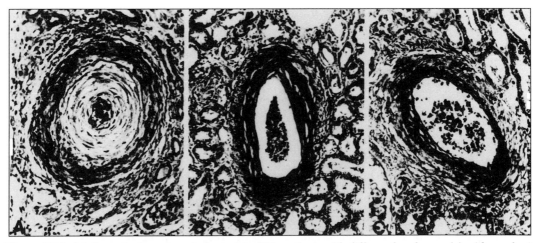

Figure 20.2. Medium sized renal cortical arteries of SSc patients with diffuse scleroderma: (*a*) with renal crisis, (*b*) without renal crisis, and (*c*) with limited scleroderma. Note the non-occlusive fibroelastotic and sclerotic intimal thickening that is seen in *b* and *c* in contrast to the severe concentric edematous myxoid intimal proliferation with almost total obliteration of the lumen in *a*. (Verhoeff-van Gieson's stain; *a* and *c* magnification × 275; *b* magnification × 175) (Reproduced with permission.)

malignant hypertension. Grossly, the capsule may show areas of infarction, hemorrhage, or even cortical necrosis. Microscopic changes are characteristically seen in the small interlobular and arcuate arteries (19). The earliest change is intimal edema, followed by an intense proliferation of intimal cells and production of mucinous ground substance composed of glycoprotein and mucopolysaccharides (20). Lymphocytes and other mononuclear cells are absent. Fibrinoid necrosis may be present either in arterial walls or in a subintimal location in small arteries and arterioles. The resulting intimal thickening in interlobular arteries leads to narrowing and often total obliteration of the lumen. In some cases the media is thickened, but more often it appears stretched and thinned. Intramural fibrin deposition or fibrin thrombi have been noted, as in other forms of malignant hypertension, but can also be seen in scleroderma patients who are not hypertensive. Adventitial and periadventitial fibrosis are seen in SRC, but are rarely noted in nonsclerodermatous malignant hypertension, making them helpful distinguishing features between the two entities (21). Large arteries may be normal or may show more typical atherosclerotic changes consistent with patient's age.

Glomerular changes are variable and include thickening and collapse of capillary loops and other ischemic changes. Irregular thickening of glomerular basement membrane may result in more loop-like lesions. Juxtaglomerular cell hyperplasia is not specific to SSc but is consistent with the marked hyperreninemia characteristic of SRC (6,9). It is most prominent when arterial narrowing is severe. Tubules appear to be secondarily affected by vascular insufficiency from arterial lumenal occlusion. Flattening and degeneration of tubular cells are the most prominent changes.

Immunoglobulins (chiefly IgM) and complement components (C3) are non-specifically deposited in small renal arteries, but discrete electron-dense deposits consistent with immune complexes are absent (7,22). Immune reactants are less frequently found in the glomeruli al-

though fibrinogen has been detected there. The nonspecificity of these findings may be attributed to gross disruption of vascular integrity and increased permeability rather than immune injury.

Most of the changes described in the previous paragraphs have also been seen in patients with scleroderma who do not have and who do not subsequently develop renal crisis (7,23). The thickening seen in the arteries of patients with limited and diffuse cutaneous disease without renal crisis is similar to that seen in renal crisis, but to a lesser degree (see Fig. 20.2). Lumenal occlusion was the most severe in SRC. Some non-renal crisis patients had extensive reduplication and proliferation of elastic fibers.

Clinical Signs and Symptoms

DEFINITION

Scleroderma renal crisis is defined as the new onset of accelerated arterial hypertension and/or rapidly progressive oliguric renal failure during the course of SSc. One should not assume that non-malignant hypertension alone without azotemia or other characteristic clinical findings is renal crisis. Likewise, urine abnormalities and/or mild azotemia in a scleroderma patient usually have other explanations and should not be considered SRC.

EPIDEMIOLOGY

Renal crisis occurs in approximately 10% of the entire scleroderma population. Interestingly, the incidence of renal crisis seems to have decreased during the last 10 years. The rate of development of SRC for patients at risk during 1972 through 1979 and 1980 through 1987 has decreased substantially. The latter time period had a significantly lower SRC frequency (9% at 5 years) than the earlier time period (22% at 5 years), with adjustment to ensure similar follow-up time. Differences between these time periods include the more extensive use of D-penicillamine and the new availability of calcium channel blockers and ACE-inhibitors. In open or retrospective studies, D-penicillamine has been associated with a decreased occurrence of renal crisis (24). Calcium channel blockers have been used extensively for peripheral Raynaud's, and ACE inhibitors have had dramatic effects in treating SRC, but there is no information concerning their ability to prevent this process.

Renal crisis is most often encountered early in the course of the disease, with 75% of SRC cases occurring less than 4 years after the first symptom attributable to scleroderma (8). However, late occurrences, even 20 years after disease onset, have been seen. Some studies indicate that Black patients are 3 times as likely as Caucasians to develop SRC, and (proportionately) males are more frequently affected than females (11), although our recent statistics do not show these associations (Table 20.1).

FACTORS PREDICTING SRC

Patients with certain clinical characteristics have a greatly increased risk to develop this complication and should be followed extremely closely for evidence of the onset of SRC (Tables 20-1 and 20.2). Patients with diffuse cutaneous scleroderma with skin thickening on the proximal extremities and/or the trunk are at greatest risk for SRC, with 20% to 25% of this patient subgroup getting SRC (25). Only 1% of patients with limited cutaneous scleroderma (previously termed the CREST syndrome) and long-standing skin changes restricted to distal extremities and/or face ever develop renal crisis. There is infrequent documentation of renal crisis in limited scleroderma patients with anticentromere antibody (26,27). Thus, the vast majority of SRC cases (75%–80%) occur in patients with obvious diffuse cutaneous changes. The rapid progression of

Table 20.1. Comparison of Clinical Charateristics in Patients with Renal Crisis and Those with Diffuse Cutaneous Scleroderma without Renal Crisis

	SRC (n = 129)	No Renal Crisis (n = 546)
Demographics		
Age	50.9	44
Symptoms less than 4 yrs (%)	75%	70%
Race, % Black	7%	8%
Sex, % Male	20%	25%
Diffuse	90%	100%
Anti-topoisomerase antibody	20%	33%
Anti-RNA polymerase III antibody	68%	44%
Anti-centromere antibody	1%	3%
Findings at Time of Renal Crisis		
BP, mean	184/108	120/74
Papilledema	11%	0%
Seizures	11%	<1%
Plasma renin activity		
24 hr protein, > 0.250gm/24	63%	9%
Hematuria, RBC > 5	38%	2%
Granular casts	29%	1%
Microangiopathic hemolytic anemia	30%	4%
Platelets < 150,000	39%	<1%
ESR > 25	63%	43%
Pericardial effusion	53%	12%
CHF/arrythmias	25%	2%

Table 20.2. Factors Occuring Prior to Onset of SRC Which May Be Helpful in Predicting SRC

Predictive of SRC	Not Predictive of SRC
Diffuse skin involvement	Prior blood pressure elevation
Rapid progression of skin thickening	Abnormal urinalysis
Disease duration < 4 years	Prior increase in serum creatine level
Anti-RNA polymerase III-antibody	Prior increase in plasma renin activity
New anemia	Pathological abnormalities in renal blood vessels
New cardiac events	Anti-SCi 70 or anticentromere antibodies
pericardial effusion	
congestive heart failure	
??Antecedent high dose corticosteroid	

skin thickening has been shown to be a good predictor of SRC (8).

Another 15% to 25% of SRC cases occur in patients who are destined to develop typical diffuse scleroderma, although they may have only minimal or even no skin changes at the time of renal crisis. There are several other distinguishing features that can be helpful in identifying those patients likely to evolve to diffuse cutaneous disease (Table 20.3). A short duration of symptoms, often less than 1 year, including polyarthritis, puffy hands and legs, carpal tunnel syndrome, and the absence of RP are a common complex of symptoms in patients with early diffuse scleroderma (28). The presence of palpable tendon friction rubs, which occur in 65% of diffuse scleroderma patients, is an extremely helpful and predictive sign, because less than 5% of limited scleroderma patients ever have this finding. Typically, limited scleroderma patients have 5 to 10 years of RP and minimal articular or systemic symptoms at initial evaluation (27).

Autoantibodies may be helpful in predicting SRC (see Table 20.1). Anti-topoisomerase antibody is a marker for diffuse cutaneous scleroderma, but within diffuse scleroderma patients alone it is not associated with an increased frequency of SRC (25). Anti-RNA polymerase III is a recently described antibody that is seen almost exclusively in diffuse scleroderma, and 24% of patients with this antibody develop SRC, in contrast to only 10% of patients with anti-topoisomerase (29). Patients with any of the features described in this paragraph should be carefully monitored for the development of SRC. These patients should be educated about their risk of developing SRC and should be taught: (a) to monitor their blood pressure at home, (b) what their normal blood pressure should be, and (c) the level of blood pressure that they should be concerned about.

Antecedent hypertension is not usually present prior to SRC. Most often there is an acute onset of markedly elevated blood pressure. The frequency of non-malignant hypertension has not been shown to be higher than in the general population (8). Although patients may develop non-malignant hypertension after the onset of disease, this condition does not predict SRC nor does it evolve to the malignant form of hypertension. Normal blood pressures have been documented within a few days prior to the onset of SRC hypertension (12).

Marked elevation of plasma renin is the hallmark of acute SRC. Often it is 10 times normal and occasionally reaches 100 times normal. Kovalchik found a rise in plasma renin activity after a cold pressor test (7), and Gavros found a rise in plasma renin activity in a few patients with mild hypertension who later developed severe hypertension (30). We did not find supine or upright plasma renins helpful in predicting the future development of renal crisis (8). There were patients who had normal renins from 1 day to 1 month prior to the acute onset of SRC, as well as patients who had elevated renins but never developed SRC (8). Since the use of ACE inhibitors interferes with the renin assay and results are often not available for weeks, the usefulness of this important finding is limited. Abnormal urinalysis and increased creatinine have also not been helpful in predicting SRC. When abnormal, these findings are usually attributable to other causes or are only transient (7,8,31).

Several non-renal abnormalities may precede SRC. Asymptomatic pericardial effusion, congestive heart failure, and/or arrhythmias have antedated renal crisis (8,14). Hyperreninemia even without hypertension may be the cause of pulmonary edema (32). Anemia, an uncommon manifestation of scleroderma, can be an early clue to renal crisis (8), particularly when microangiopathic hemolysis and thrombocytopenia are present. Careful evaluation of any anemia or thrombocytopenia is necessary to avoid falsely attributing these findings to immune mediated hemolytic anemia, drug toxicity, or other potential causes of these abnormalities. The recent (previous 2–3 months) use of high dose corticosteroid therapy (prednisone > 20mg/day) has

been reported to precede the development of SRC in a number of cases (17,18), especially those with normal blood pressure (19).

CLINICAL FINDINGS

Patients may complain of severe headache, blurred vision, or other encephalopathic symptoms with the onset of accelerated hypertension. Seizures may be an early finding, but fortunately, early and effective therapy has decreased the frequency of these events. Some patients, however, have no specific symptoms, except for nonspecific complaints of increased fatigue or just not feeling well. These must be taken seriously, particularly in those patients at high risk for SRC.

In our experience, most patients have striking elevations of blood pressure at the onset of SRC. Ninety percent have blood pressure levels greater than 150/90 mm Hg, and 30% have diastolic recordings greater than 120 mm Hg. In some cases, a normal blood pressure may be present. An increase of 20 mm Hg can result in a high blood pressure reading for that particular patient, and yet still remain in the normal range (95/60 to 140/85). Such findings should be considered very suspicious. This occurrence is called normotensive renal crisis, and it occurs in

Table 20.3. Characteristics of Limited Cutaneous and Diffuse Cutaneous Scleroderma

Limited	Diffuse
Long history of Raynaud's	Recent or absent Raynaud's
Minimal constitutional symptoms except fatigue	Acute onset with fatigue, weight loss, polyarthritis, feeling ill
Puffy fingers	Puffy fingers, hands, and lower legs
Calcinosis and telangiectasis common	Carpal tunnel syndrome
Old CREST syndrome	Tendon friction rubs
Skin thickening restricted to distal extremities/face	Skin thickening progresses up to arms, legs to trunk
Pulmonary hypertension	Renal crisis, anti-topoisomerase, and RNA polymerase III antibodies
Anti-centromere antibody	

approximately 10% of SRC patients (19). In order to make a diagnosis of normotensive SRC, other features, primarily rapidly progressive unexplained azotemia or microangiopathic hemolytic anemia, must be used. Thus, it is not surprising that microangiopathic hemolytic anemia occurs more frequently in normotensive patients than those with hypertensive SRC. Interestingly, pulmonary hemorrhage has been a life-threatening problem in several of these patients. In spite of the absence of hypertension, seizures can occur, which might then suggest thrombotic thrombocytopenia purpura, hemolytic uremic syndrome, or a similar disease. In the setting of early classic diffuse scleroderma, these other conditions are highly unlikely. A scleroderma patient who develops these findings should be treated with ACE inhibitors as if they had SRC until another diagnosis can be firmly established. Steroids and plasmapheresis have not been helpful in treating normotensive SRC patients.

Rarely, a patient will present with SRC, but with little evidence for the diagnosis of scleroderma. Careful evaluation for Raynaud's, puffy fingers, subtle skin thickening, nailfold capillary changes, scleroderma autoantibodies, and other evidence of systemic sclerosis is important.

Laboratory Findings

RENAL ABNORMALITIES

Renal failure is typically silent. Only rarely are symptoms of advanced renal insufficiency (mental confusion, nausea, vomiting) the presenting or most prominent complaints. Conversely, laboratory abnormalities indicating renal dysfunction are common. Routine urinalysis shows proteinuria (up to but usually not exceeding 2.5 g/24hr), microscopic hematuria (5–100 rbc/hpf), and often granular casts. Patients frequently present with the serum creatinine already elevated. It then rises rapidly, usually increasing by 0.5 to 1.0 mg/dl per day. Even after antihypertensive therapy has effectively controlled blood pressure it may continue to rise for several days. In some situations, serum creatinine continues to rise in spite of a persistently normal blood pressure and the patient develops renal failure. Certain patients are fortunate to be diagnosed and treated early before significant renal dysfunction has occurred. In these patients, the serum creatinine usually rises somewhat, but most often it stabilizes and then returns toward normal.

Markedly increased plasma renin activity is the rule. Values prior to ACE inhibitor therapy are often 30 to 40 times normal (9,12), which are equal to or even greater than plasma renin activity in patients with other forms of malignant hypertension. Unfortunately, the practical use of renins is very limited.

ANEMIA

Microangiopathic hemolytic anemia, which is characterized by normochromic but fragmented red blood cells, reticulocytosis, and mild thrombocytopenia, occurs in 43% of patients with SRC. The platelet count is rarely lower than 50,000/mm^3 and improves with control of blood pressure. Patients are not usually symptomatic from this process except that the anemia may precipitate congestive heart failure.

CARDIAC DECOMPENSATION

SRC may present with congestive heart failure (dyspnea, paroxysmal nocturnal dyspnea, or even pulmonary edema); serious ventricular arrhythmias (even cardiac arrest); or large pericardial effusions (14,32). This is primarily from the stress of the hypertension, effects of hyperreninemia, and from fluid overload secondary to oliguric renal failure. Control of the blood pressure promptly improves these other conditions.

RENAL ABNORMALITIES INDEPENDENT OF RENAL CRISIS

Early literature describes the occurrence of significant renal abnormalities in scleroderma patients, regardless of the presence of renal crisis. Cannon found 45% to 60% of scleroderma patients who had hypertension, proteinuria, or azotemia (2). The frequency of any renal abnormalities, including azotemia, proteinuria, hematuria, or hypertension, in our population of diffuse cutaneous scleroderma patients (Fig. 20.3) is similar to that commonly quoted in the literature (2,31, 33). Limited cutaneous scleroderma patients who rarely experience renal crisis were not included in this analysis. Some evidence of renal abnormalities was found in 353 (52%) patients with diffuse scleroderma. They were followed for a mean of 9.5 years of disease. Nineteen percent had classic scleroderma renal crisis with acute onset of hypertension and/or rapidly progressive azotemia. Mild isolated hypertension requiring medication but without typical renal crisis findings occurred in 79 (12%), and 173 (26%) had some non-SRC renal abnormality.

One hundred and five patients (15% of diffuse scleroderma patients) without renal crisis had a BUN greater than 25, or a creatinine greater than 1.2mg/dl, at some point in their illness (mean duration of disease of 9.8 years) (31). The disease course for these patients was carefully reviewed to ascertain any potential causes of the abnormality. Twenty-two had their first abnormal creatinine at the time of their terminal hospitalization. The mean greatest creatinine in this group was 1.8mg/dl. Death was most often from heart or lung failure, which resulted in decreased renal perfusion as demonstrated by an increased BUN:creatinine ratio (25:1). The deaths were not associated with either hypertension or renal failure. Increased creatinine (or BUN) in another 22 patient was explained by events including prerenal effects from severe congestive heart failure, scleroderma gastrointestinal involvement with diarrhea and/or dehydration, volume depletion from acute illness or infection, diuretics, steroids (increased BUN only), or drug reactions (Cyclosporin, D-penicillamine, non-steroid anti-inflammatory medications). Their mean greatest

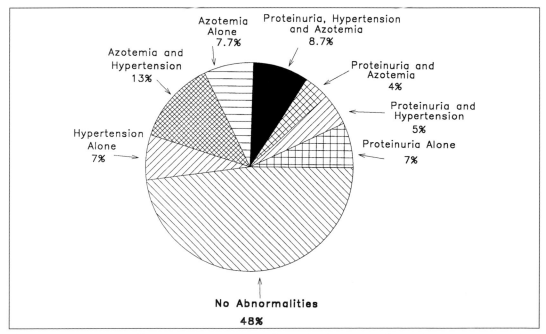

Figure 20.3. Frequency of hypertension, azotemia, and proteinuria occurring during the 9.5-year course of 675 patients with diffuse scleroderma.

creatinine was 1.7mg/dl. Transient elevation in creatinine occurred in 49 patients (Fig. 20.4). In these cases, the last recorded serum creatinine was normal, with a mean value of 1.0 mg/dl 4.9 years after the initial abnormal value. Finally, only 12 (1.8%) of all diffuse scleroderma patients had an elevation in serum creatinine, which was not easily explained by other causes. The mean value was 1.4 mg/dl at the time of the first abnormal value and 1.6 mg/dl 4.1 years later. Most patients had either pre-existing or new nonmalignant hypertension occurring after onset of scleroderma, but the increase in creatinine did not occur at time of onset of hypertension. The highest creatinine exhibited by any of these patients throughout a mean of 10 years of disease has been 2.4 mg/dl. Thus, chronic progressive azotemia independent of SRC is distinctly unusual. These patients with new hypertension and delayed azotemia may have had an aborted episode of SRC, which resulted in some mild renal dysfunction.

Proteinuria and hematuria (with or without proteinuria), are common side effects of D-penicillamine, and this toxicity accounted for 78% of the 86 patients with diffuse cutaneous scleroderma who had more than 250 mg protein in 24 hours (or +3 on dipstick) (31). Renal biopsies have shown the typical membranous glomerulonephritis associated with D-penicillamine toxicity, although in a few patients persistence of proteinuria was associated with minimal biopsy changes. After proteinuria resolved with discontinuation of D-penicillamine, in many cases (46%) the drug was able to be successfully reinstituted at a lower dose and continued for more than 3 years with urine protein maintained at less than 1 g/24hr. Other etiologies, such as bladder cancer, hemorrhagic cystitis, urinary tract infections, or congestive heart failure, were seen in seven patients. Only 12 (1.8%) of all diffuse cutaneous scleroderma patients had unexplained proteinuria (mean 400 mg/24hr), and have not developed renal crisis for a mean of 6 years from the onset of proteinuria.

Hypertension is a more difficult finding to in-

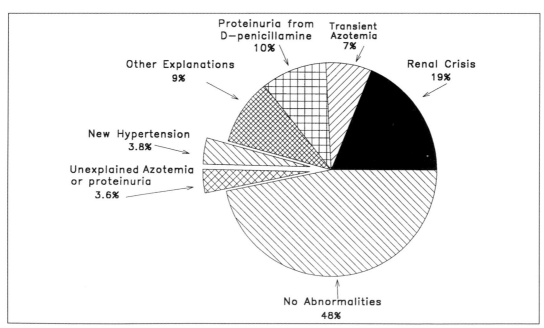

Figure 20.4. Explanations and causes of renal abnormalities in diffuse cutaneous scleroderma including renal crisis, transient azotemia, D-penicillamine proteinuria, other causes, and new unexplained abnormalities.

terpret. Twelve percent of the Pittsburgh scleroderma patients had (n = 40), or developed (n = 39), sustained hypertension, which required medication but was not associated with simultaneous proteinuria, hematuria, or azotemia. These patients have not progressed to SRC or renal failure during 6 years of follow-up, although some have developed mild azotemia with serum creatinine less than 2.0 mg/dl. Hypertension after onset of scleroderma was associated with the initiation of steroids in 61% of the patients. We believe that most of the individuals with preexisting hypertension probably have essential hypertension, which occurs in nearly 15% of the general population. With today's prompt use of ACE inhibitors for any blood pressure elevation in scleroderma patients, it is increasingly difficult to determine the significance or natural history of this type of hypertension.

Treatment

The vicious cycle of decreased blood flow, ischemia, hyperreninemia, hypertension, and further vasoconstriction almost invariably resulted in a fatal outcome prior to the availability of ACE inhibitors. Only a small minority of SRC patients (<10%) survived more than 3 months. In the late 1970s, there were several reports of survival with very aggressive control of blood pressure and, if needed, dialysis (33,34). There even was an early report of enough improvement in renal function to discontinue dialysis (34). However, drugs like minoxidil, a potent renal vasodilator, cause serious sodium retention and inhibit myocardial function. Congestive heart failure, already a threat in these severely hypertensive patients, along with potential primary scleroderma cardiac involvement, became an even greater problem to manage. Persistent, uncontrollable hypertension and resultant congestive heart failure made management even with dialysis very difficult. For a time, bilateral nephrectomy was performed to eliminate the hyperreninemia, which allowed the

blood pressure, heart failure, and dialysis to be managed more successfully (12,35).

In the late 1970s, the first ACE inhibitors became available. These drugs work by acting as competitive inhibitors of the conversion of angiotensin I to angiotensin II. They provide a "false substrate" for the converting enzyme, and thus angiotensin II is not produced. Inhibition of angiotensin II production promptly lowers blood pressure in these patients. Although angiotensin I and renin continue to accumulate, they are not biologically active and do not affect blood pressure. These drugs also proteolyze bradykinins, which, as potent vasodilators, potentially could have a role in the hypotensive effect of these agents.

Since the first exciting report of the reversal of hypertension in SRC, improved renal function, and survival of SRC by Lopez-Ovejero in 1979 (36), the use of ACE inhibitors has dramatically altered the therapy and outcome of SRC. Lopez-Overjero described two patients with impressive reversal of malignant hypertension and renal dysfunction as the result of treatment with an oral ACE inhibitor. One of these patients (case 2, a male) has been followed at the University of Pittsburgh since 1979, for a total of 14 years. He is minimally symptomatic (Raynaud's and dyspepsia), has minimal skin thickening, has been off all medication including ACE inhibitors for 4 years, and has a serum creatinine of 1.2 mg/dl. Additional series confirmed this almost miraculous response (37,38); however, not all patients' blood pressure elevation responded to an ACE inhibitor, and in some cases the drug did not prevent renal failure (39). The initial level of creatinine at the start of therapy was felt to play a major role in the final outcome. If the serum creatinine at the start of ACE inhibitors was greater than 4 mg/dl, then renal failure and dialysis were usually inevitable. If serum creatinine was less than 4 mg/dl, improvement without dialysis was more likely (39). Whitman described a patient with an initial creatinine of less than 3 mg/dl whose renal function improved enough to discontinue dialysis (39).

In our review of 108 cases of SRC seen at the University of Pittsburgh between 1972 and 1987, survival significantly improved with the use of ACE inhibitors (13). The 55 patients treated with ACE inhibitors had the typical acute onset of hypertension (mean blood pressure 180/110), but they exhibited four different patterns of response and outcomes to this agent (Figs. 20.5 and 20.6) Twenty patients developed some renal dysfunction (mean peak serum creatinine was 3.9 mg/dl), but never required dialysis. Their mean serum creatinine 1 year later was only 1.9 mg/dl. This usually continued to improve slowly and recurrence was infrequent. Fifteen patients had an early death despite aggressive therapy. This most often occurred within 3 months of onset of SRC. It was generally associated with older men, refractory hypertension, and/or congestive heart failure. Many required dialysis, but others died cardiac deaths even before renal failure occurred. The rest (20 patients) had deterioration in renal function to the extent that they required dialysis even though in most situations their blood pressure was adequately controlled. The unique feature of this group of dialysis patients is that 11 of

the 20 (55%) were successfully able to discontinue dialysis 5 to 18 months later. One year after discontinuing dialysis, these patients' mean serum creatinine was 2.1 mg/dl and continued to improve over time. Our experience since 1987 is very similar: more patients were treated with long-acting ACE inhibitors and did not experience quite so good an outcome (not statistically significant) as did the patients who were treated with captopril. Because of the increased flexibility in controlling blood pressure more rapidly, captopril should be used initially.

Although problems with vascular access or clearance in patients on hemodialysis or peritoneal dialysis have occurred, these problems generally have not been any more unmanageable in scleroderma patients than in non-scleroderma renal failure patients (26). The real possibility and hope for the return of adequate renal function, and subsequent discontinuation of dialysis, should delay any definite plans for renal transplantation. Once 18 months have passed without return of kidney function, plans for transplantation can be completed. Although a recurrence of SRC has been reported in a patient following

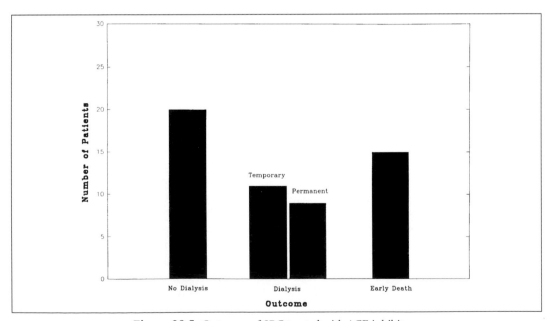

Figure 20.5. Outcome of SRC treated with ACE inhibitors.

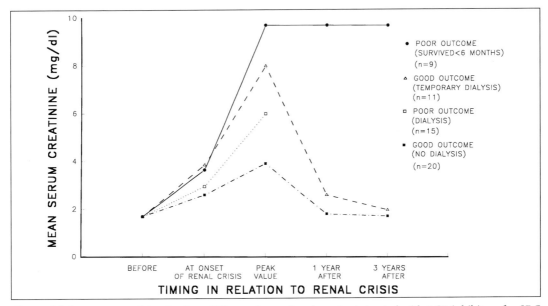

Figure 20.6. Serum creatinine levels at different time points in patients treated with ACE inhibitors for SRC grouped according to outcome.

renal transplant (40), most SRC patients do as well as other transplant patients (26).

Factors associated with early death or permanent dialysis in the ACE inhibitor SRC patients were male sex, older age, concomitant scleroderma heart disease, inability to control blood pressure within 72 hours, and a pretreatment serum creatinine greater than 3 mg/dl. Interestingly, patients who presented with extremely high blood pressures had a better outcome than those with a more moderate elevation. Perhaps this was because they came to medical attention earlier in the disease process before irreversible end organ damage had occurred.

The patients who have SRC but do not have significant hypertension, i.e., normotensive renal crisis (19), generally have a poor prognosis. Without hypertension, diagnosis is likely to be delayed. Patients with the normotensive form of SRC often have microangiopathic hemolytic anemia and widespread small blood vessel changes leading to ischemia and dysfunction of many organs. Pulmonary hemorrhage, an unusual feature of SSc or SRC, has been seen on several occasions during the course of normotensive renal crisis. It complicates the diagnosis and is a poor prognostic sign. Treatment with ACE inhibitors is indicated in normotensive SRC even if only low doses can be tolerated. This treatment regimen can reverse the process if given early enough in the course.

Survival in SRC patients treated with ACE inhibitors has dramatically improved from times when such drugs were not available (37,38). In our series, the 1-year cumulative survival rate for ACE inhibitor treated patients was 76%, in contrast to only 15% in the untreated group (Fig. 20.7). One year survivors of renal crisis treated with ACE inhibitors had 5- and 10-year survival rates similar to diffuse scleroderma patients who never had renal crisis. Although there has been a rare recurrence of the acute episode, generally it is a one time event.

Summary

Renal crisis occurs in systemic sclerosis patients with rapidly progressive diffuse cutaneous thickening early in their disease. SRC is characterized

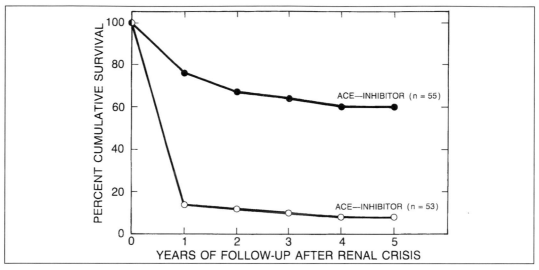

Figure 20.7. Cumulative survival of patients with SRC who were (n = 55) and were not (n = 53) treated with an ACE inhibitor. (Reproduced with permission.)

by malignant hypertension, hyperreninemia, azotemia, microangiopathic hemolytic anemia, and renal failure. This complication was almost uniformly fatal, but can now be treated successfully in most cases with ACE inhibitors. This therapy has improved survival, reduced the requirement for dialysis, and often allowed for the discontinuation of dialysis 6 to 18 months later. Prompt diagnosis and early, aggressive initiation of therapy with ACE inhibitors will result in the most optimal outcome.

References

1. Kahaleh MB, LeRoy EC. Progressive systemic sclerosis: Kidney involvement. Clin Rheum Dis 1979; 5:167–184.
2. Cannon PJ, Hassar M, Case DB, Casarella WJ, Sommers SC, LeRoy EC. The relationship of hypertension and renal failure in scleroderma (progressive systemic sclerosis) to structural and functional abnormalities of the renal cortical circulation. Medicine 1974;53:1–46.
3. Urai L, Szinay G, Nagy Z, Wiltner W. Renal function in scleroderma. Br Med J 1958;2:1264–1266.
4. Desai Y, Ghanekar MA, Siquera RD, Joshi VR. Renal involvement in scleroderma. JAPI 1990;38: 768–770.
5. Sokoloff L. Some aspects of the pathology of collagen disease. Bull NY Acad Med 1952;32:760–767.
6. Stone RA, Tisher CC, Hawkins HK, Robinson RR. Juxtaglomerular hyperplasia and hyperreninemia in progressive systemic sclerosis complicated by acute renal failure. Am J Med 1974;56:119–123.
7. Kovalchik MT, Guggenheim SJ, Silverman MH, Robertson JS, Steigerwald JC. The kidney in progressive systemic sclerosis: A prospective study. Ann Intern Med 1978;89:881–887.
8. Steen VD, Medsger TA Jr, Osial TA Jr, Ziegler GL, Shapiro AP, Rodnan GP. Factors predicting development of renal involvement in progressive systemic sclerosis. Am J Med 1984;76:779–786.
9. Fleischmajer R, Gould AB. Serum renin and renin substrate levels in scleroderma. Proc Soc Exp Biol Med 1975;150:374–379.
10. Nussbaum Al, LeRoy EC. Renal involvement in scleroderma (systemic sclerosis). In: Bacon PA, Hadler NM, eds. The kidney and rheumatic disease, London, Butterworth, 1992;17:282–296.
11. Trostle DC, Bedetti CD, Steen VD, Al-Sabbagh MR, Zee B. Renal vascular histology and morphometry in systemic sclerosis subsets: A case-control autopsy study. Arthritis Rheum 1988;31:393–400.
12. Traub YM, Shapiro AP, Rodnan GP, Medsger TA Jr, McDonald RH Jr, Steen VD, Osial TA Jr, et al. Hypertension and renal failure (scleroderma renal crisis) in progressive systemic sclerosis. Medicine 1983;62:335–352.
13. Steen VD, Costantino JP, Shapiro AP, Medsger TA Jr. Outcome of renal crisis in systemic sclerosis: Re-

lation to availability of angiotensin converting enzyme (ACE) inhibitors. Ann Intern Med 1990;113:352–357.

14. McWhorter JE, LeRoy EC. Pericardial disease in scleroderma (systemic sclerosis). Am J Med 1974;57:566–575.

15. Karlen JR, Cook WA. Renal scleroderma and pregnancy. Obstet Gynecol 1974;44:349–354.

16. Steen VD, Conte C, Day N, Ramsey-Goldman R, Medsger TA Jr. Pregnancy in systemic sclerosis. Arthritis Rheum 1989;32:151–157.

17. Lunseth JH, Baker LA, Shifrin A. Chronic scleroderma with acute exacerbation during corticotropin therapy. Arch Intern Med 1951;88:783–792.

18. Sharnoff JG, Carideo HL, Stein ID. Cortisone-treated scleroderma. JAMA 1951;145:1230–1232.

19. Helfrich DJ, Banner B, Steen VD, Medsger TA Jr. Renal failure in normotensive patients with systemic sclerosis. Arthritis Rheum 1989;32:1128–1134.

20. Fisher ER, Rodnan GP. Pathologic observations concerning renal involvement in progressive systemic sclerosis (PSS). Arch Pathol 1958;65:29–39.

21. Shapiro AP, Steen VD, Medsger TA Jr. Renal Involvement in Systemic Sclerosis. In: Schrier R, Gottschalk C, eds. Diseases of the kidney. Boston: Little, Brown and Co, 1992;73:2039–2048.

22. Lapenas D, Rodnan GP, Cavallo T. Immunopathology of the renal vascular lesion of progressive systemic sclerosis (scleroderma). Am J Pathol 1978;91:243–256.

23. Clements PJ, Paulus HE, Lachenbruch PA, Furst DE. Study of renal pathophysiology in systemic sclerosis (SSc): 10-year follow-up. Arthritis Rheum 1991;34(9):S111.

24. Steen VD, Medsger TA Jr, Rodnan GP. D-penicillamine therapy in progressive systemic sclerosis (scleroderma). Ann Intern Med 1982;97:652–659.

25. Steen VD. Epidemiology of systemic sclerosis. Rheum Dis Clin North Am 1990;16(3):641–654.

26. Donohoe JF. Nephrology Forum: Scleroderma and the kidney. Kidney Int 1992;41:462–477.

27. Steen VD, Medsger TA Jr, Rodnan GP, Ziegler GL. Clinical associations of anticentromere antibody (ACA) in patients with progressive systemic sclerosis. Arthritis Rheum 1984;27:125–131.

28. LeRoy EC, Black C, Fleischmajer R, Jablonska S, Krieg T, Medsger TA Jr, Rowell N, et al. Scleroderma (systemic sclerosis): Classification, subsets and pathogencsis. J Rheumatol 1988;15:202–205.

29. Okano Y, Steen VD, Medsger TA Jr. Novel human serum autoantibodies reactive with RNA polymerase III: A major autoantigen in systemic sclerosis with diffuse cutaneous involvement. Ann Intern Med 1993 (in press).

30. Gavras H, Gavras I, Cannon PJ, Brunner HR, Laragh JH. Is elevated plasma renin activity of prognostic importance in progressive systemic sclerosis? Arch Intern Med 1977;137:1554–1558.

31. Steen VD, Syed A, Johnson JP, Conte CL, Medsger TA Jr. Renal disease in systemic sclerosis. Arthritis Rheum 1993;36(Suppl):S131.

32. Follansbee W. The cardiovascular manifestations of systemic sclerosis (scleroderma). In: O'Rourke RA, ed. Current problems in cardiology. Chicago: Yearbook Medical Publishers, Inc, 1986:245–298.

33. LeRoy EC, Fleischmann RM. The management of renal scleroderma: Experience with dialysis, nephrectomy and transplantation. Am J Med 1978;64:974–978.

34. Wasner C, Cooke CR, Fries JF. Successful medical treatment of scleroderma renal crisis. N Engl J Med 1978;229:873–875.

35. Mitnick PD, Feig PU. Control of hypertension and reversal of renal failure in scleroderma. N Engl J Med 1978;299:871–872.

36. Lopez-Ovejero JA, Sall SD, D'Angelo WA, Cheigh JS, Stenzel KH, Laragh JH. Reversal of vascular and renal crises of scleroderma by oral angiotensin converting enzyme blockade. N Engl J Med 1979;300:1417–1419.

37. Zawada ET Jr, Clements PJ, Furst DA, Bloomer HA, Paulus HE, Maxwell MH. Clinical course of patients with scleroderma renal crisis treated with captopril. Nephron 1981;27:74–78.

38. Thurm RH, Alexander JC. Captopril in the treatment of scleroderma renal crisis. Arch Intern Med 1984;144:733–755.

39. Whitman HH 3rd, Case DB, Laragh JH, et al. Variable response to oral angiotensin converting enzyme blockade in hypertensive scleroderma patients. Arthritis Rheum 1982;25:241–248.

40. Woodhall PB, McCoy RC, Gunnells JC, Seigvler HF. Apparent recurrence of progressive systemic sclerosis in a renal allograft. JAMA 1976;236:1032–1034.

ARIANE L. HERRICK
MALCOLM I.V. JAYSON

21

Organ Involvement: Nervous System

CLINICIANS CARING FOR PATIENTS with SSc rarely suspect, or find, neurological involvement of the disease: the nervous system is not regarded as a frequent target for attack by this multisystem disease. This clinical experience finds corroboration in the findings of large series of SSc patients, now published some years ago. In 1954, Leinwand et al reported more than 150 patients with SSc and did not mention symptoms or signs of focal neurological involvement (1). In another study, of 727 patients, the only neurological disorders documented were seizures in six patients, about whom few details are given (2). Gordon and Silverstein reviewed 130 patients in 1970 and noted polyneuropathy in one patient and some form of encephalopathy in ten: the authors felt that in none of their patients did these neurological features reflect the primary pathological process of the SSc (3). More recently, Lee and colleagues conducted a prospective study of 125 patients with SSc and found four cases of carpal tunnel syndrome, and one each of peripheral neuropathy, trigeminal neuralgia, and mononeuritis multiplex (4). A recent retrospective study of 50 patients with SSc was unusual in suggesting a higher incidence of neurological abnormalities of 40%, but this figure included muscle involvement (5).

However, over the years several case reports and small series describing neurological involvement in SSc have accumulated, demonstrating that neurological involvement does occur in a proportion of patients with SSc. In addition, a number of carefully conducted studies have drawn attention to the fact that subclinical neurological involvement is not rare. As far back as 1963, one school of thought was that injury to the nervous system was the primary fault in scleroderma: skin biopsies showed degeneration and regeneration of the cutaneous nerve network in both affected and nonaffected skin (6).

In this chapter, we will review the evidence for neurological involvement in SSc. Trigeminal neuropathy, reported by several authors, is the most common form of clinically recognizable neurological involvement and is discussed first. Evidence for peripheral neuropathy is addressed next, followed by central nervous system involvement and autonomic neuropathy, this last entity becoming increasingly recognized among patients with SSc. Finally, we discuss possible pathogenic mechanisms of neurological involvement in SSc.

Cranial Nerve Involvement

Trigeminal neuropathy is now a well-recognized manifestation of SSc (4,5,7–15). The first systematic evaluation of the frequency of this problem in an SSc population was a retrospective study conducted by Farrell and Medsger in 1982 (10). Sixteen of 442 patients were found to have had trigeminal sensory complaints when comprehensive, carefully collected data on each patient were reviewed. These sixteen patients, together with 25 patients pooled from the literature, were more likely to have an overlap syndrome (34%) than the 426 patients without symptoms of trigeminal nerve involvement (5%). Generally, clinical features of SSc predated those of trigeminal neuropathy, but in seven of the 41 patients trigeminal symptoms occurred first. The problem was transient in only three patients. Most cases were bilateral, usually involving the second and third divisions of the trigeminal nerve. All three divisions were involved in 12 of the 25 cases reviewed in the literature. This was a sensory neuropathy: in no patient was there motor involvement of the trigeminal nerve, and there were no coexisting cranial nerve abnormalities. All patients had sensory impairment on testing. Comparing the 16 patients from the Pittsburgh database with trigeminal nerve involvement to those without, a higher proportion had myositis (six of 16 compared to 41 of 405), a white blood count less than $4.0 \times 10^9/l$ (three of 14 compared to 14 of 323), hypothyroidism (three of 16 compared to 10 of 401) and Sjögren's syndrome (three of 16 compared to 29 of 407). Further support for an association between trigeminal neuralgia and an overlap syndrome was that nine of 20 patients (45%) with trigeminal neuralgia had serum antibodies to ribonucleoprotein, compared to 25 of 329 patients without fifth nerve involvement (8%).

Therefore, it is clear that trigeminal neuropathy occurs in a small proportion of patients with SSc. Conversely, if a patient presents with a trigeminal sensory neuropathy, SSc is one of the underlying diagnoses to be considered. This issue was addressed by Lecky et al (11) who carefully evaluated 22 patients with chronic trigeminal sensory neuropathy. Six patients had SSc and three were felt to have mixed connective tissue disease (MCTD). Of the remaining 13 patients, nine had organ or nonorgan specific serum autoantibodies (four had an antinuclear antibody ANA of > 1:10). It is not clear in what way these patients were selected for referral to the authors.

The onset of sensory symptoms in Lecky's patients usually was gradual and if pain followed, it was not lancinating as in trigeminal neuralgia. Seven of the nine SSc/MCTD patient group had

bilateral involvement. In 14 patients pain, temperature, and light touch were affected, while light touch was spared in the other eight. The corneal reflex was depressed or absent in eleven of the 14 cases with first division sensory signs. Taste sensation was impaired in seven of the nine patients in the SSc/MCTD group. One of the patients with SSc was treated with carbamazepine and prednisolone and another with just carbamazepine—neither treatment resulted in any benefit to the patient.

Electrophysiological testing showed abnormal blink reflex recordings in three of the four SSc patients tested, and abnormal trigeminal sensory evoked potentials in all four of these patients. Histology was not available from any of the patients with SSc. One patient who did not have SSc underwent a supraorbital nerve biopsy. This procedure showed severe loss of myelinated fibres, with electron microscopy revealing increased endoneurial collagen, but no changes to blood vessel walls.

In three of the SSc/MCTD cases, trigeminal neuropathy preceded other features of connective tissue disease, barring RP. That trigeminal neuralgia can precede other features of SSc has now been noted by several authors (7–10,13).

The authors interpreted their clinical findings of absence of motor involvement, the involvement of individual branches of the trigeminal nerve, and the lack of dissociation of sensory loss as being consistent with a lesion in the trigeminal ganglion or in the proximal part of the main trigeminal division. The lack of available pathological evidence made it difficult to postulate the pathogenic mechanism of the trigeminal neuropathy.

None of the patients in the two studies described in the preceding paragraphs were thought to have cranial nerve involvement other than the trigeminal neuropathy. Teasdall et al (9) described 10 patients with SSc and trigeminal neuralgia, two of whom had myositis and two were hypothyroid. Again there was no motor trigeminal nerve involvement. In contrast to patients of other series, however, Teasdall's patients did have evidence of other cranial nerve involvement, particularly of facial nerve weakness, which was noted in five patients. Gag reflexes were impaired in three patients, tinnitus with hearing loss was present in two (interpreted by the authors as evidence of eighth nerve involvement), ninth nerve involvement was suspected in one patient, and twelfth nerve involvement in another. Three of the patients had evidence of a peripheral sensory neuropathy and two were shown to have a carpal tunnel syndrome on nerve conduction studies. Steroids were said to be unhelpful but no details were given.

Heald emphasized that a high index of suspicion of underlying disease should be maintained when a patient presents with a trigeminal neuropathy (13). His patient developed trigeminal neuropathy as early as six years before the onset of scleroderma: in the interim, further cranial nerve involvement had developed. However, the report does not clearly indicate whether this patient fulfilled the American Rheumatism Association (ARA) criteria for SSc (16).

In summary, trigeminal neuropathy has now been described in a large number of patients with SSc, and was reported in 4% of a series of 442 patients with SSc. Myositis may occur in association. Trigeminal neuropathy is a purely sensory neuropathy, and presents with slowly evolving facial numbness, sometimes progressing to pain and paraesthesia. It may be the presenting feature of SSc and often occurs early in the evolution of the disease. Its etiology is poorly understood, and clinical trials of its treatment have not been undertaken.

Peripheral Neuropathy

Many case reports of peripheral neuropathy occurring in association with SSc exist, dating back to 1954 (4,5,9,12,14,17–21). In some cases this was the only neurological manifestation of the disease, while in others there were other neurological symptoms and signs such as bilateral carpal tunnel syndrome (14), bilateral carpal

tunnel syndrome and impotence (21), trigeminal neuropathy, sometimes in association with other cranial nerve lesions (9,12). In Subenik's case, clinical features of carpal tunnel syndrome, but not of impotence or peripheral neuropathy, regressed after six months. The authors suggested that this might have been due to regression of the edema of early scleroderma, or to treatment with penicillamine (21).

Generally the neuropathy was of mixed sensory and motor type, with lower limb involvement more common than upper limb involvement. Occasionally, the neuropathy preceded the development of the classical features of SSc (19,20).

Sural nerve biopsies have been performed in a small number of patients. In the two cases reported by Di Trapani et al (19,20), light microscopy showed reduction in myelinated fibers, increased collagen production, and vascular changes with intimal thickening and adventitial edema. There were no inflammatory changes. Electron microscopic findings included hyperplasia of the Swann cell basal membranes with an increased number of filaments, active endoplasmic reticulum, and structural signs of denervation in these cells. These authors felt that their findings were in keeping with a vascular lesion as the primary pathogenic cause of the neuropathy and the increase in collagen was secondary to a microangiopathy. In Subenik's case, light microscopy of a sural nerve biopsy showed no significant abnormalities, but electron microscopy showed irregularity of the myelin sheaths and electron opaque bodies in unmyelinated fibers and in Swann cell cytoplasm (21). Sural nerve biopsy in the case of Berth-Jones et al showed a reduction in the myelinated fibres of all diameters (14), whereas no abnormality was found in the patient reported by Agarwal (12). A series of seven patients with SSc and vasculitis, referred to in the following paragraphs, included four patients with mononeuritis multiplex (22). Three patients underwent sural nerve biopsies, all of which showed vasculitis.

The entrapment neuropathy of carpal tunnel

syndrome has been described in a small number of patients, including those referred to in the preceding paragraphs who also developed peripheral neuropathy (4,5,9,14,21). It tends to be an early feature of the disease. Lee et al, reviewing 125 patients with SSc (4), found carpal tunnel syndrome in four patients, three of whom exhibited bilateral symptoms. In two patients, it was in association with active arthritis and in a third with edema of the hands. Meralgia paraesthetica associated with abdominal distension due to intestinal pseudo-obstruction has also been described in SSc (23).

Another form of peripheral nerve involvement, mononeuritis multiplex, has only rarely been described in association with SSc: five patients have been reported in the literature. The first was among the seven patients with neurological manifestations described in Lee's series (4). This patient developed mononeuritis involving the right ulnar and median nerves, and probably included the saphenous nerve. Of the four patients with mononeuritis multiplex and SSc described by Oddis et al (22), two appear to have experienced some neurological recovery on treatment with prednisolone and immunosuppressant therapy. Interestingly, three of these patients had the CREST variant of SSc and features of Sjögren's syndrome. On a similar theme, in our department two female patients with limited cutaneous SSc, both anticentromere antibody positive, have developed lateral popliteal nerve palsies (24). The first patient was aged 56 and had a 16 year history of SSc. One night she was awakened by left leg discomfort—clinical evidence indicated a lateral popliteal nerve palsy, as confirmed electrophysiologically. IgM anticardiolipin antibodies were present in a moderate titre of 36 units (normal < 3) but testing for antineutrophil cytoplasmic antibody (ANCA) was negative. Clinically she improved, but four months later she developed a further lateral popliteal nerve palsy, this time right-sided. There were no other clinical features suggestive of a vasculitis. Steroids were not prescribed, because she had osteogenesis imperfecta and severe osteoporosis.

Her symptoms lessened spontaneously. The second patient, aged 62 years and with a 9-year history of SSc, presented with a 4-day history of numbness of the lateral aspect of her right leg and "tripping up." Clinically and electrophysiologically she had a lateral popliteal nerve palsy. Again, there was no clinical evidence of vasculitis otherwise, but she was ANCA positive (cANCA 1/32) and had a moderate titre of IgG anticardiolipin antibodies of 20 units (normal < 3). This patient was already on prednisolone 10 mg daily. Azathioprine was commenced but not tolerated, and six weeks later there was some improvement in her symptoms.

Following on from these case reports, we have made a careful study of peripheral nerve function in SSc and concluded that peripheral nerve involvement of the disease is not as rare as previously thought (25). Twenty-nine patients underwent detailed clinical examination followed by motor, sensory, and sympathetic conduction studies. The quantitative sensory evaluation comprised testing of thermal sensitivity, pain and vibration threshold, and touch and two-point discrimination. Some of the results are shown in Figure 21.1. The thermal threshold was modestly increased in the hand in four patients (14%) and in the foot in five patients (18%). Heat-pain thresholds were normal in both upper and lower limbs in all patients. In only one patient was vibratory sensitivity impaired. Tactile thresholds of the fingers were raised in eight patients (28%) and of the foot in 13 patients (50%). Two-point discrimination was abnormal in 10 patients (34%).

Nerve conduction studies were abnormal in six patients, of whom five had evidence of a mild peripheral neuropathy on examination. Only one of the patients had a symptomatic neuropathy. Nerve conduction studies in two patients revealed an asymptomatic carpal tunnel syndrome. The sympathetic skin response was abnormal in four of sixteen patients who had not undergone sympathectomy.

We, therefore, demonstrated a predominantly sensory defect in a substantial proportion of

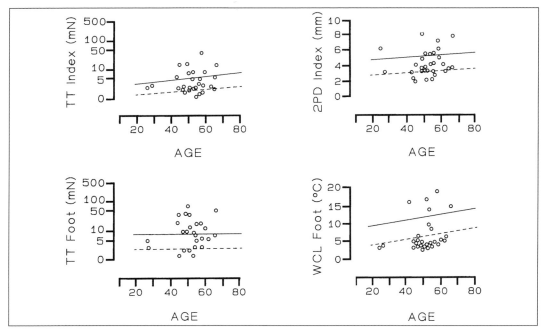

Figure 21.1. Results of quantitative sensory testing in the index finger (upper panels) and foot (lower panels) in patients with scleroderma. The broken and continuous lines indicate, respectively, the regression line with age for control subjects and the upper limit of normal. TT = tactile threshold; 2PD = two-point discrimination; WCL = warm-cold limen (thermal threshold). (Reproduced with permission from Schady, W, et al. Peripheral nerve dysfunction in scleroderma. QJM 1991;292:661.)

patients with SSc, and made the point that this is usually subclinical and worse in the feet than in the hands. The neuropathy occurred especially in patients with a longer duration of disease, in contradistinction to trigeminal neuropathy, which often occurs early in the disease. Admittedly, skin induration in patients with SSc may be in part responsible for the findings, but the nerve conduction studies did suggest that in some patients there was axonal loss in distal lower limb nerves. No firm conclusions regarding the pathogenesis of the neuropathy could be made from this study, although an obliterative microangiopathy was postulated.

Therefore, while peripheral neuropathy is an uncommon manifestation of SSc, described in only a few case reports, subclinical peripheral nerve involvement has been demonstrated in a substantial proportion of patients.

Central Nervous System Involvement

This is rare in SSc. When Gordon and Silverstein found that a significant proportion of their 18.5% of patients with neurological dysfunction had "cerebral disease," this was generally secondary to renal or cardiopulmonary involvement (3). Five of these patients had seizures (four generalized, one right-sided), of whom four were hypertensive (three with uraemia) and the fifth was hypocalcaemic following parathyroidectomy (a treatment for seizures in the 1930s). Convulsions are now a very rare manifestation of SSc, probably reflecting improved treatment of hypertension and renal failure which in former years was the major cause of mortality in this disease.

One case of subacute combined degeneration of the spinal cord secondary to vitamin B12 malabsorption as a result of gastrointestinal involvement by SSc has been described (26). Clinically, the patient had a paraparesis. Autopsy showed fibrosis of the submucosa and muscular layers throughout the gastrointestinal tract. Averbuch-Heller et al, in their retrospective series of 50 patients, diagnosed a myelopathy in four and cerebrovascular disease in three, two of whom were shown to have a cerebral infarct on CT scanning (5). There were no risk factors for cerebrovascular disease in these three female patients (age range 50–56 years), other than renal impairment in one.

Cerebral infarction caused by SSc has also been described in a case report, where autopsy findings showed not only intimal proliferation and medial thickening of the internal carotid but also inflammatory changes of the small vessels surrounding this artery (27). This was an interesting observation because, although microvascular disease is a prominent feature of SSc, vasculitis has only rarely been recognized. There have since been two other reports of cerebral vasculitis in patients with SSc. In 1979, Estey et al reported a 43-year-old woman with SSc who developed seizures and encephalopathy and had abnormalities on cerebral angiography suggestive of arteritis (28). Her clinical condition improved in the short term with steroids. More recently, Pathak and Gabor described a patient with limited cutaneous SSc who developed headaches and was found on CT scan to have had a small subarachnoid haemorrhage. She had a background of hypertension. Carotid angiography showed atherosclerotic disease but also abnormalities of several arteries said to be consistent with vasculitis (29). The patient became confused and was treated with steroids, initially with good effect, but then suffered recurrent episodes of paraesthesia and aphasia which responded to the addition of cyclophosphamide. Leptomeningeal and cerebral biopsies were normal.

On the subject of vasculitis in SSc, we observed a male patient with SSc who had vasculitis as a very prominent feature of his disease (30).

This was associated not only with central nervous involvement but also a peripheral neuropathy and myositis. His case is described in the following paragraphs because he demonstrates very well the complicated spectrum of connective tissue disease.

CASE REPORT

A 51-year-old male physician, diagnosed as having SSc four years previously, was admitted in July 1991 with a marked clinical deterioration. For 6 weeks he had had increasing difficulty walking because of muscle weakness and on admission was unable to stand, was breathless on minimal exertion, and was complaining of epigastric pain, abdominal distension and diarrhea, as well as severe Raynaud's. Previously, his disease had been characterised by widespread skin thickening, esophageal and small bowel involvement, pulmonary fibrosis, arthralgias, myositis, and complete heart block requiring a permanent pacemaker.

Drug treatment comprised prednisolone 15 mg daily. In 1987, he had been started on alpha-interferon with good effect, but he had since been lost to follow up and had stopped this treatment 6 months prior to this admission.

On examination he was cachectic, with basal crepitations, proximal muscle wasting, and impaired sensation below the knees. He went on to develop a fever.

His hemoglobin was 13.4 g/dl, white blood count raised at 35.8 X 10^9/l (this fell slightly after cefuroxime prescribed for a suspected chest infection), platelets 466 X 10^9/l, ESR 58. Serum biochemistry was essentially normal. Immunology results were as follows: ANF positive 1/20 IgG (weak homogenous), SCAT 1/256, anticentromere antibody negative, antibodies to extractable nuclear antigens (Ro, La, Scl-70, RNP, Sm) and ANCA all negative, anticardiolipin IgG positive 36 units (normal < 5), IgM low positive 6 units (normal < 3). A hydrogen breath test was strongly positive and a small bowel enema showed appearances of scleroderma. Muscle biopsy showed myositis with necrotising vasculitis (Fig. 21.2), and sural nerve biopsy also showed a vasculitis (Fig. 21.3).

His disease progressed despite treatment with an increased dosage of prednisolone, recommencement

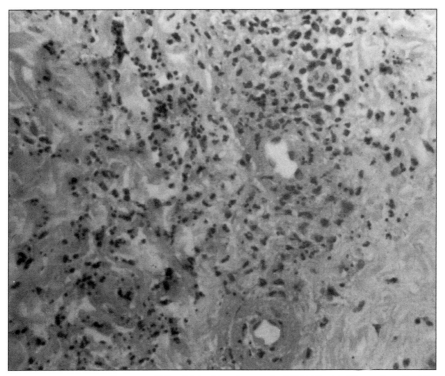

Figure 21.2. Active microvascular vasculitis within fibrotic muscle. H&E X 250. (Reproduced with permission from AJ Freemont.)

of alpha-interferon, and total parenteral nutrition. He developed bilateral wrist drop and electrophysiological testing confirmed a severe peripheral neuropathy. Pulsed cyclophosphamide was begun and also aspirin (after grand mal seizures and the suggestion of cerebral vein thrombosis on CT), but his clinical state did not improve and he died two months later after a rapid deterioration in his respiratory function.

Autopsy findings included severe myopathic change but interestingly no active myositis, and nerves showed demyelination but no acute vasculitis, although there was a mononuclear cell infiltrate intimately related to the wall of one small interstitial vessel. These findings suggested that the inflammatory component to his muscle and peripheral nerve disease responded to immunosuppressant treatment, although the patient's general condition deteriorated. It could be argued that this patient's anticardiolipin (aCL) antibodies played a role in the pathogenesis of his disease, as aCL antibodies are strongly associated with vascular disease. However, these antibodies are generally thought to be associated with thrombosis rather than with vasculitis (31), although associations of aCL antibodies and inflammatory changes in blood vessels have been reported (32–34). While at autopsy some evidence of thrombosis was found (recent thrombi in a small artery and small vein of the esophagus, small thrombi in the basal ganglia, two organising arterial thrombi in the pancreas, and recanalised previously thrombosed arteries in the kidneys), this was unlikely to have contributed significantly to the clinical progression of his disease.

In summary, central nervous system involvement is rare in SSc, but can rarely be associated at least in part with vasculitis. In turn, vasculitis is an unusual manifestation of SSc, but can occur, as evidenced by our patient who had severe vasculitis affecting peripheral nerve and muscle.

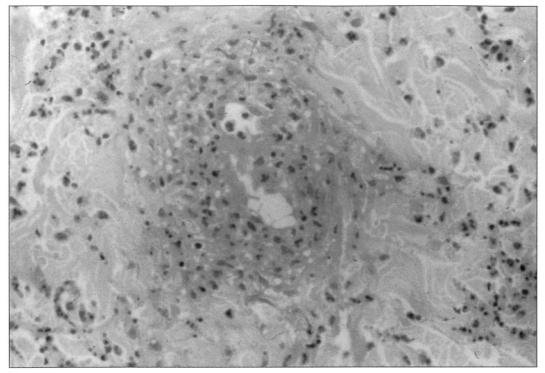

Figure 21.3. Active vasculitis within the microvasculature of a nerve sheath (H&E X 300). (Reproduced with permission from AJ Freemont.)

Autonomic Neuropathy

Autonomic neuropathy is becoming increasingly recognised in SSc. Its clinical expression was first described in 1986 by Sonnex et al in a patient with a 17-year history of SSc who developed abdominal pain, diarrhea, and marked postural hypotension. Autonomic function testing revealed both sympathetic and parasympathetic dysfunction (35). These authors went on to test sympathetic and parasympathetic function in six other patients with SSc and found evidence of parasympathetic dysfunction in three of them. None of these patients had a peripheral neuropathy.

We have performed a detailed study of autonomic function in 25 patients with SSc, 10 patients with primary RP, and 13 healthy controls (36). Two tests of cardiovascular reflexes tested efferent sympathetic function:

(a) The postural fall in blood pressure on standing (30 mmHg or more abnormal, 10 mmHg or less normal).

(b) The rise in systolic blood pressure on sustained hand grip (16 mmHg or more normal, 10 mmHg or less abnormal).

Parasympathetic function was tested in three ways, all assessing the cardiac parasympathetic nerve supply and examining changes in heart rate in response to different maneuvers:

(a) Standing. The R-R interval is measured at the 15th and 30th beat after rising from a supine position. The 30:15 ratio should be greater than 1.04.

(b) Deep breathing. Normally there is a difference in heart rate of at least 15 beats/minute between inspiration and expiration.

(c) The Valsalva maneuver. The ratio of the

longest R-R interval after the maneuver to the shortest R-R interval during the maneuver is normally 1.21 or more, whereas 1.10 or less is abnormal.

Results are summarized in Table 21.1. Significant postural hypotension occurred in none of the patients and was borderline in only two SSc patients, but the four other tests of autonomic function were significantly abnormal in the SSc group. Eighty per cent of the patients had at least three abnormal tests. Five of the patients had diffuse SSc while 20 had limited disease: abnormal results occurred in all of the diffuse subgroup and only two of the limited subgroup had only one abnormal test. There was no correlation between disease duration and the degree of autonomic failure. The results suggested that parasympathetic pathways were more affected than the sympathetic.

The results of primary Raynaud's patients were not significantly different from controls, but were intermediate between those of the SSc group and controls.

One study has addressed the issue of treatment of cardiovascular autonomic dysfunction in nine patients with RP, three of whom had SSc (37). The authors reported a trend toward normalization of results of autonomic function tests

in these nine patients following treatment with triiodothyronine. They suggested that improved tissue blood flow to ischemic neural tissue might contribute to this normalization or, alternatively, a more direct action by triiodothyronine on the autonomic system.

In view of these findings of autonomic dysfunction in SSc, it may seem surprising that these abnormalities do not find wider clinical expression and recognition. It has long been postulated that RP may be in part a result of vasomotor instability (38), although this remains far from clear. Other possible clinical reflections of autonomic neuropathy in SSc are gastrointestinal dysmotility and impotence.

Gastrointestinal involvement is common in SSc, with many patients complaining of symptoms attributable to abnormalities of esophageal and gastric emptying, and of gastric stasis.

While muscle failure accounts in large part for these problems, it may be that the myopathy is secondary to an initial neuropathy of the enteric nervous system (39). Two of eight patients with SSc undergoing upper gastrointestinal manometric studies had incoordination of pressure activity in both fasting and postprandial periods, in distinction to the hypomotility observed in most SSc patients (40). This suggested a motility response suggestive of a neuropathic rather than

Table 21.1. Results of Autonomic Function Tests in 25 Patients with SSc, 10 Patients with Primary Raynaud's Phenomenon and 13 Control Subjects

Test	SSc[b]	PRP[b]	Controls	SSc v control	SScvPRP	PRP v controls
Sustained hand grip (mmHg); N≥15	13.1(7.8)[c]	17.0(14.9)	23.2(14.1)	p = 0.05 0.1-17.2[a]	NS	NS
Heart rate on standing (30:15 ratio); N≥ 1.04	1.02(0.08)	1.23(0.10)	1.23(0.18)	p = 0.005 0.1-0.3[a]	p = 0.045 0.02-0.2[a]	NS
Valsalva ratio; N≥ 1.21	1.16(0.16)	1.47(0.20)	1.63(0.25)	p = 0.001 0.3-0.5[a]	p = 0.001 0.1-0.4[a]	NS
Deep breathing heart rate response (beats/min); N ≥ 15	7.7(5.3)	15.3(5.4)	18.8(9.0)	p = 0.001 4.0–12.8[a]	p =0.014 1.3–10.4[a]	NS

[a]Confidence intervals for the differences.
[b] SSc=systemic sclerosis; PRP=primary Raynaud's phenomenon; N=normal.
[c]Values are mean (SD)
Reproduced with permission from Klimiuk et al, 1988.

a myopathic lesion in these two patients. Abnormal rectosigmoid motility has been reported in SSc (41). Recently Leighton et al described abnormal anorectal function, especially abnormal anal sphincter resting pressures, in eight patients with SSc and altered bowel habit, fecal incontinence, or rectal prolapse (42).

Impotence has now been described in several male patients with SSc (21,43–45). In the five patients described by Lally and Jimenez, impotence was one of the presenting features of the SSc. In none of the patients was any other cause for the sexual dysfunction identified. The authors suggested two possible mechanisms: vascular changes in the small vessels of the penis, or abnormalities in neurogenic control of penile vascular tone. Impotence may be a relatively common manifestation of SSc: of ten patients with SSc six reported impotence (45).

In conclusion, autonomic neuropathy does occur in SSc and is often subclinical. It is possible that this autonomic dysfunction contributes in part to the RP, gastrointestinal manifestations, and impotence which are all features of the disease.

Pathogenesis

The pathogenesis of SSc is not known: abnormalities of connective tissue metabolism, the microvasculature, and the immune system have all been proposed. It is even less clear what mechanism is responsible for the neurological lesions. This is partly due to the dearth of histological material available.

There seem to be three possible mechanisms which, individually or collectively, may account for the different neurological problems sometimes associated with SSc. This is discounting vitamin B12 deficiency, which has only been described in the one case (26), despite the common occurrence of malabsorption in SSc. These three mechanisms are:

1. Fibrosis. In 1954, Richter (17) described thickening of the epineurium and perineurium of the peripheral nerves of a patient with scleroderma and peripheral neuropathy. While in this particular case there was thickening of blood vessel walls, there was no evidence of any infarction. It was postulated that the neuropathy resulted from compression of the myelinated fibers by the excess collagen, although Richter felt that altered vascular permeability might also contribute. The intense fibrosis noted in the sural nerve biopsies reported by Di Trapani et al (20) perhaps supports this theory of excessive fibrosis, although these authors were more in favor of a microangiopathy as being primarily responsible for the neuropathy.

2. A non-inflammatory microangiopathy affecting the blood vessels supplying neural tissue. The well-recognized and widespread changes that occur in the microvasculature of SSc (46) make this an attractive hypothesis, and one supported by Di Trapani et al, who reported, in sural nerve biopsies, changes in the vasa nervorum with intimal proliferation and adventitial edema (20).

3. Vasculitis. While this does occur in some patients with SSc, it seems unlikely that inflammatory change is responsible for most cases of neuropathy.

Further elucidation of the pathogenesis of the neuropathy will require histological studies performed prospectively, examining patients at different stages of their disease. Unfortunately, it will be difficult to conduct such studies.

Summary

Symptomatic neurological involvement is rare in SSc, and much of the relevant literature consists of case reports and small series. Trigeminal neuropathy is the most common neurological manifestation of SSc. Other cranial neuropathies, peripheral neuropathy, central nervous system involvement, and autonomic neuropathy have all been reported but less frequently. Recent years, however, have seen the more systematic evaluation of peripheral and autonomic neuropathy and suggest that subclinical neuropathy is not uncommon.

As reports of neuropathy tend to be anecdotal, no clinical trials of treatment of any of the forms of neuropathy exist and little is known about whether any particular therapy is effective. For therapy to be effective, ideally we should have some understanding of pathogenesis. Excessive fibrosis, leading to nerve compression, and microangiopathy have both been suggested. Most likely effective management of SSc neuropathy will await that of the underlying disease.

References

1. Leinwand I, Duryee AW, Richter MN. Scleroderma (Based on a study of over 150 cases). Ann Intern Med 1954;41:1003.
2. Tuffanelli DL, Winkelmann RK. Systemic scleroderma. A clinical study of 727 cases. Arch Dermatol 1961;84:359.
3. Gordon RM, Silverstein A. Neurological manifestations in progressive systemic sclerosis. Arch Neurol 1970;22:126.
4. Lee P, Bruni J, Sukenik S. Neurological manifestations in systemic sclerosis (scleroderma). J Rheumatol 1984;11:480.
5. Averbuch-Heller L, Steiner I, Abramsky O. Neurologic manifestations of progressive systemic sclerosis. Arch Neurol 1992;49:1292.
6. Pawlowski A. The nerve network of the skin in diffuse scleroderma and clinically similar disorders. Arch Dermatol 1963;88:868.
7. Beighton P, Gumpel JM, Cornes NGC. Prodromal trigeminal sensory neuropathy in progressive systemic sclerosis. Ann Rheum Dis 1968;27:367.
8. Burke MJ, Carty JE. Trigeminal neuropathy as the presenting symptom of systemic sclerosis. Postgrad Med J 1979;55:423.
9. Teasdale R, Frayha RA, Shulman LE. Cranial nerve involvement in systemic sclerosis (scleroderma): A report of 10 cases. Medicine 1980;59:149.
10. Farrell DA, Medsger TA. Trigeminal neuropathy in progressive systemic sclerosis. Am J Med 1982;73:57.
11. Lecky BRF, Hughes RAC, Murray NMF. Trigeminal neuropathy. Brain 1987;110:1463.
12. Agarwal R, Vasan RS, Singh RR, et al. Trigeminal and peripheral neuropathy in a patient with systemic sclerosis and silicosis. Clin Exp Rheumatol 1987;5:375.
13. Heald A. Progressive systemic sclerosis presenting as a case of trigeminal neuropathy. J Neurol Neurosurg Psychiatry 1989;52:918.
14. Berth-Jones J, Coates PAA, Graham-Brown RAC, Burns DA. Neurological complications of systemic sclerosis—a report of three cases and review of the literature. Clin Exp Dermatol 1990;15:91.
15. Vicente A, Herrero C, Martin E, et al. Trigeminal sensory-neuropathy in systemic sclerosis. Clin Exp Dermatol 1991;16:403.
16. Subcommittee for Scleroderma Criteria of the American Rheumatism Association Diagnostic and Therapeutic Criteria Committee. Preliminary criteria for the classification of systemic sclerosis (scleroderma). Arthritis Rheum 1980;23:581.
17. Richter RB. Peripheral neuropathy and connective tissue disease. J Neuropathol Exp Neurol 1954;13:168.
18. Kibler RF, Rose FC. Peripheral neuropathy in the "collagen diseases." Br Med J 1960;1:1781.
19. Di Trapani G, Pocchiari M, Masullo C, et al. Peripheral neuropathy in the course of progressive systemic sclerosis. Ital J Neurol Sci 1982;4:341.
20. Di Trapani G, Tulli A, La Cara A, et al. Peripheral neuropathy in course of progressive systemic sclerosis. Acta Neuropathol (Berl) 1986;72:103.
21. Subenik S, Abarbanel JM, Buskila D, et al. Impotence, carpal tunnel syndrome and peripheral neuropathy as presenting symptoms in progressive systemic sclerosis. J Rheumatol 1987;14:641.
22. Oddis CV, Eisenbeis CH, Reidbord HE, et al. Vasculitis in systemic sclerosis: Association with Sjögren's syndrome and the CREST syndrome variant. J Rheumatol 1987;14:942.
23. Kaufmann J, Canoso JJ. Progressive systemic sclerosis and meralgia paraesthetica. Ann Intern Med 1986;105:973.
24. Leichenko T, Herrick AL, Alani SM, Hilton RC, Jayson MIV. Mononeuritis in two patients with limited cutaneous systemic sclerosis. Br J Rheumatol 1994;33:594.
25. Schady W, Sheard A, Hassell A, et al. Peripheral nerve dysfunction in scleroderma. QJM 1991;292:661.
26. Bjerregaard B, Hojgaard K. Neurological symptoms in scleroderma. Arch Dermatol 1976;112:1030.
27. Lee JE, Haynes JM. Carotid arteritis and cerebral infarction due to scleroderma. Neurology 1967;17:18.
28. Estey E, Leiberman A, Pinto R, et al. Cerebral arteritis in scleroderma. Stroke 1979;10:595.
29. Pathak R, Gabor A. Scleroderma and central nervous system vasculitis. Stroke 1991;22:410.
30. Herrick AL, Oogarah P, Brammah TB, Freemont

AJ, Jayson MIV. Nervous system involvement in association with vasculitis and anticardiolipin antibodies in a patient with systemic sclerosis. Ann Rheum Dis 1994;53:349.

31. Lie JT. Vasculopathy in the antiphospholipid syndrome: Thrombosis or vasculitis, or both? J Rheumatol 1989;16:713.

32. Alarcon-Segovia D, Cardiel MH, Reyes E. Antiphospholipid arterial vasculopathy. J Rheumatol 1989;16:762.

33. Rallings P, Exner T, Abraham R. Coronary artery vasculitis and myocardial infarction associated with antiphospholipid antibodies in a pregnant woman. Aust NZ J Med 1989;19:347.

34. Reyes E, Alarcon-Segovia D. Leg ulcers in the primary antiphospholipid syndrome. Report of a case with a peculiar proliferative small vessel vasculopathy. Clin Exp Rheumatol 1991;9:63.

35. Sonnex C, Paice E, White AG. Autonomic neuropathy in systemic sclerosis: A case report and evaluation of six patients. Ann Rheum Dis 1986;45:957.

36. Klimiuk PS, Taylor L, Baker RD, Jayson MIV. Autonomic neuropathy in systemic sclerosis. Ann Rheum Dis 1988;47:542.

37. Gledhill RF, Dessein PH, Van der Merwe CA. Treatment of Raynaud's phenomenon with tri-iodothyronine corrects co-existent autonomic dysfunction: Preliminary findings. Postgrad Med J 1992;68:263.

38. Anonymous. Pathophysiology of Raynaud's phenomenon. Br Med J 1980;281:1027.

39. Cohen S, Laufer I, Snape WJ, et al. The gastrointestinal manifestations of scleroderma: Pathogenesis and management. Gastroenterology 1980;79:155.

40. Greydanus MP, Camilleri M. Abnormal postcibal antral and small bowel motility due to neuropathy or myopathy in systemic sclerosis. Gastroenterology 1989;96:110.

41. Whitehead WE, Taitelbaum G, Wigley FM, Schuster MM. Rectosigmoid motility and myoelectric activity in progressive systemic sclerosis. Gastroenterology 1989;96:428.

42. Leighton JA, Valdovinos MA, Pemberton JH, et al. Anorectal dysfunction and rectal prolapse in progressive systemic sclerosis. Dis Colon Rectum 1993;36:182.

43. Lally EV, Jimenez SA. Impotence in progressive systemic sclerosis. Ann Intern Med 1981;95:150.

44. Klein LE, Posner MS. Progressive systemic sclerosis and impotence. Ann Intern Med 1981;95:658.

45. Nowlin NS, Brick JE, Weaver DJ, et al. Impotence in scleroderma. Ann Intern Med 1986;104:794.

46. Campbell PM, LeRoy EC. Pathogenesis of systemic sclerosis: A vascular hypothesis. Semin Arthritis Rheum 1975;4:351.

GEOFFREY C. JIRANEK
JAMES E. BREDFELT

22

Organ Involvement: Gut and Hepatic Manifestations

Overview

This chapter reviews the gastrointestinal (GI) manifestations of systemic sclerosis (SSc), from the esophagus through the colon, as well as the hepatic manifestations of this disease.

SSc has frequent and diverse GI manifestations. The hallmark pathologic abnormality is atrophy of smooth muscle and fibrosis in the gut wall. The resultant failure of orderly muscle contraction can profoundly affect every segment of the digestive tract from the esophagus to the anus. An estimated 90% of patients with SSc have detectable GI involvement making it the most common visceral manifestation. Of these patients, 50% have clinically important manifestations (Table 22.1). Involvement of the gut occurs with equal frequency in diffuse and limited subtypes of SSc (1), but it occurs only rarely in the localized scleroderma syndromes (2).

Mortality from GI disease occurs less frequently than cardiopulmonary or renal disease in SSc. Nevertheless, in a large series of 264 patients with diffuse SSc who were followed for 7 years, 5% died directly from GI complications (3). Malabsorption and significant esophageal dysfunction are associated with a poorer prognosis (3).

Evidence for liver disease in patients with SSc is unusual and is identified in less than 10% of cases (4,5). Primary biliary cirrhosis (PBC) is the liver disorder identified most frequently in pa-

tients with SSc (6–8). Two additional but rare liver disorders, nodular regenerative hyperplasia of the liver and idiopathic portal hypertension, are reported only as isolated cases (9–11). These two liver disorders will result in a non-cirrhotic form of portal hypertension that can lead to the development of esophageal varices with the potential for hemorrhage and the formation of ascites. These disorders are so rare and data are so fragmentary in SSc that they will not be discussed further in this chapter.

PBC is a chronic progressive cholestatic liver disease characterized by destruction of intrahepatic bile ducts, inflammation within the portal tracts, and the development of fibrosis, leading to cirrhosis (12). Patients with PBC often will have another immune-related disease, suggesting that PBC may have an autoimmune etiology. In a study from the Mayo Clinic evaluating 113 patients with PBC, 84% of the patients had at least one other autoimmune disorder, while 41% had two or more disorders (13). Twenty of these patients (18%) had SSc or one of its variants, including nine with Raynaud's phenomenon (RP), eight with CREST syndrome, and three with classic SSc. The acronym, PACK (*P*rimary biliary cirrhosis, *A*nticentromere antibody, *C*REST syndrome and *K*eratoconjunctivitis sicca) has been proposed to identify a syndrome encompassing PBC and CREST syndrome (14). The specific autoantibody for PBC, and antimitochondrial antibody (AMA), is

453

Table 22.1. Gastrointestinal and Hepatic Manifestations Associated with Systemic Sclerosis

Esophageal dysmotility	Motor dysphagia
	Gastroesophageal reflux
Gastric dysmotility	Gastroparesis
Small bowel dysmotility	Pseudo-obstruction
	Malabsorption
	Pneumatosis cystoides intestinalis
Colorectal dysmotility	Constipation
	Pseudo-obstruction
	Pneumatosis cystoides coli
	Rectal prolapse
	Incontinence
Gut telangiectasia	Gastrointestinal hemorrhage
Liver disease	Primary buliary cirrhosis
	Nodular regenerative hyperplasia of the liver
	Idiopathic portal hyper tension

identified in 8% of patients with CREST syndrome (15).

Pathophysiology

GASTROINTESTINAL

The precise cause of smooth muscle atrophy and fibrosis of the GI tract in SSc is unknown. Abnormalities in the vascular wall, in the immune system, and in the control of collagen synthesis have been hypothesized. Small vessels are regulated by neurohumoral, inflammatory, and physical mediators. The neurohumoral mediators include acetylcholine, norepinephrine, bradykinin, arachidonic acid metabolites, endothelin, and nitric oxide. Inflammatory mediators include cytokines and physical mediators include cold temperature and trauma. These mediators along with endothelial cells, fibroblasts, and mast cells participate in complex interactions, which result in small vessel microvascular insufficiency and GI neuromuscular dysfunction and fibrosis.

Smooth muscle atrophy and fibrosis disrupt the normal, highly regulated transit of intraluminal contents. The strength of smooth muscle contractions is reduced, and propulsive force to move chyme through the bowel is diminished. Specialized areas, such as the gastric antrum (where food is broken into small particles) and the small intestine (where segmenting contractions facilitate mixing), can become dysfunctional.

Abnormalities of intestinal muscle contraction have been documented in the absence of overt pathologic changes of muscle atrophy and fibrosis (16–18). These abnormalities are thought to represent neurologic dysfunction of the myenteric plexus located between muscle layers in the gut wall. The pattern of disordered muscular hyperactivity implies neurogenic dysfunction and is thought to occur at an earlier stage in SSc than the decreased muscular activity which characterizes late SSc (19). Many patients with SSc demonstrate normal muscle contraction to direct muscle agonists, such as methacholine, but decreased contraction to agents which act through neural input to muscle, such as gastrin and edrophonium (18). Microvascular injury to neural input to muscle is a postulated mechanism of early GI dysmotility in SSc. The pathologic correlate of neural injury has yet to be reported.

HEPATIC

A vast array of immunologic abnormalities have been identified in patients with PBC (Table 22.2) (12). Most of these abnormalities are nonspecific and are likely a secondary immunologic phenomenon. The exact pathogenesis of PBC remains to be unraveled. The central theme in PBC is the presumed immune mediated destruction of intrahepatic bile ducts and the presence of AMA.

Several lines of evidence have provided a model for our understanding of the immunologic destruction of bile ducts and the possible autoimmune nature of the disease. First, aberrant expression of major histocompatibility complex (MHC) class II antigens is present on the surface of the bile duct epithelium and HLA-DR, -DQ, and -DP antigens are displayed (20,21). These MHC class II antigens are not found on normal bile duct epithelium, and only class I antigens are identified in experimental models for cholestasis (22). In the early stages of PBC, the expression of class II antigens tends to be multifocal, while its distribution becomes uniform in advanced histologic stages. These aberrant class II antigens provide a good target for activated T-lymphocytes. Assisting with this interaction is an increased expression of intercellular adhesion molecule-1 on liver tissue from patients with PBC (23).

Second, a dense aggregation of lymphocytes is invariably present within the portal tracts surrounding the injured bile ducts. In early stage disease, the T-lymphocytes, lying in close proximity to the injured bile duct epithelium, are found to be CD8+ (24,25), while the predominant T-lymphocytes found in advanced histologic stages from the livers of patients undergoing liver transplantation were CD3+, CD4+, and CD8− (26). Cytotoxic lymphocytes appear to play an important role in mediating the bile duct injury, although it is uncertain if the phenotype differences found between early and late histologic stages have importance for the functional capabilities of the T cells.

Third, a reduced generation of lymphokines (such as lymphotoxin, tumor necrosis factor, and interferon-gamma) by peripheral blood lymphocytes has been identified in patients with PBC (27,28). Additionally, the production of interleukin-2 is reduced in these patients and that may result in the diminished lymphokine formation (29). In early histologic stages when the immune responsiveness is considered at its greatest, lymphokine production was found to be reduced whereas its production was within the normal range in advanced histologic stages, especially cirrhosis (27). It is of interest that lymphokine generation is abnormally low in other autoimmune disorders (30).

The AMA, determined by indirect immunofluorescent staining of rat kidney, was first noted to be a unique autoantibody for PBC approximately 30 years ago (31,32). A family of mitochondrial antibodies has subsequently been identified (Table 22.3) (33). Recently, the M2 antibody has been shown to have a high degree of specificity and sensitivity for PBC (33). The M4, M8, and M9 antibodies are also found in PBC. While the findings are not conclusive, it has been suggested that the M4 and M8 antibodies may be associated with a more progressive disease (34,35), while the M9 antibody may be found in earlier stages of the disease (36,37).

The M2 antigen has been localized to the inner mitochondrial membrane surface of the pyruvate dehydrogenase complex (38–40). This complex has four subcomponents: E1, E2, E3, and protein X. The M2 antigen is a 70 kD protein directly linked with the E2 subunit (dihydrolipoamide acetyltransferase) (38,39). An ELISA

Table 22.2. Immunologic Abnormalities in Primary Biliary Cirrhosis

Elevated serum IgM level
Skin test anergy
Granulomas of liver and lymph nodes
Circulating immune complexes
Increased turnover of serum complement
Activated peripheral blood T and B lymphocytes
Autoantibodies
   - Antimitochondrial antibody
   - Antinuclear antibody
   - Anti-Ro antibody
   - Anticentromere antibody
   - Anti-neutrophil cytoplasmic antibody

Table 22.3. Classification of Antimitochondrial Antibodies (AMA)

AMA Type	Clinical Disease
M1	Secondary syphilis
M2	Primary biliary cirrhosis
M3	Drug-induced pseudolupus
M4	Primary biliary cirrhosis
M5	Collagen vascular diseases
M6	Iproniazid-induced hepatitis
M7	Myocarditis
M8	Primary biliary cirrhosis
M9	Primary biliary cirrhosis

assay has been developed against the E2 and protein X antigens that is highly specific for the diagnosis of PBC (41–43). In preliminary studies, the titer correlated with the histologic stage of PBC and the levels of serum bilirubin and albumin. It remains unknown what role the AMA has in either initiating or perpetuating the disease process of PBC (44,45).

Pathology

GASTROINTESTINAL

The characteristic GI abnormality in SSc is smooth muscle atrophy and fibrosis (Fig. 22.1). Smooth muscle atrophy is initially quite patchy with normal myocytes located next to areas of myocyte dropout. With progression, atrophy becomes more diffuse. The inner circular layer of the *muscularis propria* is affected more than the outer longitudinal layer. Cell contacts between myocytes are disrupted. Vacuolization of muscle, characteristic of other myopathies, is not found. Skeletal muscle is generally normal without atrophy. Fibrosis without many inflammatory cells is found in the *lamina propria* of the mucosa in the submucosa and in the *muscularis propria*. The myenteric plexus, which contains abundant nerves located between muscle layers, is usually normal although eosinophilic and mast cell infiltration has been reported. Microvascular abnormalities are frequent. Small arteries have disrupted internal elastic lining, and there is myointimal proliferation with a narrowed irregular lumen. Endothelial cells swell and proliferate with abnormal nuclei and mitochondria. The capillary basement membrane is thick and laminated (46,47).

In a large autopsy series, the frequency of

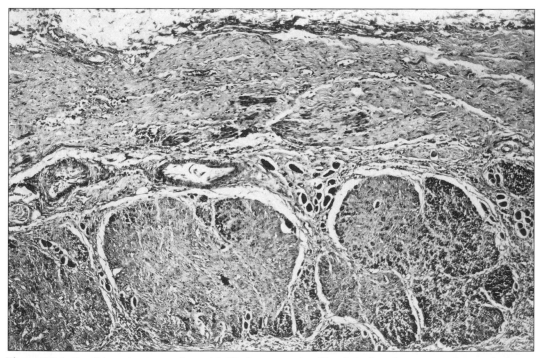

Figure 22.1. Small intestine in a patient with SSc demonstrating fibrosis in the submucosa and muscularis propria with patchy myocyte atrophy in the muscularis propria (Masson trichrome).

muscle atrophy and fibrosis of GI organs is shown in Table 22.4 (48). In the esophagus, fibrosis and smooth muscle atrophy is generally limited to the distal two-thirds, because the proximal one-third is skeletal muscle. Mucosal infiltration with polymorphonuclear leukocytes and eosinophils is frequently noted along with erosion and ulceration in the distal esophagus. Distal esophageal stricture is common and the esophagus is often dilated. Multiple wide mouth esophageal diverticula occur rarely in SSc. The stomach is infrequently dilated and gastric wall fibrosis and muscle atrophy is uncommon. Pyloric stenosis from marked fibrosis without ulceration has been rarely reported (49).

Small intestinal involvement tends to be patchy but most frequent and severe in the duodenum, intermediate in the jejunum, and least in the ileum. Dilation of bowel occurs often without lengthening or stretching the transverse folds *(valvulae conniventes)*. Uneven binding of stretched folds can provide a high-bound appearance. Large diverticula and sacculations occur at extended areas of muscle atrophy (50). Villi are generally normal but may be mildly shortened (51). Jejunal epithelial cells can have cytoplasmic condensations of cholesterol clefts and fat droplets. Fibrous encapsulation around Brunner's glands (52) and intestinal lymphangiectasia are occasionally noted. *Pneumatosis cystoides intestinalis* can occur with gas filled cysts in the submucosa or subserosa. In the colon, wide mouth "kettle drum" diverticula and sacculations are occasionally present, especially in the transverse and descending segments. The colon wall between diverticula is often rigid with thick folds. Megacolon coli can occur.

Table 22.4. Muscle Atrophy and Fibrosis in Systemic Sclerosis (Autopsy Series)

Esophagus	74%
Stomach	10%
Small Intestine	48%
Large Intestine	39%

HEPATIC

The histologic hallmark of PBC is injury to both septal and intralobular bile ducts. The so-called florid duct lesion (nonsuppurative destructive cholangitis) is the classical histologic lesion in PBC (Fig. 22.2) (53–55). Four histologic stages of PBC are defined. The stages are determined by the degree of lymphocytic infiltration within the portal tracts and the amount of developing fibrosis. It is not necessary for a florid duct lesion to be present to stage or to diagnose the disease. Stage 1 is the initial lesion and tends to be focal in nature. The portal tracts are expanded with a lymphocytic infiltrate but the limiting plate remains intact (portal hepatitis). Fibrosis usually is not present. Stage 2 lesions show erosion of the limiting plate with piecemeal necrosis (periportal hepatitis) and portal fibrosis may be found. Stage 3 disease reveals the progression of bridging necrosis, often with fibrous septa. Stage 4 disease shows the completed progression to cirrhosis. Since the histologic abnormalities, especially in the early stages, tend to be focal, it is important that the biopsy specimen contains at least 10 portal tracts to ensure that sampling error has not occurred.

Other ancillary histologic findings include granulomas, stainable copper, and Mallory hyalin (53). Granulomas are often present in early stage disease and may imply a less aggressive clinical course (56). Occasionally, the presence of granulomas may require the exclusion of sarcoidosis (57). None of these ancillary features are required for the histologic diagnosis of PBC.

Clinical Features

ESOPHAGUS: MOTOR DYSPHAGIA

Neuromuscular esophageal dysphagia is a frequent symptom in patients with SSc that results from a failure of esophageal muscle to adequately propel and empty intraluminal contents into the stomach. In health, coordinated esophageal motor activity results in primary peristalsis (the

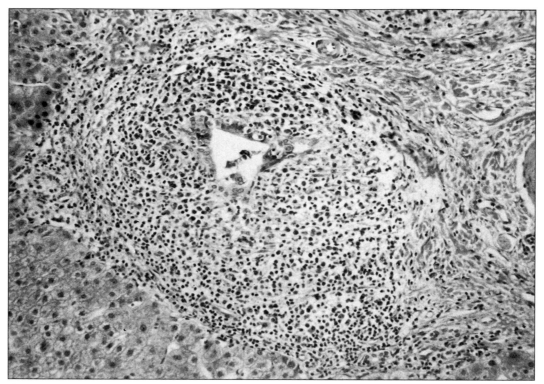

Figure 22.2. Portal triad is markedly expanded with lymphocytes. Bile duct *(center)* is undergoing an asymmetrical destruction, the "florid duct" lesion (hematoxylin and eosin, ×100).

classic "stripping" wave of contraction that proceeds distally down the esophagus initiated by swallowing) and secondary peristalsis (a similar contraction which is induced not by a swallow but by sensory stimulation from an incompletely cleared swallowed bolus or distension from gastroesophageal reflux). The lower esophageal sphincter (LES) normally remains tonically contracted but relaxes during peristalsis to facilitate esophageal emptying into the stomach. In 80% to 90% of SSc patients, abnormalities of esophageal motor activity are detectable by esophageal manometry. These include decreased strength or total absence of primary and secondary peristalsis and decreased or absent LES tone. Active simultaneous (nonperistaltic) esophageal body contraction and failure of LES relaxation on swallowing are occasionally noted (58) and are

thought to represent "early" involvement suggestive of neurologic dysfunction. When the esophageal smooth muscle is extensively atrophic and fibrotic, it is easy to conceptualize why transit is disturbed in a flaccid esophagus.

A careful history revealing that both solids and liquids produce symptoms suggests esophageal neuromuscular dysphagia. Patients may find that straightening the back and lifting the arms allows the bolus to pass. In SSc, most patients have only mild motor dysphagia because the LES tone is usually decreased. Very rare patients with SSc have more severe motor dysphagia when the LES fails to relax in a pattern similar to achalasia (58). Motor dysphagia is equally common in diffuse and limited subtypes of SSc (59). In patients with SSc, a positive antinuclear antibody (ANA) predicts worsened esophageal hypomotility (59). Some patients have minimal or no motor dysphagia symptoms despite abnormal esophageal manometry.

Oropharyngeal dysphagia (impaired passage of food from the mouth to the esophagus) was once thought to be very rare in patients with SSc, because the pharyngeal and proximal esophageal muscle is striated rather than smooth. However, dysfunction such as oral leakage, retention, penetration, aspiration, and upper esophageal sphincter incoordination occurs in up to 25% of SSc when carefully studied (60–62). The prevalence and severity is much less than esophageal body involvement. The symptoms of oropharyngeal dysphagia include a sense of food sticking in the throat, nasal regurgitation, and coughing on swallowing.

Raynaud's phenomenon (RP) correlates closely with esophageal dysfunction in patients with SSc (63–66). Esophageal motility, however, is unchanged during a cold pressor test (hand immersion in ice water) in patients with Raynaud's and SSc (67,68). Patients with Raynaud's and SSc have decreased esophageal blood flow compared to patients with Raynaud's without SSc.

ESOPHAGUS: GASTROESOPHAGEAL REFLUX

Gastroesophageal reflux is the most common clinically recognized GI abnormality in SSc. Fifty to sixty-five percent of patients with SSc have significant symptoms, such as heartburn and regurgitation, or complications related to reflux (64, 66,69–71). Heartburn (pyrosis) is described by such terms as "acid regurgitation," "sour stomach," "indigestion," and "hot chest." The patient often signifies the description with an open hand moving from the epigastric area to the throat. Temporary relief of symptoms by antacids is typical. Heartburn can occasionally result in atypical chest pains. Some of the most severe gastroesophageal reflux encountered in clinical practice occurs in patients with SSc. The correlation between symptoms and objective tests is only mod-

erate. It is not unusual to identify patients with SSc who have severe gastroesophageal reflux with extensive esophageal ulceration and yet have minimal or no symptoms.

Gastroesophageal reflux is found in equal frequency in diffuse and limited subtypes of SSc (1,59,72). Some (2,59) but not all (72) studies have indicated that the diffuse SSc subtype has very severe reflux more frequently than the limited subtype. Esophageal involvement can occur before typical cutaneous manifestations of SSc in up to 10% of cases (73). Rarely, cutaneous manifestations never develop despite typical esophageal pathology. This situation is known as systemic sclerosis sine scleroderma. Esophageal dysfunction is frequently (74,75), but not necessarily (76) progressive.

In patients with SSc, many potential abnormalities contribute to gastroesophageal reflux. First, in 30% to 50% of patients, the LES is weak and, in advanced cases, is undetectable (17). Thus, a prime barrier against reflux is lost. Second, secondary peristalsis is reduced in amplitude or may be absent. Loss of secondary peristalsis is a critically important factor disabling the esophagus to clear itself from refluxed gastric contents. In patients with SSc, the total time that acid resides in the lower esophagus correlates better with the degree of impaired peristalsis than the degree of impaired LES pressure (72). Patients with severe esophagitis and SSc have fewer but longer reflux events compared to patients with equally severe esophagitis and LES dysfunction who did not have SSc (77). Third, impaired gastric emptying may result from gastric involvement (78). In patients with SSc who have equivalent esophageal manometry, acid is found longer in the distal esophagus in those who have slower gastric emptying and less gastric myoelectric activity (79). In contrast, abnormal gastric emptying does not always predict esophagitis (2). Fourth, on rare occasions, patients with SSc may have Sjögren's syndrome as well (80). In these patients, the marked decrease in salivary secretion causes less acid neutralizing bicarbonate rich fluid to enter the esophagus. Fifth, some medications, such as calcium blockers used for Raynaud's, weaken the LES. This effect is inconsequential, however, in patients with very low or absent LES tone. Finally, acid secretion is increased in some patients with SSc (81) but studies of acid secretion in SSc have yielded inconsistent results (82).

In addition to heartburn, gastroesophageal reflux can lead to many varied complications. A stricture in the lower esophagus occurs in 40% of patients with SSc who have gastroesophageal reflux (63,83). Only 10% of patients with reflux who do not have SSc develop an esophageal stricture (84). Increased hydroxyproline is found in esophageal mucosa in patients with SSc and may explain why strictures are relatively common (85). An esophageal stricture typically causes progressive and predictable dysphagia to solid foods only. It can be quite severe and associated with weight loss because of diminished food intake. Food impaction in the stricture can present as an emergency with a distressed patient choking and coughing and unable to handle salivary secretions. Erosion and ulceration occurs in the esophagus in 60% of patients with SSc (83). Bleeding from ulceration is uncommon and perforation is quite rare, but both are potentially life threatening. A truly severe and literal form of "heart burn" has been reported in a patient with SSc who had an esophageal atrial fistula from a deep ulcer (86).

Barrett's metaplasia is a premalignant change in the mucosa of the esophagus, which is reported in increased frequency in patients with SSc (87–95). In Barrett's metaplasia, the normal squamous epithelium is replaced by columnar epithelium as a response to gastroesophageal reflux. There is migration of the squamous columnar junction from the gastroesophageal junction to a more proximal location in the esophagus. Barrett's metaplasia produces no distinctive clinical symptoms but is important because one esophageal adenocarcinoma may develop during approximately 200 patient-years. In one series of patients with SSc who had upper endoscopy, 30% were found to have Barrett's metaplasia

(95), which is higher than published rates of 4% to 13% of Barrett's in patients who had endoscopy for reflux who did not have SSc. Six patients with adenocarcinoma complicating Barrett's in SSc have been reported, but this may not be increased compared to the general population. In a retrospective study of 680 patients with SSc over an 11-year period, only one case of esophageal adenocarcinoma was found (96). Another retrospective study with 2,001 patient-years at risk found no esophageal cancer (97). Premature death in patients with SSc from other causes (3) may not allow full expression of the adenocarcinoma risk in Barrett's metaplasia.

Candida is found frequently in the esophagus in patients with SSc, especially if there are erosions, ulcerations, or stricture (83,98). Candidiasis probably results from esophageal stasis and the use of potent acid elimination medication (99). Treatment with antifungal medication, such as nystatin and fluconazole, eliminates candida in many patients with SSc, but symptoms and esophagitis are generally unchanged and candida typically recurs after antimicrobial therapy is stopped (83,99). Very rare patients with SSc may have invasive candida which would benefit from antifungal therapy.

Extra-esophageal presentations of gastroesophageal reflux are often overlooked in patients with SSc. Microaspiration of refluxed contents can lead to pulmonary infections, coughing, wheezing, and hoarseness. Chronic aspiration can lead to pulmonary fibrosis. Since pulmonary disease is a major source of morbidity and mortality in SSc, it is important to consider gastroesophageal reflux even in patients who do not complain of heartburn. A strong correlation was found in 13 patients with SSc between the amount of time when acid was in the esophagus and the total lung diffusion capacity measured by inspiring a single breath of carbon monoxide (DLCO) (99). Furthermore, 11 of these 13 patients had proximal esophagitis on upper endoscopy and 12 of 13 had laryngeal changes consistent with aspiration (99). Oropharyngeal dysfunction correlates with pulmonary dysfunction in patients with SSc (61). When esophageal dysfunction is very severe and there is extensive gastroesophageal reflux, the upper esophageal sphincter pressure is often reduced in SSc (72) in a situation where it is needed the most. Asthma is another pulmonary complication that can result from reflux. Wheezing at night, after recumbency, after meals, and occurring in mid-life without allergies all suggest the possibility of reflux. Bronchoconstriction can occur from microaspiration or through a neural reflex from stimulation of vagal afferent fibers in the esophagus. In patients with reflux, attempts to treat asthma with theophylline, beta-agonists, and anticholinergic agents can worsen bronchoconstriction since each agent lowers LES and esophageal body pressures, promoting more reflux.

STOMACH

Delayed gastric emptying has been previously reported to be infrequent in SSc (69,73,100,101). More recent studies using more sophisticated techniques demonstrate that gastroparesis is common in SSc, occurring in up to 75% of patients (78,79,83,102–104). The symptoms of delayed gastric emptying are meal related and include: early satiety, nausea, vomiting, bloating, distension, and abdominal discomfort. These symptoms are not specific to the stomach and may be attributed to the small or large intestine. Many patients with gastroparesis have symptoms previously diagnosed as "non-ulcer dyspepsia," "gastritis," "food intolerances," or "functional bowel disorder." The consequences of severe gastroparesis include dehydration, electrolyte disturbance, malnutrition, and weight loss. A succussion splash elicited 6 hours after a meal is an important physical exam finding indicative of gastroparesis. Slow gastric emptying in SSc occurs because of neuromuscular dysfunction in the vast majority of cases, but fibrous replacement of the pyloric muscle with stricture has been reported (49,105).

Gastric emptying is under complex neurohormonal control. The proximal stomach has tonic contractile activity. This activity gradually falls during feeding to accommodate a meal and is termed "receptive relaxation." The level of proximal stomach tone controls the rate of gastric emptying. The distal muscular stomach (antrum) plays an important role in solid food emptying by grinding food until it is reduced to small (2mm or less) particles, which is the maximum size that the pylorus will allow to pass through into the duodenum during feeding. During fasting, contractile activity of the stomach and small bowel is characterized by migrating motor complexes (MMC). Phase 1 of MMC has quiescent motor activity, phase 2 has irregular phasic contractile activity, and phase 3 has strong propulsive contractions in regular frequencies, which slowly sweep distally from the stomach to the distal small bowel.

In patients with SSc, solid food gastric emptying is more frequently and severely prolonged than liquid food gastric emptying (78). Most patients with bloating have delayed solid food gastric emptying, but the symptom severity does not correlate well with the magnitude of delay (78). Several patients with SSc who have delayed gastric emptying do not have significant gastroparetic symptoms. Phase 3 MMC activity during fasting is markedly reduced in patients with SSc, especially if there is gastroparesis or esophagitis (79,102,104). Incoordination of motor activity between the stomach and duodenum is common (102). During feeding, some patients have decreased amplitude and frequency of antroduodenal contractions (myopathy pattern), while others have excessive nonpropulsive tonic activity (neuropathy pattern) (104). Small (2–3 mm) particles empty normally, while cellulose empties slower than normal in patients with SSc (103).

SMALL INTESTINE

The small intestine is the second most frequently affected portion of the GI tract in SSc. Pseudo-obstruction, malabsorption, and *pneumatosis cystoides intestinalis* are important manifestations of SSc. Small bowel dysmotility is common and results in symptoms of nausea, vomiting, bloating, distension, anorexia, malnutrition (71,106), weight loss, and abdominal pain. At one extreme, dysmotility is mild with minimal symptoms, and at the other extreme, chronic intestinal pseudo-obstruction exists. Pseudo-obstruction occurs where there is such ineffective propulsion of chyme that signs and symptoms of intestinal obstruction exist in the absence of mechanical obstruction. In patients with pseudo-obstruction, the GI tract may not permit any food intake. SSc is the most common cause of chronic secondary intestinal pseudo-obstruction (107).

In SSc, some patients with symptoms of small bowel dysmotility have decreased amplitude and frequencies of duodenal contractions, presumably from muscle dysfunction due to atrophy and fibrosis (48). In other patients with SSc who do not have small bowel symptoms, a more subtle abnormality can be detected. In these patients, the baseline frequencies and velocities of propagation of slow waves are normal with normal contractions. However, instillation of normal saline into the duodenum fails to elicit the normal marked increase in slow waves and their corresponding contractions (108). This finding is consistent with the hypothesis that neurogenic defects precede symptoms and myogenic defects. Uncoordinated bursts of tonic elevations of baseline pressure are noted in patients with SSc indicative of neuropathy.

Malabsorption occurs in up to 50% of patients with SSc and is generally caused by bacterial overgrowth (59,109), although intestinal lymphangiectasis is also reported (110,111). Malabsorption appears to be more common in diffuse SSc compared to limited SSc (59), and a positive ANA is a marker for increased rates of fat malabsorption (59). Bacterial overgrowth occurs in patients with SSc because of intestinal stasis and also because of multiple or large diverticula and sacculations. Phase 3 MMCs, which are likened to a "housekeeper" sweeping down the intestine during fasting, are absent in some patients with SSc, allowing bacteria to proliferate.

Diverticula and sacculations serve as a reservoir of bacteria that fail to empty. In patients with SSc who have small bowel dysmotility and reduced or absent MMCs, the hormone motilin is increased (112). Motilin normally increases in concentration when phase 3 MMCs occur.

Small bowel bacteria deconjugate bile salts, which impedes the formation of micelles causing inefficient delivery of monoglycerides, fatty acids, and fat soluble vitamins to small bowel mucosa. Bacterial overgrowth can also damage mucosal villi reducing the absorptive surface. In intestinal lymphangiectasia, there is a block in the transfer of absorbed nutrients in the gut wall to the general circulation via the lymphatics. The clinical consequences of malabsorption and bacterial overgrowth include diarrhea, nausea, vomiting, weight loss, and malnutrition. Malabsorption of medications also occurs. For example, D-penicillamine used to treat SSc is absorbed less, and rarely not at all, in patients with SSc (113,114).

Pneumatosis cystoides intestinalis occurs occasionally in SSc in patients who typically have advanced intestinal disease (115). Bacterial overgrowth and distended small intestine are frequent coexisting conditions (116). Mucosal tears have been hypothesized to permit intraluminal gas to dissect into the wall. Gas filled cysts are most common in the ileum and generally spare the mesentery. The cysts are partly lined by epithelium and are infiltrated by macrophages and giant cells. Cysts can rupture into the peritoneum creating pneumoperitoneum (47). Many patients with *pneumatosis cystoides intestinalis,* including some with pneumoperitoneum, are asymptomatic. Symptoms can include abdominal pain, distension, and nausea, but these may be caused by underlying intestinal dysmotility. The abdomen is often nontender or has variable tenderness, but peritoneal signs are typically absent. The most important clinical feature of *pneumatosis cystoides intestinales* is recognition that the cysts are usually benign, and pneumoperitoneum is not an indication for laparotomy if there are no signs of peritonitis (117–120).

Pneumatosis cystoides intestinalis can resolve acutely or remain chronically, with cysts demonstrated for more than 1 year in some patients (118). Pneumoperitoneum can occur without pneumatosis cystoides intestinalis (121). In a large series of patients with pneumatosis cystoides intestinalis, SSc was the most common underlying disorder accounting for approximately 20% of cases (122). Pneumocystis cystoides intestinalis is associated with a poor prognosis in SSc, with four deaths in 11 patients within 6 months in one series (122).

COLON AND ANORECTUM

The colon frequently has varying degrees of slow transit dysmotility in SSc (103). Constipation is relatively frequent while obstipation and colonic pseudo-obstruction occur only occasionally, especially in the setting of megacolon (123–126). Obstruction can occur from fecal impaction (127), and there is one report of a life-threatening barium impaction as a consequence of a prior contrast study (128). Constipation can cause a stercoral ulcer, which can perforate (129). Other rarely reported colon abnormalities in SSc include: collagenous colitis (130), acute ischemia leading to stenosis (131), infarction (132), and a stenosis mimicking a carcinoma (133). Diarrhea occurs in patients with SSc but is most often related to small bowel dysfunction and malabsorption than colonic involvement.

Volvulus is reported in increased frequency in SSc and tends to occur in the transverse colon (134,135) and the sigmoid colon (126,136). Pneumatosis cystoides coli occurs less frequently that pneumatosis cystoides intestinalis but tends to occur together with similar clinical features. Large wide-mouth diverticula are common in SSc, occurring in up to 50% of patients (137). These true diverticula contain all three layers of the wall, but the muscularis layer is markedly atrophic, which allows their formation. These diverticula have a unique predilection for the antimesenteric border of the transverse and descending portions of the colon (50,100,138,

139). Diverticula form between rigid areas of the colon wall. Impaction of stool into diverticula can rarely occur causing colon obstruction, but diverticulitis and hemorrhage have not been reported. There has been one case report of colonic diverticular perforation (140). The vast majority of colon diverticula are clinically silent in SSc.

The pathophysiology of colon dysmotility is similar to other segments of the gut in SSc. Some patients do not respond to neostigmine (a direct smooth muscle stimulant) and therefore have myogenic dysfunction on the basis of atrophy and fibrosis. Many other patients respond normally to neostigmine and have normal spike potentials (the electric correlate of strength of contraction) in the basal state. With feeding, however, the normal marked increase in colon spike potentials fails to occur, indicative of neurologic dysfunction (141). Patients with SSc have low tolerances of rectal balloon distention. Greater rectosigmoid contractile activity occurs after balloon distention in SSc patients than in controls. Diarrhea in these patients correlates with more severe rectosigmoid responses to rectal balloon distention (142).

Fecal incontinence is an occasional but very distressing symptom in patients with SSc. In some cases, rectal prolapse may be an aggravating factor (143). Internal anal sphincter pressure is decreased on average in SSc and is even lower in patients with rectal prolapse and SSc (144). Some patients with SSc have absent internal anal sphincter pressure. Distention of the rectum normally causes the internal anal sphincter to relax. This rectoanal inhibitory reflex is frequently weakened or lost in SSc (144–146). Rectal capacity and compliance decrease in SSc while rectal sensory thresholds increased (146). Prolapse, internal anal dysfunction, and rectal changes are important contributors to fecal incontinence.

VASCULAR ANOMALIES

Telangiectasias are a primary feature in the CREST syndrome (147), which was originally thought to occur primarily in the limited form of

SSc. More recent studies, however, indicate that calcinosis, Raynaud's, esophageal dysmotility, and telangiectasias are equally common in the diffuse and limited subtypes of SSc (148). Telangiectasias are most notable on the skin but have been reported in the esophagus, stomach, small intestine, and colon. Bleeding can occur, most commonly in the stomach and the colon (147–152). Bleeding ranges from occult blood loss causing iron deficiency anemia (149,153) to rapid blood loss requiring emergent diagnosis and therapy.

Gastric antral vascular ectasia, also known as "watermelon stomach" (154) based on its typical endoscopic appearance of bright red streaks radiating from the pylorus in the antrum, is seen occasionally in SSc. In one large series of 45 patients with this disorder, six had SSc and more than 50% had an autoimmune or connective tissue disease (155). Blood loss from gastric antral vascular ectasia is characteristically a slow ooze. The ectasia is thought to develop as a response to injury created by loosely attached antral mucosa prolapsing through the pylorus.

LIVER

The prototypical patient with PBC is a middle-aged female whose clinical presentation is pruritus, a raised serum alkaline phosphatase, and a positive AMA. Ninety percent of patients with PBC are females with the typical age of onset between 30 and 65 years (12). PBC in the infrequent male patients resembles the disease in the female (156). The symptoms and complications of PBC vary from one patient to the next, but, with time, all patients will experience some of the complications (Table 22.5) (12). Three clinical stages of PBC may be defined.

First, the *symptomatic stage* represents the most advanced clinical stage and, in the past, as the classical clinical presentation of PBC (157). These patients will have an intense pruritus, often jaundice, fatigue, and weight loss. In almost every situation, the pruritus will precede the onset of the jaundice. The histologic stage most of-

ten will be stage 3 or 4. Many of these patients in the ensuing few years will develop complications of cirrhosis and portal hypertension.

Second, the *asymptomatic stage* is the one most commonly present at the time of diagnosis in this current era (158,159). The patients are often revealed by the inadvertent finding of an elevated serum alkaline phosphatase. The number of these patients has increased over the past two decades and parallels the widespread use of multichannel biochemical testing. The diagnosis is secured by demonstrating that the alkaline phosphatase is of liver origin in conjunction with the positive AMA and a compatible liver biopsy. The patients will lack symptoms of PBC. The serum alkaline phosphatase levels are quite variable, ranging from slightly above the upper limits of normal to 10 times elevated. The serum bilirubin is usually not increased. The histologic stage more commonly will be 1 or 2, although stage 3, or infrequently stage 4, may be found. The liver histologic stage appears to occur independent from the levels of serum alkaline phosphatase. Over the ensuing decade, the vast majority of these presently asymptomatic patients will be-

Table 22.5. Symptoms and Complications of Primary Biliary Cirrhosis

Pruritus
Jaundice
Fatigue
Weight loss
Steatorrhea
Fat soluble vitamin deficiencies
   -Vitamins A, D, E, and K
Metabolic bone disease
   -Osteopenia
   -Osteomalacia
Hypercholesterolemia
   -Xanthomas
Portal Hypertension
   -Gastroesophageal varices
   -Ascites
   -Portal-systemic encephalopathy
   -Hepatorenal syndrome
   -Hepatopulmonary syndrome
Pulmonary fibrosis
   -Pulmonary hypertension
Intra-abdominal lymphadenopathy
Hepatocellular carcinoma

come symptomatic, and progression of the histologic stage to cirrhosis will occur in approximately two-thirds of them (33).

Finally, the *preclinical stage* represents the earliest observable manifestation of PBC. These patients will have no symptoms of PBC and the serum alkaline phosphatase level will be normal. Most of these patients are uncovered during the course of an evaluation for another autoimmune disorder when a positive AMA is identified. Even though the alkaline phosphatase is normal, the liver histology will be abnormal in over 90% of these patients and will show pathognomonic changes of early PBC (45). When these patients are followed over the next 5 to 10 years, the serum alkaline phosphatase will become elevated in the vast majority and approximately 30% of them will develop symptoms (45).

For most patients with PBC, the diagnosis will be straightforward. Because the AMA has such a high specificity for the disease, it is usually not necessary to visualize the biliary tree by endoscopic retrograde cholangiopancreatography (ERCP). Cholangiography may be required in patients with atypical features, including a negative AMA, or with an inconclusive liver histology.

The long-term prognosis of patients having PBC depends upon several factors. As more patients are currently being identified with PBC who are asymptomatic and have an early histologic stage, it is becoming evident that the natural history of PBC is better measured in decades rather than in years. Initially, the prognosis may be determined by the presence or absence of symptoms. Asymptomatic patients have a quite favorable prognosis over the next 5 to 10 years, so long as they remain free of symptoms (160,161). Once symptoms do develop, the subsequent prognosis, however, becomes altered (162,163). The presence or absence of fibrosis in the initial liver biopsy will also assist in predicting histology (160). The serum bilirubin is also an important parameter, and once the serum bilirubin exceeds 6 mg/dL, mean survival is approximately 25 months (164). One study has suggested that patients with PBC and SSc or CREST syndrome

have a poorer prognosis, with the mortality directly related to the severity of the PBC (161).

Several prognostic models for PBC based upon regression analysis have been developed. The Mayo Clinic model employs the clinical and laboratory observations of patient age, serum bilirubin, prothrombin time, serum albumin, and the presence or absence of edema (165). This particular model has the distinct advantage of using readily available clinical and laboratory features and is independent of the liver histology. Other models have employed similar parameters but have also incorporated the stage of the liver histology (160,166).

Testing

ESOPHAGUS

Routine chest x-rays are occasionally abnormal with advanced esophageal involvement in SSc. A characteristic finding is air in the esophagus, not associated with an air fluid level, which is best seen on lateral views (167–169). The patient with air in the esophagus and pulmonary fibrosis should be suspected as having SSc. Barium esophagography, especially using the multiphasic cine-technique, is moderately sensitive with 33% to 75% of patients with SSc exhibiting abnormalities during this test (Fig. 22.3) (75,170, 171). Primary peristalsis is usually normal above the aortic arch, but may be absent or noted as a weak nonlumen obliterating contraction. The lower esophageal sphincter may be patulous, allowing free gastroesophageal reflux. Esophageal dilation and complications from reflux such as esophagitis, ulcer, stricture, and neoplasia can be detected. Esophageal transit can be measured quantitatively by radionucleotide scintigraphy. This test has sensitivity for esophageal dysfunction, which is roughly equivalent to manometry and somewhat better than a barium cine-esophagogram (172,173). Specificity is limited and complications from reflux are not detectable. Upper GI endoscopy (Fig. 22.4) provides the

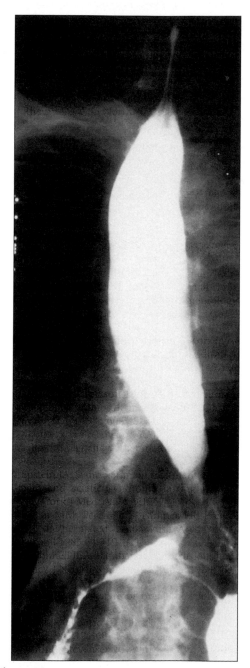

Figure 22.3. Barium esophagogram in a patient with SSc demonstrating a dilated esophagus which during fluoroscopy was flaccid.

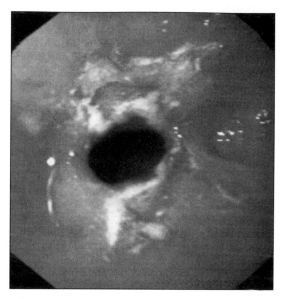

Figure 22.4. Endoscopic view of the distal esophagus in a patient with SSc demonstrating a dilated esophagus with a benign ulcerated stricture.

most accurate means to detect complications of reflux including esophagitis, ulceration, stricture, Barrett's neoplasia, esophageal neoplasia, and laryngeal changes suggestive of aspiration. Peristalsis and lower esophageal sphincter tone can be assessed only subjectively using this technique.

Esophageal manometry is the most sensitive test, detecting esophageal dysfunction in up to 87% of patients with SSc (71). It quantifies reduced lower esophageal sphincter tone and decreased amplitude of esophageal body contractions and nonperistaltic sequences that typify SSc (Fig. 22.5) (70,75). Esophageal body dysfunction appears to precede lower esophageal sphincter dysfunction (16) when patients are followed for several years. Impaired lower esophageal sphincter tone and diffuse esophageal contraction are rarely detected manometric abnormalities that are noted in "early" esophageal involvement suggestive of neurologic dysfunction (58). Manometric abnormalities of aperistalsis and decreased lower esophageal sphincter tone are not specific for SSc and are reported in other connective tissue diseases such as systemic lupus erythematosus, rheumatoid arthritis, polymyositis, polyarteritis nodosa, mixed connective tissue disease, and psoriatic arthritis (64,68,174). The same pattern can be found in patients without connective tissue disease (175).

Twenty-four-hour esophageal pH monitoring can be performed with a small pH probe positioned 4 cm above the lower esophageal sphincter. This quantifiable test has high sensitivity in detecting reflux and predicts erosive esophagitis (2,83,176). Intraesophageal high frequency ultrasound probes provide images of the esophageal wall delineating mucosa, submucosa, and muscularis propria layers (177). Increased echogenicity correlates well with increased fibrosis *in vitro*. Good correlation has been found between ultrasound changes in the esophageal body muscularis propria, esophageal body manometry, and 24-hour esophageal pH monitoring. The

correlation, however, between the ultrasound images of lower esophageal sphincter and manometry of the sphincter was low. When gastroesophageal reflux is suspected as a cause of pulmonary dysfunction from occult aspiration of gastric contents, a radionucleotide test can be performed after ingestion of an oral test meal of ^{99}Tc sulfur colloid. Delayed radionucleotide activity over the lateral thoracic area is a specific but not very sensitive finding indicative of aspiration (99).

In general, there is fair to good correlation between all the techniques used to detect esophageal abnormalities in SSc. A barium cine-esophagogram is a logical first test to evaluate patients with SSc because it is well tolerated, has fairly good sensitivity, and can detect esophagitis and reflux complications. Upper endoscopy can be performed if there is a need to determine the severity of esophagitis and assess for complications more accurately. If the barium study is

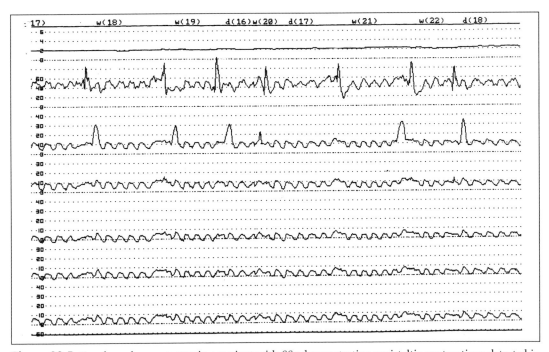

Figure 22.5. Esophageal manometry in a patient with SSc demonstrating peristaltic contractions detected in the proximal esophagus *(top two leads)* but no contractions whatsoever in the more distal esophagus *(bottom four leads)*. The small variation of baseline is due to respiration.

normal, then esophageal manometry, radionu-cleotide scintigraphy, and 24-hour esophageal pH studies are more specialized tests that can be performed because they are more sensitive tests for esophageal dysfunction in SSc. If esophageal manometry is normal, the rest of the GI tract is generally not involved with SSc.

STOMACH

When gastric involvement in SSc is particularly severe, barium upper GI series can reveal a dilat-ed stomach with retention of previously ingested food (49). It is insensitive in detecting mild to moderate gastric dysfunction. Radionucleotide scintigraphy is a well tolerated and sensitive test to assess gastric motor dysfunction. Delayed gas-tric emptying is reported in 50% to 75% of SSc patients, making it much more common than pathologic studies would indicate (48,78). Virtu-ally all patients who have postprandial nausea, vomiting, and bloating have slow emptying, while many patients without such symptoms have slow emptying as well. Gastroduodenal manometry is a sensitive but less well tolerated test to detect gastric motor dysfunction (104).

SMALL INTESTINE

Radiographic evaluation of the small intestine with plain films and barium contrast studies is the primary test to survey the small bowel in pa-tients with SSc (Fig. 22.6). The duodenum is of-ten dilated, with one series reporting an average diameter of 4.7 cm (178) (normal up to 3.0 cm). The proximal small intestine tends to be affected more than the distal small intestine (137,179), with a dilated hypoperistaltic pattern (49,100) and stasis or flocculation of barium. Two addi-tional radiographic findings characterize SSc in-volvement and serve to distinguish it from other small intestinal dysmotility disorders: "packed valvulae" and sacculations. "Packed valvulae" (179) is relatively specific for SSc (180) and oc-curs when the circular muscle is affected more than the longitudinal muscle causing the small

intestine to dilate without separation of the *valvulae conniventes*. Sacculation (181) occurs less commonly than "packed valvulae" but is more typical of SSc than other dysmotility syn-dromes (180). Transient nonobstructive intus-susception occurs in up to 17% of patients with SSc (117,180). Small bowel contrast studies are abnormal in 40% to 60% of patients with SSc (50,71,139,178). *Pneumatosis cystoides intesti-nales* and pneumoperitoneum usually are detect-ed by plain abdominal films, although abdomi-nal CT scanning is more sensitive (Fig. 22.7). Manometry is used primarily in the very proxi-mal small intestine.

Malabsorption can be detected by analysis of a 72-hour collection of stool on a 5-day stan-dardized diet. Bacterial overgrowth can be diag-nosed from properly collected jejunal aspirate that is serially diluted and cultured for a variety of aerobic and anaerobic bacteria exceeding 10^5 organisms per cubic centimeter. This test is the "gold standard" but is difficult to perform ade-

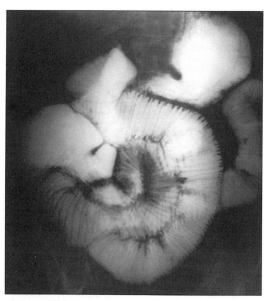

Figure 22.6. Barium upper gastrointestinal series in a patient with SSc demonstrating dilated proximal small intestine with normal sized valvulae which are packed close together.

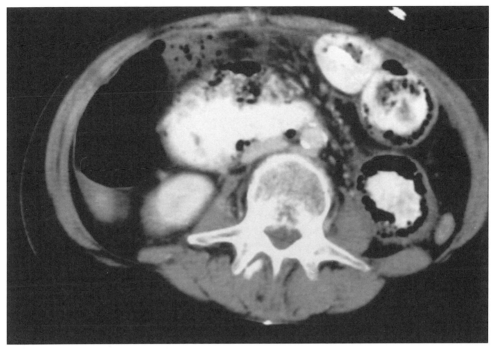

Figure 22.7. CT scan of the abdomen with oral contrast in a patient with SSc demonstrating air in the wall of two dilated contrast filled loops of small bowel *(pneumatosis cystoides intestinalis).*

quately. If available, the ^{14}C-D-Xylose breath test is a relatively simple test with excellent sensitivity and specificity for diagnosing bacterial overgrowth (112). Delayed gastric emptying can lower the sensitivity of the test. Increase serum unconjugated bile acids indicate small bowel dysfunction in SSc (182).

COLON AND ANORECTUM

Colon dysfunction is generally evaluated by plain x-rays and barium contrast studies. In SSc, the colon can be dilated and hypotonic or atonic with diverticulosis and sacculations (137,183). Pneumatosis is occasionally encountered in the colon as it is in the small intestine. Anorectal dysfunction is generally assessed with anorectal manometry. Prolapse can be detected by physical examination (Fig. 22.8), although a barium defecatory proctogram can be used to identify occult prolapse.

HEPATIC

The diagnosis of PBC is generally straightforward, based on the AMA and a liver biopsy, as previously discussed. The AMA will be positive in 95% of patients with PBC, and an AMA titer of 1:80 or greater is highly predictive for the presence of PBC (44,45). A normal cholangiogram may be needed in patients with atypical features.

Treatment

ESOPHAGUS

In general, there are no convincing data that systemic therapy for SSc halts the progression of visceral GI involvement (74), despite a few anecdotal improvements in esophageal motility with reserpine (184), captopril (185) and immunosuppression with plasmapheresis (186). Therefore, the treatment of GI dysfunction of SSc

Figure 22.8. Rectal prolapse with an atonic anal sphincter in a patient with SSc.

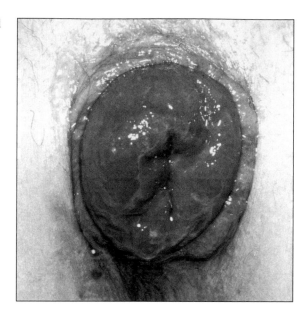

centers on specific manifestations and not the underlying etiology.

Gastroesophageal reflux in the setting of SSc often requires very aggressive therapy. Raising the head of the bed, not eating before recumbency, avoiding tight clothing, and losing weight if overweight are important but sometimes neglected measures to reduce reflux. Coffee, chocolate, peppermint, onions, garlic, alcohol, and foods high in fat should be minimized because they can decrease lower esophageal sphincter tone. H_2 blockers reduce heartburn and improve esophagitis in most patients with SSc (187,188) but do not reduce dysphagia. When H_2 blockers are stopped, pretreatment symptoms promptly recur. Proton pump inhibitors, such as omeprazole 20 mg to 40 mg per day, are much more potent inhibitors of acid secretion than H_2 blockers (189) and reliably reduce acid in the distal esophagus in SSc (190). Omeprazole is more effective than H_2 blockers in treating severe esophagitis in SSc (191). Metoclopramide (10 mg q.i.d.) is a prokinetic agent that blocks noradrenergic inhibitory nerves and enhances the response to acetylcholine. In SSc, it increases lower esopha-

geal sphincter pressure (192,193) and increases gastric emptying (193). It has minimal benefit in improving esophageal transit, augmenting esophageal body pressures, and restoring peristalsis (193). While it reduces gastroesophageal reflux, multiple central depressant and antidopaminergic side effects limit its use. Cisapride (10–20 mg q.i.d.) is a newer prokinetic agent that releases acetylcholine in the myenteric plexus and has fewer side effects than metoclopramide. It decreases heartburn and regurgitation by augmenting lower esophageal sphincter tone and improving gastric emptying (194–196). Cisapride restores and strengthens peristalsis only minimally (197). Erythromycin is a motilin agonist (188) that increases gastric contractions and lower esophageal sphincter tone and is of potential benefit in SSc (189).

Neuromuscular dysphagia is best treated by eating in the upright position. Prokinetic medications appear to be of limited benefit (193, 194). A single report of improved benefit from transcutaneous nerve stimulation (200) was not confirmed in a follow-up study (201). Dysphagia caused by stricture can be approached endoscopically to first rule out a neoplasm and second to assist with dilatation. Refractory strictures are rarely encountered and require resective surgery.

Calcium channel blockers and anticholinergics can potentially worsen gastroesophageal reflux. Diltiazem has been reported to have less of an affect on the lower esophageal sphincter than does nifedipine (202). Patients with SSc are at high risk for pill-induced esophagitis (quinidine, tetracycline, doxycycline, potassium chloride, aspirin, nonsteroid anti-inflammatory drugs, iron, etc.) because of abnormal peristalsis. Patients should carefully swallow fluids before and after pills and avoid recumbency after ingestion.

Antireflux surgery has been performed for severe gastroesophageal reflux refractory to medical therapy, but postoperative severe dysphagia is a potential major problem (203). A "loose" fundoplication around a 46 French bougie has been suggested to decrease the severity of dysphagia, but only short follow-up results are available (204). Others have proposed esophageal resection with bowel interposition, because the recurrent rate of esophagitis is often very high (205) for standard antireflux procedures.

STOMACH

In patients with SSc and gastroparesis, metoclopramide can normalize gastric emptying in some but not all patients (117,193). Erythromycin (250 mg t.i.d.) normalizes gastric emptying in some of these patients and reduces nausea, vomiting, and abdominal pain when used for 4 weeks (206). Cisapride (10 mg q.i.d.) for 1 month has been shown to improve solid and liquid gastric emptying and improve gastroparetic symptoms (194).

SMALL INTESTINE

Malabsorption in patients with SSc as a result of bacterial overgrowth can be treated with antibiotics with occasional success (207–209), as demonstrated by decreased diarrhea and fat in the stool. Bacterial resistance commonly becomes a problem in this chronic condition where prolonged and repeated use of antibiotics is often necessary. Antibiotics (such as tetracycline 250 mg q.i.d., amoxicillin with clavulanic acid 500 mg t.i.d., cephalothin 250 mg q.i.d., or metronidazole 250 mg t.i.d. plus an antibiotic that covers aerobes) are given by mouth in 7- to 10-day courses. Some patients then go into remission for months. Other patients, however, require a rotating antibiotic for 7 to 10 days each month. Still others may require prolonged therapy for up to a couple of months. Although pancreatic secretion is decreased in one-third of patients with SSc (210), clinically relevant pancreatic insufficiency causing malabsorption is quite rare (211) and readily treated with oral enzymes.

The standard prokinetic drugs (metoclopramide, cisapride, and erythromycin) should, in theory, treat the underlying dysmotility in SSc. Unfortunately, these drugs have had only anecdotal success in improving symptoms of small bowel dysmotility and malabsorption (102). A single study reported restoration of normal small bowel motility and elimination of bacterial overgrowth in five patients with SSc and severe malabsorption when given octreotide 50 μg subcutaneously at bedtime (112). Octreotide, a long-lasting analog of somatostatin, caused an average of 3.6 migrating motor complexes to occur in 3 hours of small bowel recordings when previously there were no such complexes. Breath hydrogen testing to detect overgrowth decreased from an average of 25 ppm to 4 ppm. This normalization of breath hydrogen exceeds the results achieved with the use of antibiotics for bacterial overgrowth. Octreotide given for 1 month improved the diarrhea, bloating, nausea, and vomiting in these patients. Octreotide must be given only in the fasting state to induce small bowel motility.

Treatment of pseudo-obstruction and severe small intestinal failure refractory to prokinetic medications is difficult. The diet should be restricted to a lactose-free, low fiber diet, and the fat content can be partially replaced with medium chain triglycerides. Some patients require monthly intramuscular injections of vitamin B$_{12}$ and oral supplementation with fat and water soluble vitamins, calcium, and iron. In general, laparotomy and surgery should be avoided if at all possible, because adhesions can create diagnostic difficulties distinguishing pseudo-obstruction from mechanical obstruction in the future. Resection of isolated segments of dysfunctional bowel is rarely helpful, because SSc typically causes diffuse and progressive gut dysfunction. There are rare patients with severe intestinal failure in whom all medical and dietary therapy is unsuccessful. These patients often require total parenteral nutrition and sometimes a venting enterostomy (212–214). Long-term survival is reported, but severe complications such as central venous thrombosis and sepsis can occur (213). In the future, small bowel transplantation may be an increasingly viable option.

Pneumatosis cystoides intestinalis and pneumoperitoneum should be treated nonoperatively if there are no signs of peritonitis. Because gas cyst formation in SSc generally results from bacterial fermentation of carbohydrate, which is absorbed and trapped in the gut wall, medical treatment involves elimination of dietary carbohydrates. Oxygen therapy and hyperbaric oxygen promotes cyst resolution by reducing the partial pressure of other gases in venous blood and enhancing diffusion of these gases from the cysts into surrounding tissue. Antibiotics to decrease gas forming bacteria may be useful but inconsistent results are reported. For most asymptomatic patients with SSc and *pneumatosis,* reduction of carbohydrates such as lactose, sorbitol, fructose, and fiber will permit resolution of the cysts. For some symptomatic patients, however, oxygen therapy and antibiotics are useful.

COLON AND ANORECTUM

Constipation in patients with SSc can be treated with osmotic agents, such as milk of magnesia and stimulant laxatives, if needed. Renal failure precludes the use of magnesium because exces-

sive accumulation can occur. Fiber and lactulose may be useful, but if small bowel dysmotility is present, then abdominal pain and distention can worsen. Prokinetic agents, such as metoclopramide, cisapride, and erythromycin, have not been reported to improve colonic dysfunction in SSc.

Anorectal dysfunction can be treated with occasional benefit with anorectal biofeedback. Loperamide and fiber are generally useful for treating incontinence but may worsen stomach and small bowel symptoms. If rectal prolapse is present, surgical repair may be of benefit (144,146).

LIVER

The treatment for PBC can be directed toward two separate therapeutic pathways. First, general supportive measures can be provided to the patient. Second, specific treatment directed toward PBC may also be considered.

General supportive measures would include management of pruritus, correction of fat-soluble vitamin deficiencies, and management of metabolic bone disease (12,215–218). The pruritus of PBC can be a particularly troublesome symptom. Antihistamine derivatives are of little or no benefit. Fortunately, most patients do respond to the use of cholestyramine. In those patients who are intolerant of this agent or who do not benefit from it, changing to colestipol or rifampin may be useful. The principal fat-soluble vitamins requiring correction are usually vitamins D and K. Vitamin D is particularly important for its presumed role in the osteopenia often found in PBC patients.

Many agents have been evaluated as a specific treatment of PBC. These agents have focused on modifying one of several factors present in PBC and have had one of the following treatment properties: anti-inflammatory, immunosuppressive, antifibrogenic, or anticholestatic. The ultimate goal in the treatment of PBC would be to improve or reverse symptomatology, improve biochemical abnormalities, stabilize or improve the histologic stage, prolong survival, and have an acceptable safety profile. More recently, the following four agents have been evaluated: colchicine, cyclosporin A, ursodcoxycholic acid (ursodiol), and methotrexate.

Colchicine was evaluated because it may retard the formation of fibrosis, which is an inevitable occurrence in PBC. Three prospective, double-blind trials of colchicine have been completed (219–221). In general, colchicine improved biochemical features of serum bilirubin, albumin, and cholesterol, but the histologic stage and survival were not altered.

Cyclosporin A was evaluated in three clinical trials (222–224). In all studies, biochemical parameters were improved and histologic improvement was found in one study (222). A high frequency of side effects, particularly hypertension and renal toxicity, precludes recommendation for its use.

Ursodiol has been studied for its potential in reducing levels of endogenous, toxic bile acids within hepatocytes, which occur as a consequence of prolonged cholestasis. It has also been recently shown that ursodiol will favorably modify the display of the aberrant class I and II HLA antigens on bile duct epithelium (225,226). Several prospective trials using ursodiol in PBC have been reported, employing a dose of 10 to 14 mg/kg/day (227–231). Biochemical improvement has been shown to occur in all studies. In one study, an improvement in the mean histologic score was noted in the ursodiol-treated patients whose initial serum bilirubin level was less than 2 mg/dL (231). Ursodiol does not, however, appear to improve overall survival or the requirement for liver transplantation. No adverse side effects have been identified.

Methotrexate is the final agent evaluated for the treatment of PBC. The preliminary results from an open-label trial suggested a favorable response to methotrexate (232). One reservation for the use of methotrexate in PBC is its known hepatotoxicity, with the formation of fibrosis as its principal feature (233). Currently, a multi-center trial comparing ursodiol with the combination of ursodiol and methotrexate is underway.

The main limiting factor in all of the clinical trials for PBC is the duration of treatment. Because the natural history of PBC is probably several decades in length, the relative brevity of these trials, limited to 2 to 4 years, makes it difficult to interpret what long-term benefits, if any, might occur from any of the study medications.

Nevertheless, there remains a very definitive treatment for advanced PBC, namely liver transplantation. Liver transplantation will be reserved for those patients developing complications of portal hypertension and progressive jaundice. Application of the Mayo Clinic model may be useful in defining those patients whose 12- to 14-month survival is greatly altered (165). Studies have shown that patients with an advanced stage of PBC will benefit from liver transplantation and that their survival after transplantation is similar to other forms of liver disease (234,235). The AMA remains present in the patient's serum after liver transplantation, and histologic evidence for PBC may be found in the liver biopsy histology (236,237).

References

1. Furst DC, Clements PJ, Saab M, Sterz MG, et al. Clinical and serologic comparison of 17 chronic, progressive systemic sclerosis (PSS) and 17 CREST syndrome patients matched for sex, age, and disease duration. Ann Rheum Dis 1984;43: 794–801.
2. Zaninotto G, Peserico A, Costantini M, et al. Esophageal motility and lower esophageal sphincter competence in progressive systemic sclerosis and localized scleroderma. Scand J Gastroenterol 1989;24:95–103.
3. Altman RD, Medsger TA, Bloch DA, Michel PA. Predictors of survival in systemic sclerosis (scleroderma). Arthritis Rheum 1991;34:403–413.
4. Bartholomew LG, Cain JC, Winkleman RA, Bagenstoss AH. Chronic disease of the liver associated with systemic sclerosis. Am J Dig Dis 1964; 9:43.
5. Clarke AK, Galbraith RM, Hamilton EBD, Williams R. Rheumatic disorders in primary biliary cirrhosis. Ann Rheum Dis 1978;37:42.
6. Reynolds TB, et al. Primary biliary cirrhosis with

scleroderma, Raynaud's phenomenon and telangiectasia. Am J Med 1971;50:302.

7. Murray-Lyon IM, et al. Scleroderma and primary biliary cirrhosis. Br Med J 1970;3:258.

8. Hirakata M, et al. Coexistence of CREST syndrome and primary biliary cirrhosis. Serologic studies of two cases. J Rheumatol 1988;15:1166.

9. Russell ML, Kahn HJ. Nodular regenerative hyperplasia of the liver associated with progressive systemic sclerosis: A case report with ultrastructural observation. J Rheumatol 1983;10:748.

10. McMahon RFT, Babbs C, Warnes TW. Nodular regenerative hyperplasia of the liver, CREST syndrome and primary biliary cirrhosis: An overlap syndrome? Gut 1989;30:1430.

11. Umeyama K, et al. Idiopathic portal hypertension associated with progressive systemic sclerosis. Am J Gastroenterol 1982;77:645.

12. Kaplan MM. Primary biliary cirrhosis. N Engl J Med 1987;316:521.

13. Culp KS, et al. Autoimmune associations in primary biliary cirrhosis. Mayo Clin Proc 1982;57:365.

14. Powell FC, Schroeter AC, Dickson ER. Primary biliary cirrhosis and the CREST syndrome: A report of 22 cases. QJM 1987;62:75.

15. Fregeau DR, et al. Autoantibodies to mitochondria in systemic sclerosis. Arthritis Rheum 1988;31:386.

16. Treacy WL, Baggenstoss AH, Slocumb CH, Code CF. Scleroderma of the esophagus. A correlation of histologic and physiologic findings. Ann Intern Med 1963;59:351–356.

17. Atkinson M, Summerling MD. Esophageal changes in systemic sclerosis. Gut 1966;7:402–408.

18. Cohen S, Fisher R, Lipshutz W, et al. The pathogenesis of esophageal dysfunction in scleroderma and Raynaud's disease. J Clin Invest 1972;51:2663–2668.

19. Bortolotti M, Pinotti R, Sarti P, Barbara L. Esophageal electromyography in scleroderma patients with functional dysphagia. Am J Gastroenterol 1989;84:1497–1502.

20. Ballardini G, et al. Aberrant expression of HLA-DR antigens on bile duct epithelium in primary biliary cirrhosis: Relevance to pathogenesis. Lancet 1984;2:1009.

21. Spengler U, et al. Differential expression of MHC class II subregion products on bile duct epithelial cells and hepatocytes in patients with primary biliary cirrhosis. Hepatology 1988;8:459.

22. Calmus Y, et al. Cholestasis induces major histocompatibility complex class I expression in hepatocytes. Gastroenterology 1992;102:1371.

23. Ayres RCS, et al. Intercellular adhesion molecule-1 and MHC antigen on human bile ducts: Effect of proinflammatory cytokines. Gut 1993;34:1245.

24. Pape GR, et al. Involvement of the cytotoxic/suppressor T cell subset in liver tissue injury of patients with acute and chronic liver disease. Gastroenterology 1983;85:657.

25. Yamada G, et al. Ultrastructural and immunocytochemical analysis of lymphocytes infiltrating bile duct epithelium in primary biliary cirrhosis. Hepatology 1986;6:385.

26. Krams SM, et al. Analysis of hepatic T lymphocytes and immunoglobulin deposits in patients with primary biliary cirrhosis. Hepatology 1990;12:306.

27. Pape GR, Spengler U, Hoffmann RM, Jung M-C. Pathogenesis of primary biliary cirrhosis. In: Krawitt EL, Wiesner RH, eds. Autoimmune liver disease. New York: Raven Press, 1991.

28. Spengler U, et al. T lymphocytes from patients with primary biliary cirrhosis produce reduced amounts of lymphotoxin, tumor necrosis factor and interferon-gamma upon mitogen simulation. J Hepatol 1992;15:129.

29. Menendez JL, et al. Deficient interleukin-2 responsiveness of T lymphocytes from patients with primary biliary cirrhosis. Hepatology 1992;16:931.

30. Kroemer G, Wick G. The role of interleukin-2 in autoimmunity. Immunol Today 1989;10:246.

31. Walker JG, Doniach D, Raitt IM. Serological tests in the diagnosis of primary biliary cirrhosis. Lancet 1965;1:827.

32. Klatskin G, Kantor FS. Mitochondrial antibodies in primary biliary cirrhosis and other diseases. Ann Intern Med 1972;77:533.

33. Berg PA, Klein R. Heterogeneity of antimitochondrial antibodies. Semin Liver Dis 1989;9:103.

34. Berg PA, Klein R, Lindenburn-Fotinos J. Antimitochondrial antibodies in primary biliary cirrhosis. J Hepatol 1986;2:123.

35. Weber P, et al. Characterization and clinical relevance of a new complement-fixing antibody (anti-M8) in patients with primary biliary cirrhosis. Hepatology 1986;6:553.

36. Klein R, et al. Antimitochondrial antibody profiles determined at early stages of primary biliary cirrhosis differentiate between a benign and a progressive course of the disease. J Hepatol 1991;12:21.

37. Klein R, et al. The antimitochondrial antibody anti-M9—A marker for the diagnosis of early primary biliary cirrhosis. J Hepatol 1988;6:299.

38. Gershwin ME, MacKay IR, Sturgess A, Coppel RL.

Identification and specificity of a cDNA encoding the 70 dk mitochondrial antigen recognized in primary biliary cirrhosis. J Immunol 1987;138:3525.

39. Surh CD, et al. Antimitochondrial antibodies in primary biliary cirrhosis recognize cross-reactive epitope(s) on protein X and dihydrolipoamide acetyltransferase of pyruvate dehydrogenase. Hepatology 1989;10:127.

40. Briand J-P, et al. Multiple autoepitope presentation for specific detection of antibodies in primary biliary cirrhosis. Hepatology 1992;16:1395.

41. Yeaman SF, et al. Primary biliary cirrhosis identification of two major MS mitochondrial autoantigens. Lancet 1988;1:1067.

42. Van de Water J, et al. Detection of autoantibodies to recombinant mitochondrial proteins in patients with primary biliary cirrhosis. N Engl J Med 1989;320:1377.

43. Leung PSC, et al. Use of designer recombinant mitochondrial antigens in the diagnosis of primary biliary cirrhosis. Hepatology 1992;15:367.

44. Berg, PA, Klein R. Antimitochondrial antibodies in primary biliary cirrhosis. Scand J Gastroenterol 1988;23:103.

45. Mitchison HC, et al. Positive mitochondrial antibody but normal alkaline phosphatase: Is this primary biliary cirrhosis? Hepatology 1986;6:1279.

46. Russell ML, Friesen D, Henderson RD, Hanna WM. Ultrastructure of the esophagus in scleroderma. Arthritis Rheum 1982;25:1117.

47. Stafford-Brady FJ, Kahn HJ, Ross TM, Russell ML. Advanced scleroderma bowel: Complications and management. J Rheumatol 1988;15:869–874.

48. D'Angelo WA, Fries JF, Masi AD, Shulman LE. Pathologic observations in systemic sclerosis (scleroderma). Am J Med 1969;46:428–440.

49. Peachey R, Creamer B, Pierce J. Sclerodermatous involvement of the stomach and the small and large bowel. Gut 1969;10:285–289.

50. Heinz ER, Steinberg AJ, Sackner MA. Roentgenographic and pathologic aspects of intestinal scleroderma. Ann Intern Med 1963;59:822.

51. Hendel L, Kobayasi T, Petri M. Ultra structure of the small intestinal mucosa in progressive systemic sclerosis (PSS). Acta Pathol Microbiol Immunol Scand 1987;95:41–46.

52. Rosson RS, Yesner R. Per oral duodenal biopsy and progressive systemic sclerosis. New Engl J Med 1966;272:391–394.

53. Ludwig J, Dickson ER, McDonald GSA. Staging of nonsuppurative destructive cholangitis (syndrome of primary biliary cirrhosis). Virchows Arch 1978;379:103.

54. Kanel GC, Korula J, eds. Atlas of liver pathology. Philadelphia: WB Saunders, 1992.

55. Portmann B, MacSween RNM. Diseases of the intrahepatic bile ducts. In: MacSween RNM, Anthony PP, Scheuer PJ, eds. Pathology of the liver. Edinburgh:Churchill Livingston, 1987.

56. Lee RG, et al. Granulomas in primary biliary cirrhosis: A prognostic feature. Gastroenterology 1981;81:983.

57. Keeffe EB. Sarcoidosis and primary biliary cirrhosis. Am J Med 1987;83:977.

58. Park RHR, McKillop JH, Belch JJF, et al. Achalasia-like syndrome in systemic sclerosis. Br J Surg 1990;77:46–49.

59. Äkesson A, Wollheim FA. Organ manifestations in 100 patients with progressive systemic sclerosis: A comparison between the CREST syndrome and diffuse scleroderma. Br J Rheumatol 1989;28:281–286.

60. Rajapakse CNA, et al. Pharyngoesophageal dysphagia in systemic sclerosis. Ann Rheum Dis 1981;40:612–614.

61. Montesi A, Pesaresi A, Cavalli ML, et al. Oral pharyngeal and esophageal function in scleroderma. Dysphagia 1991;6:219–222.

62. Takebayashi S, Matsui K, Ozawa Y, et al. Cervical esophageal motility: Evaluation with US in progressive systemic sclerosis. Radiology 1991;179:389–393.

63. Cohen S. Motor disorders of the esophagus. N Engl J Med 1979;31:184.

64. Stevens MB, Hookman Q, Siegel CI, et al. Aperistalsis of the esophagus in patients with connective tissue disorders and Raynaud's phenomenon. N Engl J Med 1964;270:1218–1222.

65. Hurwitz AL, Duranceau A, Postlethwait RW. Esophageal dysfunction and Raynaud's phenomenon in patients with scleroderma Am J Dig Dis 1976;21:601–606.

66. Turner R, Lipshutz W, Miller W, et al. Esophageal dysfunction in collagen disease. Am J Med Sci 1973;285:191–199.

67. Klein HA, Wald A, Graham TO, et al. Comparative studies of esophageal function in systemic sclerosis. Gastroenterology 1992;102:1551–1556.

68. Tsianos AB, Drosos AA, Chiras CD, et al. Esophageal manometric findings and autoimmune rheumatic diseases: Is scleroderma esophagus a specific entity? Rheumatol Int 1987;7:23–27.

69. Tuffanelli DL, Winkelmann RK. Systemic scleroderma. A clinical study of 727 cases. Arch Dermatol 1961;84:359.

70. Clements PJ, Kadell B, Oppoliti A, Ross M.

Esophageal motility in progressive systemic sclerosis (PSS). Dig Dis Sci 1979;24:639–644.

71. Poirier TJ, Rankin GB. Gastrointestinal manifestations of progressive systemic scleroderma, based on a review of 364 cases. Am J Gastroenterol 1972;58:30–44.

72. Yarze JC, Varga J, Stampfl D, et al. Esophageal function in systemic sclerosis: A prospective evaluation of motility and acid reflux in 36 patients. Am J Gastroenterol 1993;88:870–876.

73. Kinder RR, Fleischman R. Systemic scleroderma: A review of organ systems. Int J Dermatol 1974; 13:362–395.

74. Hendel L, Stentoft P, Aggestrup S. The progress of esophageal involvement in progressive systemic sclerosis during D-Penicillamine treatment. Scand J Rheumatol 1989;18:149–155.

75. Garrett JM, Winkelmann RK, Schlegel JF, Coade CF. Esophageal deterioration and scleroderma. Mayo Clin Proc 1971;46:92–96.

76. Dantas RO, Meneghelli UG, Oliveria RB, Villanova MG. Esophageal dysfunction does not always worsen in systemic sclerosis. J Clin Gastroenterol 1993;17:281–285.

77. Murphy JR, McNally P, Peller P, et al. Prolonged clearance is the primary abnormal reflux parameter in patients with progressive systemic sclerosis and esophagitis. Dig Dis Sci 1992;37:833–841.

78. Maddern GJ. Horowitz M, Jamieson GG, et al. Abnormalities in esophageal and gastric emptying and progressive systemic sclerosis. Gastroenterology 1984;87:922–926.

79. Bortolotti M, Turba E, Tosti A, et al. Gastric emptying and inter-digestive antroduodenal motility in patients with esophageal scleroderma. Am J Gastroenterol 1991;86:743–747.

80. Osial TA, et al. Clinical and serologic study of Sjögren's syndrome in patients with progressive systemic sclerosis. Arthritis Rheum 1983;26:500–508.

81. Äkesson A, Äkesson B, Gustafson T, Wollheim F. Gastrointestinal function in patients with progressive systemic sclerosis. Clin Rheumatol 1985; 4:441–448.

82. Bettarello A, Neves DP, Zaterka S. Progressive systemic sclerosis: I. Gastric secretory pattern. Am J Dig Dis 1967;12:804–807.

83. Zamost BJ, Hirschberg J, Ippolidi et al. Esophagitis in scleroderma. Prevalence and risk factors. Gastroenterology 1987;92:421.

84. Palmer ED. Subacute erosive ("peptic") esophagitis. Clinical study of one hundred cases. Arch Intern Med 1984;94:364–374.

85. Hendel L. Hydroxyproline in the esophageal mucosa of patients with progressive systemic sclerosis during omeprazole-induced healing of reflux esophagitis. Aliment Pharmacol Ther 1991;5: 471–480.

86. Lambert DR, Llaneza PP, Gaglani RD, Lach RD, et al. Esophageal-atrial fistula. J Clin Gastroenterol 1987;9:384–389.

87. Cameron AJ, Payne WS. Barrett's esophagus occurring as a complication of scleroderma. Mayo Clin Proc 1978;53:612.

88. Halpert RD, Laufer I, Thompson JJ, Reccko PJ. Adenocarcinoma of the esophagus in patients with scleroderma. Am J Rheumatol 1983;140: 927–930.

89. Niv Y, Abu-Avid S, Yellin A, Lieberman Y. Barrett's epithelium and esophageal adenocarcinoma in scleroderma. Am J Gastroenterol 1988;83:792–793.

90. McKinley M, Sherlock P. Barrett's esophagus with adenocarcinoma and scleroderma. Am J Gastroenterol 1984;79:438–439.

91. Dill JE. Barrrett's epithelium in scleroderma. Gastrointest Endosc 1983;29:296–297.

92. Sprung DJ, Gibb, SP. Dysplastic Barrett's esophagus in scleroderma. Am J Gastroenterol 1985;80: 518–522.

93. Agha FP, Dabich L. Barrett's esophagus complicating scleroderma. Gastrointest Radiol 1985;10: 325–329.

94. Anderson M, Seymour EQ. Association of Barrett's esophagus and scleroderma. South Med J 1987;80:764–765.

95. Katzka DA, Reynolds JC, Saul SH, et al. Barrett's metaplasia and adenocarcinoma of the esophagus and scleroderma. Am J Med 1987;82:46–52.

96. Segel MC, Campbell WL, Medsger TA, Roumm AD. Systemic sclerosis (scleroderma) and esophageal adenocarcinoma: Is increased patient screening necessary? Gastroenterology 1985;89: 485–488.

97. Abu-Shakra M, Guillemin F, Lee P. Cancer in systemic sclerosis. Arthritis Rheum 1993;36:460–464.

98. Hendel L, Svejgaard E, Walsoe I, et al. Esophageal candidosis and progressive systemic sclerosis: Occurrence, significance and treatment with fluconazole. Scand J Gastroenterol 1986;23:1182–1186.

99. Johnson DA, Drane WE, Curran J, et al. Pulmonary disease in progressive systemic sclerosis: A complication of gastroesophageal reflux and occult aspiration? Arch Intern Med 1989;149: 589–593.

100. Gondos P. Roentgen manifestations in progressive systemic sclerosis (diffuse scleroderma). Am J Roentgenol 1960;84:235.

101. Goldgraber MB, Kirsner JB. Scleroderma of the gastrointestinal tract: Review. Arch Pathol 1957; 64:255.

102. Rees WD, Leigh RJ, Christofides ND, et al. Interdigestive motor activity in patients with systemic sclerosis. Gastroenterology 1982;83:575–580.

103. Madsen J, Hendel L. Gastrointestinal transit times of radiolabeled meal in progressive systemic sclerosis. Dig Dis Sci 1992;37:1404–1408.

104. Greydanus MP, Camilleri N. Abnormal postcibal, antral, and small bowel motility due to neuropathy or myopathy in systemic sclerosis. Gastroenterology 1989;96:110–115.

105. Hirakata M, Akizuki M, Okano Y, Hama N, et al. Pyloric stenosis in a patient with progressive systemic sclerosis. Clin Rheumatol 1988;7:394–397.

106. Lundberg AC, Åkesson A, Åkesson B. Dietary intake and nutritional status in patients with systemic sclerosis. Ann Rheum Dis 1992;51:1143–1148.

107. Faulk DL, Anuras S, Christensen J. Chronic intestinal pseudo-obstruction. Gastroenterology 1978;74:922–931.

108. Di Marino AJ, Carlson G, Myers A, et al. Duodenal myoelectric activity in scleroderma. Abnormal responses to mechanical and hormonal stimuli. N Engl J Med 1973;289:1220–1223.

109. Cobden I, Axon T, Ghonein AT, et al. Small intestinal bacterial growth in systemic sclerosis. Clin Exp Dermatol 1980;5:37–42.

110. Greenberger NJ, Dobbins WO, Ruppert RD, Jesseph JE. Intestinal atony in progressive systemic sclerosis (scleroderma). Am J Med 1968;45: 301–308.

111. Van Tilburg AJP, Van Blankenstein M, Verschoor L. Intestinal lymphangiectasia and systemic sclerosis. Am J Gastroenterol 1988;83:1418–1419.

112. Soudah HC, Hasler WL, Owyang C. Effect of octreotide on intestinal motility and bacterial overgrowth and scleroderma. N Engl J Med 1991;325: 1461–1467.

113. Hendel L, Ammitzboll T, Kreuzig F, et al. Bioavailability of D-Penicillamine in a patient with gastrointestinal progressive systemic sclerosis. Scand J Rheumatol 1986;15:91–94.

114. Ammitzboll T, Hendel L, Kreuzig F, Asboe-Hansen G. Bioavailability of D-penicillamine in relation to gastrointestinal involvement of generalized scleroderma. Scand J Rheumatol 1987;16: 121–126.

115. Gompels BM. *Pneumatosis cystoides intestinalis*

116. Meihoff WE, Hirschfield JS, Kern F. Small intestinal scleroderma with malabsorption and *pneumatosis cystoides intestinalis*. Report of three cases. J Am Med Assoc 1968;204:854–858.

117. Cohen S, Laufer I, Snape W, et al. The gastrointestinal manifestations of scleroderma: Pathogenesis and management. Gastroenterology 1980; 79:155–166.

118. Ritchie M, Caravelli J, Shike M. Benign persistent pneumoperitoneum in scleroderma. Dig Dis Sci 1986;31:552–555.

119. Brandt LJ, Bernstein LH. Spontaneous pneumoperitoneum with *pneumatosis cystoides intestinalis* in a patient with connective tissue disease. Am J Gastroenerol 1978;69:494–500.

120. Hoover EL, Cole GD, Mitchell LS, et al. Avoiding laparotomy in nonsurgical pneumoperitoneium. Am J Surg 1992;164:99–103.

121. Battle WM, McLean GK, Brook JJ, et al. Spontaneous perforation of the small intestine due to scleroderma. Dig Dis Sci 1979;24:80–84.

122. Sequeira W. *Pneumatosis cystoides intestinalis* in systemic sclerosis and other diseases. Sem in Arthritis Rheum 1990;19:269–277.

123. Srinivas V. Sclerodermatomyositis with mega colon, small bowel involvement and impaired lung function. Proc R Soc Med 1976;69:263–264.

124. Shamberger RC, Crawford JO, Kiakham SE. Progressive systemic sclerosis resulting in megacolon. JAMA 1983;250:10063–10065.

125. Ferreiro JE, Busse JC, Saldana MJ. Megacolon in a collagen vascular overlap syndrome. Am J Med 1986;80:307–311.

126. Brandwein M, Schwartz IS. Megacolon and volvulus complicating progressive systemic sclerosis. Mt Sinai J Med 1988;55:343–345.

127. Davis RP, Hines JR, Flinn WR. Scleroderma of the colon with obstruction. Dis Colon Rectum 1976; 126:704–713.

128. Thompson MA, Summers R. Barium impaction as a complication of gastrointestinal scleroderma. J Am Med Assoc 1976;235:1715–1717.

129. Robinson JC, Teitelbaum SL. Stercoral ulceration and perforation of the sclerodermatous colon. Dis Colon Rectum 1974;17:622–632.

130. Esselinckx W, Brenard R, Colin J, Malange M. Juvenile scleroderma and collagenous colitis. The first case. J Rheumatol 1989;16:834–836.

131. Lorentzen M, Hoffmann J. Scleroderma of the colon presenting with acute abdominal symptoms. Acta Chir Scand 1984;150:511–512.

132. Edwards DA, Lennard-Jones JE. Diffuse systemic

sclerosis presenting as infarction of the colon. Proc R Soc Med 1960;53:877–879.

133. Sacher P, Buchmann P, Burger H. Stenosis of the large intestine complicating scleroderma and mimicking a sigmoid carcinoma. Dis Colon Rectum 1983;26:347–348.

134. Budd DC, Nirdlinger EL, Sturtz DL, et al. Transverse colon volvulus associated with scleroderma. Am J Surg 1977;133:370–372.

135. Javors BR, Sorkin NS, Flint GW. Transverse colon volvulus: A case report. Am J Gastroenterol 1986; 81:708–712.

136. Fraback RC, Kadell BM, Nies KM, et al. Sigmoid volvulus in two patients with progressive systemic sclerosis. J Rheumatol 1978;5:195–198.

137. Kemp-Harper RA, Jackson DC. Progressive systemic sclerosis. Br J Radiol 1965;38:825–834.

138. Ballard JL, Snyder CR, Jansen GT. The gastrointestinal manifestations of generalized scleroderma. South Med J 1969;62:1243.

139. Olmsted WW, Madewell JE. The esophageal and small bowel manifestations of progressive systemic sclerosis. Gastrointest Radiol 1976;1:33.

140. Janson MI, Somon PR, Grough J, et al. Spontaneous bowel perforation in intestinal scleroderma. Postgrad Med J 1972;48:56–58.

141. Battle WM, Snape WJ, Wright S, et al. Abnormal colonic motility in progressive systemic sclerosis. Ann Intern Med 1981;94:749–752.

142. Whitehead WE, Taitelbaum G, Wigley FM, Schuster MM. Rectosigmoid motility and myoelectric activity in progressive systemic sclerosis 1989;96: 428–432.

143. D'Angelo G, Stern HS, Myers E. Rectal prolapse in scleroderma: Case report and review of the colonic complications of scleroderma. Can J Surg 1985;28:62–63.

144. Leighton JA, et al. Anorectal dysfunction and rectal prolapse in progressive systemic sclerosis. Dis Colon Rectum 1993;36:182–185.

145. Hamel-Roy J, Devroede G, Arhan P, et al. Comparative espohageal and anorectal motility in scleroderma. Gastroenterology 1985;88:1–7.

146. Chiou AWH, Lin JK, Wang FM. Anorectal abnormalities in progressive systemic sclerosis. Dis Colon Rectum 1989;32:417–421.

147. Allende HD, Ona FW, Noronha AI. Bleeding gastric telangiectasia: Complications of Raynaud's phenomenon, esophageal motor dysfunction, sclerodactyly and telangiectasia (CREST) syndrome. Am J Gastroenterol 1981;75:354–356.

148. Kesson A, Willheim FA. Organ manifestations in 100 patients with progressive systemic sclerosis: A comparison between the CREST syndrome and diffuse scleroderma.

149. Baron M, Srolovitz H. Colonic telangiectasias in a patient with progressive systemic sclerosis. Arthritis Rheum 1986;29:282–285.

150. Marshall JB, Moore GF, Settles RH. Colonic telangiectasias in scleroderma. Arch Intern Med 1980;140:1121.

151. Rosekrans PCM, de Rooy DJ, Bosman FT, et al. Gastrointestinal telangiectasia as a cause of severe blood loss in systemic sclerosis. Endoscopy 1980; 12:200–204.

152. Kolodny M, Baker WG. CREST syndrome with persistent gastrointestinal bleeding (calcinosis, Raynaud's phenomenon, sclerodactyly and telangiectasia). Gastrointest Endosc 1976;15:16–17.

153. Holt JM, Wright R. Anemia due to blood loss from telangiectasias of scleroderma. Br Med J 1967;3:537–538.

154. Jabhar M, Roeleen C, Lough J, et al. Gastric antral vascular ectasia: The watermelon stomach. Gastroenterology 1984;87:1165–1170.

155. Gostout CJ, Viggiuno TR, Ahlquist DA, et al. The clinical and endoscopic spectrum of the watermelon stomach. J Clin Gastroenterol 1992;15: 256–263.

156. Lucey MR, Neuberger JM, Williams R. Primary biliary cirrhosis in men. Gut 1986;27:1373.

157. Sherlock S, Sheuer PJ. The presentation and diagnosis of 100 patients with primary biliary cirrhosis. N Engl J Med 1973;289:674.

158. Fleming CR, Ludwig J, Dickson ER. Asymptomatic primary biliary cirrhosis. Mayo Clinic Proc 1978;53:587.

159. James O, Macklon AF, Watson AJ. Primary biliary cirrhosis—A revised clinical spectrum. Lancet 1981;1:1278.

160. Roll J, Boyer JL, Barry D, Klatskin G. The prognostic importance of clinical and histologic features in asymptomatic primary biliary cirrhosis. N Engl J Med 1983;308:1.

161. Beswick DR, Klatskin G, Boyer JL. Asymptomatic primary biliary cirrhosis. Gastroenterology 1985; 89:267.

162. Balasubramaniam K, et al. Diminished survival in asymptomatic primary biliary cirrhosis. Gastroenterology 1990;98:1567.

163. Mitchihson HC, et al. Symptom development and prognosis in primary biliary cirrhosis. Gastroenterology 1990;99:778.

164. Shapiro JM, Smith H, Schaffner F. Serum bilirubin: A prognostic factor in primary biliary cirrhosis. Gut 1979;20:137.

165. Dickson ER, et al. Prognosis in primary biliary cirrhosis: Model for decision making. Hepatology 1989;10:1.

166. Christensen E, et al. Beneficial effect of azathio-

prine and prediction of prognosis in primary biliary cirrhosis. Final results of an international trial. Gastroenterology 1985;89:1084.

167. Dinsmore RE, Goodman D, Dreyfuss JR. The air esophagogram: A sign of scleroderma involving the esophagus. Radiology 1966;87:348.

168. Kraus A, Alarcon-Segovia D. Air esophagogram and intestinal pseudo-obstruction in a patient with scleroderma. J Rheumatol 1991;18:897–899.

169. House AJS, Griffiths GJ. The significance of an air esophagogram visualized on conventional chest radiographs. Clin Radiol 1977;28:301.

170. Campbell WL, Schultz JC. Specificity and sensitivity of esophageal motor abnormality in systemic sclerosis (scleroderma) and related diseases: A cintiradiographic study. Gastrointest Radiol 1986;11:218–222.

171. Clements JL, Abernathy J, Weens HS. Corrugated mucosal pattern in the esophagus associated with progressive systemic sclerosis. Gastrointest Radiol 1978;3:119.

172. Drane WE, Karvelis K, Johnson DA, et al. Progressive systemic sclerosis: Radionuclide esophageal scintigraphy and manometry. Radiology 1986;160:73–76.

173. Geatti O, Shapiro B, Fig LM, et al. Radiolabeled semi-solid test meal clearance in the evaluation of esophageal involvement in scleroderma and Sjögren's syndrome. Am J Phys Imaging 1991;6:65–73.

174. DeMerieux P, Verity A, Clements PJ, Paulus HE, Esophageal abnormalities and dysphagia in polymyositis and dermatomyositis. Clinical, radiologic and pathologic features. Arthritis Rheum 1983;26:961–968.

175. Schneider HA, Yonker RA, Longley S, et al. Scleroderma esophagus: A nonspecific entity. Ann Intern Med 1984;100:848–850.

176. Stentoft P, Hendel L, Aggestrup S. Esophageal manometry and pH probe monitoring in the evaluation of gastroesophageal reflux in patients with progressive systemic sclerosis. Scand J Gastroenterol 1987;22:499–504.

177. Miller LS, Liu J, Klenn BJ, et al. Endoluminal ultrasonography of the distal esophagus in systemic sclerosis. Gastroenterology 1993;105:31–39.

178. Bluestone R, MacMahon M, Dawson JM. Systemic sclerosis and small bowel involvement. Gut 1969;10:185–193.

179. Horowitz AL, Myers MA. The "hide-bound" small bowel of scleroderma: Characteristic mucosal fold pattern. Am J Roentgen Radiol Ther Nucl Med 1973;119:332–334.

180. Rohrmann CA, Ricci MD, Krishnamurthy S,

Schuffler MD. Radiologic and histologic differentiation of neuromuscular disorders of the gastrointestinal tract: Visceral myopathies, visceral neuropathies, and progressive systemic sclerosis. Am J Rheumatol 1984;143:933–941.

181. Queloz JM, Woloshin HJ. Sacculation of the small intestine and scleroderma. Radiology 1972;105:513.

182. Stellaard F, Sauerbruch T, Luderschmidt C, et al. Intestinal involvement in progressive systemic sclerosis detected by increased unconjugated serum bioassets. Gut 19987;28:446–450.

183. Cassada WA, Armstrong RH, Neal M. Involvement of the gastrointestinal tract by progressive systemic sclerosis. South Med J 1968;61:475–481.

184. Willerson JD, Thompson RH, Hookman P, et al. Reserpine in Raynaud's disease and phenomenon. Short term response to intra-arterial injection. Ann Intern Med 1970;72:17–27.

185. Koffel KK, Greenberger NJ, Miner PB. Esophageal motor dysfunction and progressive systemic sclerosis: Improvement after captopril treatment. Gastroenterology 1985;88:1451A.

186. Äkesson A, Wollheim FA, Thysell H, et al. Visceral improvement following combined plasmapheresis and immunosuppressive drug therapy in progressive systemic sclerosis. Scand J Rheumatol 1988;17:313–323.

187. Pctrokubi RJ, Jeffries GH. Cimetidine vs antacids in scleroderma with reflux esophagitis. Gastroenterology 1979;77:691–695.

188. Hendel L, Aggestrup S, Stentoft P. Long-term ranitidine and progressive systemic sclerosis (scleroderma) with gastroesophageal reflux. Scand J Gastroenterol 1986;21:799–805.

189. Klinkenberg-Knol EC, Jansen JMBJ, Festin HPM, et al. Double-blind multicentered comparison of omeprazole and ranitidine in the treatment of reflux esophagus. Lancet 1987;1:349–351.

190. Shoenut JP, Wieler JA, Micflikier AB. The extent and pattern of gastroesophageal reflux in patients with scleroderma esophagus: The effect of low-dose omeprazole. Aliment Pharmacol Ther 1993;7:509–513.

191. Hendel L, Hage E, Hendel J, Stentoft P. Omeprazole in the long term treatment of severe gastroesophageal reflex disease in patients with systemic sclerosis. Aliment Pharmacol Ther 1992;6:565–577.

192. Ramirez-Mata M, Ibanez G, Alarcon D. Stimulatory effect of metoclopramide on the esophagus and lower esophageal sphincter of patients with PSS. Arthritis Rheum 1977;20:30–44.

193. Johnson DA, Drane WE. Curran J, et al. Metoclopramide response in patients with progressive

systemic sclerosis. Effect on esophageal and gastric motility abnormalities. Arch Intern Med 1987;147:1597–1601.

194. Horowitz M, Maddern GJ, Maddox A, et al. Effects of cisapride on gastric and esophageal emptying and progressive systemic sclerosis. Gastroenterology 1987;93:311–315.

195. Kahan A, Amor B, Menkes CJ, et al. Cisapride in the treatment of esophageal abnormalities and systemic sclerosis. Arthritis Rheum 1989;32:5120.

196. Kahan A, Chaussade S, Gaudric M. Effect of cisapride on gastroesophageal dysfunction and systemic sclerosis: A controlled manometric study. Br J Clin Pharmacol 1991;31:683–687.

197. Limburg A, Smit A, Kleibeuker JH. The effects of cisapride on esophageal motor function of patients with progressive systemic sclerosis or mixed connective tissue disease. Digestion 1991; 49:156–160.

198. Peeters T, Matthijs G, Depoortere I, et al. Erythromycin is a motilin receptor agonist. Am J Physiol 1989;257:G470–G474.

199. Kahan A, Chaussade S, Michopoulos S, Samama J. Erythromycin and esophageal abnormalities in systemic sclerosis. Arthritis Rheum 1991;52:116.

200. Kaada B. Successful treatment of esophageal dysmotility and Raynaud's phenomenon in systemic sclerosis and achalasia by transcutaneous nerve stimulation. Increase in plasma VIP concentration. Scand J Gastroenterol 1987;22: 1137–1146.

201. Mearin F, Zacchi P, Armengol JR, et al. Effect of transcutaneous nerve stimulation on esophageal motility in patients with achalasia and scleroderma. Scand J Gastroenterol 1990;25:1018–1023.

202. Jean F, et al. Effects of diltiazem versus nifedipine on lower esophageal sphincter pressure in patients with progressive systemic sclerosis. Arthritis Rheum 1986;29:1054–1055.

203. Henderson RD, Pearson FG. Surgical management of esophageal scleroderma. J Thorac Cardiovasc Surg 1987;66:286–292.

204. Orringer MB, Dabich L, Zarafonedis CJD, et al. Gastroesophageal reflux in esophageal scleroderma: Diagnosis and implications. Ann Thorac Surg 1976;21:601–606.

205. Mansour KA, Malone CE. Surgery for scleroderma of the esophagus. A 12 year experience. Ann Thorac Surg 1988;46:513–514.

206. Dull JS, Raufman JP, Zakai MD, et al. Successful treatment of gastroparesis with erythromycin in a patient with systemic sclerosis. Am J Med 1990; 89:528–530.

207. Salen G, Goldstein F, Wirtz CW. Malabsorption in intestinal scleroderma: Relation to bacterial flora and treatment with antibiotics. Ann Intern Med 1966;64:834–841.

208. Alpert LI, Warner RRB. Systemic sclerosis. Case presenting with tetracycline responsive malabsorption syndrome. Am J Med 1968;45:468–473.

209. Kahn IJ, Jeffries GH, Sleisenger MH. Malabsorption in intestinal scleroderma. Engl J Med 1966; 274:1339–1344.

210. Dreiling DA, Soto JM. The pancreatic involvement in disseminated "collagen" disorders. Studies of pancreatic secretion in patients with scleroderma and Sjögren's "disease." Am J Gastroenterol 1976;66:546.

211. Grief JM, Wolfe WI. Idiopathic calcific pancreatitis, CREST syndrome and progressive systemic sclerosis. Am J Gastroenterol 1979;71:177–182.

212. Levien DH, Fiallos F, Barone R, Taffet S. The use of cyclic home hyperalimentation for malabsorption in patients with scleroderma involving the small intestine. J Parenterol Enterol Nutr 1985;9: 623–625.

213. Ng SC, Clements PJ, Berquist WE, et al. Home central venous hyperalimentation in 15 patients with severe scleroderma bowel disease. Arthritis Rheum 1989;32:212–216.

214. Grabowskii G, Grant JP. Nutritional support in patients with systemic scleroderma. J Parenteralol Nutr 1989;13:147–151.

215. Kaplan MM, et al. Fat-soluble vitamin nutrition in primary biliary cirrhosis. Gastroenterology 1988;95:787.

216. Herlong HF, Recker RR, Maddrey WC. Bone disease in primary biliary cirrhosis: Histologic features and response to 25-hydroxyvitamin D. Gastroenterology 1982;83:137.

217. Hodgson SF, et al. Bone loss and reduced osteoclastic function in primary biliary cirrhosis. Ann Intern Med 1985;103:855.

218. Matloff DS, et al. Osteoporosis in primary biliary cirrhosis—the effects of 25-hydroxyvitamin D treatment. Gastroenterology 1982;83:97.

219. Kaplan MM, et al. A prospective trial of colchicine for primary biliary cirrhosis. N Engl J Med 1986; 315:1448.

220. Warnes TW, et al. A controlled trial of colchicine in primary biliary cirrhosis: Trial design and preliminary report. J Hepatol 1987;5:1.

221. Zifroni A, Schaffner F. Long-term follow-up of patients with primary biliary cirrhosis on colchicine therapy. Hepatology 1991;14:990.

222. Wiesner RH, et al. A controlled trial of cyclosporin in the treatment of primary biliary cirrhosis. N Engl J Med 1990;322:1419.

223. Minuk GY, et al. Pilot study of cyclosporin A in

patients with symptomatic primary biliary cirrhosis. Gastroenterology 1988;95:1356.

224. Lombard M, et al. Cyclosporin A treatment in primary biliary cirrhosis: Results of a long-term placebo-controlled trial. Gastroenterology 1993; 104:519.

225. Calmus Y, Gane P, Rouger R, Poupon R. Hepatic expression of class I and class II major histocompatibility complex molecules in primary cirrhosis: Effect of ursodeoxycholic acid. Hepatology 1990;11:12.

226. Tox U, et al. Differences in the effect of ursodeoxycholic acid and chenodeoxycholic acid on the expression of HLA-molecules on human primary hepatocytes. Hepatology 1993;18:176A.

227. Poupon RE, et al. A multicenter controlled trial of ursodiol for treatment of primary biliary cirrhosis. N Engl J Med 1991;324:1548.

228. Leuschner U, et al. Ursodeoxycholic acid in primary biliary cirrhosis: Results of a controlled double-blind trial. Gastroenterology 1989;97:1268.

229. Batta AK, et al. Effect of long-term treatment with ursodiol and clinical and biochemical features and biliary bile acid metabolism in patients with primary biliary cirrhosis. Am J Gastroenterol 1993;88:691.

230. Lindor KD, et al. Ursodeoxycholic acid (UDCA) is beneficial therapy for patients with primary biliary cirrhosis (PBC) (abstract). Hepatology 1992; 16:91A.

231. Combes B, et al. A randomized, double-blind, placebo-controlled trial of ursodeoxycholic acid (UDCA) in primary biliary cirrhosis (abstract). Hepatology 1993;18:171A.

232. Kaplan MM, Knox TA. Treatment of primary biliary cirrhosis with low-dose methotrexate. Gastroenterology 1991;101:1332.

233. Zimmerman JH, Maddrey WC. Toxic and drug-induced hepatitis. In: Schiff L, Schiff ER, eds. Diseases of the liver. 7th ed. Philadelphia: JB Lippincott, 1993.

234. Markus BH, et al. Efficacy of liver transplantation in patients with primary biliary cirrhosis. N Engl J Med 1989;320:1709.

235. Esquivel CO, et al. Transplantation for primary biliary cirrhosis. Gastroenterology 1988;94:1207.

236. Polson RJ, et al. Evidence for disease recurrence after liver transplantation for primary biliary cirrhosis. Gastroenterology 1989;97:715.

237. Balan V, et al. Histologic evidence for recurrence of primary biliary cirrhosis after liver transplantation. Hepatology 1993;18:1392.

23

Organ Involvement:
Sexual Function and Pregnancy

THE PRESENCE of a systemic disease such as scleroderma or systemic sclerosis (SSc) (the terms will be used interchangeably in this chapter) may have profound effects on all aspects of someone's life. Sexual function in males and females is invariably affected to varying degrees. Gynecologic, fertility, breast, and pregnancy issues occurring in persons with SSc (both male and female) are discussed in this chapter. Additional coverage will be given to medications as they relate to these concerns, including breast feeding. Brief mention will also be made of the musculoskeletal syndromes that may cause pain and problems during pregnancy.

Non-Pregnancy Issues

FEMALE ISSUES

Gynecologic Concerns

In a recently reported study of sexuality, my colleagues and I have recorded complaints of vaginal dryness, dyspareunia, and menstrual irregularities, especially at the time of SSc onset. Additionally, occasional linear mucosal erosions in the vaginal vault were seen, and were sometimes mistaken for herpetic lesions (1). Czirjak et al, in a case control study of 61 patients with SSc (sixty females) and age- and sex-matched controls, noted that menstrual bleeding disturbances (metropathy and/or menorrhagia) were significantly higher in the SSc cases than in controls (p < .001). None of 15 SSc cases reported coagulopathies and/or thrombocytopenia (2). Premature menopause was noted in 4 of 60 SSc patients (2). In a study of 27 women with SSc, Serup and Hagdrup could find no statistically significant difference in age at menopause for SSc (47.8 years) versus 6000 published regional controls (47.3 years) (3). Another study reported that menopause occurred early in SSc (1).

A few isolated case reports of histopathologic changes in the uterine cervix consistent with scleroderma have been recorded (4,5). Steanlever and Ng's large review of the post-mortem histologic changes in the uterine cervix in SSc patients, however, found histologic changes consistent with SSc in only one of fifty-five specimens (6). Ballou (7) reported one case of local scleroderma of the genital area, similar to Steanlever's (6) description.

Only seven cases of ovarian carcinoma in association with SSc were found in the literature (8–11). All of these cases were adenocarcinomas and, in four of them, the SSc was diagnosed within one year of the ovarian carcinoma.

Summary. Menstrual abnormalities, vaginal dryness, and early menopause, occur occasionally in SSc, but their incidence is *not* clearly higher than controls. Direct sclerodermatous involvement of the female genital tract is rare.

Breast, Female

Few reports exist concerning the breast in scleroderma patients. The breasts are often spared the skin changes found elsewhere on the body, for reasons that are not clear.

Breast cancer does not appear to be more common in scleroderma than nonscleroderma patients, but it is fascinating to note that more than twenty cases have been reported in which SSc onset has occurred in close temporal proximity to breast cancer onset (8,9,12–15).

Women may suffer massive breast enlargement and hyperprolactinemia during d-penicillamine therapy (16). The breast enlargement of one SSc woman responded to danazol (17).

Summary. The breasts are often spared in SSc, but whether the incidence of breast cancer is increased remains controversial.

Sex Hormones

Sex hormones may play a role in immunological functioning. In SSc the female to male ratio is greater during the child bearing ages and equalizes with increasing age (18), suggesting that sex hormones may have an etiopathogenic or permissive role. One study of age at menopause of females with SSc versus nondisease controls found no significant difference (3), whereas a second found early menopause in SSc (1).

A study of relationships of menstrual cycle phase to symptoms of rheumatoid arthritis has found symptoms to be greater in the pre- than post-ovulatory phase (19). Menstrual cycle phase changes were reported by women with scleroderma, but with varying patterns (1).

Summary. No coherent data exists relating to the role of sex hormones, or abnormal hormonal levels, in SSc.

MALE ISSUES

Impotence

Impotence (inability to attain and/or maintain penile erection) may occur in men with scleroderma (20–23), and male erectile dysfunction may occur as an early manifestation of SSc (20). In one study (22), six of ten men with scleroderma were impotent, contrasted with none of ten age-matched male controls who had rheumatoid arthritis. In three reports (20–22), neurologic, psychiatric, and hormonal causes of impotence were not present. Levels of a variety of hormones were normal, including serum testosterone, free testosterone index, follicle stimulating hormone, luteinizing hormone, prolactin, estradiol, thyroxine, and thyrotropin. Nowlin's group (22) did show markedly low penile blood pressures in four of six patients, two of whom had lower extremity claudication and diminished ankle blood pressures, findings suggestive of large vessel disease.

Jimenez and Lally (23) reported five patients with erectile dysfunction from a clinic population of 43 male patients with scleroderma (12%). Since the initial study (20), three additional cases of male impotence were discovered (by the same investigators) among 11 new male scleroderma cases (27%).

Causes potentially contributing to impotence in scleroderma are noted in Table 23.1. Several authors (20–23) have speculated that impotence might result from disease of the nervous system, including autonomic nervous system dysfunction, and disease of the circulation. All the reported cases had erectile dysfunction, not loss of libido, which is the more common cause of impotence in the general population. Nowlin (24)

Table 23.1. Potential Cause of Loss of Libido in Systemic Sclerosis (Male and Female)

1. Body image-related depression
2. Fatigue/malaise
3. Muscle weakness/myopathy
4. Pain (primary arthralgias)
5. Restrictions of range of motion/contractures
6. Itching
7. Decreased oral and vaginal aperture
8. Neuropathy/neuralgias
9. Gastrointestinal disturbances (reflux, emesis)
10. Lung involvement/shortness of breath
11. Cardiac involvement/fear
12. Renal involvement
13. Medications
14. Vaginal dryness/dyspareunia

reported one SSc male patient who had loss of libido, normal potency, bilateral gynecomastia, bilateral testicular atrophy, normal testosterone levels, and elevated gonadotropin levels.

I can add one case of a male with generalized morphea, coup de sabre, and linear scleroderma who did not suffer erectile dysfunction. This patient suffered from infertility, as a result of a combination of a sperm liquefaction and motility disorder. These abnormalities may have been related to a lifelong series of experimental drug therapies or to the SSc disease process.

Klein reported an SSc patient with erectile dysfunction who was treated with implantation of a penile prosthesis (25). Varga, Lally, and Jimenez noted no success treating impotence in SSc with oral yohimbine, and reported that they were trying intramuscular and intrapenile papaverine (26). The latter has worked in one of my own SSc patients with erectile dysfunction (unpublished, anecdotal data).

Varga et al (26) also examined testicular tissue in three SSc patients and found changes similar to those reported by Middleton (27). One of those patients exhibited testicular fibrosis, poor spermatogenesis, and thickening of the basement membrane of the seminiferous tubules.

Summary. Male impotence certainly occurs in SSc and may occur frequently, although no large studies of this problem have been published. Erectile dysfunction probably occurs between 12% and 27% of cases. Treatment success is reported anecdotally.

Male Breast

In the male, gynecomastia is a reported complication of two known scleroderma therapies: d-penicillamine (16) and low dose methotrexate (28).

BOTH SEXES

Expressions of sexuality for men and women, whether for the purpose of reproduction and/or intimacy, are mentally, emotionally, and physically demanding. Lack of sexual education, which is inadequate for most of the population,

allows little room for the average person to compensate for the mental, emotional, and physical demands of a chronic illness such as SSc. SSc may be a problem primarily of older adults when contrasted with the younger onset of systemic lupus, but the concept that there is a decrease in sexual function and/or desire after both male and female climacteric is more myth than reality (29). Sexual desire may increase, decrease, or remain the same but sexual counseling should provide factual information and supportive guidance so full sexual potential may be reached (29,30). Studies done with arthritis patients (although not specifically SSc patients) find that when patients are given the opportunity to discuss their sexuality, they express a wide range of problems about pain and fatigue, sexual opportunity, sexual image, sexual drive, sexual competence, sexual expression, and sexual function (30–32). A sex counseling study comparing attitudes of disabled versus nondisabled subjects revealed that disabled subjects preferred to be counseled by a physician rather than a psychologist or social worker, and they exhibited greater anxiety toward the issue of sex (33). A model for human sexuality rehabilitation, called PLISSIT (34), was first designed for spinal cord injuries but may be adapted for SSc. PLISSIT is an acronym describing a four-level approach to sexual concerns:

Permission-(**P**)—an authority figure, such as a physician, gives permission, or provides a comfortable opportunity, to discuss sexuality as a matter-of-fact routine part of rehabilitation;

Limited Information-(**LI**)—the authority figure transmits specific information from his/her expertise with regard to the patient's disease and sexual functioning;

Specific Suggestions-(**SS**)—problem solving occurs after completing an evaluation of a couple's sexual functioning;

Intensive Therapy-(**IT**)—sexuality exercises are designed for patient and partner (34).

Most physicians can treat sexual concerns on the first three levels, while experts in sexual rehabilitation may be needed for the fourth level (34). To augment teaching and to enhance discussions, pamphlets and articles are available through the Arthritis Foundation and the United Scleroderma Foundation. Some of these materials contain appropriate illustrations. Communication among physician, patient, family, and allied health workers is truly the keystone to dealing with this delicate area of concern.

Summary

No data specific to sexual functioning in SSc appear to have been published. General guidelines for discussion of sexual function are presented, including PLISSIT (Permission, Limited Information, Specific Suggestions, Intensive Therapy).

Pregnancy Issues

PLANNING

Health care providers involved in the care of SSc patients must address issues related to sexuality, contraception, and pregnancy as early as possible in the SSc process. Otherwise, ill-conceived and uninformed concepts may guide patients through these most important issues. Warnings given about not becoming pregnant while taking certain medications are not enough. Contraceptive issues should be dealt with directly, and the form of birth control should be tailored to the patient's needs (e.g., use of diaphragm and condoms may be difficult for contractured scleroderma hands). Oral contraceptive use should be discussed as should all other forms of contraception.

FERTILITY

Fertility is an issue for both sexes with SSc. There is a paucity of information on male fertility. In women, the fertility rate may be crudely determined by counting the number of pregnancies. Since SSc may occur when only a few years of fer-

tility remain, adjusted fertility rates are important in the assessment of SSc, because adjusted rates allow for consideration of years of potential fertility from a given point. In this discussion, the term "abortion" means the spontaneous termination of pregnancy occurring prior to 20 weeks of gestation, while the term "stillbirth" means spontaneous termination of pregnancy occurring after 20 weeks of gestation.

Before the 1980s, reports concerning SSc and pregnancy made repeated reference to how rarely the association of SSc and pregnancy was mentioned anecdotally in the medical literature or in large surveys, especially for those women within the child bearing ages (35–38). The inference was drawn that scleroderma patients suffer decreased fertility, but not complete sterility.

Giordano et al, in 1985, reported a retrospective study of pregnancies in SSc patients from the University of Naples, Italy (39). They compared 86 women with SSc to 86 healthy control women. Only six of the 86 scleroderma patients had had no pregnancies, which was not significantly different than the four of 86 healthy controls who had not had pregnancies (39). The remaining 80 SSc patients had experienced 299 pregnancies, compared to 82 healthy controls with 332 pregnancies. On the other hand 50 of 299 SSc pregnancies versus 32 of 332 healthy control pregnancies experienced spontaneous abortion (39).

Wilman reported that, of 155 case control pairs, women destined to develop SSc had twice the rate of spontaneous abortion and three times the rate of fertility problems prior to the onset of SSc (as measured by no successful pregnancy by the age of 35) compared to the control women (40). Age of menarche was similar for both groups (12.8 for SSc) as was contraceptive use (36% for SSc). Leinwald has also written of reduced fertility in SSc (36), and Orabona described ovarian atrophy (41). Siamopoulou-Mavridou (42) also found a higher rate of spontaneous abortion prior to scleroderma onset when contrasted with healthy controls ($p < .05$), but this was per pregnancy and did not remain statistically significant when the incidence per woman was studied. Fertility rates were comparable to healthy controls (42).

A large study of reproductive function prior to the onset of scleroderma was done using a postal questionnaire (43). The study involved 204 women with scleroderma, 233 women with primary Raynaud's phenomenon (RP), and 189 healthy women from a population register (36). Results were analyzed by the use of odds ratios estimating the relative risk of developing scleroderma; each reproductive variable was compared to the risk in the comparison groups. The results indicated that women with scleroderma were more likely than healthy women to have had a delay in conception equal to or greater than one year (OR 2.6), or to be infertile (OR 2.3), but no differences were seen when SSc women were compared to the group with primary RP (36). Self reports of maternal ill health during pregnancy were similarly increased in women with scleroderma when compared to the healthy women (OR 2.1), but not when compared to the women with RP (43). The three groups showed no difference in early fetal loss, but there were more perinatal losses in the scleroderma group than the other two groups. There were also a greater proportion of live births of low birth weight. These reports suggest that reproductive function before onset of scleroderma may be impaired, which suggests that there may be a negative impact of prodromal immunologic and/or vascular changes. A third possible explanation may be related to the increased chromosomal breakage rate recently reported in scleroderma (37).

A study of 54 cases of RP compared to controls noted a higher incidence of infertility in the Raynaud's group. The authors postulated that RP may parallel internal organ vasospasm/vasculopathy and thereby affect menstruation, menopause, and pregnancy (38).

One case was reported of a woman with clinical and histologic features of morphea associated with spontaneous abortion, thrombocytope-

nia, cerebral infarct, and circulating anticoagulant (44). A study of autoantibodies in SSc and other autoimmune disorders during pregnancy found elevated IgG anticardiolipin antibody levels in only 11% of 28 SSc patients (13% rheumatoid arthritis (RA), 26% systemic lupus erythematosus (SLE)), and only one of the five anticardiolipin positive patients had recurrent fetal loss (44,45). While pregnancy loss was high for SSc in this study (44,45), no significant correlation was noted between pregnancy loss and the finding of antibodies to SSA and/or to SSB, and of cardiolipin antibodies. Although the differences were not statistically significant, anticentrome antibodies, anti-Scl-70, and Jo-1 antibodies were more frequent in those with at least one pregnancy loss (45). In the same study of 28 women with SSc (45), 78% of 81 pregnancies occurred before disease onset, and a high pregnancy loss rate (33%) was noted.

In a study by Kaufman et al, mixed connective tissue disease patients demonstrated a normal fertility rate unaltered by disease. Reduced parity and increased fetal wastage both before and after onset of disease were also noted (46). A second study showed no remarkable differences in these rates prior to disease onset (42).

Summary

Patients with SSc have some delay in conception, may have decreased fertility, possibly have an increased incidence of spontaneous abortion, and probably have increased perinatal losses. There is probably an increased incidence of pre-term and low birth weight infants in SSc (see following paragraphs). Interestingly, these may relate to the presence of RP rather than SSc. For clear answers, larger, stratified prospective studies will be needed.

In conclusion, despite compelling evidence that SSc will affect the chances of conception and pregnancy outcome, outcome in any individual case cannot be predicted. Further, the diversity of possible SSc clinical findings will require larger series, stratified by extent of involvement and pregnancy outcome, to enhance our ability to predict outcome.

PREGNANCY

General Effects of SSc on Pregnancy and Pregnancy on SSc

Eno's report, in 1937, was the first in the English language literature to describe pregnant women with scleroderma; there was no maternal mortality and only one intrauterine death (47). In 1964, Gunther (48) and DeCarle (49) were the first to describe multiple pregnancies (three pregnancies in a single SSc patient in each report). However, it was Johnson (50), also in 1964, whose study of 36 instances of concomitant scleroderma and pregnancy (Table 23.2) described enough cases from which to draw inferences. Johnson noted that in 39% of the cases, the scleroderma did not change during pregnancy, in 22% the scleroderma was clinically improved, and in 22% the scleroderma worsened (third trimester edema with persistence and progression of sclerodermatous skin changes) (50). In 17% of the cases, the onset of scleroderma occurred during pregnancy (50). Although there was no maternal mortality, one stillbirth and three spontaneous abortions occurred (all occurred in the same patient). In 1968, Slate (51) described a very high rate of spontaneous abortion (Table 23.2), 13 of 17 pregnancies, but Donaldsen (37,38) in a discussion of the same paper, reported results of a questionnaire of pregnant SSc patients in the Seattle area in which only three of 17 scleroderma pregnancies ended in spontaneous abortion; in 13 of 17 instances the mothers suffered no worsening of the disease process. It should be noted that the majority of cases in Slate's report (51) were from Los Angeles County hospitals where a poor prognosis among indigent patients is not unexpected.

Nineteen additional pregnancies not recorded in Table 23.2 have been reported in 13 case reports (35,36,47–49,52–59). In all cases, episiotomies and Caesarian sections healed. Scleroderma worsened in four (one maternal death),

improved or remitted in three, and remained unchanged in twelve. Twelve of 19 infants lived; the remainder were stillborn or died in the immediate postpartum period. A complete gamut of pregnancy-related problems were seen including toxemia, abruptio placenta, and premature rupture of membrane. The reports through 1970 indicated that scleroderma remained unchanged or improved in the majority of cases, and maternal mortality was low. However, fetal deaths (combining abortion, stillbirth, and perinatal death) were high (33% or 29 of 88 combining pre-1970 data from Table 23.2 and references 35,36,47–49,52–59). Live birth babies were often premature or of low birth weight. Examination of placentae, fetuses, and newborns detected no evidence of sclerodermatous changes (as referenced previously), except for two of 88 cases (47,56) with changes described as sclerodermatous lasting only for weeks to a month.

Leinwand, in 1954, noted that six of 108 women with SSc seen over a 14-year span at New York University Hospital experienced their first scleroderma symptoms shortly after delivery (36). Two of those patients developed RP during the fifth month of pregnancy, and developed full-blown SSc several months after delivery. Since that report, numerous SSc cases have been reported in which SSc onset has occurred during or shortly after a pregnancy (60).

The past twenty-five years have brought about remarkable improvements in the care of premature infants and neonates. These changes are reflected by improved outcome for pregnancy in SSc in more recent reports (7,60–65) (Table 23.2).

In an important study comparing scleroderma pregnancies to pregnancies in rheumatoid arthritis and neighborhood controls, Steen et al (66) found an increase in preterm births and small full-term babies prior to and after the onset of SSc. Maternal and fetal mortality were not increased in SSc contrasted with controls (66). Maternal SSc remained unchanged in 88% of 133 pregnancies, and maternal pregnancy complications such as placenta previa, infection, or uter-

Table 23.2. Pregnancy After Developing Systemic Sclerosis: Studies with More than 3 Patients

Author/ Reference	Year	Number of Pregnancies	Mean Maternal Age	Change in SSc		(<38wks) Toxemia	Spontaneous Prematurity	(<20wks) Perinatal Abortion	Maternal Death	Death
Johnson (50)	1964	36	27 yo	Better No change Worse	8 14 14	3	NDA[a]	3	1	NDA
Slate (51)	1968	17	26 yo	NDA		1	2	13	2	1
Donaldson 2 separate reports (37,39)	1964, 1968	17	26 yo	No change Worse	13 4	1	4	1	2	0
Weiner (60)	1986	21	23 yo	Better Worse No change Onset with pregnancy	1 3 15 2	1	4	1	2	0
Black (67)	1989	12	NDA	Better Worse No change Onset with pregnancy	0 8 3 1	3	NDA	4	2	1
Steen (66)	1989	19[b] 114[c]	25 yo	No change	117	13	2 18[d]	3[d] 5[d]	0[d] 0	1

[a]NDA, No Data Available
[b]Diffuse Systemic Sclerosis
[c]Limited Scleroderma
[d]No increased frequency contrasted with rheumatoid arthritis or normal controls.

ine bleeding were not increased above the control levels (66).

McHugh (45) found reproductive loss (spontaneous abortion plus stillbirth) after scleroderma onset to be 83% of 18 pregnancies; however, 13 of his 15 reported reproductive losses were from a single woman who had had 15 first trimester pregnancy fetal deaths, 13 occurring after SSc onset (45). Black (67) reported 12 diffuse SSc pregnancies, noting that maternal SSc progressed in eight of 12, had its onset in three of 12 and maternal death in one case. However, as Silman (68) states, case reports may be biased toward problem outcomes, and small numbers make interpretation of data hazardous. Examples of this would be to draw inferences from Meyer's three cases of abruptio placenta in a single scleroderma patient (69), or the 13 reproductive losses in the one woman in McHugh's series (45).

Summary. Although data are incomplete and conflicting, it appears that more patients remain stable (approximately 40%–60%) than worsen (approximately 20%) or improve (approximately 20%). Anecdotal reports indicate some increased incidence of disease onset immediately after pregnancy, but the data are uncontrolled and subject to much bias. There is probably an increased incidence of pre-term and low birth weight infants in SSc, similar to other connective tissue diseases.

Individual Organ Considerations

Musculoskeletal Complaints. A wide variety of musculoskeletal and neurologic problems have been associated with pregnancy (Table 23.3). Pregnant SSc patients are more susceptible than the general population to many of these problems (e.g., carpal tunnel syndrome (CTS) and osteoporosis (70,71)).

CTS has been found in a small percent of SSc patients (70) and may be expected to occur in a slightly larger percentage during pregnancy. However, no study examining the simultaneous occurrence of pregnancy, SSc, and CTS has been reported. CTS associated with pregnancy occurs in the second or third trimester and may develop in 20% of normal pregnancies (72,73). Splinting and carpal canal injections may be tried. Surgery for CTS should be avoided during pregnancy, because CTS and tenosynovitis often resolve after parturition (72–74). It is of note that both syndromes may not improve until breast feeding is stopped (74).

Leg cramps (75), usually nocturnal, are as common as CTS, frequently occurring in the second half of pregnancy, and usually respond to calcium supplementation. Low back pain may occur from a variety of causes (Table 23.2), and occurs in one-half to two-thirds of all pregnant women, most often in the later stages of pregnancy (73,76–81). A trochanteric belt or a lumbosacral corset modified with an abdominal panel may be particularly helpful. Osteoporosis along with bone resorption is well described in SSc (71) and may be even more common because of the additive effects of osteoporosis from pregnancy (82,83). Meralgia paresthetica has also been described in both SSc (91) and, separately, in pregnancy (73,92).

Table 23.3. Musculoskeletal Problems and Pregnancy[a]

1. Carpal tunnel syndrome	(72, 73)
2. De Quervains tenosynovitis	(74)
3. Back pain/pelvic pain	(73, 76–81, 84, 129)
a. Strain	
b. Sciatica	
c. Herniated disc	
d. Osteitis condensans ilii	
e. Osteitis pubis	
f. Bursitis	
g. Relaxin induced SI joint laxity	
4. Muscle cramps	(75)
5. Fatigue	
6. Postpartum cervical myofascial pain syndrome	(85, 130)
7. Osteoporosis	(82, 83)
8. Stress fracture	(86, 131)
9. Coccyx fracture	(87, 132)
10. Scoliosis progression	(88, 133)
11. Transient osteoporosis	(89, 134)
12. Meralgia paraesthetica	(73)
13. Intercostal neuralgia	(73, 90, 135)

[a]References 72–83, 84–90, 129–135

Summary. Carpal tunnel syndrome, leg cramps, and low back pain are common in SSc but no controlled comparisons relative to normal populations are available. Osteoporosis has also been described.

Gastrointestinal. Two thirds of patients with SSc have gastrointestinal problems: decreased oral aperture, xerostomia, dysphagia, pyrosis, spontaneous emesis, alteration of bowel habits, and/or malabsorption. During pregnancy smooth muscle tone decreases, resulting in an increase of pyrosis in scleroderma patients that is far worse than what would be expected with gestation alone (93). Additionally, delayed gastric emptying causes early satiety and onset of, or aggravation of, malabsorption (93). This may result in a need for supplemental fat soluble vitamins (94).

Summary. The frequent gastrointestinal difficulties in SSc patients, particularly pyrosis and delayed gastric emptying, probably become even more problematic during pregnancy.

Cardiovascular. Although pregnancy brings about shifts in blood volume (increases 50% above baseline, peaking at 30–32 weeks), RBC mass (increases 20%–40%), cardiac output (increases 40% above baseline by 20th week), and blood pressure (decreases), problems with cardiac arrhythmias are rarely associated with adverse maternal or fetal outcomes (95,96). Cardiovascular drugs and anesthetics should be used with special care, being especially watchful for hypotension and cardiac failure, which can occur with calcium channel blocking agents (96). However, one woman with SSc who had lost four of six previous pregnancies had a successful pregnancy with a healthy infant, having taken nifedipine 30–60 mg/day for treatment of a foot ulcer during her entire pregnancy (97). Congestive heart failure in the peripartum period related to renal disease and/or pulmonary disease may have a more ominous prognosis (7,98,99), although occasional good outcomes have been reported (99).

Summary. Cardiac arrhythmias are rare and medications are as problematic as for pregnancies in general. The effects of renal and pulmonary disease on cardiovascular function require careful attention.

Thyroid Disorders. Thyroid disorders are found more often than would be expected by chance alone in scleroderma. Special consideration should be given to medical, surgical, and anesthetic management of thyroid disease in pregnancy (100).

Pulmonary Disease. The immediate postpartum period of SSc patients who have caesarian section may, rarely, be complicated by pulmonary edema (101) and/or pulmonary hypertension (98). These changes have usually occurred in association with preexisting subclinical lung disease. Even so, patients with SSc and preexisting (pre-pregnancy) pulmonary fibrosis (47,62) and pulmonary hypertension (102) have had successful outcomes. Aspiration pneumonia during delivery in the puerperium (51), or even several weeks postpartum, remains a significant risk (103).

Summary. Post-partum pulmonary edema and, especially, aspiration pneumonia need to be avoided and special attention is needed even for several weeks after delivery.

Peripheral Gangrene. One case report detailed a patient who experienced the onset of RP during pregnancy and who developed gangrene of the fingers in the 32nd week of gestation (104). The case was managed with multiple drugs but successful outcome was attributed to nifedipine, repeated stellate ganglion bupivacaine blocks, and careful local care (104). Another case has been reported of an SSc patient with Raynaud's whose pregnancy was complicated by sepsis, disseminated intravascular coagulation, shock, retained placenta, and development of gangrene of all four extremities (105). This unfortunate patient also developed post partum renal failure.

Thompson et al (62) and Younker et al (98) pointed out several useful techniques for treating Raynaud's during delivery. These techniques are reviewed in the *Anesthesia* and *Management of Delivery* sections of this chapter.

Summary. Peripheral gangrene is apparently a very rare problem in SSc during pregnancy.

Renal Disease. Renal failure complicating scleroderma pregnancy was first reported in 1968 by Fear (106) and again in 1970 and 1973 by Sood (107) and Karlen (108). Since accelerated hypertension and proteinuria also can herald eclampsia as well as scleroderma renal crisis, it is frequently very difficult to know which process is paramount. In the three single case reports, the patients were Caucasian primigravidas with no prior clinical renal disease. Between weeks 27 and 31 they developed what appeared to be pre-eclampsia with proteinuria and hypertension. All progressed to renal failure and subsequently died. At post mortem they had sclerodermatous changes in the kidney. Only one of three infants survived. Accelerated hypertension (renal crisis) is a poor prognostic sign for mother and fetus (63,98,105,109). In the last 15 years, however, similar cases have documented lower maternal and fetal mortality (62,102,110–112). There is also a report of the successful outcome in a woman with preexistent (pre-pregnancy) SSc and renal disease (61,102,112,113).

Steen et al (68) found no increase in the frequency of pregnant versus nonpregnant renal crisis, preeclampsia, or hypertensive pregnancy. However, the few cases of renal crisis in pregnancy had a poor prognosis. The authors recommend that women with early, rapidly progressive, diffuse skin thickening, who appear to be at higher risk for renal crisis with or without pregnancies, avoid becoming pregnant (66).

The keys to successful management of pregnancies in SSc with renal disease are careful monitoring of weight, proteinuria, and blood pressure weekly, or even daily, along with judicious use of medications (62,97,102,110–112) including captopril, if necessary (66,113). Subsequent dialysis, and even renal transplant, may reduce maternal mortality (110), but overall maternal and fetal mortality in reported cases of renal failure complicating SSc pregnancy remains high (61).

Mention should also be made of a case with a successful outcome of SSc and twin pregnancy that was complicated by an obstructive uropathy due in part to a rigid abdominal wall and polyhydramnios (99).

Summary. Renal failure is probably not increased during pregnancy, but if it occurs has a very poor prognosis for mother and infant. Aggressive therapy appears warranted (angiotensin converting enzyme (ACE) inhibitors and evacuate the uterus).

CREST. The analysis of seven women with CREST syndrome undergoing 20 pregnancies (60) indicates that outcome depends more on overlapping diseases that may be present in association with CREST. In CREST unassociated with other disorders, worsening of telangiectasias and Raynaud's was observed; CREST with mixed connective tissue disease (MCTD) had worsening of telangiectasias, Raynaud's, arthralgias, one case of preclampsia and one of toxemia. Finally, CREST with primary biliary cirrhosis had a poor prognosis with high fetal and neonatal loss (60).

Medication Use During Pregnancy

No drug can ever be considered 100% safe for use during pregnancy or for use while breast feeding (Table 23.4). Relative risks of medications are different for the fetus (penetration of the maternal-fetal circulation) (114) and the breast-feeding newborn (passage into breast milk) (115). Also, relative risks of medication change at different stages of fetal development (5,104,116). Furthermore, lack of human trials of medications during pregnancy, for obvious reasons, may leave us dependent on animal studies, which often do not reflect the human situation.

Salicylate. Salicylic acid and acetylsalicylic acid are teratogenic in animals (114,116–118). The prostaglandin inhibiting effects of aspirin may result in anemia, peripartum maternal hemorrhage, prolongation of labor, prolongation of pregnancy, fetal hemostatic problems, fetal intracranial hemorrhage, and premature closure of the patent ductus arteriosus (114,116,118–121). Most studies suggest that salicylates should be discontinued at least 1 week before the predicted date of delivery and should be used in as low a dose as possible during the pregnancy.

Nonsteroidals. Nonsteroidals are also teratogenic in animals (114) but have not proven to be so in humans. Since they are prostaglandin inhibitors, all the hematologic and reproductive problems associated with aspirin may theoretically occur with all nonsteroidals (114,116,117, 122). Therefore, discontinuation at least 1 to 2 weeks prior to the estimated date of delivery is recommended to avoid platelet inhibition and other effects on labor and delivery.

Acetaminophen. Acetaminophen, in standard therapeutic doses, is not associated with human teratogenicity or other adverse effects to the fetus (119,122) and may be recommended for analgesia. Liver toxicity to the fetus could occur with overdosing (119).

Corticosteroids. Corticosteroids demonstrate fetal damage in animals but in humans appear to be safe at low doses (113,114,123). Descriptions in the literature of a large series of patients using steroids during pregnancy showed anecdotal risks of fetal adrenocortical insufficiency and cleft lip/palate (123,124). It is also important to supplement maternal corticosteroids during delivery, if they have been given in the year prior to delivery (117). Scleroderma patients have undergone successful pregnancy while taking corticosteroids (125). Since prednisone does not cross the placenta, it is the preferred corticosteroid in pregnancy.

Penicillamine. Most reports on the use of penicillamine are anecdotal and are for Wilson's disease (51). Fetal problems have included a generalized connective tissue defect similar to cutis laxa, vitamin B6 deficiency (rarely), placental transfer of antibody to acetylcholine receptors, and one minor ventricular septal defect (62,116, 117). Normal children have been born to mothers taking penicillamine for Wilson's disease (117). Lyle (126) reviewed 27 SSc pregnancies of mothers using d-penicillamine and found only one infant with problems: the previously mentioned minor ventricular septal defect. However, should pregnancy occur while taking penicillamine, the advice from several authors is that the drug be withdrawn slowly (61,114). Penicillamine should not be started during pregnancy.

Colchicine. Colchicine is a known teratogen. Its use should be avoided during pregnancy (111,114).

Cytotoxic and Antimetabolite Drugs. Cyclophosphamide and methotrexate may be both teratogenic and mutagenic, and steps should always be taken to prevent pregnancies while patients are on these drugs (116,117,127). While successful uncomplicated pregnancies have been reported, fetal risk appears to be very high (114, 116,117,127).

Cyclosporin. Cyclosporin A crosses the placenta. While anecdotal reports of successful use in pregnancy exist, more information is needed (128,129).

Antiarrhythmics. Cardiac arrhythmias occur in scleroderma and may be worsened during the hemodynamic changes occurring during pregnancy. The approach to therapy in pregnant patients must include special consideration in drug selection with regard to adverse fetal effects (130). A successful pregnancy has been reported in a woman with SSc who had a previously poor obstetric record, and who was taking nifedipine 30 mg/day during the pregnancy (97).

ACE Inhibitors. ACE inhibitors have been a boon to the treatment of scleroderma renal disease and hypertension in pregnancy (131). Reports of fetal abnormalities with the use of captopril or enalapril during pregnancy are rare, but this risk must be carefully considered when deciding on their risk:benefit ratio.

Two reports of captopril use during SSc resulted in successful maternal and neonatal outcomes despite renal crisis (66,113). One of the two women did have agranulocytosis as a complication of the captopril (113).

Psychotropics. Tricyclic antidepressants and benzodiazepines are occasionally given to rheumatic disease patients. Since birth defects and, for benzodiazepines, a neonatal abstinence syndrome have been reported, the drugs should be avoided during pregnancy (132).

Table 23.4. Medication Use During Pregnancy and Breast Feeding[a]

	Pregnancy	Breast Feeding
Salicylates	May complicate delivery. Contraindicated at dose > 650 mg or in late pregnancy.	Risk considered small at low dose (<650 mg). Possible metabolic acidosis at high dose (2.4g/day).
Nonsteroidals	May complicate delivery. Contraindicated at high dose or in late pregnancy.	Presence in breast milk varies with drug. Relative contraindication in PDR. Ibuprofen may be safest.
Acetaminophen	Considered safe in therapeutic dose range, but unsafe at high doses.	—
Corticosteroids	Considered safe at low dose (<15mg prednisone a day), risky at higher doses.	May be safe at low doses (<7.5 mg of prednisone a day).
Penicillamine	Birth defects reported—do not use.	Contraindicated—found in trace amounts of breast milk.
Colchicine	Teratogen—do not use.	Contraindicated.
Cytotoxic/ Antimetabolites	Teratogenic and mutagenic—do not use.	Contraindicated—found in breast milk.
Cyclosporin	Dose dependent inhibition of fetal growth— do not use.	Found in breast milk, contraindicated.

[a]No drug is ever considered safe during pregnancy or breast feeding.

Summary. The use of medications in pregnant women with SSc is no different than for healthy pregnant women. Care is necessary. Successful pregnancies have been reported for women on nearly all of these drugs, but this does not imply that these medications are safe to use. Cutis laxa has been reported in an infant whose mother used D-penicillamine. Colchicine is teratogenic, while methotrexate and cytotoxics clearly increase the risk of teratogenicity and mutagenesis. Data on cyclosporin are not known, although cyclosporin crosses the placenta. ACE inhibitors are used for SSc renal disease during pregnancy.

Considerations When Anesthesia Is Necessary

A variety of anesthetic concerns arise for the SSc patient undergoing surgery (133,134); these same concerns are germane to the delivery of the pregnant scleroderma patient as well. Two existing reviews (62,98) delineate the problems and propose solutions (133,134).

Management of Delivery

RP necessitates a warm delivery room environment, warmed intravenous fluids, warm compresses for the extremities, and the consideration of regional anesthesia (epidural block) to provide peripheral vasodilation and increased skin perfusion of the lower extremities (110,121,127, 134). Because the beta blockers may aggravate RP, careful selection of agents for treatment of hypertensive problems is equally important (104, 105). Vascular access may be difficult in patients with SSc. Large veins should be accessed prophylactically to provide for potential emergency situations. Use of a Hickman catheter may be necessary (62,98). Catheterization with a Swan-Ganz catheter (102) may be necessary to assist with fluid management and for monitoring problems with systemic hypertension, pulmonary hypertension, myocardial perfusion, and renal perfusion (62,98,102,104,125). Catheter placement in peripheral arteries (e.g., radial, brachial) should be avoided because of possible vasospasm (62). Endotracheal intubation may be difficult because of decreased size of the oral aperture and nares (52,98). Avoidance of aspiration, a major contributing factor to poor outcome, has led some to suggest awake intubation to preserve the gag reflex, and others to view this as another reason for regional anesthesia (62). Intubation with endoscopic guidance may help guard against aspiration (98). Bleeding from oral, nasal, and/or upper airway telangiectasias may occur rarely (62). There may also be enhanced sensitivity to any anesthetic agent because of impaired internal organ function (62, 98,104,105). Complicating Sjögren's syndrome necessitates careful hydration of airways and of any gases given. Protection of the eyes involved with xeroophthalmia is also advisable (62,104). Caesarian section may be done since the skin will heal appropriately. Careful consideration of the aforementioned problems and of cardiovascular, gastrointestinal, pulmonary, and renal factors is essential before deciding on this method of delivery (62,98,102,105).

Summary. Large vein access, prophylactically, is recommended. Avoidance of aspiration is strongly suggested, including possible early intubation with endoscopic guidance. Finally warmth and good airway hydration are required. This will require a team approach to delivery.

POST-PARTUM CONSIDERATIONS

General

The postpartum period may be fraught with as many difficulties as pregnancy itself. Infant care for a woman with hand, wrist, and elbow contractures is extremely difficult. Combinations of disease factors and pregnancy factors can leave the new SSc mother with little strength or energy to care for a newborn infant. Help from spouse, family, friends, and, if possible, hired professionals is critical. Support systems must be established prior to delivery. The possibility of premature delivery should be considered. Breast feeding and medication are discussed below.

Medications When Breast Feeding

Many drugs are excreted in human breast milk, even when taken as usual doses. Several are excreted in doses sufficient to produce pharmacologic effects in a nursing infant (115,117).

Plasma salicylate concentrations of 24 mg/dl were found in a breast-fed child with metabolic acidosis, whose mother was taking 2.4 grams of aspirin a day (115,117). Nonsteroidals, as weak acids, do not achieve high concentrations in breast milk, but there is a dearth of reported clinical information (117). If nonsteroidals are used, those with short half-lives and inactive metabolites, such as ibuprofen and flurbiprofen, are preferred. Glucocorticoids enter breast milk; however, in doses of 15 mg of prednisolone a day or less, they are probably safe (115,117). Alkylating agents and antimetabolites should not be used during breast feeding (115,117). Although penicillamine is protein-bound and only small amounts are found in breast milk, its potential for renal and bone marrow toxicity preclude its use (115,117). Cyclosporin is transferred to breast milk (129) and therefore should not be used during lactation.

Conclusions

A team approach for the treatment of the SSc patient should be tailored to address the individual problems and needs of each patient. Recognition and education with regard to male impotence and female breast and gynecologic concerns are also important. Decisions about pregnancy must be made on a case-by-case basis and should involve education and planning. Should a decision be made to proceed with a pregnancy, early involvement of specialists in high risk obstetrics, high risk perinatology, and anesthesia is indicated. Following delivery, sclerodermatous skin heals well from episiotomy and Caesarian section (135). Anticipation and preparation for premature and/or low birth weight infants must be made (66). Postpartum maternal and infant care issues are important. Use of medications during pregnancy and breast feeding are discussed in previous paragraphs.

Successful SSc pregnancies do occur despite the possibility of reduced fertility and disease-related complications. While childbirth may not be essential, its profound societal, familial, psychologic, and religious impact must be considered and may lead the physician to encourage pregnancy despite its dangers. The best outcomes will be those where ongoing discussion and education are provided for patient and family.

References

1. Bhadauria S, Moser D, Clements PJ, Singh RR, Lachenbruch PA, Pitkin RM, Weiner SR. Genital tract abnormalities and female sexual function impairment in systemic sclerosis. Am J Obstet Gynecol 1995;172:580–587.
2. Czirjak L, Bokk A, Csontos G, Lorincz G, Szegedi G. Clinical findings in 61 patients with progressive systemic sclerosis. Acta Derm Venereol 1989; 69:533–538.
3. Serup J, Hagdrup HK. Age at menopause of females with systemic sclerosis. Acta Derm Venereol 1983;63:71–73.
4. Bellucci MJ, Coustan DR, Plotz RD. Cervical scleroderma: A case of soft tissue dystocia. Am J Obstet Gynecol 1984;150:891–892.
5. Eno E. Pregnancy in a patient suffering with scleroderma. Am J Obstet Gynecol 1987;33:514–515.
6. Stenlever MA, Ng ABP. Scleroderma of the uterine cervix. Am J Obstet Gynecol 1970;107:965–966.
7. Ballou SP, Morley JJ, Kushner I. Pregnancy and systemic sclerosis. Arthritis Rheum 1984;27:295–298.
8. Duncan SC, Winkelmann RK. Cancer and scleroderma. Arch Dermatol 1979;115:950–955.
9. Roumm AD, Medsger TA. Cancer and systemic sclerosis. An epidemiologic study. Arthritis Rheum 1985;28;1336–1340.
10. Young R, Towbin B, Isern R. Scleroderma and ovarian carcinoma. Br J Rheumatol 1990;29:314.
11. Jacobsen BB, Pendersen M, Herting SE. Generalized scleroderma. Report on a case associated with acute nephropathy, haemolytic anemia and malignant ovarian tumor. Acta Med Scand 1972; 192:107–111.
12. Lee P, Alderdice C, Wilkinson S, Keystone EC, Urowitz MB, Gladman DD. Malignancy in progressive systemic sclerosis—association with breast carcinoma. J Rheumatol 1983;10:665–666.
13. Talbott JH, Barrocas M. Progressive systemic sclerosis (PSS) and malignancy, pulmonary and non pulmonary. Medicine 1979;58:182–207.
14. Neto RPD, Steinberg A, Kron SD, Rachmann R. Breast carcinoma in a patient with scleroderma. Postgrad Med 1968;44:161–166.
15. Forbes AM, Woodrow JC, Verbov JL, Graham RM. Carcinoma of breast and scleroderma: Four further cases and a literature review. Br J Rheumatol 1989;28:65–69.
16. Frantz AG, Wilson JD. Endocrine disorders of the breast. In: Wilson JD, Foster DW, eds. Williams textbook of endocrinology, 7th ed. Philadelphia: WB Saunders, 1985;402–421.
17. Kahl LE, Medsger TA, Klein E. Massive breast enlargement in a patient receiving d-penicillamine for systemic sclerosis. J Rheumatol 1985;12:990–991.
18. Masi AT. Chapter 2. Clinical-epidemiological perspective of systemic sclerosis (scleroderma). In: Jayson MIV, Black CM, eds. Systemic sclerosis: scleroderma. New York, John Wiley & Sons, Ltd, 1988;15–16.
19. Letman NS. Relation of menstrual cycle phase to symptoms of rheumatoid arthritis. Am J Med 1983;74:957–960.
20. Lally EV, Jiminez SA. Impotence in progressive systemic sclerosis. Ann Intern Med 1981;95:150–155.
21. Klein LE, Posner MS. Progressive systemic sclerosis and impotence. Ann Intern Med 1981;95:658–659.
22. Nowlin NS, Brick JE, Weaver DJ, Wilson DA, Judd HL, Lu JKH, Carlson HE. Impotence in scleroderma. Ann Intern Med 1986;104:794–798.
23. Jiminez SA, Lally EV. Impotence in progressive systemic sclerosis. Ann Intern Med 1982;96:125–126.
24. Nowlin S, Zwillich SH, Brick JE, Carlson HE. Male hypogonadism in scleroderma. J Rheumatol 1985;12:605–606.
25. Klein LE, Posner MS. Progressive systemic sclerosis and impotence. Ann Intern Med 1981;95:658–659.
26. Varga J, Lally EV, Jiminez SA. Chapter 18: Endocrinopathy and other visceral organ involvement in progressive systemic sclerosis. In: Jayson MIV, Black CM, eds. Systemic sclerosis: scleroderma. New York, John Wiley & Sons, Ltd, 1988; 267–278.
27. Middleton WS. Diffuse systemic sclerosis. Ann Intern Med 1962;57:183–188.
28. Paine DWD, Leek JC, Jakle C, Robbins DL. Gynecomastia associated with low dose methotrexate therapy. Arthritis Rheum 1983;26:691–692.
29. Gruis ML, Wagner NN. Sexuality during the climacteric. Postgrad Med 1979;65:197–200.

30. Cohen M. Sexuality and the arthritic patient—how well are we doing? J Rheumatol 1987;14:403–404.
31. Baum J. A review of the psychological aspects of rheumatic disease. Semin Arthritis Rheum 1982;11:352–361.
32. Hamilton A. Sexual problems in arthritis and allied conditions. Int Rehabil Med 1981;3:38–42.
33. Florian V. Sex counseling: Comparison of attitudes of disabled and nondisabled subjects. Arch Phys Med Rehabil 1983;64:81–89.
34. Madorsky JGB, Dixon TP. Rehabilitation aspects of human sexuality. West J Med 1983;139:174–176.
35. Spellacy WN. Scleroderma and pregnancy. Obstet Gynecol 1964;23:297–300.
36. Leinwand I, Duryee AW, Richter MN. Scleroderma (based on a study of over 150 cases). Ann Intern Med 1954;41:1003–1037.
37. DeCarle DW. Pregnancy associated with scleroderma (Discussion by Donaldson LB). Am J Obstet Gynecol 1964;89:359–361.
38. Slate WG. Scleroderma and pregnancy (Discussion by Donaldson LB). Am J Obstet Gynecol 1968;101:340–341.
39. Giordano M, Valentini G, Lupoli S, Giordano A. Pregnancy and systemic sclerosis. Arthritis Rheum (letter) 1985;28:237–238.
40. Silman AJ, Black C. Increased incidence of spontaneous abortion and infertility in women with scleroderma before disease onset: A controlled study. Ann Rheum Dis 1988;47:441–444.
41. Orabona ML, Albono O. Systemic progressive sclerosis (or visceral scleroderma). Acta Med Scand 1958;333(suppl):5–170.
42. Siamopoulou-Mavridou A, Manoussakis MN, Mavridis AK, Moutsopoulos HM. Outcome of pregnancy in patients with autoimmune rheumatic disease before the disease onset. Ann Rheum Dis 1988;47:982–982.
43. Englert H, Brennan P, McNeil D, Black C, Silman AJ. Reproductive function prior to disease onset in women with scleroderma. J Rheumatol 1992;19:1575–1579.
44. Freeman WE, Lesher JLL, Graham Smith J. Connective tissue disease associated with sclerodermoid features, early abortion and circulating anticoagulant. J Am Acad Dermatol 1988;19:932–938.
45. McHugh NJ, Reilly PA, McHugh LA. Pregnancy outcome and autoantibodies in connective tissue disease. J Rheumatol 1989;16:43–46.
46. Kaufman RL, Kitridou RC. Pregnancy in mixed connective tissue disease: Comparison with systemic lupus erythematosus. J Rheumatol 1984;9:549–559.
47. Eno E. Pregnancy in a patient suffering from scleroderma. Am J Obstet Gynecol 1987;33:514–517.
48. Gunther RE, Harer BW. Systemic sclerosis in pregnancy—report of a case. Obstet Gynecol 1964;24:98–100.
49. DeCarle DW. Pregnancy associated with scleroderma. Case report of a patient with three successful pregnancies. Am J Obstet Gynecol 1964;89:356–361.
50. Johnson TR, Banner EA, Winkelman RK. Scleroderma and pregnancy. Obstet Gynecol 1964;23:467–469.
51. State WG, Graham AR. Scleroderma and pregnancy. Am J Obstet Gynecol 1968;101:335–341.
52. Winkelman E. Scleroderma and pregnancy. Clin Obstet Gynecol 1965;8:280–285.
53. Tischler S, Zarowitz H, Daichman I. Scleroderma and pregnancy. Obstet Gynecol 1957;10:457–459.
54. Guttmacher A. A case of severe scleroderma with successful delivery. Urol Cutan Rev 1943;47:107–108.
55. Casten GG, Boucek RJ. The use of relaxin in the treatment of scleroderma. JAMA 1958;166:319–329.
56. Etterich M, Mall M. Sklerodermic und schwangeschaft. Gynaecologia 1955;135:236–242.
57. Hayes GW, Walsh CR, D'Alesandro EE. Scleroderma in pregnancy: Report of a case. Obstet Gynecol 1962;19:273–274.
58. Hoffman JB, Diamond B. Scleroderma treated with steroids through pregnancy: Caesarian section and puerperium. Postgrad Med 1961;30:498–501.
59. Maymon R, Fejgin M, Ben-Aderet N, Bahary C. Scleroderma and pregnancy. Acta Obstet Gynecol Scand 1989;68:469–470.
60. Weiner SR, Brinkman CR, Paulus HE. Scleroderma, CREST syndrome and pregnancy. Arthritis Rheum 1986;29(suppl):51.
61. Scarpinato L, MacKenzie AH. Pregnancy and progressive systemic sclerosis. Case report and a review of the literature. Clev Clin Q 1985;52:207–211.
62. Thompson J, Conklin KA. Anesthetic management of a pregnant patient with scleroderma. Anesthesiol 1983;59:69–71.
63. Mor-Yosel S, Navot D, Rabinowitz R, Schenker JG. Collagen diseases in pregnancy. Obstet Gynecol Surv 1984;39:837–844.
64. Knupp MZ, O'Leary JA. Pregnancy and scleroderma. J Fla Med Assoc 1971;58:28–30.

65. Goplerud CP. Scleroderma. Clin Obstet Gynecol 1983;26:587–591.

66. Steen VD, Conte C, Day N, Ramsey-Goldman R, Medsger TA Jr. Pregnancy in women with systemic sclerosis. Arthritis Rheum 1989;32:151–157.

67. Black CM, Stevens WM. Scleroderma. In: Pregnancy in patients with rehumatoid diseases. Rheum Dis Clin North Am 1989;15:193–212.

68. Silman AJ. Pregnancy and scleroderma. Am J Report Immunol 1992;28:238–240.

69. Meyer CJ. Three recurrent abruptions of the placenta in a patient with scleroderma. Proc Rud Vich Med Soc NY 1970;28:65–68.

70. Lee P, Bruni J, Sukenik S. Neurological manifestations in systemic sclerosis (scleroderma). J Rheumatol 1984;11;480–483.

71. Lovell CR, Jayson MIV. Joint involvement in systemic sclerosis. Scand J Rheumatol 1979;8:154–160.

72. Gould JS, Wissinger HA. Carpal tunnel syndrome in pregnancy. South Med J 1978;71:144–145.

73. Donaldson JO. Neuropathy in neurology of pregnancy. Philadelphia: WB Saunders Co, 1978; 23–55.

74. Schumacher HR, Dorwart BB, Korzeniowski OM. Occurrence of De Quervain's tendinitis during pregnancy. Arch Intern Med 1985;1457:2083–2084.

75. Hammar N, Larsson L, Tegler L. Calcium treatment of leg cramps in pregnancy. Acta Obstet Gynecol Scand 1981;60:345–347.

76. Mantle MJ, Greenwood RM, Currey HLF. Backache in pregnancy. Rheumatol Rehabil 1977;16: 95–101.

77. Epstein JA. Symposium on treatment of low back pain and sciatic syndrome during pregnancy. New York J Med 1959;59;1757–1768.

78. LeBan MM, Perrin JCS, Latimer FR. Pregnancy and the herniated lumbar disc. Arch Phys Med Rehabil 1983;64:319–321.

79. O'Connell JEA. Lumbar disc protrusions in pregnancy. J Neurol Neurosurg Psychiat 1960;23:139–141.

80. Sands RX. Backache of pregnancy. Obstet Gynecol 1958;12:670–676.

81. Avital F, Shapiro DF. Back pain in pregnancy. Spine 1987;12:368–371.

82. Smith R, Stevensen JC, Winearls CG, Woods CG, Wordsworth BP. Osteoporosis of pregnancy. Lancet 1985;1:1178–1180.

83. Dent OE, Friedman M. Pregnancy and idiopathic osteoporosis. J Quart Med 1965;34:341–357.

84. MacLennan AH, Nicolson AR, Green RC. Serum relaxin in pregnancy. Lancet 1986;2:244–245.

85. Habbell SL, Thomas M. Post partum cervical myofascial pain syndrome: Review of four patients. Obstet Gynecol 1985;65:565–567.

86. Spalin SH. Stress fracture in pregnancy. Orthop Rev 1985;14:87–89.

87. Milgrom C, Liebergaldi M. The fracture of the coccyx as a complication of normal delivery. Orthop Rev 1984;60:60–61.

88. Carr WA, Moc JH, Winter RB, Lonstein JE. Treatment of idiopathic sclerosis in the Milwaukee brace. J Bone Joint Surg Am 1980;62A:599–612.

89. Beaulieu JG, Razzano CD, Levine RD. Transient osteoporosis of the hip in pregnancy. Clin Orthop 1976;115:165–168.

90. Pleet AB, Massey EW. Intercostal neuralgia of pregnancy. JAMA 1980;243:768–769.

91. Kaufman J, Canoso JJ. Progressive systemic sclerosis and meralgia paresthetica. Ann Intern Med 1986;105:973.

92. Kitchen C, Simpson J. Meralgia paresthetica: A review of 67 patients. Acta Neurol Scand 1972;48: 547–555.

93. Calhoun BC. Gastrointestinal disorders in pregnancy. In: Medical complications during pregnancy. Obstet Gynecol Clin North Am 1992;19: 733–742.

94. Maymon R, Fejgin M. Scleroderma in pregnancy. Obstet Gynecol Surv 1989;44:530–543.

95. Raymond R, Underwood DA, Douglas DS. Cardiovascular problems in pregnancy. Cleve Clin J Med 1987;54:95–104.

96. Sullivan JM, Ramanathan KB. Management of medical problems in pregnancy—severe cardiac disease. N Engl J Med 1985;313:304–308.

97. Wilson AGM, Kirby JDT. Successful pregnancy in a woman with systemic sclerosis while taking nifedipine. Ann Rheum Dis 1990;49:51–52.

98. Younker D, Harrison B. Scleroderma and pregnancy. Anesthetic considerations. Br J Anaesth 1985;57:1136–1139.

99. Moore M, Saffran JE, Baraf HSB, Jacobs RP. Systemic sclerosis and pregnancy complicated by obstructive uropathy. Am J Obstet Gynecol 185;153: 893–894.

100. Burrow GN. The management of thyrotoxicosis in pregnancy. N Engl J Med 1985;313:562–565.

101. Hoffman JB, Diamond B. Scleroderma treated with steroids through pregnancy, caesarian section and puerperium. Postgrad Med 1967;30: 498–504.

102. Baethge BA, Wolf RE. Successful pregnancy with scleroderma renal disease and pulmonary hypertension in a patient using angiotensin converting enzyme inhibitors. Ann Rheum Dis 1989;48:776–778.

103. Luiz DA, Moodley J, Naicker SN, Pudifin D. Pregnancy in scleroderma. A case report. S Afr Med J 1986;69:642–643.
104. Aorech OM, Golan A, Pausky M, Langer R, Caspi E. Raynaud's phenomenon and peripheral gangrene complicating scleroderma in pregnancy—diagnosis and management. Br J Obstet Gynecol 1992;99:850–857.
105. Smith CA, Pinals RS. Progressive systemic sclerosis and postpartum renal failure complicated by peripheral gangrene. J Rheumatol 1982;9:455–458.
106. Fear RE. Eclampsia superimposed on renal scleroderma: A rare cause of maternal and fetal mortality. Obstet Gynecol 1968;31:69–74.
107. Sood SV, Kohler HG. Maternal death from systemic sclerosis. J Obstet Gynecol (Brit Com) 1970;77:1109–1112.
108. Karlen JR, Cook WA. Renal scleroderma and pregnancy. Obstet Gynecol 1974;44:349–354.
109. Palma A, Sanchez-Palencia A, Armos JR, Milan JA, Fernandez-Sanz J, Llach F. Progressive systemic sclerosis and nephrotic syndrome. Arch Intern Med 1981;141:420–521.
110. Ehrenfeld M, Licht A, Stessman J, Yanko L, Rosenmann E. Postpartum renal failure due to progressive systemic sclerosis treated with chronic hemodialysis. Nephron 1977;18:175–181.
111. Altieri P, Cameron JS. Scleroderma renal crisis in a pregnant woman with late partial recovery of renal function. Nephrol Dial Transplant 1988;3:677–680.
112. Sivanesaratnam V, Chong HL. Scleroderma and pregnancy. Aust NZ J Obstet Gynecol 1982;22:123–124.
113. Watson MA, Radford NJ, McGrath BP, Swintin GW, Agar JM. Captopril induced agranulocytosis in systemic sclerosis. Aust NZ J Med 1981;11:79–81.
114. Needs CJ, Brooks PM. Antirheumatic medications in pregnancy. Br J Rheumatol 1985;24:282–290.
115. Needs CJ, Brooks PM. Antirheumatic drugs during lactation. Br J Rheumatol 1985;24:291–297.
116. Cecere FA, Persellin RH. The interaction of pregnancy and the rheumatic diseases. Clin Rheum Dis 1981;7:747–769.
117. Byron MA. Prescribing in pregnancy: Treatment of rheumatic disease. Brit Med J 1987;294:236–238.
118. Tanaka S. Effects of salicylic acid and acetyl salicylic acid on the fetuses and offspring of rats. Teratology 1972;6;1121.
119. Niederhoff H, Zahradnick H. Analgesics during pregnancy. Am J Med 1983;(suppl):117–120.
120. Stone D, Siskind V, Heinonen OP. Aspirin and congenital malformations. Lancet 1976;1:1373–1375.
121. Corby DG. Aspirin in pregnancy: Maternal and fetal effects. Pediatrics 1978;62:930–945.
122. Rudolph AM. Effects of aspirin and acetaminophen in pregnancy and the newborn. Arch Intern Med 1981;141:358–363.
123. Bongiovanni AM, McPadden AJ. Steroids during pregnancy and possible fetal consequences. Fertil Steril 1960;11:181–186.
124. Warrell DW, Taylor R. Outcome for the foetus of mothers receiving prednisolone during pregnancy. Lancet 1968;1:117–118.
125. Wagoner RD, Holley KE, Johnson WJ. Accelerated nephrosclerosis and postpartum acute renal failure in normotensive patients. Ann Intern Med 1968;69:237–248.
126. Lyle WH. Penicillamine in pregnancy. Lancet 1978;1:606–607.
127. Coates A. Cyclophosphamide in pregnancy. Aust NZ J Obstet Gynecol 1970;10:33–34.
128. Lewis GJ. Successful pregnancy in a renal transplant recipient taking cyclosporin A. Br Med J 1983;286:603–605.
129. Flescher SM. The presence of cyclosporin in body tissues and fluids during pregnancy. Am J Kidney Dis 1985;5:60–63.
130. Rotmensch HH, Elkayam U, Frishman W. Antiarrhythmic drug therapy during pregnancy. Ann Intern Med 1983;98:487–497.
131. Mehta N, Modi N. ACE inhibitors in pregnancy. Lancet 1989;1:96–97.
132. Guze BH, Guze PA. Psychotropic medication use during pregnancy. West J Med 1989;151:290–298.
133. Davidson-Lamb RW, Finlayson MCK. Scleroderma complications encountered during dental anesthesia. Anesthesia 1977;32:893–895.
134. Eisele JM, Reetan JA. Scleroderma, Raynaud's phenomenon and local anesthesia. Anesthesiology 1971;34:386–387.
135. Pitkin RM. Autoimmune disease in pregnancy. Semin Perinatal 1977;1:161–168.

ROBERT P. ROCA
FREDERICK M. WIGLEY

24

Psychosocial Aspects

Systemic sclerosis (SSc), or SSc, is an unpredictable, disfiguring, and often painful disease for which there are few effective treatments. As such, it is a demoralizing disease, and patients often experience considerable emotional distress as they struggle to meet the many challenges it imposes. Problems in adjustment are therefore both common and understandable, and patients experiencing such difficulties benefit from empathic attention.

At the same time, persons with SSc may develop distinct syndromes of cognitive and attentional disturbance (i.e., delirium) or profound, pervasive sadness associated with self-reproach and loss of interest in activities (i.e., major depression). In such cases, it is critical to make the correct diagnosis and to institute appropriate treatment; medical approaches to evaluation and management, not empathy alone, are necessary.

The understanding and management of psychiatric disorders among persons with SSc thus requires two approaches: the empathic and the medical. Each approach has its methods, strengths, and weaknesses. The empathic approach relies on the ability of clinicians to put themselves "in the shoes" of their patients and understand emotionally how persons in such a predicament could feel sad, or angry, or otherwise distraught. The medical approach relies on clinicians' knowledge of psychiatric diagnosis and treatment and on their skill in performing a mental status examination. The empathic approach emerges from the question "Why is this individual experiencing distress in these particu-

lar circumstances?" and thus ensures that the unique aspects of an individual's predicament are taken into account. In contrast, the medical perspective follows from the question "Do the observed signs and symptoms constitute a syndrome with a defined clinical course, response to treatment, and prognosis?" and thus ensures that the benefits of diagnostic classification and the findings of systematic diagnosis-based clinical investigation are brought to bear on the case. This two-pronged approach to formulation underlies everything that follows. We will first present a method for obtaining a basic psychiatric history and performing a mental status examination. We will then review psychiatric disorders associated with SSc. Finally, we will discuss the "normal" emotional response to SSc and consider approaches that physicians may use to help patients handle this disease.

Psychiatric History and Mental Status Examination

The main component of the basic psychiatric history is the history of the current symptomatology (e.g., tearfulness, confusion) as described by the patient and, if possible, by a family member or close friend. Inquiry should be made regarding past psychiatric symptomatology and past treatment for emotional problems by any sort of practitioner. A family history of psychiatric illness or treatment should be sought. Finally, a special effort should be made to discover

501

evidence of substance abuse, especially alcoholism; a brief standardized approach, such as the CAGE Questionnaire, is helpful for this purpose (1) (Table 24.1). The remainder of the psychiatric history overlaps with the complete general medical history.

The principal purpose of the mental state examination is to demonstrate the presence or absence of current psychiatric symptomatology in the realms of belief, perception, mood, and cognition. In most cases, a few questions suffice to elicit information about each domain. Fixed, false beliefs, or delusions, are usually persecutory in content and, when present, are very disturbing and therefore often readily described by patients. When such beliefs are suspected but not volunteered, the clinician may elicit them by asking a question such as "Have you felt that you are in danger in any way or that you need to be on guard?." False perceptions, or hallucinations, occur principally in the auditory and visual realms and are also often described spontaneously by patients. When such symptoms are suspected but not volunteered, the clinician may plainly ask patients if they are "hearing voices" or "seeing visions." Such questions are usually well accepted by patients and may afford great relief to persons who are hallucinating and are afraid to tell anyone for fear that their complaints will be misunderstood. While not diagnostically specific, hallucinations and delusions are important psychiatric symptoms and should prompt psychiatric consultation. Psychiatric symptomatology

among persons with SSc is most often in the realm of mood, and it is by means of the mental state examination that the clinician establishes the presence of the most important disorder of mood—major depression. Depression will be discussed later in this chapter. For now, it is enough to say that the clinician may screen for disorders of mood by asking a few direct questions (e.g., "How have your spirits been holding up?") or by having patients fill out a self-report depression survey, such as the Beck Depression Inventory (2). Scores of 18 or higher suggest depression of at least moderate severity.

Cognitive disorder is uncommon in patients with SSc, because the disease process does not directly involve the CNS. When present, delirium is the chief cognitive disorder found among persons with SSc and is generally a consequence of drug toxicity or severe end-organ compromise (e.g., respiratory failure). It is the subject of further discussion later in this chapter. The detection of delirium depends on the demonstration of cognitive impairment in the presence of disturbed attention and concentration. While gross impairments are obvious to informal observation, subtle deficits go undetected unless the clinician employs a more thorough approach to cognitive assessment. The Mini-Mental State Examination (3) (Table 24.2) is a reliable, well-validated approach to cognitive assessment that can be administered and scored in less than 5 minutes.

Perfect performance earns 30 points, and scores below 24 suggest the presence of delirium or dementia. False positives are most common among the poorly educated and the elderly (4).

Table 24.1. CAGE Questionnaire

1. Have you ever felt you should CUT DOWN on your drinking?
2. Have people ANNOYED you by criticizing your drinking?
3. Have you ever felt bad or GUILTY about your drinking?
4. Have you ever had a drink first thing in the morning to steady your nerves or get rid of a hangover (i.e., taken an EYEOPENER)?*

*NOTE: If two questions are answered affirmatively, the probability of alcoholism is high.
Modified from Buschbaum et al. Screening for drinking disorders in the elderly using the CAGE questionnaire. J Am Geriatr Soc 1992;40: 662–665.

Psychiatric Disorders in Scleroderma

Psychiatric disorders among rheumatology patients are of three general types: (*a*) disorders caused by the physiological effects of the illnesses themselves; (*b*) disorders caused by the physiological effects of treatment; and (*c*) psychological reactions to the illnesses.

Table 24.2. Mini-Mental State Examination

Maximum Score	
	Orientation
5	What is the (year)(season)(date)(day)(month?)
5	Where are we(city)(state)(county)(hospital)(floor)?
	Registration
3	Name three objects: one second to say each. Ask the patient for all three after you have said them. Give one point for each correct answer. Repeat them until all three are learned. Count trials and record number.
	Attention and calculation
5	Serial sevens backward from 100 (stop after five answers). Alternatively, spell WORLD backward.
	Recall
3	Ask for the three objects repeated above. Give one point for each correct answer.
	Language and praxis
2	Show a pencil and watch, and ask subject to name them.
1	Ask the patient to repeat the following: "No ifs, ands, or buts."
3	(Three-stage command): "Take this paper in your right hand, fold it in half, and put it on the floor."
1	"Read and obey the following: Close your eyes."
1	"Write a sentence."
1	"Copy this design" (interlocking pentagons).

Modified from Folstein et al. The "Mini-Mental State": A practical method for grading the cognitive state of patients for the clincain. J Psychiatr Res 1975; 12: 189–198.

Systemic lupus erythematosus (SLE), the best studied of rheumatologic diseases from this point of view, is an excellent example of an illness in which all three types are seen (5). Delirium, major affective disorders, and schizophrenia-like syndromes may occur in SLE patients as a result of direct or indirect effects of SLE on the brain; in such cases, the cornerstone of psychiatric treatment is medical treatment for SLE and/or its complications. At the same time, pharmacologic treatments for SLE, especially corticosteroid therapy, may themselves cause serious psychiatric symptomatology, especially major affective disorders. In these cases, alteration of the treatment regimen, if possible, is the treatment of choice; otherwise, symptomatic treatment with psychotropic medications is generally required. Finally, persons with SLE face disappointment, pain, uncertainty about the future, and many other demoralizing challenges and circumstances. While these emotions are readily understandable and not qualitatively abnormal, they may become a source of great discomfort and a cause of excess disability, and in such cases they warrant and usually benefit from psychotherapy.

Patients with SLE thus may develop psychiatric disorders as a result of medical, iatrogenic, or psychogenic processes, and each calls for different therapeutic approaches. The psychiatry of SSc has not been so thoroughly studied. Nevertheless, there is evidence that all three types of psychiatric disorders occur among these patients as well. As distinct SSc-related psychiatric disorders are discussed below in terms of the current psychiatric nomenclature, it will become clear that psychiatric manifestations are in some cases direct or indirect products of SSc itself, in some cases side effects of treatment, and in some cases maladaptive psychological responses to an often devastating illness.

DISORDERS OF MOOD: MAJOR DEPRESSION

Clinical Manifestations, Prevalence, and Etiology

Major depression is a clinical syndrome characterized by low mood, diminished vitality (i.e., anergy, disinterest in activities, impaired capacity for pleasure), and self-dissatisfaction (i.e., self-criticism, self-blaming). Disturbances in sleep and appetite are common. Without treatment, symptoms generally persist for months, carrying with them marked functional disability (6) and the risk of suicide.

The formal diagnostic criteria for major depression are shown in Table 24.3. The diagnosis is made when at least five of these symptoms (including low mood or loss of interest in activities) are persistently present over the course of at least 2 weeks (7). Clinicians often worry that the so-called "somatic" symptoms (e.g., loss of appetite, insomnia, loss of energy) are nonspecific and may be endorsed by medically ill persons who are not depressed. In fact, the presence of such symptoms rarely confounds the diagnosis. As long as the "psychological" or "cognitive affective" (8) symptoms are also present, the inclusion of the somatic symptoms generally does not produce false-positive diagnoses of major depression (9).

There are few studies of the prevalence of depression among persons with SSc. Roca et al (10) found that 17% of outpatients with SSc had self-reported depressive symptomatology of moderate or high severity; this is comparable to the prevalence rates found among persons with other chronic diseases (11).

There is a single case report of a major depressive syndrome in a 63-year-old woman with clinical SSc, confirmatory serum serologies, inflammatory cerebrospinal fluid abnormalities (e.g., lymphocytosis, elevated protein), and magnetic resonance imaging findings suggestive of "ischemia due to vascular lesions" (12). The authors propose that this is the first documented case of "depression as a cerebral manifestation of scleroderma." While this is an intriguing possibility, the relationship between the depressive disorder and the general medical findings in this case is uncertain, because the authors provide no information about the treatment the patient received or the longitudinal course of clinical and immunological findings during follow-up. In the absence of such validating data, it is difficult to rule out the possibility that this case simply documents the chance co-occurrence of SSc and a common psychiatric condition.

It is tempting to believe that serious depression in persons with SSc is typically a response to exacerbations of disease activity. As reasonable as this appears, there is evidence that it may not be true. Roca et al (10) found little correlation between the severity of depressive symptoms and most medical indices of SSc disease severity (e.g., pulmonary function, skin score). Instead, depression was much more strongly correlated with aspects of personality (e.g., neuroticism) and with perceived social support. Similarly, Moser (13) demonstrated strong correlations between emotional distress and such variables as "hardiness" and satisfaction with social support. Taken together, these studies suggest that psychosocial factors may be more important than medical factors in the etiology of depression in SSc. Others have reached similar conclusions about depression in persons with rheumatoid arthritis (14).

Table 24.3. Diagnosis of Major Depression ($\geq$5 symptoms for $\geq$2 weeks)

Sleep disturbance
Loss of Interest[a]
Inappropriate guilt
Loss of energy
Depressed mood[a]
Poor concentration
Change in appetite
Psychomotor retardation or agitation
Suicidality or passive wish for death

[a]Loss of interest or depressed mood must be present.
Modified from American Psychiatric Association. Diagnostic and Statistical manual of Mental Disorders, 3rd ed. Revised. Washington, DC: American Psychiatric Association, 1987.

Treatment

Given the importance of psychosocial factors in the etiology of depression in SSc, disease education and counseling have an important place in the treatment of depression among persons with SSc. For clinicians who are interested in conducting such treatment themselves, there are many publications available that provide practical guidelines regarding the performance of psychotherapy by primary care physicians (15,16).

At the same time, major depression is the principal indication for antidepressant medication, and SSc patients with major depression suffer unnecessarily when pharmacologic treatment is passed over simply because it "makes sense" for them to be depressed.

Many antidepressant drugs are currently available (Table 24.4). Each is effective in 65% to 70% of cases of major depression. All patients do not respond to every drug, and there is no reliable way of selecting the most effective agent in an individual case. The side effects of these drugs differ appreciably; therefore, drug selection often involves choosing the agent with the most favorable side effect profile. Because patients with SSc often have esophageal reflux and disturbances in gastrointestinal motility, they are often poorly tolerant of drugs with high levels of anticholinergic activity. For this reason, newer nontricyclic compounds such as trazodone, fluoxetine, sertraline, paroxetine, and bupropion may be preferable to the less expensive but more strongly anticholinergic tricyclics (e.g., amitriptyline, nortriptyline, imipramine, doxepin). Furthermore, there is some recent evidence that the serotonergic activity of many of these newer agents, fluoxetine in particular, may have direct beneficial effects on vascular hyperreactivity in Raynaud's phenomenon (RP) (17).

Case 1: A 38-year-old woman was referred for psychiatric treatment because of depression. She first developed signs of SSc at age 16 and now had esophageal dysmotility, type III skin changes, and severe pulmonary disease (DCO 25% of predicted). She described pervasively low mood, poor energy, diminished interest in her usual activities, and profound self-dissatisfaction. She related much of this symptomatology to her SSc, but recognized that she was depressed and that depression might be compromising her ability to deal with her illness. Fluoxetine 20 mg daily was prescribed, and she was seen in psychotherapy 2 or 3 times per month. She reported vivid dreams—a common side effect of fluoxetine therapy—but no other troublesome treatment-emergent symptoms. The dose was increased slowly to 40 mg per day over the next 6 weeks. In the meantime, her pulmonary symptomatology progressed and she became oxygen-dependent.

Table 24.4. Psychotropic Drugs

	Common Brand Names	Usual Daily Dose
Antidepressants		
Amitriptyline	Elavil	50–200 mg
Nortriptyline	Pamelor	25–100 mg
Imipramine	Trofranil	50–150 mg
Doxepin	Sinequan	25–150 mg
Trazodone	Desyrel	150–300 mg
Fluoxetine	Prozac	20–40 mg
Sertraline	Zoloft	50–100 mg
Paroxetine	Paxil	10–30 mg
Bupropion	Wellbutrin	200–300 mg
Antipsychotic Drugs		
Halperidol	Haldol	1.0–15 mg
Thiothixene	Nuvane	6–15 mg
Benzodiazepines		
Lorazepam	Ativan	2–6 mg

Her exercise tolerance continued to decline, and she acquired a motorized cart to enhance her ability to get around independently. Despite the progression of her disease and functional incapacity, her mood and energy improved and she regained her enthusiasm for activities she had formerly enjoyed. She helped organize a family vacation, arranging by telephone to replenish her oxygen supply as she traveled. She said that her quality of life was better than it had been for years, despite the marked progression of her illness. At the time of my last visit with her prior to her death of respiratory failure, she wore a T-shirt with the inscription: "Wouldn't you know it. Now that I'm finally getting my head together, my body is going to hell."

DISORDERS OF MOOD: ADJUSTMENT DISORDERS AND MILD CHRONIC DEPRESSION

Clinical Manifestations and Etiology

Adjustment disorders are excessive or otherwise maladaptive reactions to life stresses. They bear a clear temporal relationship to troubling life circumstances, usually significant losses or disappointments. In most cases the predominant mood is depression, but the formal features of a major depression are lacking. As a rule, the mood disturbance resolves as the patient "adjusts" to the precipitating loss or disappointments. Occasionally depression persists, and if it lasts for at least two years, then the appropriate diagnosis is "dysthymia"—a mild chronic depression that is often associated with chronic illness, persistent psychosocial stress, personality disorder, and other enduring states and circumstances that interfere with access to life's gratifications.

Persons with SSc face many demoralizing losses and disappointments as a consequence of their disease. Changes in physical, especially facial, appearance may prompt concerns about attractiveness. Loss of capacity to function normally at home and at work may diminish a patient's sense of personal value and importance. Furthermore, fears about the progression of disease and disability may generate an undercurrent of tension that surfaces as irritability and impatience, compromising interpersonal relationships that are ultimately critical to patients' long-term well-being.

While it is not surprising that these illness-associated difficulties often lead to discouragement, they are more demoralizing to some patients than to others, suggesting that nonmedical factors affect the vulnerability of individuals to adjustment problems in the face of illness. One such factor is personality. Histrionic persons, for example, tend to be particularly concerned with physical attractiveness and may be especially distressed by changes in facial appearance. Compulsive persons tend to be overly devoted to work and may have particular difficulty accepting a reduction in work hours. Another relevant factor is the adequacy of the patient's social support system—as perceived by the patient. Inadequate perceived social support has been found to be correlated with depression among women with rheumatoid arthritis (18) and among outpatients with SSc (10,13).

Treatment

The aim of treatment is to help patients achieve a healthy adjustment to illness and to promote the restoration of morale. This effort has two components: a **cognitive task** and a **relational task**. The cognitive task involves developing a working understanding, or formulation, of the case and using this understanding to assist the patient in problem-solving. This begins with identifying the most demoralizing aspects of a patient's life circumstances, but also requires considering how aspects of a patient's personality and/or social support system might render him or her particularly vulnerable to the precipitating circumstances. Once such a working formulation is developed, it is possible to help the patient discover ways, within the constraints of personality, of coming to grips with demoralizing losses and disappointments. The demoralizing circumstances so often entail losses of activities and roles that had sustained the patient's sense of personal worth; therefore, counseling often focuses on helping him or her become more open-minded and flexible regarding possible sources of self-esteem.

The second component of treatment—the relational task—is to promote the development of "expectant trust," an attitude on the part of the patient that the physician is caring, competent, committed, and confident that the patient can improve (i.e., make a satisfactory adjustment to illness) (19). This begins with a willingness on the part of the physician to listen empathically (i.e., to put oneself in the patient's shoes) and to permit the responsible expression of all varieties of emotions, including anger, fear, and hopelessness. The physician's willingness to accept patients' expressions of distress is often in itself a source of great relief to patients, assisting them in the processes of working through such feelings and freeing themselves to move on to constructive, problem-solving behaviors.

Case 2: A 48-year-old man with SSc was referred for psychiatric treatment one year after retirement. He had no past psychiatric history. He had been a successful business executive who had enjoyed working and playing golf until chronic fatigue and sclerodactyly forced him to give up these activities. He complained that he was unable to do what he enjoyed most and that he did not much enjoy what he was able to do (e.g., read, watch television). He spent more time around his family than he ever had but found that they did not welcome his advice; they often seemed to regard him as intrusive and "annoying." Furthermore, he believed that his impotence—determined to be organic in origin—was complicating his relationship with his wife. As a result of these problems, he felt "depressed and overwhelmed," that he was "simply existing, going through the motions." His appetite was fair and his sleep adequate. He was not self-blaming and did not wish for death. He did not meet criteria for major depression, but he was clearly severely demoralized by the circumstances of his illness. Increasing his vulnerability to adjustment problems were his compulsive personality traits (e.g., his inability to be flexible and develop new interests, his tendency to be self-righteous and controlling in his dealings with his family) and his dissatisfaction with the social support available from his family. His mood improved rapidly in response to empathic listening and a resolution to work on improving his relationship with his wife and identifying gratifying new projects.

PSYCHOLOGICAL FACTORS AFFECTING THE PHYSICAL CONDITION

Psychological stresses may precipitate exacerbations of physical symptomatology related to objective SSc-related organic pathology. These are categorized as instances of "psychological factors affecting a physical condition," a formal diagnostic entity in the current psychiatric nosology. One example is stress-induced RP. Another is stress-induced exacerbation of dysphagia in a patient with SSc-related esophageal disease. Appropriate treatment usually entails psychotherapy aimed at helping the patient recognize the relationship between physical symptoms and psychological factors and assisting him or her deal more effectively with the precipitating stress(es).

Case 3: A 44-year-old woman with SSc involving the skin and the gastrointestinal tract was being treated effectively for depression with fluoxetine. She had chronic dysphagia but managed to nourish herself adequately using liquid dietary supplements. During a routine visit she acknowledged that she had recently been having greater difficulty swallowing and that she had been using Tylox to "relax (her) throat" sufficiently to permit her to drink. She reported that her symptoms were especially troublesome during the week and virtually absent on weekends. On further reflection she recognized that her swallowing difficulties coincided with the work week and had begun shortly after a new employee had been added to the staff. She felt that the new employee was interested in displacing her, and she dreaded being in her presence. She was also upset that her boss appeared insensitive to her feelings about the new employee. Over the course of the session she came to understand that the recent exacerbation of her dysphagia was precipitated by anxiety and anger stirred up by these events in the workplace. Treatment involved nonpharmacologic, psychotherapeutic approaches to helping her express and manage her feelings about her boss and new coworker.

Delirium

Clinical Manifestations. Delirium is a clinical syndrome characterized by cognitive impairment in the presence of disturbances in attention and concentration. The terms "acute encephalopathy," "confusion," and "acute confusional state" are roughly synonymous. Disorientation, memory impairment, disorganized speech, and other signs of cognitive dysfunction occur in a patient who is clearly somnolent or, in less obvious cases, impaired in his or her ability to sustain or shift attention. The syndrome usually develops over a period of hours or days and may last for weeks, often with a waxing and waning course characterized by nocturnal agitation, daytime drowsiness, and occasional periods of apparent lucidity. Delirium is a clinical diagnosis and does not require confirmation by laboratory testing of any kind; however, delirious patients usually have nonfocal slowing of the background rhythm on the electroencephalogram (EEG).

Causes. Delirium is almost never "functional" or "psychogenic." It is nearly always the product of one or several medical, surgical, or neurological conditions or their treatments. Serious infections, metabolic derangements, uremia, trauma, cardio- and cerebrovascular disorders, respiratory failure, and drug toxicity are but a few of the more common causes of delirium. Among patients with SSc, respiratory failure and drug toxicity are probably the principal causes. In fact, the SSc process does not directly effect the CNS. However, patients with SSc may develop the typical clinical and EEG manifestations of delirium in the absence of an identifiable secondary cause. In one reported case, the clinical and EEG signs of delirium cleared twice in response to a course of corticosteroids (20). This suggests that some patients with clinical SSc may have inflammatory CNS disease (e.g., vasculitis) perhaps secondary to an associated autoimmune process. Delirium in the SSc patient should prompt a vigorous search for potentially treatable secondary consequences of organ failure or its treatments.

Treatment. The most important therapy for delirium is treatment of the underlying medical condition(s). When appropriate treatment is provided, full recovery occurs in the great majority of cases. It is common, however, for clinical delirium to persist for days or even weeks after rational treatment has been initiated. In such cases, symptomatic measures are often required to ameliorate agitation, insomnia, and psychotic manifestations such as delusions and hallucinations. Since delirious patients are usually disoriented and frightened, they nearly always benefit from frequent reorientation to their surroundings and the identities of those around them. It is also helpful to reassure patients that they are safe, that their confusion is a symptom of their illness, not a sign that they are "going crazy," and that they will recover. In addition, they may also benefit from well-selected and targeted psychopharmacologic interventions. Paranoid delusions and auditory and visual hallucinations generally respond to antipsychotic, or neuroleptic, medications such as haloperidol or thiothixene, often in relatively low dosages. Haloperidol may be given in a dose of 1 to 2 mg po or IM every 1 to 2 hours

until the symptoms are eradicated or safely under control. The total dose required for control may then be given over the course of 24 hours in scheduled doses. Frequent reassessment is required to monitor for the response of target symptoms and for the emergence of significant side effects (e.g., oversedation, dystonia). Short-acting benzodiazepines (e.g., lorazepam) may be preferable to neuroleptics in the treatment of simple insomnia or agitation unaccompanied by delusions or hallucinations.

BEHAVIORAL DISORDERS: SEXUAL PROBLEMS

Although there has been little empirical study of sexuality among persons with SSc, clinical experience suggests that sexual problems are common and disturbing complications of this disease. Case 2 shows that they may serve as the focal difficulty in a marriage and thereby destabilize the most critical relationship in a patient's social support network. It is important to ask about sexual problems and to address them in a straightforward manner once they are identified.

Erectile Dysfunction

Men with SSc may lose the ability to achieve normal erections and to ejaculate, often without loss of sexual interest (21). These symptoms may occur early in the course of the disease and be preceded by a phase during which erections are painful. Sclerotic changes in penile vasculature and autonomic neuropathy have been proposed as causes, but no pathogenetic mechanism has been proven. Furthermore, the case reports do not definitively rule out psychological causes of erectile dysfunction, since psychological evaluations and/or studies of nocturnal penile tumescence were not performed, and behavioral forms of sex therapy were not undertaken. Men should be asked if they have difficulty achieving or maintaining erections and, if so, how often and under what circumstances these difficulties occur. If patients have normal sleep-associated nocturnal erections or normal erections in certain sexual contexts (e.g., masturbation) but not in others, then there are probably important underlying nonorganic or psychological factors, and the patient will probably benefit from referral to a behaviorally-oriented expert in the treatment of sexual disorders. On the other hand, if erections fail to occur under all sexual circumstances and sleep-associated nocturnal erections cannot be documented, then vascular and/or neurogenic causes are likely, and referral to a urologist may be most appropriate.

Loss of Sexual Interest

Loss of sexual interest is the "final common pathway" for many different kinds of problems. Nonspecific, systemic manifestations of SSc, such as generalized fatigue, may transform sexual activity, formerly a source of enjoyment, into a burdensome obligation. Focal painful symptoms affecting the hands (e.g., ulceration), face (e.g., diminished oral aperture), genitalia (e.g., reduced vaginal lubrication, painful erections), and other end organs may render sex uncomfortable and unenjoyable. The conviction that one is unattractive or otherwise sexually undesirable diminishes one's willingness to initiate sex (sometimes due to fear of rejection) or even respond to the initiative of others ("He doesn't want me; he just feels sorry for me."). Moreover, major depression is characteristically accompanied by loss of sexual interest.

The clinical approach to loss of interest depends on the cause. When it is caused by major depression, antidepressant medications are usually effective. When generalized fatigue is the cause, it is helpful for the couple to arrange for privacy early in the day or whenever energy is most adequate. When pain interferes with sexual interest and enjoyment, then specific measures to treat the painful conditions (e.g., vaginal lubricants) or changes in the mechanics of sexual activity (e.g., digital stimulation rather than vaginal penetration) may be helpful. Consultation with an expert in the treatment of sexual problems may greatly assist couples in their adaptation to SSc-related sexual difficulties.

THE "NORMAL" RESPONSE TO SCLERODERMA

For many reasons, SSc is a highly distressing disease for patients. Diagnosis is often delayed for months or years. Myalgias, arthralgias, pigmentary skin changes, puffy fingers, fatigue, and other nonspecific constitutional symptoms may precede by months other more obvious signs of SSc. Such symptoms often baffle clinicians, and many patients have seen many physicians before the diagnosis is confirmed. This experience undercuts patients' confidence in the medical profession and engenders anger, suspiciousness, sadness, fear, and anxiety—feelings that are often not volunteered by the patient and may contaminate the doctor-patient relationship.

Scleroderma is usually progressive and often involves the heart, lungs, and kidneys, but the course is highly variable. Patients are chagrined to learn that they cannot be cured and are further upset to discover that their prognosis cannot be predicted with accuracy. They are also distressed to find that disease activity is often difficult to assess; patients may have pain or loss of function as a consequence of tissue injury without evidence that the disease is still biologically "active." This often leads to misconceptions about the goals and expectations of treatment and may prompt feelings of despair and futility.

Scleroderma is also an uncommon disease. At the time of diagnosis most patients have never heard of SSc and have never known anyone with the disease; therefore, they may feel isolated and freakish. They have no frame of reference for their symptoms and no means of anticipating the challenges that lie ahead. The fact that SSc is rare also means that patients' family physicians usually have little or no experience managing the illness. As a result, patients often must leave their community and their usual health care system to find expert help.

Scleroderma affects every aspect of the patient's life. Unlike persons with a "silent" chronic disease (e.g., hypertension), SSc patients must cope on a daily basis with uncomfortable symptoms and physical limitations. Intolerance to cold temperatures often forces patients to change their lifestyles. They may not be able to participate in family activities, particularly outdoor events. Hand contractures interfere with dressing and other self-care activities. All these behavioral adjustments may frustrate and embarrass patients. Losing the capacity to function fully in their social roles (mother, husband, wife, etc.) is particularly demoralizing. Women of childbearing age may be additionally stressed by the desire to have children.

Scleroderma is disfiguring, a distressing but rarely discussed characteristic of the disease. Deformity and contractures of the fingers are extremely common, and these changes concern patients greatly because the hands are readily visible to others. Facial SSc, telangiectasia on the face, furrowing of the skin around the mouth, and decreased oral aperture also disturb most patients.

There is no cure for SSc, and there are few treatments that offer any potential of altering the disease process. Patients repeatedly hear the message that "nothing can be done" and that the disease is progressive over time. Physicians often feel helpless and transmit these feelings to the patient. It is not uncommon to hear patients say, "My doctor does not know what else to do for me; he says he doesn't know much about SSc." This is frightening and demoralizing news. Experimental medications or unproven treatments may be the only therapeutic options. Patients will use diets, herbs, vitamins, and other unconventional therapeutic methods in desperate efforts to heal themselves.

References

1. Buschbaum DG, Buchanan RG, Welsh J, Centor RM, Schnoll SH. Screening for drinking disorders in the elderly using the CAGE questionnaire. J Am Geriatr Soc 1992;40:662–665.
2. Beck AT, Ward CH, Mendelson M, et al. An inventory for measuring depression. Arch Gen Psychiatry 1961;4:53–63.
3. Folstein MF, Folstein SE, McHugh PR. The "Mini-Mental State": A practical method for grading the cognitive state of patients for the clinician. J Psychiatr Res 1975;12:189–198.
4. Anthony JC, LeResche L, Niaz U, et al. Limits of the "Mini-Mental State" as a screening test for dementia and delirium among hospital patients. Psychol Med 1982;12:397–408.
5. Perry S, Miller F. Psychiatric aspects of systemic lupus erythematosus. Systemic lupus erythematosus, 2nd ed. pages 845–863.
6. Wells KB, Stewart A, Hays RD, Burman MA, Rogers W, Daniels M, Berry S, Greenfield S, Ware J. The functioning and well-being of depressed patients: Results from the medical outcomes study. JAMA 1989;262:914–919.
7. American Psychiatric Association. Diagnostic and statistical manual of mental disorders, 3rd ed. revised. Washington, DC: American Psychiatric Association, 1987.
8. Cavanaugh S, Clark DC, Gibbons RD. Diagnosing depression in the hospitalized medically ill. Psychosomatics 1983;24:809–815.
9. Kathol RG, Noyes R, Williams J, Mutgi A, Carroll B, Perry P. Diagonsing depression in patients with medical illness. Psychosomatics 1990;31:434–440.
10. Roca RP, Wigley FM, White B. Depression in systemic sclerosis. Presented at the 146th Annual Meeting of the American Psychiatric Association, San Francisco, May 25, 1993.
11. Katon W, Sullivan MD. Depression and chronic medical illness. J Clin Psychiatry 1990;51:6(supp) 3–14.
12. Muller N, Gizycki-Nienhaus B, Gunther W, Meurer M. Depression as a manifestation of Scleroderma: Immunological findings in serum and cerebrospinal fluid. Biol Psychiatry 1992;31:1151–1156.
13. Moser DK, Clement PJ, Brecht ML, Weiner SR. Predictors of psychosocial adjustment in systemic sclerosis. Arthritis Rheum 1993;36:1398–1405.
14. Peck JR, Smith TW, Ward JR, Milano R. Disability and depression in rheumatoid arthritis. Arthritis Rheum 1989;32:1100–1106.
15. Roca RP, Schmidt CW, Barker LR. Psychotherapy in ambulatory practice. In: Barker LR, Burton JR, Zieve PD, eds. Principles of ambulatory medicine, 4th ed. Baltimore: Williams & Wilkins, 1995.
16. Stuart MR, Lieberman A. The fifteen-minute hour. Applied psychotherapy for the primary care physician. New York: Praeger Scientific, 1986.
17. Bolte MA, Avery D. Case of fluoxetine-induced remission of Raynaud's phenomenon—a case report. Angiology 1993;44:161–163.
18. Goodenow C, Reisine ST, Grady KE. Quality of social support and associated social and psychologi-

cal functioning in women with rheumatoid arthritis. Health Psychol 1990;9:266–284.

19. Frank J. Persuasion and healing, revised ed. Baltimore: Johns Hopkins University Press, 1974.

20. Wise TN, Ginzler EM. Scleroderma cerebritis, an unusual manifestation of progressive systemic sclerosis. Dis Nervous Sys 1975;36:60–62.

21. Lally EV, Jimenez SA. Impotence in progressive systemic sclerosis. Ann Intern Med 1981;95:150–153.

IV

Treatment

PHILIP J. CLEMENTS
DANIEL E. FURST
JAMES R. SEIBOLD
PETER A. LACHENBRUCH

25

Controlled Trials: Trial Design Issues

AS IS DISCUSSED elsewhere in this book, there are NO therapies that have been proven to modify the course of systemic sclerosis (SSc), with the possible exception of angiotensin converting enzyme (ACE) inhibitors in SSc subjects with acute renal crisis (1). Even in 1994, only one agent was FDA-approved in the United States for any single clinical complication or feature of SSc (potassium aminobenzoate for skin thickening), and this agent has recently come under challenge by the Food and Drug Administration (2).

The impediments to drug development in SSc are many and include a low level of interest by the pharmaceutical industry, the absence of a clear unifying mechanism of disease deserving specific therapy, and the absence of uniform and agreed upon standards for design and conduct of clinical trials.

Well-designed randomized, controlled prospective trials of adequate size and duration have been lacking. As our understanding of the disease process increases, new plausible opportunities for intervention will be presented. This chapter focuses on the basic issues of trial design for these future trials (Table 25.1). Improved understanding of the natural history of disease and increased study of potential outcome measures suggest that a reliable and relatively uniform approach to the study of SSc is now possible (3).

Basic Standards for SSc Drug Trials

CRITERIA FOR THE DIAGNOSIS OF SSc.

The American College of Rheumatology (ACR) preliminary criteria for the diagnosis of SSc were published in 1980 (4). Subjects are considered to have SSc if they meet either the major criterion of proximal scleroderma (defined as cutaneous sclerosis proximal to the metacarpal-phalangeal or metatarsal-phalangeal joints of the hands or feet), or at least two of the three minor criteria (sclerodactyly, digital pitting scars or the loss of subcutaneous tissue of the fingertips, and/or chronic interstitial pulmonary change on chest X-ray). In comparison to control populations of systemic lupus erythematosus (SLE), inflammatory muscle disease and isolated Raynaud's phenomenon (RP), these criteria were 91% sensitive and 99% specific. It is recognized that many patients with SSc do not fulfill classification criteria and that there are many non-SSc disorders in which proximal skin thickening is a prominent clinical feature (e.g., scleredema, eosinophilic fasciitis). Most recent studies of SSc have adhered to the ACR classification criteria but have required additional criteria to eliminate confounding disorders.

Table 25.1. Basic Standards for SSc Drug Trials

1. Criteria for diagnosis of SSc
2. Thorough knowledge of SSc natural history
3. Relevant, reliable outcome measures
4. Appropriate patient population
5. Eliminiation of bias
6. Confounding variables
7. Sample size calculations
8. Duration of trial
9. Biologic markers of disease activity
10. Rationale for treatment

THOROUGH KNOWLEDGE OF SSc NATURAL HISTORY

A number of generalizations about the overall course of disease can be made by data that are presently available. Since the skin is the largest organ in the body and the most accessible for study, it has been natural to use skin involvement to make predictions about survival and about what may occur in the visceral organs. In discussing natural history, we will focus on the following items: the distribution of skin thickening, the evolution of skin thickening (as assessed by skin thickness scoring) over time, how long the patient has had SSc, and the likelihood of organ involvement over time.

Rodnan et al pioneered the use of clinical palpation to estimate semiquantitatively skin thickness in multiple areas of the body as an overall measure of skin involvement in scleroderma (5). His rating of local thickness by clinical palpation correlated well with the weight of uniform core skin biopsies, although not with the weights of desiccated tissue shards and hydroxyproline content (5). Rodnan assessed 26 body areas by clinical palpation (0 normal, 1+ slight, 2+ mild, 3+ moderate, 4+ severe) and proposed a semiquantitative Total Skin Score (0–104 maximum) (6). Clements et al and Kahaleh et al have also described semiquantitative skin scoring techniques for assessing tethering and/or thickness in multiple body areas (7, 8).

Investigator consensus in recent years has simplified the Rodnan skin score to include 17 body areas and a rating scale of 0 to 3 (9). This modified-Rodnan (m-Rodnan) skin score more accurately reflects body surface area, eliminates certain body areas felt to be clinically difficult to assess reliably (toes, neck, back), and has been validated in a previous study (10).

The extent and distribution of cutaneous thickening reflect prognosis and the likelihood of visceral involvements. In two studies, the summed score of the semiquantitative skin scoring techniques has been shown to correlate inversely with survival; that is, high skin scores (both as an independent predictor and also as a reflection of visceral involvement) correlate with poor survival (7,11). The distribution of cutaneous sclerosis on the body has also been reported to predict survival. As cutaneous sclerosis moves centrally to involve the trunk, survival declines significantly (12–15).

Medsger described the course of skin thickness score in 2 subsets of SSc patients: (*a*) patients with *diffuse* cutaneous SSc who have thickening of skin proximal and distal to elbows and/or knees, with or without facial involvement, but often with truncal involvement; and (*b*) patients with *limited* cutaneous SSc who have skin thickening limited to skin areas distal to, but not proximal to, elbows and/or knees, with or without facial involvement (15, 16). In early diffuse SSc, the extent and severity of cutaneous thickening tends to progress rapidly, with a peak in skin score in some studies at approximately 2 to 3 years (17). Thereafter, skin score plateaus for a time, and then slowly decreases (17). Clements et al found that individuals with diffuse cutaneous scleroderma entering a therapeutic drug trial tended to have stable skin scores in their first year of follow-up and significant decreases over the subsequent 2 to 3 years (18). The rate of softening was independent of disease duration. In Clements' and Medsger's studies, patients with limited cutaneous thickening or tethering maintained low skin scores, which changed little over many years (17, 18).

Few patients with SSc receive no therapy, and the true natural history of skin involvement remains incompletely defined. Patients with diffuse SSc most typically manifest worsening skin involvement early, while later the disease is more typically stable or improving (15, 17, 19). However, there is considerable heterogeneity of clinical course within either group. While spontaneous improvement in later disease might be seen as a source of "placebo" effect, so might the disease course in those patients with early disease in whom spontaneous arrest of skin progression occurs. Additional prospective data are needed to define these effects.

Although it is not possible to predict with any precision the course of visceral involvement in an individual patient by observing what happens in the skin, we can make some generalizations from studies on large populations of SSc patients (15, 19). If patients with SSc are going to have significant heart, lung, and/or kidney involvement, these complications usually appear within the first 3 to 5 years (20–22). Thereafter, new visceral involvements tend to occur less frequently and to progress very slowly, if at all. Severe heart or kidney involvement tend to occur primarily in diffuse SSc, while severe lung involvement occurs equally in limited and diffuse SSc (15, 19–22). Most patients with limited SSc tend to have smoldering problems with RP, cutaneous ulcerations, esophageal and gastrointestinal problems, and only late develop serious visceral complications (i.e., pulmonary artery hypertension, biliary cirrhosis) (15, 19).

Therefore, knowing the natural history sets the stage for discussing which therapeutics may be of help to which patients in whatever phase and whatever duration of disease they have. Patients with early diffuse disease are more likely to have shortened survival, progressive skin thickening, and early accrual of severe visceral involvement (15, 19); thus, they constitute a group in which more aggressive experimental and potentially dangerous treatments might be offered. This is the group most likely to need a disease-modifying drug that could soften skin, prevent organ involvement, and thereby prolong survival. In contrast, late diffuse and early and late limited SSc tend not to develop *de novo*, rapidly progressive, or severe cutaneous or visceral involvement (15, 19). Rather, they may have problems with pulmonary or pulmonary vascular disease, RP, cutaneous ulcers, and GI problems, which makes them good candidates for studies of vasodilators for RP and cutaneous ulcers, and anti-reflux and promotility drugs for gastrointestinal (GI) tract dysfunction. Patients with skin thickening in a diffuse distribution at the time they are evaluated (be it early or late in their course) may be appropriate candidates for therapies that soften the skin (18).

RELEVANT, RELIABLE OUTCOME VARIABLES

The subject of which outcome variables are appropriate for scleroderma trials has recently been reviewed (23). Formalized guidelines detailing appropriate variables for remission-inducing therapies for scleroderma trials have also been proposed by a committee composed of representatives of the American College of Rheumatology, Food and Drug Administration (FDA), and the National Institutes of Health (NIH) (24). Key outcomes and disease specific organ systems from which to draw outcome variables are presented in Table 25.2.

Emphasis should be placed on the use of methods that give results on a continuous scale, rather than ones that give results on a discrete/dichotomous scale. Trials relying on dichotomous variables tend to require more patients to

Table 25.2. Key Organ Systems and Outcomes from Which to Draw Outcome Variables

1. Survival
2. Skin
3. Organs
   A. Heart
   B. Lungs
   C. Kidneys
   D. Gastrointestinal
   E. Musculoskeletal
4. Raynaud's
5. Functional
6. Global

demonstrate differences than do trials relying on continuous variables.

Survival

Experience has suggested that the mortality rate in SSc is significant, even when patients are studied early in their disease. A recent prospective experience, in which patients were initially seen within one year of onset, revealed that 8% of patients died within 1 year of symptom onset while 25% and 32% died at 3 and 5 years, respectively, after onset (25).

Many scleroderma visceral complications are known to affect prognosis. Bennett et al and Medsger et al demonstrated that heart, lung, and kidney involvement adversely affected outcome (12, 26). Even in the absence of heart, lung, or kidney involvement, however, Medsger's study demonstrated that the diagnosis of SSc, *per se*, adversely affected outcome (26). Bennett, Giordano, Barnett, and Medsger, with their groups, have, in addition, suggested that cutaneous sclerosis on the central areas of the body (i.e., trunk) is associated with shortened survival (12–15). Clements et al showed that a high skin tethering score (and therefore extensive cutaneous sclerosis and thickening) was independently associated with shortened survival (7). Future studies that propose to show improvement in survival must, therefore, take into account the influence of extensive and centrally located skin disease, as well as significant heart, lung, or kidney involvement, at entry (i.e., at the time of randomization patients might be stratified based upon extensive skin, heart, lung, or kidney involvement).

Skin (Cutaneous)

Although extent and severity of skin involvement underlies the classification of SSc and has parallels with both accrual of visceral involvement and survival, it remains controversial whether or not skin, *per se*, is an adequate measure of outcome or merely an accessible clinical surrogate marker. Skin involvement is symptomatic (pain, burning, pruritus), cosmetically disfiguring, and interferes with local joint motion. Individuals with high skin scores have more difficulty with simple tasks of daily living than do individuals with low skin scores (27–29). However, an individual in whom treatment resulted in improvement of skin concomitantly with worsened lung or gastrointestinal function might fairly question physician definitions of successful outcome.

A number of devices and techniques have been proposed to quantitate the degree of skin involvement: devices that pinch, stretch, compress, and depress; ultrasound; and radiographic. Although some of these techniques have shown promising reliability, they have not enjoyed wide use. Semiquantitative skin scoring does appear to be reproducible and reliable (9, 30, 31). Several recent studies have quantitated the inter- and intra-observer error associated with the modified Rodnan skin score (9, 30, 31). In one study, the *inter*-observer error (mean ± within patient standard deviation) was 17.7 ± 4.6 and, in a follow-up study, *intra*-observer error (mean ± within patient standard deviation) was 20.7 ± 2.45 (9, 31). This compares favorably to reported *inter*-observer measures of ARA (18.2 ± 7.8) and Ritchie (16.1 ± 5.9) joint counts used in rheumatoid arthritis trials (32).

As noted above, significant changes in cutaneous thickening occur in diffuse SSc (i.e., rapid increases in the first 2–3 years of SSc followed by slow decreases in the years thereafter), while little change in cutaneous thickening occurs in patients with limited SSc (15, 18, 19). Therefore, trials of therapy that propose to alter skin thickness or tethering should recruit patients who are capable of showing significant changes (i.e., patients who have diffuse skin involvement and/or have high skin thickness scores at the time of entry), and should avoid patients with limited cutaneous involvement (i.e., patients whose skin involvement is not likely to change significantly no matter how long they are studied) (18).

Methods for mapping and quantitating the "areas" of cutaneous thickening, similar to the "rule of nines" for burns, have been reported in SSc trials (30, 33). The method was derived from the dermatology experience in which areas of skin involved by psoriasis are quantitated. Brennan et al recently reported that the skin area score is a less reliable method for quantitating skin involvement than is the skin thickness score, in part because the variability increased considerably with increasing percentages of skin involvement (30).

Other indirect methods have been described for quantitating skin involvement (Table 25.3). Physical methods have included measurements of grip strength and of oral aperture; goniometric measurements of finger flexion at distal interphalangeal (DIP), proximal interphalangeal (PIP), and metacarpophalangeal (MCP) joints of the fingers; measurement of flexion contractures; photocopies of palm prints; and measurement of cutaneous oxygen pressure (23, 34–40). Skin elasticity measurements have employed suction cups, Pierard tonometry, and clinical assessments of mobility (36, 39–43). Skin biopsy specimens have been examined by routine histopathology, uniform diameter core biopsy specimens have been weighed, and quantitative measurements of hydroxyproline in skin biopsies have been described (5, 44). High frequency ultrasound, B mode ultrasound, and soft tissue radiographs also have been described (45–49). Since use of most of these techniques is limited to assessment of one or two small areas of the body, they fail to give a global assessment of skin involvement and thereby risk the problem of sampling error. In addition, the techniques have not been well standardized (i.e., multiple investigators at multiple centers might not be able to employ them reliably). In short, they have not become popular methods for multi-center trials. For the moment, semiquantitative skin scoring seems to be the major cutaneous assessment technique.

Visceral Involvement

If change in visceral organ involvement or the onset of new organ involvement is sought, it should be sought at a time when organ system involvement is likely to occur. Steen et al presented data showing that if severe organ involvement is going to occur, it usually does so within 3 to 5 years of scleroderma onset (15, 20, 21). This suggests that the onset and the most rapid progression of organ involvement occurs in the first few years. Therefore, only patients who are at risk of developing new, severe organ involvement (i.e., SSc of less than 12–18 months duration) should be entered into trials for which the primary objective is to assess the onset or modification of heart, lung, or kidney involvement. If patients are entered late rather than early in their course (>3–5 years after SSc onset), then SSc organ involvement will tend to occur and to worsen more slowly, and more years and more patients will be needed to demonstrate a difference in the courses.

Renal Involvement. The natural history of renal scleroderma, including its treatment with ACE inhibitors, must be taken into account in trial design. Renal crisis usually occurs in the first 5 to 6 years of SSc (approximately 90%), occurs more frequently in diffuse SSc (approximately 70%–80%), and is routinely treated with ACE inhibitors (1, 20). It is easier to assess the onset of new renal disease than it is to assess the effect of a non-ACE inhibiting therapy (i.e.,

Table 25.3. Other Methods for Assessing Skin Involvement in SSc

Modality	Measurements
• Physical	Grip strength
	Oral aperature
	Finger flexion
	Hand extension
	Palm prints
	Contractures
	Cutaneous hypoxia
	Percent skin area involved
• Skin elasticity	Suction cup
	Pierard tonometer
	Bachman skin mobility
• Biopsy	Weight
	Pathology
	Amount of hydroxyproline
• Ultrasound/x-ray	High frequency ultrasound
	B-mode ultrasound
	Soft tissue radiographs

organ involvement" might be a more useful outcome measurement of visceral involvement than measurement of changes in organ function once dysfunction has occurred (6). This outcome variable is applicable primarily for early diffuse SSc patients, because organ system involvement tends to occur early in diffuse SSc (15, 19). One set of criteria for organ system involvement (derived from the ongoing High-Dose vs Low-Dose Penicillamine Trial) that could be used to determine the new onset of organ involvement is shown in Table 25.4. Other criteria for organ involvement could be employed.

Raynaud's Phenomenon

RP is present in more than 90% of individuals with SSc and is typically an early symptom. A therapy to prevent its onset is not theoretically possible, because vascular injury is probably already present at initial clinical presentation. The clinical impact of RP includes the pain of individual episodes, the loss of tactile sensitivity and hand function in cold environments, and the major sequela of digital ulcerations and frank ischemic injury.

A uniform approach to assessing RP is lacking. A variety of non-invasive vascular testing modalities have been used but have not been standardized among centers and are expensive and notoriously non-reproducible. Clinical measures include continuous variables such as frequency of daily episodes recorded in patient diaries and patient ratings of the impact of Raynaud's on daily function (58). Dichotomous variables include healing and prevention of discrete ischemic ulcerations. Inter-observer variability in assessing whether or not an individual ulcer is healed is high, and photographic or videotaped documentation techniques lack standardization. Multicenter studies of Raynaud's are rendered problematic by differences in climate and ambient temperature. Crossover studies of Raynaud's are rendered problematic by seasonal change (i.e., active treatment begun in winter with placebo crossover in spring and vice versa).

Functional and Global Assessments

Global and functional indices have been reviewed by Pope, who found in her review of multiple previous scleroderma studies that global and functional indices are capable of demonstrating change over time and are therefore worthwhile in clinical trials (23). Techniques that use Lickert or visual analog scales are preferred.

Few functional indices have been validated in scleroderma. Several reports have assessed the reliability and validity of the Health Assessment Questionnaire (HAQ and its 8 domains) in scleroderma (27–29). The 20-item HAQ-disability scale is the most widely used technique in scleroderma and is a reasonable choice for future studies. Other functional indices might be appropriate but have not been tested to date.

Patient assessment of outcome is of increasing importance to regulatory agencies. Additional study of self-assessment techniques is clearly needed in SSc. The ideal measurement would be reproducible, yet sensitive to change, and would relate patient function to the disease process.

Review of Recommended Outcome Variables

The methodology incorporated into the High-Dose vs Low-Dose Penicillamine trial (which began in January, 1991) took into account much of

Table 25.4. Sample Criteria for Organ Involvement in SSc[a]

A. Renal
   - Creatinine clearance >2 SD below mean of age and sex-adjusted normal values
   - Serum creatinine. U.L.N.[b] (>2 SD above normal mean)
   - Urine protein >300 MG/24 hrs
B. Pulmonary
   - DLCO ≤70% of predicted
   - FEVI, FVC or TLC ≤75% of predicted
   - Interstitial fibrosis (chest x-ray)
C. Cardiac
   - Arrhythmia requiring medication
   - Pericarditis
   - Cardiomegaly, C.H.F.
D. Musculoskeletal
   - CPK ≥2 Times U.L.N.
   - Ritchie articular index ≥5

[a]High-dose vs low-dose d-pen ion SSc
[b]U.L.N., upper limit of normal

what has been discussed in previous paragraphs (3). The group of outcome variables for that trial can serve as minimal measures for evaluating outcome (Table 25.5). The continuous variables being measured include: modified Rodnan skin score, joint tenderness count, CPK, serum creatinine, 24-hour urine protein, 24-hour urine creatinine clearance, diffusing capacity, total lung capacity, and HAQ-disability scale. The dichotomous variables are the new onset of organ involvement, cardiomegaly, presence of interstitial markings on chest x-ray, and survival. Laboratory assessment of gastrointestinal and cardiac involvement were felt to be too expensive and not sensitive enough to include in this multi-center trial.

Pope has presented her recommendations for potential response parameters for future scleroderma trials (Table 25.6) based on the ability of the parameter to change over a 1- to 3-year period (23). Only two measurements were considered likely to change and be worthwhile: skin score and global assessment. Secondary measurements (those uncertain to show changes over 1–3 years) included functional, physical, change in percent predicted diffusing capacity, new onset of renal disease, and survival.

An ACR-FDA-NIH committee has established guidelines for testing potential disease modifying therapies for future scleroderma trials (Table 25.7) (24). Disease modification is defined by a treatment's ability to improve survival

Table 25.5. Outcome Variables in High-Dose vs Low-Dose Penicillamine Trial

A. Primary outcome variables
  1. Survival
  2. New onset of renal disease
  3. Skin score (modified rodnan)
B. Secondary outcome variables
  1. Chest x-ray (cardiomegaly, interstitial change)
  2. Joint tenderness count
  3. CPK
  4. 24-hour urine protein
  5. 24-hour creatinine clearance
  6. DLCO, TLC, FVC
  7. HAQ disability scale

Table 25.6. SSc Response Parameters—Pope[a]

1. Primary (most likely to show changes)
  • Skin score
  • Global
2. Secondary (uncertain to show changes)
  • Functional
  • Physical (grip, oral, finger flexion)
  • Change in % predicted DLCO
  • New onset renal crisis
  • Survival

[a]Raynaud's not mentioned.

Table 25.7. SSc Response Parameters—ACR Committee on Design and Outcomes in Clinical Trials in Systemic Sclerosis[a]

1. Survival
2. Organ
  • Kidneys: Serum creatinine, blood pressure
  • Lungs: DLCO, FVC
  • Heart: ejection fraction (echo-cardiogram), serious arrhythmia requiring therapy
  • Skin: skin score
  • Gut: Pseudoobstruction, malabsorption requiring total parenteral nutrition
3. Global
  • Health status instrument (i.e., HAQ-disability scale)
  • Patient and physician global assessment
  • Body weight or body mass index

[a]Raynaud's not mentioned.

and prevent organ dysfunction. Survival is an outcome by itself. Prevention of organ dysfunction can be monitored by organ-specific laboratory or examination procedures: creatinine clearance and blood pressure for renal disease; diffusing capacity and forced vital capacity for pulmonary involvement; ejection fraction on echocardiogram and need for treatment of serious arrhythmias for cardiac involvement; skin score for cutaneous involvement; and onset of pseudoobstruction and malabsorption requiring total parenteral nutrition for gastrointestinal involvement. The Committee was unable to define specific recommendations for measurement of musculoskeletal involvements because it felt that there were no established reliable measures for evaluating outcomes in this area. Useful global measures include health status instruments (i.e., HAQ disability scale), patient and physician global assessments, and body weight or body mass index.

The above recommendations are for testing drugs that may modify disease. The Committee plans to develop guidelines for organ-specific treatments which are to be directed at improving function in specific organs.

APPROPRIATE PATIENT POPULATION

The objectives of the study dictate which patients should be included and excluded. If survival is the endpoint, then logic dictates that the patients most likely to show differences in survival are the patients who have very early diffuse scleroderma (say, less than 12–18 months duration at entry at a time that patient death can still be prevented). For the same reason, prevention of new organ involvement would also require patients who have very early diffuse scleroderma (also less than 12–18 months). Conversely, if the objective of the study is to show that treatment softens skin, then patients who have diffuse cutaneous sclerosis at the time of entry (regardless of duration) might be reasonable candidates, because they have the capacity to show softening of skin (18). If healing of cutaneous ulcers is the endpoint, then patients who have digital ulcers are the ones who should be included.

ELIMINATION OF BIAS

Trial Design

In his review of the influence of study design on drug trial outcome (59), Colditz divided study designs into 6 basic categories (Table 25.8). His analysis suggested that the randomized, double-blind trial design (parallel or cross-over) is the most rigorous test for determining treatment efficacy (59). This design is less likely to show bias in favor of the new treatment than are non-randomized controlled trials, which in turn are less likely to show such bias than are trials of active treatments against historical controls or of observational trials.

In their analysis of cardiac disease in SSc

Table 25.8. Classification of Drug Study Designs (Colditz)

1. Randomized controlled trial
   A. Parallel
   B. Cross-over
2. Non-randomized controlled trial
   A. Parallel
   B. Cross-over
3. Active treatment against historical controls
4. Observational

patients in the chlorambucil vs placebo trial, Clements et al reported that patients who had entered the trial but then withdrew within 6 months (either because they did not take study medication or for reasons other than adverse effects, such as unreliability, or "didn't want to continue") had a significantly different outcome than did patients who remained in the trial for greater than 6 months (60). Patients who "chose not to be followed" in the context of the trial had a much higher mortality rate over the next few years than those who continued in the drug trial. This single variable (continuing the trial vs withdrawing within the first 6 months) was the most significant predictor of survival (60). This illustrates the hazards of using such patients (dropouts or "discards," if you will) as a "control" group for a drug-treated group.

Blinding is the ideal, with a double blind being the usually required method. If a characteristic trait of treatment requires it (i.e., an event might unblind the patient and/or observer), then an independent masked observer should be used. Alternatively, an endpoint that is not subject to observer bias (such as survival) could be used as the primary outcome measure.

Randomization of control and treated patients is mandatory. Patient randomization should occur after drug wash-out is complete and just before the patient is to begin the study. In any randomized trial, patients should not be permitted to change the randomization choice by opting out of the randomized choice and then being entered into the other treatment arm. An intent-to-treat (or "last observation carried forward") analysis should be performed in conjunction with the analysis of "completers," because the intent-to-treat analysis reduces the bias introduced into the analysis when patients who are not doing well are excluded from the analysis. Within the randomization schedule, patients might be pre-stratified by important organ involvements (i.e., patients with a severe degree of cardiac involvement might be randomized separately so that there is even distribution between the treatment groups). In a multi-center trial, stratification by center should be done to account for center effects, and the analysis should account for this stratification. Conversely one should beware of over-stratification because the size of treatment groups may be too small to be analyzable.

Controls

Different types of controls are acceptable for scleroderma drug trials (Table 25.9). Until such time as a treatment is identified that modifies the outcome of scleroderma, placebo controlled trials are preferred. Once a treatment has been shown to alter outcome, active controls can be compared to a new treatment in future trials (although statistical power considerations may mandate very large patient numbers). A "sham" should be considered for treatments that involve procedures that would be difficult to blind (i.e., photopheresis).

Dose response trials are a reasonable alternative to a two-arm placebo-controlled trial. If this design is used, a minimum of 3 doses (including the maximum effective and the least effective or placebo doses) should usually be included. The 3-dose-response design requires that the sample size be increased by only a few patients over the 2-arm study. Cross-over designs are less feasible for disease modifying trials because the length of time required to show disease modification is too long to make a cross-over design feasible. Cross-over designs are more suitable for studies of organ-specific protocols where results can be achieved within several months (i.e., H2-blockers, anti-inflammatory drugs, promotility drugs). One could consider a placebo or no-treatment washout between arms to minimize carry over effects.

CONFOUNDING VARIABLES

Exclusion criteria homogenize the patient group into specific diagnostic categories and eliminate patients who are so ill that they cannot be helped or who would adversely weigh against a definitive outcome. Other medications that might influence the outcome of therapy should also be excluded or controlled for. Pregnancy, unprotected child-bearing potential, recent drug and alcohol abuse, unreliability, and chronic debilitating diseases that make it difficult to evaluate the outcome should be excluded. Sample exclusions from the High-Dose vs Low-Dose Penicillamine Trial are shown in Table 25.10.

SAMPLE SIZE CALCULATIONS

Tables 25.11 and 25.12 show sample size calculations based on skin score (an outcome variable which is a continuous variable) and on survival (an outcome variable which is dichotomous). The natural history of skin involvement in SSc must be taken into account when calculating sample sizes, because the natural history of the disease may make the endpoint a moving, or in some instances an unattainable, target. Preliminary data or experience is critical in making assumptions about effect size or expected changes in outcome variables during the trial. Some available skin score data suggest that the average

Table 25.9. Controls for SSc Drug Trials

1. Placebo-control (preferred)
2. Sham (preferred for procedures)
3. Active control
4. Dose-response
   - Minimum of 3 doses
   - May include placebo or minimum effective dose
   - Should include maximum effective dose
5. Cross-over
   - Best for organ-specific
   - Not so good for disease modification or prevention of new organ involvement

Table 25.10. Exclusion Criteria for SSc DMARD Trials-I

1. SSc 2° environmental exposure
2. SSc in overlap
3. Significant internal organ damage
   A. Renal:
      • Serum creatinine ≥2MG%
      • Renal crisis
   B. Lungs:
      • FVC ≤50% predicted
      • DLCO ≤40% predicted
   C. Heart:
      • Ejection fraction ≤40%
      • ? Arrhythmias requiring Rx
   D. Gut:
      • Pseudoosbstruction
      • ? Malabsorption requiring antibiotics
4. Other therapy which might influence outcome
   A. Current:
      • Steroids (>10mg/day of prednisone)
      • Ace-inhibitors (sulfhydryl-containing)
      • ? Prostaglandin analogs
   B. Previous:
      • Penicillamine within past 6 months or having taken it for more than 3 months
      • Other potential DMARDS within past 3–6 months
5. Other conditions
   A. Chronic debilitating diseases
   B. Pregnancy or unprotected childbearing potential
   C. Recent drug/alcohol abuse
   D. Unreliability

early diffuse SSc patient will have a modified-Rodnan skin thickness score of about 21 at entry, and that over the next year there will be minimal change downward (final skin score in the controls of 19). If the active drug is expected to be mildly effective, the treatment group might show a change from 21 to 18 over the course of 1 year, which is only 1 unit difference compared to the 19 in the control group (Table 25-11). If 0.8 power is acceptable, then 1,029 patients would be needed per group. Needless to say, this would be an impossible study. If, on the other hand, the treatment group is expected to have a drop in skin score from 21 down to 15 (or a difference of 4 between the final skin score in the treatment [15] vs control [19] group), then 64 patients in each group will be needed. An even more effective treatment might show a final skin score in the active treatment group of 13 with a difference between control and treatment group of 6. In that case (with a power 0.8), 29 subjects per group would be required.

Steen and group's penicillamine study of 1982 showed a 2-year survival in the penicillamine group of 93% and the comparison group of 75% (6): the mortality rate in the control group was four times that in the control group (a hazard ratio of 4, Table 25-12). Therefore, a controlled trial of penicillamine would need 52 subjects per group in a 2-year study (assuming a power of 0.8). If a treatment were expected to be even

Table 25.11. Sample Size Calculations Based on Skin Score (SKSC)*

SKSC	Final SKSC		Difference Between CTRL and Treatment	No. Needed/Group	
At Entry	CTRL	Treat		Power of 0.8	Power of 0.9
21	19	18	1	1029	1379
21	19	17	2	257	345
21	19	16	3	114	153
21	19	15	4	64	86
21	19	14	5	41	55
21	19	13	6	29	38

* Assume: 1) Entry SKSC of 21 ± 8
         2) Control decreases by 2 in first year.
         3) Alpha = 0.05

Table 25.12. Power Calculations for Survival (D-PEN)[a]

| Hazard ratio | Subjects needed per group | |
	Power 0.8	Power 0.9
2.0	205	274
2.8	91	122
4.0	52	69
5.6	33	44
8.0	23	31

[a]Assume 2-year survival for D-PEN of 93% for untreated of 75%; Alpha = 0.05.

more effective, mortality in the treatment group might be 1/8th that of the control group (hazard ratio of 8, Table 25-12). In that instance, only 23 subjects would be needed per group for a 2-year trial.

Unless a very effective treatment is discovered, however, such large differences are rarely found. Trials should generally be designed to detect moderate differences, i.e., hazard ratios of 2 or so, and effect sizes of 0.5 to 0.6 where:

$$\text{Effect size} = \frac{(\text{mean change first treatment} - \text{mean change control treatment})}{\text{standard deviation}}$$

An important distinction to make is that some changes which are statistically significant are not medically meaningful. Table 25.13 shows those changes that are considered to be medically meaningful by a consensus of clinicians (24). Although there is little information to corroborate that patients themselves would agree with this set

of medically meaningful changes, there is reasonable consensus among investigators that if a treatment were to show this degree of change in an organ system, that would be a medically meaningful change.

DURATION OF TRIAL

The duration of a trial depends on the objective(s) and the outcome variables studied. Data are available which suggest that, even in early diffuse scleroderma, the mortality rate at 3 years is approximately 25%. If we have a therapy which cuts that mortality rate by 50% to 75%, we would need to study a group of early diffuse scleroderma patients for at least 3 years to be able to demonstrate a difference in outcome in the two groups (assuming an adequate sample size). Prevention of onset of new organ involvement also would probably require 3 or more years of study in a group of early diffuse SSc patients.

A study of RP, on the other hand, could require as little as 3 to 6 months duration (assuming the trial was started and completed in the cooler winter months). Alternatively, a study that followed patients with RP for 1 year (all patients going through hot and cold seasons) might be acceptable, and would be expected to facilitate demonstrating efficacy for RP. A study in which the goal is to soften skin should concentrate on diffuse patients, and should plan to follow them for at least 12 months to ensure that they will be able to show a lasting difference between the control and the treatment group.

Table 25.13. Medically Meaningful Changes in SSc

Response Parameters	Medically Meaningful Change
Skin Score	≥30% (in diffuse SSc)
Serum creatinine	≥70% baseline
FVC	≥15% baseline
DLCO	≥15% baseline
Left ventricular ejection fraction	≥10% baseline
Blood pressure	≥20 mm systolic or ≥10 mm diastolic (on 2 different occasions)

BIOLOGIC MARKERS OF DISEASE ACTIVITY AND RATIONALE

A cohesive theory of pathogenesis of SSc needs to fully address the evidence of immune activation, the phenomenon of extracellular collagen and matrix accumulation, and the progressive nature of vascular injury, all three of which are ubiquitous in all forms of the disease (15, 19). Much of this text is dedicated to the advances in the descriptive biology of these effects and to enumerating the remarkable spectrum of accompanying laboratory abnormalities.

A true surrogate marker of disease would be one that reflected the essence of the disease process and that, in serial assay, strongly paralleled or predicted disease outcome. There is no such test presently available. Potential areas for further investigation are listed in Table 25.14 and include markers of new collagen production (serum levels of the aminoterminal propeptide of Type III collagen); measurements of endothelial injury and response (endothelin-1, Factor VIII/von Willebrand factor antigen, thrombospondin and beta-thromboglobulin and other measures of platelet activation); measurements of T cell activation and turnover (serum levels of soluble interleukin-2 receptors, soluble CD4 and soluble CD8); and measurements of various pro-inflammatory and profibrotic cytokines (interleukin-6, TNF-alpha, etc.).

A major difficulty in assessing the value of any of these proposed assays is the lack of any correlative prospective clinical study (with a few exceptions: e.g., serum interleukin-2 receptor levels). The overwhelming majority of reports of candidate markers have derived from point prevalence surveys of local scleroderma populations. Studies frequently contrast findings in limited vs diffuse cutaneous scleroderma but do not offer data that permit comparison of assay results with subsequent clinical outcome. The same precepts of study design listed above that segregate disease by classification, duration, and severity need be applied to these tests and prospective interventional trials need to include pilot efforts to validate these measures.

Independent of the scientific value of inter-relating a test abnormality with clinical outcome is the promise of biologic markers for serving as outcome measures for pilot trials. The definitive long term disease modifying trial described above is labor-intensive and expensive. One can safely predict that few trials of this magnitude will be undertaken in the future without some preliminary pilot data suggesting a reasonable chance of success. Short term improvement in a surrogate marker reasonably related to both

Table 25.14. Biologic Measures of SSc Disease Activity

Process	Variable
• Collagen turnover	• Serum aminoterminal peptide of α (III) collagen
• Endothelial cell damage	• Circulating factor VIII antigen
• Immune activation	• Serum interleukin-2 receptor
	• Soluble CD4
	• Soluble CD8
	• Endothelin-1
	• Thrombospondin
	• β-Thromboglobulin
	• Platelet activation
• Cytokines	• Interleukins 1, 2 & 6
	• TGF-β
	• TNF-α
	• Platelet derived growth factor
	• β-1 integrins

disease process and disease outcome would likely be sufficient in this regard.

Reporting Requirements

In this section we discuss aspects of reporting the study results. Sometimes, suggestions will lead to a longer manuscript than an editor will publish. When substantial shortening is required, the material may be made available to interested readers as a technical report or a protocol document. As Friedman et al state, "The investigator has an obligation to review critically his study and its findings and to present sufficient information so that readers can properly evaluate the trial" (61).

INTRODUCTION

In this section, a short description of the study with its goals clearly enunciated is helpful to the reader. A statement of the hypotheses being tested, or quantities being estimated is useful. Results of other relevant studies should be discussed. The importance of the study to clinical practice may be indicated (this can also appear in the discussion section).

METHODS AND MATERIALS

A complete description of the patient population including the source (hospital, survey, multiple sources, etc.), the entry and exclusion criteria, any stratification that might be used, and variables being measured. A discussion of standardization methods (i.e., inter- and intra-observer or test variability; investigator training sessions) is useful, although this may be difficult to publish.

The therapeutic intervention, if any, should be discussed: manufacturer, dosages, and schedule stated. If rules for stopping the trial are being used, they should be described.

Comparative studies should be randomized. The randomization procedure should be clearly described including any stratification (restric-tions on the randomization). Similarly, studies should be blinded to prevent bias in the evaluation. This is especially important in studies in which the outcome may be subjective. Thus, in evaluating a therapy using skin scores, the scorers should not know the status of the patient being evaluated. This may require special procedures (a blinded observer) for some studies (e.g., photopheresis). If these standard approaches have not been used, then the alternative approach must be justified.

The statistical methods should be described. In particular, statistical transformations (i.e., converting to logarithms), if needed, should be discussed. Many methods are available for determining the best transformation. Responses that are expressed as percentages are usually equivalent to taking logarithms of the original data (for example, considering the change in a response as a percentage is equivalent to using the log of the ratio of the first and last responses). The analytic methods often include t-tests, analysis of variance, and survival analysis. A discussion of the assumptions made in these methods can appear here, although this again may be difficult to publish. It may be given as part of the technical report. Published or not, this should be discussed between the statistician and the investigator (the statistician may be a full member of the research group or a consultant—in any event, examination of the assumptions is a needed part of the analysis). Inappropriate analyses are sometimes discovered by this process. It is better to find them before attempting publication.

RESULTS SECTION

The organization suggested here should be adapted to the needs of the study. The outcomes of the study can be considered by first describing the groups at baseline. If randomization has been successful, there will be few large differences in the groups at baseline. Next, the time course of the patients can be presented. This can be graphical (be careful of graphs that look like plates of spaghetti and don't communicate much) or numerical (change scores, slopes of within patient lines). Patients who drop from the study need to be noted and their reasons for dropping analyzed. These may be due to death, toxicity of the therapy, moving to another location, etc. The toxicities (side effects) of the drug, and their frequency, should be described.

The analyses must account for strata, such as gender, clinical center, risk group. There are often differences among centers which must be accounted for. In the extreme case, if all of the treatment difference is due to an excellent result at one center, this may be due to the outstanding skill of one group or a failure of the protocol at one or more centers. Results can be presented in tabular form. Tables of means and standard deviations abound. Other descriptions of data are becoming popular and may provide more information when data are not normally distributed. These include the "five number summary," consisting of the minimum and maximum values, and the 25th, 50th, and 75th percentiles. These are less useful when the sample size is less than 20. Tables of tests of hypotheses can be combined with these. However, tables consisting only of p-values (or p < .05, NS, etc.) should be avoided, because they convey far less information about the study.

In most studies, there are multiple responses evaluated and many "looks" at the data. This leads to problems of multiple testing, which may roughly be defined as the loss of interpretability of p-values. If a number of hypotheses are tested at the 0.05 significance level, the overall probability of rejecting a true null hypothesis can be far greater than 0.05. The most desirable solution is to select a few hypotheses *at the time of the study design*, and use a test procedure that accounts for the number of hypotheses being tested. Such a procedure is not valid after the data have been examined. This should not be construed as a prohibition from exploring the data for interesting relationships. It merely says that the latter "significant" results are suspect because they were the most significant ones from this data set discovered *post hoc*.

DISCUSSION/CONCLUSIONS

Interpreting the results to others is crucial. Many readers will not be expert in SSc and will be susceptible to over enthusiasm. Caution is advised. Explaining the limitations of the study, need for further research, etc., are especially helpful to readers.

Conclusions

This chapter has addressed the features that we feel should be included in a definitive trial of disease-modifying therapy for SSc (and to a lesser extent, of organ-specific therapy). Improved clinical descriptions, improved understanding of natural history, and long overdue studies of the accuracy and reproducibility of outcome measurements suggest that truly reliable trial design is now a reality in scleroderma. This does not mean that such trials will be conducted. Clinical studies of adequate sample size and duration that permit assessment of dose response relationships and include measurements of visceral status are extremely expensive ($2–$5 million) and funding for such studies has been lacking. The effects of health care reform on the pharmaceutical industry are increasing their focus on "high-impact" therapies for the more common human disorders and are secondarily diminishing their focus on less common diseases like scleroderma. An increasingly small share of the federal research dollar is directed to patient-oriented research.

The challenges to the community of clinical researchers in scleroderma are many. We need first and foremost, consensus as to what constitutes disease modification so as to minimize confusion in both potential sponsors and regulatory agencies. We need collaborative efforts that offer sponsors efficient and timely recruitment of appropriate subjects. One such group, the Scleroderma Clinical Trials Consortium, has begun to do so in the United States. Harmonization of drug development among Europe, the United

States, Australia, and the Pacific Rim will offer new opportunities for collaboration. Laboratory researchers should seek to interact with their more clinical colleagues to permit more rapid and reliable testing and validation of proposed biologic markers. Adequate studies are within our collective reach.

References

1. Steen VD, Costantino JP, Shapiro AP, Medsger TA Jr. Outcome of renal crisis in systemic sclerosis: Relation to availability of angiotensin converting enzyme (ACE) inhibitors. Ann Intern Med 1990; 113:352–357.
2. Clegg DO, Reading JC, Mayes MD, Seibold JR, Harris C, Wigley FM, Ward JR, et al. Comparison of aminobenzoate potassium and placebo in the treatment of scleroderma. J Rheumatol 1994;21: 105–110.
3. Seibold JR, Furst DE, Clements PJ. Why everything (or nothing) seems to work in the treatment of scleroderma. J Rheumatol 1992;19:673–676.
4. Subcommittee for Scleroderma Criteria of the American Rheumatism Association Diagnostic and Therapeutic Criteria Committee. Preliminary criteria for the classification of systemic sclerosis (scleroderma). Arthritis Rheum 1980;23: 581–590.
5. Rodnan GP, Lipinski E, Luksick J. Skin thickness and collagen in progressive systemic sclerosis (scleroderma) and localized scleroderma. Arthritis Rheum 1979;22:130–140.
6. Steen VD, Medsger TA Jr, Rodnan GP. D-penicillamine therapy in progressive systemic sclerosis (scleroderma). Ann Intern Med 1982;97:652–658.
7. Clements PJ, Lachenbruch PA, Ng SW, Simmons M, Sterz M, Furst DE. Skin score. A semiquantitative measure of cutaneous involvement that improves prediction of prognosis in systemic sclerosis. Arthritis Rheum 1990;33:1256–1263.
8. Kahaleh MB, Suttany GL, Smith EA, Huffstutter JE, Loadholt CB, LeRoy EC. A modified scleroderma skin scoring method. Clin Exp Rheumatol 1986;4:367–369.
9. Clements PJ, Lachenbruch PA, Seibold JR, Zee B, Brennan P, Silman P, Allegar A, et al. Skin thickness score in systemic sclerosis (SSc): An assessment of inter-observer variability in three independent studies. J Rheumatol 1993;20:1892–1896.
10. Ramsden MF, Goldsmith CH, Lee P, Sebalt R, Baer P. Clinical assessment of scleroderma: Observer variation in five methods. Arthritis Rheum 1986; 29:S61.
11. Medsger TA Jr, Steen VD, Ziegler G, Rodnan G. The natural history of skin involvement in progressive systemic sclerosis. Arthritis Rheum 1980; 22:720–721.
12. Bennett R, Bluestone R, Holt PJL, Bywaters EGL. Survival in scleroderma. Ann Rheum Dis 1971;30: 581–588.
13. Giordano M, Valentini G, Migliaresi S, Picillo V, Vatti M. Different antibody patterns and different prognoses in patients with scleroderma with various extent of skin sclerosis. J Rheumatol 1986;13: 911–916.
14. Barnett AJ, Miller MH, Littlejohn GO. A survival study of the patients diagnosed with scleroderma over 30 years (1953–1983): The value of a simple cutaneous classification in the early stages of the disease. J Rheumatol 1988;15:276–283.
15. Medsger TA Jr. Systemic sclerosis (scleroderma), localized forms of scleroderma, and calcinosis. In:McCarty DJ, Koopman WJ, eds. Arthritis and allied conditions. Philadelphia: Lea & Febiger, 1993;1253–1292.
16. LeRoy EC, Black C, Fleischmajer R, Jablonska S, Krieg T, Medsger TA Jr, Rowell N, Wollheim F. Scleroderma (systemic sclerosis): Classification, subsets, and pathogenesis. J Rheumatol 1988;15: 202–205.
17. Medsger TA Jr. Progressive systemic sclerosis. Clin Rheum Dis 1983;9:655–670.
18. Clements PJ, Lachenbruch P, Furst D, Paulus H. The course of skin involvement in systemic sclerosis (SSc) over 3 years in a trial of chlorambucil versus placebo. Arthritis Rheum 1993;36:1575–1579.
19. Seibold JR. Scleroderma. In: Kelley WN, Harris ED, Ruddy S, Sledge CB, eds. Textbook of rheumatology. Philadelphia: WB Saunders, 1993;1113–1143.
20. Steen VD, Medsger TA Jr, Osial TA, Ziegler GL, Shapiro AP, Rodnan GP. Factors predicting development of renal involvement in progressive systemic sclerosis. Am J Med 1984;76:779–786.
21. Steen VD, Conte C, Owens G, Medsger TA Jr. Severe restrictive lung disease in systemic sclerosis (SSc). Arthritis Rheum 1994;37:1283–1289.
22. Steen VD, Medsger TA Jr. Epidemiology and natural history of systemic sclerosis. Rheum Dis Clin North Am 1990;16:1–10.
23. Pope JE, Bellamy N. Outcome measurement in scleroderma clinical trials. Semin Arthritis Rheum 1993;23:22–33.
24. White B, Bauer EA, Goldsmith LA, Hochberg MC, Katz LM, Korn JH, Lachenbruch PA, et al. Guidelines for clinical trials in systemic sclerosis (sclero-

derma). I. Disease-modifying interventions. American college of rheumatology committee on design and outcomes in clinical trials in systemic sclerosis (scleroderma). Arthritis Rheum 1995;38: 351–360.

25. Bulpitt KJ, Clements PJ, Lachenbruch PA, Paulus HE, Peter JB, Agopian MS, Singer JZ, et al. Early undifferentiated connective tissue disease. III. Outcome and prognostic indicators in early scleroderma (systemic sclerosis). Ann Intern Med 1993;118:602–609.

26. Medsger TA Jr, Masi AT, Rodnan GP, Benedek TG, Robinson H. Survival with systemic sclerosis (scleroderma): A life table analysis of demographic and clinical factors in 309 patients. Ann Intern Med 1971;75:369–376.

27. Poole JL, Steen V. The use of the Health Assessment Questionnaire to determine physical disability in systemic sclerosis. Arthritis Care Res 1991;4: 27–31.

28. McCloskey DA, Patella SJ, Seibold JR, Iloprost Study Group. Health Assessment Questionnaire (HAQ) in systemic sclerosis (SSc). Arthritis Rheum 1990;33:S206.

29. Clements PJ, Lachenbruch PA, Seibold JR, Furst DE, Investigators in the High-Dose vs Low-Dose Penicillamine (D-pen) in SSc Trial. Health Assessment Questionnaire (HAQ) in patients with early, diffuse cutaneous systemic sclerosis (SSc). Arthritis Rheum 1994;37:S260.

30. Brennan P, Silman A, Black C, Bernstein R, Coppock J, Maddison P, Sheeran T, et al. Reliability of skin involvement measures in scleroderma. Br J Rheumatol 1992;31:457–460.

31. Clements PJ, Lachenbruch PA, Seibold JR, White B, Weiner S, Martin R, Weinstein A, et al. Inter- and intra-observer variability of total skin thickness score (modified-Rodnan) in systemic sclerosis (SSc). J Rheumatol 1995;22:1281–1285.

32. Eberl DR, Fasching B, Rahfls V, Schleyer I, Wolf R. Repeatability and objectivity of various measurements in rheumatoid arthritis. Arthritis Rheum 1976;19:1278–1286.

33. Rook AH, Freundlich B, Jegasothy BV, Perez MI, Barr WG, Jimenez SA, Rietschel RL, et al. Treatment of systemic sclerosis with extracorporeal photochemotherapy. Results of a multicenter trial. Arch Dermatol 1992;128:337–346.

34. Binnick SA, Shore SS, Corman A, Fleischmajer R. Failure of dimethyl sulfoxide in the treatment of scleroderma. Arch Dermatol 1977;113:1398–1402.

35. Beckett VL, Conn DL, Fuster V, Osmundson PJ, Strong CG, Chao EYS, Chesebro JH, et al. Trial of platelet-inhibiting drug in scleroderma. Double-

blind study with dipyridamole and aspirin. Arthritis Rheum 1984;27:1137–1143.

36. Scherbel AL. The effect of percutaneous dimethyl sulfoxide on cutaneous manifestations of systemic sclerosis. Ann NY Acad Sci 1983;411:120–130.

37. Bluestone R, Graham R, Holloway V, Holt PJL. Treatment of systemic sclerosis with D-penicillamine: A new method of observing the effects of treatment. Ann Rheum Dis 1970;29:153–159.

38. Silverstein JL, Steen VD, Medsger TA Jr, Falanga V. Cutaneous hypoxia in patients with systemic sclerosis (scleroderma). Arch Dermatol 1988;124: 1379–1382.

39. Gibson T, Grahame R. Cyclofenil treatment of scleroderma—a controlled study. Br J Rheum 1983;22:218–223.

40. Guillevin L, Chouvet B, Mery C, DeGery A, Thivolet J, Godeau P, Delbarre F. Treatment of progressive systemic sclerosis using factor XIII. Pharmatherapeutica 1985;4:76–80.

41. Blöm-Bülow B, Oberg K, Wollheim FA, Persson B, Jonson B, Malmberg P, Bostrom H, Herbai G. Cyclofenil versus placebo in progressive systemic sclerosis. A one-year double-blind crossover study of 27 patients. Acta Medica Scand 1981;210:419–428.

42. Ballou SP, Mackiewicz A, Lysikiewicz A, Neuman MR. Direct quantitation of skin elasticity in systemic sclerosis. J Rheumatol 1990;17:790–794.

43. Bachman DM. Quantifying skin mobility in scleroderma. Arch Dermatol 1961;83:598–605.

44. Gruber BL, Haufman LD. A double-blind randomized controlled trial of ketotifen versus placebo in early diffuse scleroderma. Arthritis Rheum 1992;34:362–366.

45. Dykes PJ, Marks R. Measurement of skin thickness. A comparison of two in vivo techniques with a conventional histometric method. J Invest Dermatol 1977;69:275–278.

46. Black MM. A modified radiographic method for measuring skin thickness. Br J Dermatol 1969;81: 661–666.

47. Bliznak J, Staple TW. Roengenographic measurement of skin thickness in normal individuals. Radiology 1975;116:55–60.

48. Äkesson A, Forsberg L, Hederstrom E, Wollheim F. Ultrasound examination of skin thickness in patients with progressive systemic sclerosis (scleroderma). Acta Radiol (Diagn) 1986;27:472–477.

49. Myers SL, Cohen JS, Sheets PW, Bies JR. B-mode ultrasound evaluation of skin thickness in progressive systemic sclerosis. J Rheumatol 1986;13: 577–580.

50. Greenwald GI, Tashkin DP, Gong H, Simmons M, Duann S, Furst DE, Clements PJ. Longitudinal

changes in lung function and respiratory symptoms in progress systemic sclerosis: Prospective study. Am J Med 1987;83:83–92.

51. Steen VD, Graham G, Conte C, Owens G, Medsger TA Jr. Isolated diffusing capacity reduction in systemic sclerosis. Arthritis Rheum 1992;35:765–770.

52. Peters-Golden M, Wise RA, Hochberg MC, Stevens MB, Wigley FM. Carbon monoxide diffusing capacity as predictor of outcome in systemic sclerosis. Am J med 1982;73:385–394.

53. Wells AU, Cullinan P, Hansell DM, Rugens MB, Black CM. Newman-Taylor AJ, du Bois RM. Fibrosing alveolitis associated with systemic sclerosis has a better prognosis than lone cryptogenic fibrosing alveolitis. Am J Respir Crit Care Med 1994; 149:1583–1590.

54. Steen VD. Systemic sclerosis. In: Cannon GW, Zimmerman GA, eds. The lung in rheumatic disease. New York: Marcel Dekker, 1990;279–302.

55. Kostis JB, Seibold JR, Turkevich D, Masi AT, Grau RG, Medsger TA Jr, Steen VD, et al. Prognostic importance of cardiac arrhythmias in systemic sclerosis. Am J Med 1988; 84:1007–1015.

56. Zamost BJ, Hirschberg J, Ippoliti AF, Furst DE, Clements PJ, Weinstein WM. Esophagitis in scleroderma: Prevalence and risk factors. Gastroenterology 1987;92:421–428.

57. Clements PJ, Furst DE, Campion DS, Bohan A, Harris R, Levy J, Paulus HE. Muscle disease in progressive systemic sclerosis: Diagnostic and therapeutic considerations. Arthritis Rheum 1978;21: 62–71.

58. Wigley FM, Wise RA, Seibold JR, McCloskey DA, Kujala G, Medsger TA Jr, Steen VD, et al. A multicenter placebo-controlled double-blind study of intravenous iloprost infusion in patients with Raynaud's phenomenon secondary to systemic sclerosis (SSc). Ann Intern Med. 1994;129:199–206.

59. Colditz GA, Miller JN, Mosteller F. How study design affects outcomes in comparisons of therapy. I: Medical. Stat Med 1989;8:441–454.

60. Clements PJ, Lachenbruch PA, Furst DE, Paulus HE, Sterz MG. Cardiac score: A semiquantitative measure of cardiac involvement which improves prediction of prognosis in systemic sclerosis. Arthritis Rheum 1991;34:1371–1380.

61. Friedman LM, Furberg CD, DeMetds DL. Fundamentals of clinical trials. Boston: John Wright, PSG, Inc, 1981;205.

JAMES R. SEIBOLD
DANIEL E. FURST
PHILIP J. CLEMENTS

26

Treatment of Systemic Sclerosis by Disease Modifying Agents

No therapies have proven to be effective in the treatment of systemic sclerosis (SSc). This is, in the main, attributable to the lack of understanding of the etiology and pathogenesis of a disease from which an ideal and specific treatment might be derived. Discussed elsewhere in this text are many remarkable advances in the descriptive pathobiology of SSc. Although our basic understanding of the disease remains incomplete, sufficient data are available to suggest many rational approaches to intervention.

There may well be partially effective therapies for this disease, which might include drugs that have already been studied. Many agents have been tested in scleroderma but few reliably designed trials of sufficient size and duration have been performed (1). Few trials have employed clear definitions of outcomes and fewer yet have assessed whether or not the outcomes are, in fact, clinically meaningful. It is rare for past trials to have included sufficiently homogeneous study populations and few have offered generalizable results.

Past our lack of understanding of disease pathogenesis, there are numerous other impediments to the development and study of potential disease-modifying treatments for scleroderma. Prominent among these have been a general lack of agreement by both the investigative community and regulatory authorities as to what constitutes true *modification* of disease. An unfortunate result of this lack of consensus has been a relative dearth of interest in the disease by the pharmaceutical industry.

This chapter will, in part, review and critique past and ongoing approaches to "disease-modifying" therapy. However, the student of scleroderma needs to consider this presentation from several sometimes conflicting standpoints. There is an inevitable tendency for scientifically based therapies to be chosen based on some aspect(s) of *disease process*, whereas assessment of effectiveness is based on measures of *clinical outcome*.

Definitions of Outcome

Potential outcome measures in scleroderma are many (Table 26.1). Guidelines for clinical trials of disease-modifying interventions in SSc have been proposed (2), and elsewhere in this text is a specific discussion of the issues of trial design that are necessary to fulfill these guidelines (3).

A truly effective disease-modifying therapy for SSc should enhance survival and/or reduce disability and co-morbidity from the disease. The available clinical data and simple common sense equate these effects with the behavior of internal organ involvement. Patients with heart, lung, and kidney involvement fare less well in terms of survival and functional status (4,5) than do patients without these complications. Thus, the least to be expected from a disease-modifying therapy should be a clinically meaningful effect

Table 26.1. Potential Measures of
Outcome in Systemic Sclerosis

Survival
Hospitalization
Disability
Patient self-assessment
Functional capacity
Organ-related morbidity
Cost of care

on these important visceral complications. Goals of treatment (in addition to improved survival) might include: (1) prevention of internal organ involvement, (2) arrest of or slowing of deterioration of function in previously involved organs, and/or (3) improvement in the function of previously involved organs (including the skin). A positive effect in any of these would likely improve patient survival and/or functional status.

Modification of disease should not be confused with the many remarkable advances in palliative and supportive therapy available to the individual with scleroderma and which are discussed in other chapters of this text.

Overall survival from SSc is improving (4) in large measure because of these ancillary improvements in clinical care. Most prominent is the availability of specific therapy for the accelerated hypertension of scleroderma, "renal crisis" (5). Lessened use of corticosteroids, improved therapies for esophageal dysfunction, better drugs for Raynaud's phenomenon (RP), and other advances have, in part, contributed to improvement in more global measures of outcome including disability, co-morbidity, and survival.

As in other areas, surrogate markers of response have often been used. A change in a surrogate marker is thought, hopefully, to reflect a change in disease outcome. In cardiovascular disease, for example, decreasing blood pressure is taken as a surrogate marker for decreasing the incidence of strokes and myocardial infarctions. In SSc, a prime surrogate marker that has been used for many years is a change in the degree of skin thickness or tethering. It is only recently that this surrogate marker has been shown to actually reflect

survival (6). Thus, studies examining changes in skin involvement may well be reflecting changes in outcome.

Measures of Disease Process

Both the etiology and pathogenesis of SSc are complex. A cohesive hypothesis of disease causation needs to address three principal yet not clearly overlapping areas of knowledge of disease process (Table 26.2). The most ubiquitous abnormalities are the disruption of the microvasculature and fibrotic arteriosclerosis of the small artery. These features are present in all forms of the disease and are detectable from the earliest recognizable stages of illness (7). Once disease is established, the early extravascular tissue lesions feature the ingress of a complex array of immigrant inflammatory cell populations. Paracrine and autocrine effects of growth factor/cytokine produced by these cells are likely responsible for the activation of hyperproliferative and hypersecretory matrix-producing cells (7). The net effect is accumulation of collagen, glycosaminoglycan, fibronectin, adherence molecules, and edema. The patient and physician recognize the result as the tightened and thickened skin for which the disease is named. See Chapter 13 for a more complete synthesis of the above hypothesis.

Opportunities for intervention include (a) specific or nonspecific suppression or inhibition of tissue immune activation and inflammation, (b) abrogation of progressive structural vascular injury, (c) reduction of secondary tissue ischemia through vasodilatation, and (d) approaches that either reduce accumulation of extracellular matrix or accelerate tissue remodeling in previously affected areas. Ultimately uncovering the etiologic agent/process will lead to interventions that will prevent these disease processes altogether.

Table 26.2. Processes in Systemic Sclerosis
Amenable to Intervention

Fibrosis
Immune activation
Vascular integrity

Rational Therapeutics in Scleroderma

The goal of therapy in scleroderma is to meld a scientifically rational choice of drug, which is based on some well-defined aspect of the disease process, into a clinical protocol with reproducible measures of disease outcome. This has proved to be, and is likely to remain, more difficult than might be expected. An ideal therapy that halted all secondary fibrosis of skin and viscera might not alter vascular features nor reverse tissue atrophy. Similarly, a predictably effective agent for vasospastic features would, in turn, not necessarily alter tissue fibrosis or inflammation.

We currently lack any therapies that predictably affect any of the three major pathogenic aspects of scleroderma: vasculopathy, immune activation, and fibrosis. Thus, we have not been able to dissect through clinical experience which of these processes is key in determining ultimate disease outcome. Clear demonstration of a reproducible biologic action may not parallel measures of clinical outcome or of patient satisfaction. As an example, a patient in whom drug therapy was useful for skin thickening might not recognize her/his situation as improved if she/he still suffered from intractable intestinal complaints or recurrent digital ulcerations. Similarly, a patient in whom skin tightening was progressive and severe and refractory to treatment might, in turn, either accept or not accept as successful a therapy that prevented visceral complications.

The Impact of Disease Duration and Classification/Disease Type

The paramount consideration in the interpretation of clinical trials and in the design of studies of new therapies is the remarkable heterogeneity of the course of SSc. Disease modification implies either prevention of bad outcomes or improvement in previous complications. Patients with scleroderma face differing levels of risk of bad outcomes based on their disease classification or disease type (i.e., limited versus diffuse) as well as on their duration of disease (8,9).

There are remarkably few published data that confirm and quantify the effects of disease duration. Nonetheless, there is near consensus among experienced clinical researchers of scleroderma that the risk of the progressivity of diffuse disease is strongly related to duration (i.e., early versus late) (1,8,9). It is generally accepted that patients with early (i.e., first 1–3 years from disease onset) diffuse scleroderma are at risk for worsening of skin involvement during which time risk of new visceral complications is highest (7–9). Patients in the early years of limited scleroderma experience a disease course in which skin involvement is minimally progressive and in which risk of visceral embarrassment is negligible. During the later years, diffuse scleroderma is associated with stable or improving skin thickening and slow worsening of previously involved internal organs, but a much diminished risk of development of new internal complications. The later years of limited scleroderma may be associated with the onset and inexorable worsening of important visceral changes in the forms of accelerated pulmonary artery hypertension or primary biliary cirrhosis. Table 26.3 outlines the impact of classification and of disease duration on the definition of the therapeutic agenda.

In general, inclusion of heterogeneous patient populations is particularly true of older reported studies. The critical reader should attempt to discern what potential impact patient selection may have had on reported results. Hallmark questions for interpretation of published trials include:

1. Are the patients reported of the same classification of disease (i.e., diffuse versus limited)? If not, are they presented in other stratified subgroups for analysis, such as early versus late or heart involvement versus no heart involvement?
2. Are the reported patients reasonably uniform in terms of disease duration (i.e., early versus late)?
3. How ill were the patients at entry (i.e., diffuse versus limited; heart, lung, or kidney disease)?

Table 26.3. Clinical Phenomenology and Rational Therapeutics in Scleroderma

Goal of Therapy	Applicable Study Population
Prevent new visceral involvement	Early (0–3 yrs) diffuse scleroderma
Reverse established visceral involvement	
Interstitial lung disease	Early and late, diffuse and limited
	Define by pulmonary function & presence or absence of alveolitis
Pulmonary hypertension	Later (10 yrs+) limited scleroderma
Gastrointestinal	Define by presence and severity
Cardiac	Define by presence and severity
Reverse established skin involvement	Diffuse scleroderma >1–2 yr duration defined by extent of skin involvement

4. Are the measures of outcome a reasonable reflection of treatment goals for the population under study? That is, measuring survival in a group of late limited patients may not be an appropriate outcome in a trial of H2 blockers for reflux but would be appropriate in a group of early diffuse patients treated with methotrexate.

5. Are the specific measures of outcome applicable to risks faced by the study population? That is, diffuse patients with high skin scores should be enrolled in a study designed to show improvement in skin thickening.

6. Is the duration of intervention appropriate for the outcome being studied (i.e., 3–4 years duration of trial to influence survival; 1 year for improving skin thickening)?

7. Are potential confounding clinical variables addressed (i.e., cigarette smoking, malabsorption, race, age, corticosteroid use)?

The Impact of Disease Process on Approach to Therapy

Current consensus is that immune activation and cytokine release or effects on the vascular endothelium precede fibrosis in SSc (see Chapter 13). Evidence includes the clinical appearance of local skin edema and erythema at early stages of disease. Nonspecific laboratory measures of T cell activation and turnover including soluble CD8, and soluble interleukin-2 receptor levels appear to correlate with disease progressivity (10, 11). Similarly, bronchoalveolar lavage studies reveal evidence of inflammatory alveolitis preceding interstitial fibrosis (12). Other authors point to the effects on the vascular endothelium prior to fibrosis, raising the possibility that a "vasculopathy" precedes fibrosis (see Chapter 8).

It follows that therapies directed against the immune system would be most appropriately directed at patients with early progressive disease. This approach might best be viewed as one of prevention of fibrosis and atrophy. In the individual at later stages of disease, the rationale for aggressive immune-oriented therapy is less clear. While modification of disease is perhaps still possible, the degree and pace of effect would be predicted to be smaller and slower. The late hidebound patient would be best enrolled in a study of therapy that facilitated tissue remodeling, were such a therapy available. The essence of this approach is one of reversal versus prevention.

Specific Therapies

In the discussion that follows, emphasis is placed on randomized controlled trials, if they are available, with the exceptions of interferon-gamma, penicillamine, and cyclosporin. Table 26.4 outlines the study design issues that need to be considered in examining controlled studies. Tables

26.5 and 26.6 outline how the randomized controlled trials that are reviewed in this section fulfill the requirements of study design which would enable one to have confidence in the results.

PREVENTION OF FIBROSIS BY INTERFERENCE WITH COLLAGEN METABOLISM

As fibrosis is clearly a major source of both disability and mortality in SSc, many therapies have been utilized to attempt to decrease fibrosis. As in the rest of this chapter, the emphasis in this section will be on controlled trials in these areas. The principal controlled trials aimed at decreasing fibrosis are those including the use of col-

chicine, cyclofenil, dimethylsulfoxide (DMSO), ketotifen, N-acetylcysteine (NAC), aminobenzoate potassium (POTABA™), and stanozolol (8, 13–27). Penicillamine and interferon-gamma are also discussed, although controlled trials are not yet available for either of these therapies (23,35).

Table 26.4. Study Design Issues to Measure Response

(1)	Patient selection
(2)	Patient comparability
(3)	Prevention of bias
	a. randomization
	b. control
(4)	Valid measures of response
(5)	Sufficient duration
(6)	Sufficient numbers

Table 26.5. General Trial Characteristics for Controlled Trials in SSc

Ref	Therapy	N/gp	Trial Type[1]	Disease[2] Type	Mean Disease Duration (yrs)	Study Duration (Mos.)
42	Aldomet & Propoanolol/placebo	14/14	P, DB	?	6.7	24
28	Apheresis/no rx	11/5	P, SB	?	<4	3
29	Chlorambucil/placebo	33/32	P, DB	M	7.4	36
13	Colchicine/placebo	7	X, DB	?	?	3
14	Colchicine/placebo	11/8	P, DB	?	?	12
15	Colchicine/placebo	28	X, DB	?	Males: 3 Females: 8	9
16	Cyclofenil/placebo	27	X, DB	D	6	6
17	Cyclofenil/placebo	11	X, DB	M	12.5	4
18	DMSO/Placebo	95/45	P, DB	?	9.3	3
36	Dipyridimol & aspirin/placebo	14/13	P, DB	?	?	12
37	Factor XIII/Placebo	25	X, DB	D	?	3
30	5-flurouracil/placebo	33/37	P, DB	M	5	6
38	Iloprost/placebo	64/67	P, DB	M	12	2.2
40	Ketanserin/placebo	12/12	P, DB	?	3.8	6
19	Ketotifen/placebo	12/12	P, DB	D	3.25	6
20	NAC/placebo	11/11	P, DB	M	11	12
32	Photochemo/d-Pen	31/25	P, SB	?	1.8	6
21	Potaba/placebo	72/74	P, DB	D	8.6	0.9
43	Spironolactone/placebo	34/37	P, DB	?	?	9
22	Stanozolol/placebo	41	X, DB	?	13.75	6
34	Total lymphoid irradiation/no rx	6/6	P, Open	D	3.7	12
31	Methotrexate/placebo	15/10	P, DB	?	?	6

[1]P = parallel; X = crossover; DB = double-blind; SB = single blind
[2]D = diffuse; M = mixed; ? = not defined

Table 26.6. Design Characteristics of Controlled Trials in SSc

Ref	Therapy	Uniform Dis Type[1]	Responsive Patients[2]	Patient Comparability	Random-ization	DB/SB[6]	Outcome vs Process[3]	Sufficient Duration[4]	Sufficient Numbers[5]
42	Aldonet & Propamanolol	?	N	Y	Y	DB	O+P	Y	N
28	Apheresis	?	Y	N	Y	SB	P	N	Y
29	Chlorambucil	Y	N	Y	Y	DB	P	Y	Y
13	Colchicine	?	?	?	Y	DB	P	N	N
14	Colchicine	?	?	?	Y	DB	P	N	N
15	Colchicine	?	?	?	Y	DB	?	N	N
16	Cyclofenil	Y	N	?	Y	DB	O+P	N	N
17	Cyclofenil	N	Y	Y	Y	DB	P	N	N
18	DMSO	Y	Y	Y	Y	DB	P	Y	Y
36	Dipyridimol & Aspirin	?	?	?	Y	DB	P	Y	N
37	Factor XIII	Y	Y	?	Y	DB	P	N	N
30	5-fluorouracil	?	N	Y	Y	DB	O+P	N	?
38	Iloprost	?	Y	Y	Y	DB	P	Y	Y
40	Ketanserin	?	N	Y	Y	DB	O+P	N	N
19	Ketotifen	Y	Y	Y	Y	DB	P	N	N
20	N-acetyl-cysteine	N	N	Y	Y	DB	O+P	Y	N
32	Photochemo.	?	Y	Y(?)	Y	SB	P	N	Y
21	Potaba	?	N	Y(?)	Y	DB'	P	N	Y
43	Spironolactone	?	?	?	Y	DB	P	N	N
22	Stanozolol	?	N	?	Y	DB	P	N	N
34	Total lymphoid irradiation	Y	Y	?	Y	Open	P	Y	Y
31	Methotrexate	?	Y	?	Y	DB	P	N	N

Y = yes; N=no; ? = undefined
[1] or analysis by disease type (limited or diffuse)
[2] Y = disease duration ≤ 3 years plus measures allowing response; N = disease duration 5 years or more plus measures not responsive or not validated; ? = unknown
[3] O = Outcome such as function, survival; P = process or surrogate such as skin induration, renal or pulmonary fctn etc.
[4] Sufficient defined as ≥ 1 year
[5] Authors' estimate if no power analysis was done
[6] DB = double blind; SB = single blind

Colchicine

Three controlled trials have been done utilizing colchicine (13–15). *In vitro*, colchicine inhibits pro-collagen secretion from fibroblasts, interferes with collagen deposition, and increases collagen degradation. Unfortunately, none of the trials were published in their entirety; as a result, there are insufficient data to come to any decision or conclusion with regard to the utility of this therapy. For example, Alarcon-Segovia's study examined 14 patients in a three month, double-blind, cross-over trial versus placebo (13). Fourteen patients completed the crossover, with nine "improving" on colchicine, while only three "improved" during the placebo arm. The number of patients obviously is too small, the trial is too short, and the disease duration and extent of skin involvement of patients is not known. Finally, measures of clinical outcome were not well defined. Similar problems existed for the study of Urutia and Sabah (14) (published only in abstract), who examined 19 patients (very few details of response were given), and Steigerwald, who examined 28 patients in a 9-month cross-over study of colchicine versus placebo (15). In all cases, there was a trend toward improvement on colchicine, but very few of the study design elements necessary for a credible trial were outlined in any of the publications.

Cyclofenil

Cyclofenil has been examined in two controlled studies (16,17). Cyclofenil, a weak estrogen that inhibits sulfate incorporation, was tested at doses of 200 mg tid in two placebo-controlled, crossover trials of 6 and 4 months' duration, respectively. Blöm-Bülow et al (16) examined 38 patients with an average disease duration of 6 years whose disease type (diffuse versus limited) was not detailed. Three of the cyclofenil patients discontinued therapy because they developed elevated liver function tests. During the cyclofenil arm, 13 of the remaining 35 patients also had elevated liver function tests. A large number of measurements were done, including a suction cup apparatus used to measure skin tethering,

but none showed a drug effect except physician "overall" response. Gibson and Grahame tested 11 patients in a 4-month cross-over trial (17). Only six of the 11 patients completed the study, because four patients discontinued the trial secondary to liver function abnormalities on cyclofenil and one died of scleroderma renal disease. Thus, in the latter study, no statistical analysis was possible. In both studies, cyclofenil did not prove to be effective, but the short duration and small numbers involved in these studies precluded any positive or negative conclusions.

Dimethyl Sulfoxide (DMSO)

The best study of DMSO was performed by Williams et al (18). This double-blind trial compared topical 0.85% normal saline, 2% DMSO, and 70% DMSO over 3 months in the treatment of hand ulcers of patients with SSc (18). There were 31 saline-treated controls, 47 2% DMSO-treated patients, and 47 70% DMSO-treated patients; disease type was not well outlined and mean disease duration was 119 months. There was 50% improvement in open ulcers in 38% of the control patients, 38% of the 2% DMSO-treated patients, and 43% of the 70% DMSO-treated patients (not significant). It was thought that double blinding would be impossible secondary to the garlicky odor imparted to the breath by metabolism of DMSO: 14% of the saline-treated patients, 16% of the 2% DMSO-treated patients, and 64% of the 70% DMSO-treated patients were noted to have a "garlicky odor," thus preserving the study blind. Power calculations revealed a 90% power to detect a 72% difference between any two groups. It would have taken 212 patients to detect a 30% difference. Thus, this study suffered from too few patients, a relatively short treatment period and some lack of disease definition. It nevertheless indicates that DMSO is unlikely to be effective in treating the ulcers of patients with SSc.

Ketotifen

Ketotifen is a mast cell membrane stabilizer with H_1-anti-histamine effects, thus potentially decreasing mast cell activation of fibroblasts in scleroderma. Gruber and Kaufman published the only controlled double-blind study of ketotifen versus placebo in SSc (19). Ketotifen 6 mg a day was examined in 24 patients (12 patients per group) who had SSc of 31 months' duration and probably had diffuse disease. The 6-month placebo-controlled study showed no significant improvement in clinical parameters, pulmonary function tests, or mast cell response. The small number of patients aside, the fact that this dose of ketotifen had no effect on mast cell suppression unfortunately precluded the possibility that the importance of this mechanism in SSc could be tested *and* precluded any conclusion with respect to the efficacy of ketotifen in SSc.

N-acetylcysteine

N-acetylcysteine is thought to act by reducing disulfide bonds, inhibiting dermal inflammation, and decreasing migration inhibition factor (20). An early, small (11 patients per group), 1-year, double-blind trial compared N-acetylcysteine (NAC) 9 grams per day to a matched placebo in a mixed group of SSc patients whose mean disease duration was 11 years. Twenty-one clinical parameters plus a number of immunological parameters were tested. The study suffered because there were too few patients, subgroups of patients were poorly defined prior to entry, and patients had long-standing disease. The study was nevertheless instructive by showing that patients with long-standing disease tended to change little (even in the placebo group) although it was unsuccessful in showing any effect of NAC.

Potassium Aminobenzoate (POTABA™)

Clegg et al tested aminobenzoate potassium (POTABA™) versus placebo in 146 patients during a 48-week double-blind study (21). Disease duration in these patients averaged 102 months, and it is not clear what disease types (diffuse versus limited) were included. Withdrawal rate in this study was very high (48% of the patients on POTABA™ and 20% of the placebo-treated patients). Ultimately, only five of 72 POTABA™-treated patients (7%) and nine of 74 placebo-treated patients (13%) rated a 30% improvement in skin score (not significant). Other disease measures also did not differ between the groups. This admirable attempt at a well done trial failed, in part, because there was such a large number of dropouts and there was no intent to treat analysis (only "completer" analysis was published). In addition, patients with disease of long duration and mixed diseases type were recruited (i.e., many patients with late limited disease were mixed with patients with early and/or diffuse disease).

Stanozolol

Because stanozolol stimulates the fibrinolytic system, it was hypothesized to be of potential therapeutic value in treating RP and SSc. Twenty-four patients were treated in a 6-month double-blind cross-over study (22). Seventeen patients completed the study. Dermal fibrosis was examined but there was no change. Among the placebo-treated patients, the skin fibrosis score remained at approximately 17, while it dropped from approximately 15 to 13 in the stanozolol-treated group (as indicated in a figure from the study) and this drop was not significant. This study, like those before it, tended to suffer from short duration and small numbers. The type of disease evaluated (limited versus diffuse) was also not detailed. On the other hand, a well-defined examination of fibrinolysis was undertaken. Fibrinolysis activity improved, although no clinical change was noted.

D-penicillamine

Among the uncontrolled studies of interference with collagen metabolism, those involving D-penicillamine are the most well known. D-penicillamine was originally developed as a chelating agent for conditions such as Wilson's disease. It has demonstrable lathyritic effects through interfering with cross-linking of extracellular collagen. A retrospective report from the University of Pittsburgh reviewed the clinical course of a number of patients receiving D-penicillamine and compared it with matched populations receiving other therapies (23). Their retrospective data suggested that 750 to 1000 mg per day D-penicillamine reduced new visceral involvement, improved survival, and decreased skin involvement. Other prospective but uncontrolled observations by the same group compared 152 patients to 80 patients receiving a variety of other therapies (7). Improved 5-year survival (80% on D-penicillamine versus 60% on other treatments) was once more corroborated (8). The study populations represented probands followed with disease duration of 2 to 6 years, making them patients with later disease and raising the possibility that the results are confounded by the inevitable problems arising from uncontrolled studies. Currently, a prospective controlled study of D-penicillamine is underway in the United States (1).

Interferon-gamma

Interferon-gamma has striking effects on collagen production by dermal fibroblasts in culture, including a strong dose-related inhibition of collagen synthesis, which persists for several generations of tissue culture subpassage (24,25). Three uncontrolled pilot efficacy trials have been conducted in a homogeneous population of early diffuse systemic sclerosis. In these studies, there were inconsistent but notable clinical effects on skin thickening and hand function. The sporadic occurrence of scleroderma renal crises suggested a potential deleterious effect on vascular features of disease (26,27). Interestingly, in animal models of pulmonary hypertension with hypoxemic damage, interferon-gamma is associated with lessening of both intimal and medial vascular damage. Unfortunately, there appear to be no current plans to conduct a prospective and controlled investigation of this potential therapy.

PREVENTION OF FIBROSIS BY IMMUNE SUPPRESSION

A variety of immunosuppressive agents have been studied in controlled trials in systemic sclerosis, including apheresis, chlorambucil, 5-fluorouracil, methotrexate, extra corporeal photochemotherapy (photophoresis), and total lymphoid irradiation (28–32). In addition, an open controlled pilot experience with cyclosporin has been reported (35).

Apheresis

Weiner et al reported, in abstract, a randomized comparison of five patients who were treated with plasmapheresis, six patients who were treated with lymphoplasmapheresis, and five patients who were not treated (28). Disease duration was less than 4 years and patients had SSc (not further defined). They were followed for 3 months. Skin scores improved by 10 out of a possible 58 in the lymphoplasmapheresis group and were statistically less in the other two groups. No differences in internal organ involvement were found, although physician and patient global assessments improved more in the treatment than control groups. This encouraging report was never published as a complete article. It suffers from relatively small numbers and undefined disease type, but it did recruit patients with early disease and certainly deserves further testing.

Chlorambucil

Furst et al examined chlorambucil versus placebo in a 3-year, parallel, randomized, double-blind trial of 65 patients (29). Ten organ systems were examined as indices and a change per unit time analysis was done, allowing for a power of greater than 0.80 for the indices. There were 33 chlorambucil-treated patients and 32 placebo-treated patients. No statistically significant or clinically significant differences between drug and placebo were found (18). Unfortunately, the patients had longer duration of disease (mean: 7.4 years) and a mixed population of patients was used (approximately 63% diffuse disease and 37% limited disease).

5-fluorouracil (5-FU)

5-fluorouracil was studied in a 6-month double-blind trial in patients of 5 years' disease duration

(30). The protocol required 12 mg/kg IV 5-FU for four doses, then 6 mg/kg every 2 days, followed by 12.5 mg/kg weekly. Based on a mean original Rodnan skin thickness score of 29 (from a maximum of 104), 28% of the 26 5-FU patients had a greater than 30% improvement in skin score compared to none of the 20 placebo-treated patients (P < 0.001). Global function also favored the 5-FU group. On the other hand, hematologic toxicity occurred in 46% of the 5-FU patients and only 5% of the placebo patients. The authors stated that they felt 5-FU gave a "modest" benefit to patients with SSc but that 5-FU was a toxic medication.

Methotrexate

Van den Hoogen et al compared 15 mg oral methotrexate to placebo over a period of 6 months (31). At the end of that time, patients on placebo were given methotrexate if they were doing poorly and those on 15 mg methotrexate had their dose raised to 25 mg methotrexate weekly. Thus, comparisons could be made only up to 6 months. From the published abstract, it is difficult to tell whether the blind was somehow broken in order to allow a decision on which patients received 15 or 25 mg methotrexate after 6 months. The skin thickness scores decreased by approximately 10% in the methotrexate-treated group but remained essentially unchanged in the placebo-treated patients. Four of 15 methotrexate patients had a reduction of their skin score by greater than 30% compared to one of ten in the placebo-treated patients. This small study, reported thus far only in abstract, failed to show any effect of methotrexate; however, it is not clear whether the patients had early disease, and the number of patients was small.

Photopheresis

A controversial study by Rook et al tested extracorporeal photochemotherapy in SSc (32). Extracorporeal photochemotherapy is a form of immunotherapy in which 8-methoxy-psoralen (which coats T cells and possibly macrophages) is given to patients. The drug on white cells is

then activated extracorporeally by ultraviolet light (PUVA). This treatment apparently results in removal of T cells by the spleen. The study was a 10-month, single-blind examination of infusions of autologous white blood cells treated extracorporeally with PUVA for 2 consecutive days each month versus D-penicillamine up to 750 mg qd. Commendably, mean disease duration was short (1.83 years) and all patients had diffuse SSc. While the skin score improved by at least 15% in 21 of 31 PUVA-treated patients, only 8 of 25 patients treated with D-penicillamine improved by 15% by 6 months (P < 0.02). Unfortunately, by 10 months this difference had disappeared. These very encouraging results were tempered by the very small change that was observed in the skin score, a possible lack of randomization of patients, and at least the appearance of a conflict of interest of the principal investigator who is said to hold a patent on the photochemotherapy procedure (33).

Total Lymphoid Irradiation

An open, controlled study of total lymphoid irradiation has been conducted with six patients. Control patients were those not treated for the duration of the trial (12 months) (34). Despite immunosuppression, no detectable benefit was found and there was a suggestion that pulmonary and gastrointestinal deterioration accelerated.

Cyclosporin

Cyclosporin acts by binding with a specific intracellular carrier protein (cyclophilin) and subsequently inhibiting calcineurin phosphatase activity in lymphocytes, with the result of diminished interleukin-2 production. Although limited by an apparent mechanism-based toxicity on endothelium, and the fact that cyclosporin is associated with hypertension and diminished renal function, open pilot experiences suggest potential disease-modifying benefits. The only trial with a control or comparison group was that of Clements et al who reported ten patients (9 with diffuse cutaneous scleroderma) with <60 months of SSc who received cyclosporin for 48 weeks (35). The course of these ten patients was compared to the first 48-week course of 13 matched diffuse SSc patients (also with <60 months of SSc) who had received placebo in a previous chlorambucil versus placebo trial (29). Skin thickening decreased significantly in the cyclosporin treated patients but not in the placebo comparison group. Pulmonary and cardiac involvement remained unchanged in both groups. The trial deficiencies included small numbers of patients and the lack of a concurrent control group. Although cyclosporin's efficacy should be tested in a larger, double-blind placebo controlled trial, there are currently no plans for such a trial.

Trials of immunosuppression in SSc have been marred by some of the factors which, it has been learned, may confound results. Importantly, patients with early and diffuse SSc need to be recruited to these studies. Furthermore, studies with small numbers of patients have low statistical power which often confuses rather than clarifies results of therapeutic trials.

MODIFICATION OF DISEASE THROUGH VASOACTIVE DRUGS

Controlled trials approaching treatment of the vasculopathy found in SSc include trials of dipyridamole plus aspirin, Factor XIII, carboprostacyclin (Iloprost), ketanserin, propranolol/methyldopa (Aldomet™), and spironolactone (36–43).

Dipyridamole Plus Aspirin

The trial by Beckett et al was an early and commendable attempt at a double-blind randomized trial in SSc (36). Dipyridamole 75 mg tid and aspirin 325 mg tid were used versus placebo for 1 year. The rationale in this trial included the presence of activated platelets in patients with SSc; thus, the use of dipyridamole and aspirin would theoretically prevent platelet activation and endothelial damage. Raynaud's phenomenon, creatinephosphokinase, x-ray changes and a skin induration index (maximum of 24) were mea-

sured. A 12.5% improvement in the skin induration index was defined as significant improvement. Three of 13 patients on placebo improved by this amount, while none of 14 drug-treated patients did so. The negative results in this trial are inconclusive because the number of patients was small, and the type and duration of disease utilized in this trial are unknown.

Factor XIII

Factor XIII was used in a study of SSc because it was thought to intercollate into the collagen and make the collagen more easily cleared by macrophages. This very short trial was only of 3 weeks' duration with a 6-week observation period, followed by a cross-over (37). Twenty-five patients with diffuse disease of a mean of 2.67 years' duration were included. Several approaches were used to measure response. Among these, a Leichert scale of disease activity and an 11-point functional scale both favored Factor XIII over placebo (P < 0.05). At the end of the trial, the Factor XIII period was preferred by 20 of 25 patients, while the placebo period was preferred by only 3 of those patients. This encouraging trial is severely limited by its very short duration so that long-term effects on function or "disease modification" are unknown.

Carboprostacyclin (Iloprost)

Iloprost is a prostacyclin analog and, therefore, is a vasodilator. One hundred thirty-one patients (many with digital ulcers) who had SSc of 12 years' duration were given 5 daily IV Iloprost infusions in a double-blind placebo-controlled trial and were followed by observations for up to 9 weeks (38). Two of seven measures examining aspects of Raynaud's phenomenon (RP) plus the physician's overall rating improved more in the Iloprost-treated patients than in the placebo-treated patients (P < 0.05). This suggestive result, despite the long disease duration in these patients, is leading toward another trial of this medication, although an oral formulation is being used (39).

Ketanserin

Ketanserin is a serotonin blocker. This drug could, theoretically, decrease vasoreactivity and prevent perivascular fibrosis. A 12-patient-per-group, 6-month, double-blind, placebo-controlled study examined ketanserin (40–80 mg/day) versus placebo in patients whose disease duration was a mean of 3.8 years (40). Eighteen response measures were examined, including a number relating to visceral organ systems (all examined by visual analog scale), oral aperture, activities of daily living, and a physician global assessment. The only statistically different measure was the physician global assessment, and this difference (occurring in 1:18 measures) could be found by chance alone. This study is commendable in that disease duration was relatively short and a functional index was used, thus attempting to examine a useful and direct outcome measure. Unfortunately, the number of patients was small, the trial duration was short, and the type of disease examined was unknown. An incompletely reported 1-year, double-blind trial of ketanserin versus placebo in 151 patients failed to confirm benefit in RP and demonstrated no effects on skin or visceral involvement (41).

Propranolol/Methyldopa (Aldomet™)

Fries et al directly examined the effect of antihypertensive agents on skin, serum creatinine, health assessment questionnaire, and overall disease (42). The skin induration measures were limited and not well validated. About two-thirds of the 28 patients entering the study completed the 24-month placebo-controlled trial. Disease type (diffuse versus limited) and skin scores were not defined and mean disease duration was approximately 6.7 years. There was no discernible effect of antihypertensive therapy on SSc. The small number of patients, lack of disease definition, and long disease duration all mitigate against finding any differences, even if the treatment were effective.

Spironolactone

This double-blind 9-month trial of spironolactone involved 34 spironolactone-treated and 37 placebo-treated (43) patients. There was approximately a 50% dropout rate and there was no definition of response. This, plus the small number of patients, precluded the possibility of drawing any conclusion from this trial.

SYNTHESIS AND CONCLUSIONS

Professor Eric Bywaters has said, "No drug has been proven totally ineffective until it has been used for scleroderma." This survey of the better research to date sadly confirms his view. On the other hand, the controlled experience in these trials has led to a better definition of the study design and inclusion/exclusion criteria mostly likely to result in definitive conclusions. For example, it has become more clear that, despite the difficulty, uniform disease (often diffuse), short duration of disease (probably less than 3 years), and sufficient numbers (despite the difficulty) are necessary prerequisites for definitive trials in disease modification for scleroderma. There are some indications that the general approaches outlined above may yet yield positive results. For example, further trials of immunosuppressive agents, such as alkylating agents, 5-fluorouracil, apheresis, and, possibly, photophoresis, are justifiable. Likewise, studies of immunomodulators, such as cyclosporin and methotrexate, need to be completed. Among the vasoactive trials, Factor XIII and iloprost appear to be worthy of further study.

Successful drug development in SSc will per force be driven by the highest quality laboratory and clinical science. Breakthroughs will doubtless be incremental. Demonstration of benefit in early progressive diffuse disease might lead to extended studies in other clinical circumstances. An agent that enhances tissue remodeling might initially focus on later established fibrosis and then be extrapolated to studies of progressive early disease.

References

1. Seibold JR, Furst DE, Clements PJ. Why everything (or nothing) seems to work in the treatment of scleroderma. J Rheumatol 1992;19:673–676.

2. White B, Bauer EA, Goldsmith LA, et al. Guidelines for clinical trials in systemc sclerosis (scleroderma):I. Disease-modifying interventions. Arthritis Rheum 1995;38:351–360.

3. Clements PJ, Furst DE, Seibold JR, Lachenbruch PA. Trial design issues. In: Clements PJ, Furst DE, eds. Systemic sclerosis. Baltimore:Williams & Wilkins, 1995, 515–534.

4. Silman AJ. Scleroderma and survival. Ann Rheum Dis 1991;50:267–269.

5. Altman RD, Medsger TA, Bloch DA, Michel BA. Predictors of survival in systemic sclerosis (scleroderma). Arthritis Rheum 1991;34:403–413.

6. Clements PJ, Lachenbruch PA, Ng SW, Simmons M, Sterz M, Furst DE. Skin score, a semiquantitative measure of cutaneous involvement that improves prediction of prognosis in systemic sclerosis. Arthritis Rheum 1990;33:1256–1263.

7. Seibold JR. Scleroderma. In: Kelley WN, Harris ED, Ruddy S, Sledge CB, eds. Textbook of rheumatology. Philadelphia:WB Saunders, 1989;1215–1244.

8. Steen VD. Systemic sclerosis. Management. In: Klippel JH, Dieppe PA, eds. Rheumatology. St. Louis:Mosby, 1994;6.10.1–6.10.8.

9. Steen VD, Medsger TA, Osial TA, et al. Factors predicting the development of renal involvement in progressive systemic sclerosis. Am J Med 1984;76:779–786.

10. DeGiannis D, Seibold JR, Czarnecki M, et al. Soluble interleukin-2 receptors in patients with systemic sclerosis. Clinical and laboratory correlations. Arthritis Rheum 1990;33:375–380.

11. LeRoy EC, Smith EA, Kahaleh MB, et al. A strategy for determining the pathogenesis of systemic sclerosis. Is transforming growth factor beta the answer? Arthritis Rheum 1989;32:817–825.

12. Äkesson A, Scheja A, Lundin A, Wollheim FA. Improved pulmonary function in systemic sclerosis after treatment with cyclophosphamide. Arthritis Rheum 1994;37:729–735.

13. Alarcon-Segovia D. Colchicine. Clin Rheum Dis 1979;5:294–302.

14. Urrutia A, Sabah D. Tratamiento de la sclerosis systemica progresiva con colchicina. Estudio preliminar (abstract). Proceedings of II congreso internacional de rheumatologia del conosur Santiago de Chile, 1980;53.

15. Steigerwald JC. Colchicine vs. placebo in the treatment of progressive systemic sclerosis (scleroderma). In: Black CM, Meyers AR, eds. Scleroderma. New York:Gower Medical Pubishing, 1985;415–417.

16. Blöm-Bülow B, Oberg K, Wollheim FA, et al. Cyclofenil vs. placebo in progressive systemic sclerosis. Acta Med Scand 1981;210:419–428.

17. Gibson T, Grahame R. Cyclofenil treatment of scleroderma-controlled study. Br J Rheum 1983;22:218–223.

18. Williams HJ, Furst DE, Dahl SL, et al. Double-blind multi-center controlled trial comparing topical dimethylsulfoxide and normal saline for treatment of hand ulcers in patients with systemic sclerosis. Arthritis Rheum 1985;28:308–314.

19. Gruber BL, Kaufman LD. A double-blind, randomized controlled trial of ketotifen vs. placebo in early diffuse scleroderma. Arthritis Rheum 1991;34:362–366.

20. Furst DE, Clements PJ, Harris R, et al. Measurement of clinical change in progressive systemic sclerosis: A one-year double-blind, placebo controlled trial of N-acetylcystine. Ann Rheum Dis 1979;38:356–361.

21. Clegg DO, Reading JC, Mayes MD, et al. Comparison of aminobenzoate potassium and placebo in the treatment of scleroderma. J Rheumatol 1994;21:105–110.

22. Jayson MIV, Holland CD, Keegan A, et al. A controlled study of stanozolol in primary Reynaud's phenomenon and systemic sclerosis. Ann Rheum Dis 1991;50:40–47.

23. Steen VD, Medsger TA, Rodnan GP. D-penicillamine therapy in progressive systemic sclerosis (scleroderma). A retrospective analysis. Ann Intern Med 1982;97:652–659.

24. Rosenbloom J, Feldman G, Freundlich B, Jimenez SA. Inhibition of excessive scleroderma fibroblast collagen production by recombinant gamma-interferon. Arthritis Rheum 1986;29:837–842.

25. Duncan MR, Berman B. Persistence of a reduced-collagen producing phenotype in cultured sclderoderma fibroblasts after short term exposure to interferons. J Clin Invest 1987;79:1318–1322.

26. Freundlich B, Jimenez SA, Steen VD, et al. Treatment of systemic sclerosis with recombinant interferon-gamma. A Phase I/II trial. Arthritis Rheum 1992;35:1134–1142.

27. Kahan A, Amor B, Menkes CJ, Stauch G. Recombinant interferon gamma in the treatment of systemic sclerosis. Am J Med 1989;87:273–277.

28. Weiner SR, Kono DH, Osterman HA, et al. Preliminary report on a controlled trial of apheresis in the treatment of scleroderma. (Abstract). ARA meeting, Washington DC, 1987;S27.

29. Furst DE, Clements PJ, Hillis S, et al. Immunosuppression with chlorambucil versus placebo, for scleroderma: Results of a three-year, parallel, randomized, double-blind study. Arthritis Rheum 1989;32:582–593.

30. Casas JA, Saway PA, Villareal I, et al. Five fluorouracil in the treatment of scleroderma: A randomized, double-blind, placebo controlled international collaborative study. Ann Rheum Dis 1990; 49:926–928.

31. Van den Hoogen FAJ, Boerbooms AMT, Vanlier HJJ, et al. Methotrexate in systemic sclerosis: Preliminary 24-week results of placebo controlled double-blind trial (Abstract). Arthritis Rheum 1993;36:S217.

32. Rook AH, Freundlich B, Jegasothy BV, et al. Treatment of systemic sclerosis with extra corporeal photochemotherapy. Results of a multi-center trial. Arch Dermatol 1992;128:337–346.

33. Fries JF, Seibold JR, Medsger TA. Photopheresis for scleroderma? No! J Rheumatol 1992;19:1011–1013.

34. O'Dell JR, Steigerwald JC, Kennaugh RC, et al. Lack of clinical benefit after treatment of systemic sclerosis with total lymphoid eradiation. J Rheumatol 1989;16:1050–1054.

35. Clements PJ, Lachenbruch PA, Sterz M, et al. Cyclosporine in systemic sclerosis: Results of a 48-week open safety study in 10 patients. Arthritis Rheum 1993;36:75–83.

36. Beckett VL, Conn DL, Fuster V, et al. Trial of platelet-inhibiting drugs in scleroderma. Double blind study with dipyridamole and aspirin. Arthritis Rheum 1984;27:1137–1143.

37. Guillevin L, Chouvet B, Mery O, et al. Treatment of progressive systemic sclerosis using factor XIII. Pharmaco Therapeutica 1985;4:76–80.

38. Wigley FM, Wise RA, Seibold JR, et al. Intravenous iloprost infusion in patients with Raynaud phenomenon secondary to systemic sclerosis. A multicenter, placebo-controlled, double-blind study. Ann Intern Med 1994;120:199–206.

39. Belch JJF, Capell HA, Cooke ED, et al. Oral iloprost as a treatment for Raynaud's syndrome: A double-blind multicenter placebo controlled study. Ann Rheum Dis 1995;54:197–200.

40. Ortonne JP, Torzuolt C, Dujordin P, et al. Ketanserin in the treatment of systemic sclerosis: A double-blind controlled trial. Br J Dermatol 1989; 120:261–266.

41. Seibold JR, Clements PJ, Lachenbaruch PA, et al. Prospective, controlled trial of ketanserin vs placebo in systemic sclerosis (SSc). Arthritis Rheum (in press).

42. Fries JF, Wasner C, Brown J, et al. A controlled trial of anti-hypertensive therapy in systemic sclerosis (scleroderma). Ann Rheum Dis 1984;43:407–410.

43. Altmeyer P, Goerz G, Hammer H, et al. Spironolactone treatment in scleroderma—A double-blind therapy study. Dermatologica 1985;171(5): 374–375.

FARRUKH ZAIDI
ROY D. ALTMAN

27

Therapy of Systemic Sclerosis with Unproven Remedies

SYSTEMIC SCLEROSIS (SSc), or scleroderma, is a connective tissue disease (1) characterized by fibrosis with subsequent atrophy and scarring of the skin, synovium, muscles, and some internal organs. Clinically, the disease is characterized by skin thickening caused by excessive accumulation of connective tissue. The pathogenesis of SSc is poorly understood; however, on histopathology, SSc is characterized by excessive fibroblast activity with collagen deposition in numerous organs associated with a number of microvascular abnormalities.

The study of SSc is complex. The disease is quite variable in its presentation and rate of progression. There are different subgroups of the disease that have different disease outcomes in terms of organ involvement and total morbidity. Hence, therapeutic trials need to recognize and subset the variants of SSc in order to properly interpret their results.

Wigley (2) and Seibold et al (3) pointed out some of the challenges involved in the investigation of treatments for SSc. The relevant points are listed in Table 27.1.

In view of all the problems in the investigation of therapeutic modalities, the lack of effective and proven treatment modalities, and the potential for a disabling disease, a number of novel and varied therapies have been attempted over the years, only a few of which are reported in the medical literature. The following paragraphs contain our review of the recent medical literature regarding some of the unproven treatment options for SSc (Table 27.2).

We have included most of the reports published during a 20-year period. We have not included a multitude of remedies that may be popular in different areas of the world, but have not been published at least in abstract form. It is appreciated that any list of nontraditional or unproven remedies will be incomplete. It is also appreciated that a program listed as a nontraditional or unproven remedy does not imply effectiveness or lack of effectiveness, simply that adequate information is not available and its value is as yet unproven.

Interferon

SSc is a disease characterized by excessive collagen deposition. The rationale leading to the use of the lymphocyte product, interferon gamma (IFN-γ), came from findings indicating that *in vitro*, this lymphokine can inhibit collagen production by normal human dermal fibroblasts (4) and can also modulate the excessive collagen biosynthesis characteristic of fibroblasts from patients with SSc (5). It was also found to have a number of immunoregulatory functions that could potentially have beneficial effects on the immunological abnormalities in SSc (6) (see Chapter 11).

Kahan et al (7) performed a pilot study examining the effects of IFN-γ on 10 selected patients with SSc of varying disease duration. The patients were treated with intramuscular injections of recombinant IFN-γ daily for 6 months. The

Table 27.1. Difficulties in Clinical Research Related to Systemic Sclerosis

A. Population
   1) Systemic sclerosis is an uncommon disease
   2) Patient selection for trials difficult
   3) Patient access to the research team is increasingly restricted
B. Disease
   1) Incomplete understanding of pathogenesis
   2) Individual patients have variable clinical courses of disease
   3) Disease subsetting does not adequately reduce the diversity of the individual variation in clinical course of disease
   4) The natural history of the illness often involves a plateau effect after a few years of disease
   5) Following the plateau there is often a variable rate and extent improvement in skin disease
   6) Medication related improvement in therapy of overall disease may be difficult to measure because of continued development of more effective therapy of related complications of systemic sclerosis (e.g. more effective therapy of hypertension, esophageal dysmotility, Raynaud's disease)
   7) There is no effective way to consistently diagnose early disease
C. Measurements
   1) No reliable clinical or laboratory tools adequately follow the disease course
   2) Although skin scores have good intra-observer reliability, inter-observer variability is much greater
   3) Changes in skin scores inconsistently reflect change in extent of internal organ disease (e.g. pulmonary, gastrointestinal, renal)
   4) Placebo response rate is difficult to calculate (e.g. Raynaud's phenomenon)
   5) Demonstration of an alteration in course of disease from baseline may require years
   6) Demonstration of differences from a control group may require hundreds of patients

Table 27.2. Unproven Remedies in Systemic Sclerosis (Scleroderma)

AGENTS OF INTEREST
   Cyclofenil
   Dextran
   Dimethylsulfoxide
   Extracorporeal Photochemotherapy
   Factor XIII
   5-Fluorouricil
   Gamma Interferon
   Ketanserin
   Ketotifen
   N-Acetylcysteine
   Paraaminobenzoic Acid
   Recombitant Tissue Plasminogen Activator

AGENTS WITH LESSER OR NO MEDICALLY PUBLISHED LITERATURE
   Anti-tuberculous Medications
   Benoxaprofen
   Estrogens (other)
   Griseofulvin
   Isotretinoin
   S-Adenosine Methionine
   Salazopryrin
   Stanazolol
   Superoxide Dismutase
   Thymopentin

initial dose of 10 μg was increased at 10-day increments to reach a maintenance dose of 100 μg, which was maintained for 5 months. The clinical parameters monitored were total skin score (0–4 for 26 anatomic sites and a possible score of 104), maximal oral opening, range of motion of wrists and elbows, grip strength, functional index, Raynaud's phenomenon (RP), digital ulcers, dyspnea, dysphagia, heartburn, arthralgia, patient/ physician overall assessment, electrocardiogram, echocardiogram, pulmonary function tests, chest x-rays, and serological tests. Nine of the 10 patients completed the study. The tenth had worsening of disease and renal failure requiring dialysis within 6 weeks. At 6 months, with improvement in the skin and musculoskeletal system in the remaining 9 patients. There was improvement in total skin score by ≧10 points (5), improved opening of the oral aperture (4), increased range of motion of joints (4), and improved grip strength (5). The improvement was noted within 2 to 3 months. There was also improvement in dysphagia and increased creatinine clearance. Adverse reactions included low grade fever (3) and a sustained, stable leukopenia/lymphopenia. The authors concluded that IFN-γ may be beneficial in the treatment of cutaneous SSc and some aspects of visceral SSc. Although the study was limited by its small sample size and the lack of a control group, it generated further interest in the use of IFN-γ in SSc.

Hein et al (8) performed an open label trial of recombinant IFN-γ on 14 patients with 4 to 10 years of SSc. Patients received 50μg subcutaneously once daily, initially 5 days per week for 2 weeks, then once daily 2 to 3 times a week for 12 months. They monitored skin score with pulmonary, cardiac, hepatic, renal, and esophageal function. Nine of the 14 patients completed the trial. There was improvement in skin score in five of the nine patients, usually noted within 3 to 4 months and sustained for the 1 year trial. Of the seven patients with pulmonary involvement, there was no deterioration in total lung capacity (TLC) or carbon monoxide diffusion capacity (DLCO); the authors felt that the pulmonary disease process had been arrested or partially reversed, though changes were not statistically significant. There were no changes in cardiac, renal, hepatic, esophageal, or serologic parameters. As with Kahan et al (7), there was no control group; however, the study did confirm the impression of improved cutaneous disease during IFN-γ therapy by Kahan et al (7) without confirming the leukopenia.

Freundlich et al (9) described the results of an 18-week open label study in which they enrolled 18 patients with diffuse cutaneous SSc. Of the patients completing the 3 times a week injections of IFN-γ for 18 weeks, six patients received "low dose" (0.1mg/m²) and 8 received "high dose" (0.5mg/m²) IFN-γ. Four failed to complete the study because of renal crisis (2), myocardial infarction (1), and a severe flu like syndrome (1). Another patient developed renal crisis at week 16, but was included in the final data analysis. There was an improvement in skin score in 12 of 14 patients, with a worsening in skin score in two patients. No factors were identified to account for the difference between responders and nonresponders, and no improvement was noted in other organ system involvement. There was a trend favoring skin area score improvement in the high dose versus the low dose group. A "center effect" was demonstrated as skin scores dropped in one center and did not change in another. This indicated a potential systematic bias in the study. The most common adverse reactions were febrile reactions and flu like symptoms, which were severe enough to warrant discontinuation of therapy in one patient. Of concern was the occurrence of renal crisis in three patients; the role of interferon in precipitating renal failure was unclear. A tendered explanation was that the patients were in the early stages of severe SSc and at increased risk of renal crisis (10). The influence of advanced age in these patients may have been a contributing factor.

Unemori et al (11) studied dermal fibroblasts from seven patients with SSc who had been treated with relaxin and IFN-γ individually, and then in combination. Both relaxin and IFN-γ reduced expression of the collagen gene. There was an additive effect when the drugs were used in combination. Further study was encouraged.

Although IFN-γ has been the most extensively studied interferon, several of its properties may not be very desirable in SSc: (*a*) induction of macrophage activation, class II antigen expression on cells including fibroblasts and endothelial cells (12); (*b*) IL-2 receptor expression (13); (*c*) IgG Fc receptor expression on both monocyte and monocyte-like cell lines (14); and (*d*) increased ICAM expression on endothelial cells (13).

In view of the above, Stevens et al (15) elected to use interferon alpha (IFN-α) in an open label pilot trial. The authors felt that patients with early onset illness and rapid progression of skin disease were most likely to show measurable change within the confines of the study, and studied 19 patients with diffuse cutaneous SSC (dsSSc) of less than 3 years duration. Each patient was treated with recombinant IFN-α intramuscularly or subcutaneously 3 times weekly: 3×10^6 units for 1 month, 6.0×10^6 units for 2 months, and 9.0×10^6 units for the remainder of the 6 month trial. Clinical parameters that were monitored included the following: (*a*) skin score (scale 0–3 at 20 anatomic sites, maximum score 60); (*b*) grip strength; (*c*) measurement of digital contractures; (*d*) Ritchie index; (*e*) assessment of muscle weakness; and (*f*) overall physicians assessment of response to therapy. A multitude of laboratory tests were obtained, including aminoterminal procollagen Type III peptides (P-III-NP) felt to be elevated in SSc (16), pulmonary function tests, echocardiograms, and dermal punch biopsies for histology and fibroblast culture for an estimation of collagen synthesis. The results were based on the 14 of 19 patients completing the study. The 5 withdrawals were for concomitant medical illnesses, except for one case where muscle pain and weakness were thought to be related to the IFN-α, because symptoms resolved when the drug was stopped. A few other patients developed flu-like symptoms, but they were not severe enough to warrant discontinuation of therapy.

The authors reported that there was a decrease in skin score in four patients at 6 months (p > .05) and a decrease in skin score of 10% or more in seven patients (p > .05). Grip strength remained unchanged, but there was a reduction of 4 mm in the distance between the finger tip and mid palmar crease (p value unknown). There was essentially no change in pulmonary function, and one patient developed renal disease. The physicians' overall assessment was: improvement in seven patients (50%); deterioration in five (36%); and unchanged in two. Four of 7 pretreatment biopsies from "uninvolved" skin showed early inflammatory features with no inflammation after treatment. The 7 skin biopsies taken from "involved" skin showed no pre- or post-treatment differences. There was a reduction in type I collagen synthesis in the 7 "uninvolved" skin biopsy cultures and a nonsignificant reduction of collagen synthesis in "involved" skin biopsy cultures. P-III-NP was stable or decreased in nine of 13 (67%) interferon-treated patients with a decrease in only one of eight (13%) disease-matched historical controls.

The authors felt the modest improvement in skin score and lack of progression in several other parameters were encouraging. The authors felt the change in biochemical parameters were suggestive of an effect of IFN-α on collagen synthesis, and that this was more marked in early disease, as evidenced by changes in clinically "uninvolved skin." It is difficult to draw conclusions from this study, given the open label short duration, small number of patients, and modest clinical benefit in overall assessment (i.e., 50%). It was noted that improvement in biochemical indices may or may not translate into clinical benefit.

These studies support the impression that IFN-α may have a benefit on the skin manifestations of scleroderma. However, it has become clear that large scale, placebo-controlled studies are still needed to clarify the questions of efficacy and safety.

Dimethyl Sulfoxide

Dimethyl sulfoxide (DMSO) is a versatile compound with numerous industrial and medicinal uses. A considerable amount of literature has been generated during the past 30 years on the types of pharmacologic actions of this compound, including several studies on the efficacy of DMSO in SSc with variable degrees of success (Table 27.3). The pharmacological actions of DMSO are diverse, and the effects of DMSO in SSc are thought to be the result of a combination of analgesic, vasodilatory, and membrane penetrating actions (17), as well as effects on collagen metabolism (18) and prostaglandin synthesis (19).

Scherbel et al reported encouraging results in a preliminary report on the use of DMSO on 10 patients with SSc (20), and expanded his group to 42 patients (21). The patients, whose ages ranged from 20 to 69 years, were treated with DMSO for 2 to 23 months. An investigator devised a system based on cutaneous and systemic manifestations, which graded the severity of the disease as mild (18), moderate (19), and severe (5). Ischemic digital ulcers were present in 19 of 42 patients. Measurements included grip strength, ability to flex fingers, frequency of RP, healing of ulcers, and increased growth of hair on hands and forearms. DMSO was applied by the following methods: (*a*) topical application of 30% to 60% DMSO, increased in some instances to 100% DMSO; (*b*) immersion of hands and wrists in 50% DMSO for ten non-responders to topical application; and (*c*) subcutaneous DMSO in nine patients with circumscribed and interstitial calcinosis, tendon contractures, and capsular adhesions who had not responded adequately to topical DMSO.

Good or excellent response to therapy was

Table 27.3. Treatment of Systemic Sclerosis with Dimethyl Sulfoxide (DMSO)

Author	No. of patients	Duration of Trial	Objective Paramenters	Results
Scherbel (14)	42	3–23 months	• Grip strength • Frequency of Raynaud's • Ability to flex fingers • Ulcer healing • Urine hydroxyproline • Skin biopsy (21 pts)	• 62% showed good or excellent response to treatment. 3 out of these 26 went into remission • 38% showed fair or poor response to therapy.
Tuffanelli (15)	24	2–5 months	• Size & number of ulcers • Tightness & thickness of skin • Joint mobility • Skin biopsy in 3 patients	• No clinical or histological difference between treated & untreated extremity.
Engel (16)	20	1 year	• Healing of ulcers • Joint mobility • Skin biopsy	• All patients showed improvement in increased mobility, healing of ulcers & relief of pain. • "Most" patients showed histological evidence of improvement. • No effect on systemic disease.
Binnick (18)	24	3–9 months	• Range of motion (goniometer) • Skin induration • Cutaneous ulcers • Skin temperature	• No significant improvement noted in any of the clinical parameters studied. • 13% showed minimal ↓ induration. • 17% showed ↑ induration.
Williams (19)	84	12 weeks	• Number, size & location of digital ulcers • Pain from ulcers on a VAS.	• No significant difference between normal saline, 2% DMSO & 70% DMSO. • No significant improvement in pain in the 70% DMSO group.

noted by 26 of 42 patients, with subsequent "complete remission" in three patients. Skin ulcers healed in 12 of 19 patients within 3 to 6 weeks. Those remaining patients treated with immersion all had complete healing of ulcers. Major histochemical alterations were seen on skin biopsies, with increased acid mucopolysaccharide in the treated area thought to be collagen breaking down and returning to the mucopolysaccharide moiety phase. The authors concluded that DMSO was effective in the treatment of cutaneous manifestations of scleroderma. It is noted that most of the patients who responded had mild disease; only two patients classified as having severe disease responded to therapy.

This initial study triggered an interest in the use of DMSO in SSc. Intrigued by the results of Scherbel's study and pressured by his patients, Tuffanelli (22) conducted a trial on 24 patients with extensive cutaneous SSc. Patients used 90% DMSO topically on one extremity, using the other extremity as a control in a 2 to 5 month study. Tuffanelli monitored tightness and thickness of the skin, size and number of cutaneous ulcers, arthralgias, and joint mobility. There was no detectable difference between the treated and untreated extremity, clinically or histologically. It was concluded that, under the conditions of the study, DMSO was not beneficial for the cutaneous manifestations of SSc. The issue of systemic absorption of DMSO with bilateral effects was not addressed.

Engel (23) studied 90% DMSO applied topically twice daily for 1 year in 20 patients with varying severity of SSc. There was clinically significant improvement in cutaneous disease in all patients as judged by healing of ulcers, improved joint mobility, and relief of pain with motion. However, systemic disease was not influenced and three patients died during treatment as a result of severe systemic SSc. The authors reported that even the patients who died had some improvement in the severity of their skin disease. Histologic changes observed were thickening of the epidermis, reappearance of previously flattened rete pegs, and some loosening of dense collagen. This study further promoted the use of DMSO in SSc with the hypothesis that the longer duration of therapy was of value; however, there was no control group. The mechanism of pain relief was thought to be blockage of pain conduction by DMSO (24). It was not entirely clear how ulcer healing occurred, but it was thought that DMSO-induced vasodilation and increased blood flow may have played a role.

Binnick (25) et al studied 24 patients with varying disease severity and duration of SSc. The patients were treated with 70% topical DMSO by painting and immersion techniques for one arm, using the contralateral arm as a partial control with 5% DMSO. They monitored range of motion, skin induration, and digital ulcers over 3 to 8 months of treatment. Perhaps DMSO provided a local analgesic effect, as the ulcers were less tender after DMSO in 10 of 16 patients with ulcers. However, ulcer healing was unaffected; no significant improvement was noted overall and no difference was noted between the arms. Although it could be argued that systemic absorption may have a bilateral effect, the authors felt that a higher concentration locally should have demonstrated some beneficial effects. The authors concluded that DMSO applied topically did not have a beneficial effect on the cutaneous or vascular manifestations of scleroderma, and that the results of their study were more valid than earlier reports, because objective parameters of response to therapy were used.

One of the largest studies, conducted by Williams et al (26), specifically recorded digital ulcers in a double-blind, 3-month study of DMSO treatment of 84 patients that were randomly divided into three treatment groups: (*a*) normal saline (N = 31), (*b*) DMSO 2% (N = 25), (*c*) DMSO 70% (N = 28). Each patient was instructed to soak only the more severely affected hand and wrist in the study solution 3 times daily. Patients were monitored for the total number of ulcers, the location of ulcers, the size of ulcers, ulcer pain, the presence or absence of infection, and the amount of characteristic (DMSO) breath odor.

The total number of ulcers in all three groups remained unchanged. Interestingly, there was a reduction in the size of the ulcers in the treated extremity in all three groups. There was a trend toward improved pain in the patients receiving 70% DMSO. It was suggested that soaking of the hand 3 times a day had a beneficial effect, regardless of the solution used. The most significant adverse reactions were skin reactions including cracking, blistering, and sloughing; eight of the nine patients with this reaction were in the DMSO 70% group. The authors concluded that DMSO 70% applied by immersion technique was not effective for the treatment of digital skin ulcers. This study was unique because for the first time the trial was randomized, double-blind, and placebo controlled. Previous studies have been hesitant to use a placebo group, because DMSO causes a characteristic breath odor which makes blinding difficult. However, it was observed by the investigators that even 2% DMSO, which is thought to possess minimal therapeutic benefit (27), also gave rise to the same type of odor, and was felt that there was enough odor in other treatment groups to prevent unblinding.

Interest in DMSO for treating SSc has recycled for over 20 years. There has been considerable interest in the lay press, spurring research interest. Despite these cycles of interest, the information available suggests that DMSO is ineffective in SSc.

5-Fluorouracil

The use of 5-fluorouracil (5-FU) in the treatment of systemic sclerosis was initially suggested by Casas et al (28). These investigators observed improvement in skin manifestations of SSc in a patient who had received chemotherapy including 5-FU as treatment for breast cancer. They also observed beneficial effects of topical 5-FU in a patient with plantar fibrosclerosis. These observations prompted them to use 5-FU in 12 women with SSc. The patients' ages ranged from 24 to 60 years, with a mean disease duration of 65 months. The total skin score for these patients was studied by Medsger et al (29), while Casas et al conducted a serial evaluation for vascular and visceral involvement, including chest radiographs, urinary creatinine clearance, electrocardiogram, and esophageal imaging studies. The patients had systemic disease with esophageal, pulmonary, and/or cardiac involvement. Patients received 4 or 5 doses of 5-FU, 12.5 mg/kg/day intravenously, followed by 4 additional doses of 5-FU at 8 to 10 mg/kg every 2 days, followed by a weekly maintenance dose of 10 to 20 mg/kg intravenously for 1.5 to 20 months (9 of 12 received at least 6 months of therapy).

Improvement in skin scores was noted as early as 1 to 2 weeks after treatment was started, and seemed to be related to the severity of disease and its duration, i.e., the worse the symptoms and the shorter the duration, the more beneficial the treatment. Esophageal and pulmonary function seemed to respond to treatment. Reappearance or worsening of skin lesions occurred within a few weeks in two patients who stopped the drug. Side effects included mild self-limited upper gastrointestinal symptoms and a mild transient leukopenia that resolved when the interval between dose of 5-FU was increased. Interpretation of the results are limited because the study was neither blinded nor controlled. Despite these limitations, the authors felt that 5-FU was beneficial to cutaneous and visceral SSc based on improvement in all patients and reappearance of disease in those in whom the drug was stopped. Larger scale trials were recommended. The authors speculated that the mechanism of action of 5-FU in SSc was that 5-FU could prevent the differentiation of endothelial and periendothelial cells into fibroblasts and thus the active deposition of collagen.

Malaviya et al (30) conducted a similar trial on 11 patients with SSc who had failed various therapies. They used a smaller dose of 5-FU than that used earlier. These authors reported a high incidence of serious side effects including a syndrome of severe weakness, diarrhea, mucosal ulcerations, and erythematous lesions on the face in three patients, one of whom developed septicemia and shock. Other patients developed thrombocytopenia, leukopenia, emesis, and increased skin pigmentation. Although their trial was too short to assess any long term potential beneficial effects of 5-FU, they did conclude that 5-FU was toxic and a modification of the dose and schedule should be entertained for future trials.

Encouraged by the results of their earlier study, Casas et al (31), conducted a double-blind, placebo-controlled, 6 month, randomized trial of 5-FU on 70 age and sex matched patients with SSc, 33 of whom were randomized to receive placebo. Assessments and dosing schedule of 5-FU were similar to their original trial. 5-FU was reduced by 25% if leukopenia, anemia, or severe nausea/vomiting occurred. Improvement was observed in the 5-FU group for total skin score, patients' global assessment, and Raynaud's score. No improvement was noted in visceral disease. The most common side effects from 5-FU were gastrointestinal followed by hemocytopenias; these side effects responded to 5-FU dose reduction. The authors concluded that in the short term 5-FU provided modest benefit in cutaneous SSc, but no improvement could be demonstrated in functional status or visceral disease. It was noted that the modest benefit was accompanied by a high incidence of side effects. It was not clear from this trial whether a longer treatment program or treatment limited to patients with disease duration less than 2 years would have different results.

The value of 5-FU in SSc remains unproven. Considering the toxicity of 5-FU and the limited value demonstrated to date, it does not appear that this drug will receive much interest in the future.

Extracorporeal Photochemotherapy

Extracorporeal photochemotherapy (ExPht) is a form of immunotherapy in which peripheral blood leukocytes treated with 8-methoxypso-ralen are exposed to ultraviolet A light irradiation and reinfused into the patient. This process leads to suppression of pathogenic T cell clones, suggesting that ExPht may act as an immune response modifier (32).

An ExPht program was originally used by Edelson (33) et al for cutaneous T cell lymphoma, where they reported improvement in survival rates, even in patients with advanced disease. Subsequent reports (34,35) showed use of ExPht in autoimmune disease, including (34) Malamista et al reporting efficacy in rheumatoid arthritis (RA) (33). In addition, marked clinical improvement was reported in two patients with SSc undergoing ExPht (36).

Encouraged by these preliminary results, a multicenter trial was conducted in patients with SSc of recent onset. This investigation compared ExPht with D-Penicillamine in a randomized, single blind, parallel group, 12 month trial (37). Monthly disease activity was assessed with measurements of skin thickness, area of skin involvement, oral aperture, right and left hand closure, pulmonary function tests, skin biopsies, and routine hematologic, electrolyte, and liver function tests. Patients that were randomized to ExPht (N = 25) received treatment for 2 consecutive days every 4 weeks. Patients that were randomized to D-Penicillamine (N = 31) received 750 mg daily for 6 months. Corticosteroids, colchicine, paraaminobenzoic acid (PABA), and griseofulvin were not permitted during the study.

By 6 months, 68% of patients receiving ExPht showed at least a 15% improvement in skin score, with worsening in 9.7%; skin score improved in 32% of those on D-penicillamine and 32% worsened. By 10 months, improvement in skin score was seen in 69% of those on ExPht and 50% of those on D-penicillamine; worsening skin score was observed in 10% of those receiving ExPht and 16% of those on D-penicillamine. Seven patients discontinued D-penicillamine between the 6 and 10 month visit; five of seven had worsening skin disease. There was no change in pulmonary function tests in either group. Skin biopsies improved in 18 of 24 patients, with return to more delicate and widely spaced collagen bundles correlating with the improvement in skin score. None of the patients in the ExPht group had to withdraw because of side effects.

The authors concluded that ExPht was safe and effective in the treatment of the cutaneous manifestations of SSc. Although not studied, they suggested the possibility of an additive effect of ExPht in combination with other treatments (38).

In a critical editorial, Fries et al (39) pointed out the following with regard to the ExPht study just described: the study did not attempt to achieve a standard 25% reduction in skin score; a 15% improvement in 69% of the ExPht group versus 50% of the D-penicillamine group at 10 months was modest at best, and of lesser importance in light of the lack of improvement in visceral disease; the cost of therapy was high; and there were problems with the data which included lack of documentation of randomization visit frequency and dosage adjustment, discrepancies between study case record reports and source documents, and evidence of inclusions of patients with either long standing disease or inappropriate classification (limited scleroderma). Information is further clouded by a potential conflict of interest that was reported, because one of the investigators holds a patent to the photophoresis machine. There is concern that the flaws in study design and performance are great enough to obviate drawing any conclusions from this trial.

At this time, there is need for a large multicenter trial to clarify the potential efficacy of ExPht in SSc. There have been several delays in the initiation of such a trial. Until such a trial has been completed, ExPht remains an unproven therapy.

Recombinant Tissue Plasminogen Activator

The rationale to use recombinant tissue plasminogen activator (TPA) in SSc stems from studies on the pathogenesis of SSc indicating that early changes of SSc involve injury to the endothelial cells of the involved vascular compartments. So called "circulating factors" may have a role in the fibrosis that ensues (40–42). In relation to this, SSc is associated with coagulation abnormalities, thrombotic episodes, fibrin deposition, increased rate of fibrinogen breakdown, and altered regulation of plasminogen activator and plasminogen activator inhibitors (43–45).

It was in this context that Fritzler and Hart (46) first described a patient with SSc who benefited from TPA therapy. TPA is produced by recombinant DNA technology. It is a potent thrombolytic agent that acts by converting clot-bound plasminogen to plasmin. Fibrin within the thrombus then undergoes proteolytic digestion (47). TPA has been used in patients with coronary vascular occlusion where it has been shown to reduce infarct size, improve cardiac function, and decrease mortality (48). Fritzler and Hart's patient was a 44-year-old woman who had SSc for 15 years. Her disease was characterized by severe RP, digital ulceration, distal digital tuft resorption, and calcinosis cutis. She had diffuse cutaneous SSc, but did not have evidence of cardiac, pulmonary, or renal disease. When she developed a sudden onset of pain in both arms, she was diagnosed as having an acute myocardial infarction. This resulted in treatment with recombinant TPA infusion over a 4-hour period, followed by a heparin infusion. Within hours of starting therapy, she reported dramatic improvement in her RP but no comment was made on her arm pain. Over the ensuing 4 to 6 weeks, she also reported progressive softening of the skin and healing of her skin ulcers. During an 18 month follow-up period, her modified scleroderma skin score changed from 44 to 38, and RP remained mild. Although a spontaneous remission in scleroderma is well known (49), it was felt that the temporal relationship of recombinant TPA administration suggests a therapeutic effect.

In a pilot study, Kliminik et al (50) treated four patients with SSc and digital ischemia who had not responded to vasodilator therapy with two different regimens of recombinant TPA. The patients improved both clinically and with increased blood flow.

Encouraged by these results, these same investigators, using TPA, conducted a randomized, placebo-controlled, double-blind trial on 10 patients with limited cutaneous SSc and digital ischemia (51). They assessed global status, digital ischemia by skin color, temperature, digital pitting, and ulceration at intervals during the 2-day infusion and up to 1 month afterward. Objective skin blood flow measurements also included recording skin temperature, ultrasound Doppler, and transcutaneous oxygen and carbon dioxide. The five patients receiving placebo infusions were given TPA infusions after 1 week. The authors reported that during the infusion, there were significant changes from baseline in the skin blood flow measurements and patient assessment of pain, limb temperature, and body temperature by a 10 cm visual analog scale. Also, significant fibrinolytic effects were seen during the infusion, but neither effect was sustained nor observed after the infusions (Table 27.4). When compared to those receiving placebo, the TPA group improved in whole body warmth, laser Doppler measurements of blood flow, skin temperature, and fibrinolytic measurements. After 5 days, however, there were no differences between the groups.

It was concluded that in digital ischemia secondary to SSc, recombinant TPA had short term benefit on the microcirculation. The limitations of the study included the small sample size and a mode of TPA administration that was different than conventional methods. The authors felt that additional studies involving larger numbers of patients using alternative TPA administration regimens would be useful.

There can be no argument with the above conclusion. At present, there is not enough information to change recombinant TPA from an unproven remedy.

Ketanserin

Raynaud's phenomenon (RP) is almost universal in patients with SSc. Serotonin and the 5-hydroxytryptamine (5-HT) pathway may be involved in peripheral vasospastic disease (52,53). Subcutaneous administration of 5-HT precipitates vasoconstriction in SSc patients. 5-HT has been linked to fibrosis (54), increased cell proliferation, and collagen accumulation of fibroblasts in culture. Ketanserin is an antagonist of 5-HT at its receptor sites on vascular smooth muscle, platelets, and bronchial tissue (55). It blocks 5-HT-induced platelet aggregation and vasoconstriction.

Seibold et al (56) performed an open-label pilot study of ketanserin in 30 patients with RP: (*a*) five patients with idiopathic RP; (*b*) seven patients with systemic lupus erythematosus (N = 6) or rheumatoid arthritis (N = 1); (*c*) 18 patients with SSc (diffuse cutaneous N = 9, limited cutaneous N = 9); and (*d*) eight volunteer normal controls. All were given oral ketanserin 60 mg/ day for the first week, with an increase to 120

Table 27.4. Recombinant Tissue Plasminogen Activator in Systemic Sclerosis Measurements of Fibrinolysis[a]

TEST	BASE	DAY0	DAY1	NORMAL
Euglobulin clot lysis time (min)	208	37	196	173
Fibrin Plate lysis area (mm^2)	106	383	105	100
Fibrinogen blood level (mg/dl)	285	237	255	267
Plasminogen blood level (% normal)	109	73	95	104
Antiplasmin (% activity)	92	54	76	111

[a]Modified with permission from Klimiuk et al (44); only mean or median values presented. Blood obtained using an indwelling venous cannula under resting conditions.

mg/day for the following 3 weeks. All medications with potential vasodilatory actions were discontinued except corticosteroids. Colchicine, nonsteroidal antiinflammatory drugs, and D-Penicillamine were continued. The severity of RP was assessed from the patient's estimate of frequency of attacks per day, physician assessment of severity of digital tip ulcerations, and patients rating of pain. All patients had a reduction in attacks of RP; however, the reduction was more impressive in the SSc group. Patients reported marked or moderate improvement in global assessment in 83% of those with SSc and 33% of those with RP. All nine patients with hand edema had improvement or "remission." There was rapid healing of digital ulceration in the seven patients with ulcerations during the treatment period. Ketanserin therapy improved digital blood flow by plethysmography in all groups of patients with RP, although the greatest increase occurred in the SSc group. When patients were cold-challenged, blood flow was preserved only in the SSc group while on ketanserin. The authors felt that ketanserin may be a useful treatment option in patients with SSc and ischemic digital ulcerations.

Altamore et al (57) subsequently performed an uncontrolled 10-patient, 10 month trial with ketanserin 60 mg/day for SSc. Response was assessed by the patients' subjective evaluation of RP and by plethymography. Six of the 10 patients reported improvement in RP.

Ortonne et al (58) performed a small, double-blind, placebo-controlled trial with ketanserin for 6 months on 24 patients with predominantly cutaneous SSc. Patients were without hepatic or renal disease and entered into the study after washout from confounding drugs. The ketanserin (N = 14) group received 40mg/day for 2 weeks, followed by 80mg/day for the remainder of the 6 months. In this study with negative results, there were no differences observed between the ketanserin and placebo groups in any of several functional parameters that were measured.

Two of the above studies were uncontrolled. Even though initial results were encouraging,

larger scale controlled studies are needed. Until then, ketanserin remains an unproven therapy.

Dextrans

Dextrans of varying molecular weights have been used in the treatment of peripheral vascular disorders. Low molecular weight dextran improves blood flow in the microcirculation by having a disaggregating effect on erythrocytes (59), reducing whole blood viscosity (60), and/or increasing intravascular volume leading to increased venous return and cardiac output (61). Clinical trials with dextrans are summarized in Table 27.5.

Since digital ischemia caused by intimal thickening of small vessels and microthromboses are so common in patients with SSc, there have been several trials of dextrans in SSc.

Holti (62) tested Dextran 40 in 12 patients with SSc. Ten of the 12 patients reported significant improvement in digital blood flow by improvement in skin temperature (63), relief of pain, and healing of ulcers.

Kantor and Katz (64) treated four SSc patients with continuous 48-hour infusions of Dextran 40 10% in normal saline. Although no objective parameters were used, the "general clinical opinion" was improvement in peripheral circulation and softening of skin.

Kirk and Dixon (65) studied 10% low molecular weight dextran in an average of four 48-hour infusions, at 3 to 5 week intervals, in six SSc patients with SSc and digital ischemia including digital ulcerations. In a complex design, four patients were randomized to receive dextran or saline in a blinded fashion. Response was assessed by history, grip strength, range of motion in joints, and digital blood flow by changes in finger tip temperature. Transient improvement in digital blood flow and skin temperature were present for some of the infusions. The patients were subjectively better after the dextran infusions and half of them felt better after saline. Skin disease continued to progress. Visceral disease

Table 27.5. Treatment of Systemic Sclerosis with Dextran

Author	No. of. Patients	Duration of Trial	Objective Parameter	Results
Holti (55)	12	5–12 weeks	• Digital blood flow by skin temperature • Healing of ulcers	• 83% improved; $\uparrow$ blood flow, healing ulcers and $\downarrow$ pain.
Kantor and Katz (57)	4	2 days	• None	"General Clinical Opinion" of definite improvement in peripheral circulation & softening of skin
Fountain (58)		6 weeks	• Digital pulse recording	400% $\uparrow$ pulse amplitude with 6% HMWD[a] 430% $\uparrow$ in pulse amplitude with 10% LMWD[b]
Kirk and Dixon (59)	6	12–20 weeks	• Grip strength • Joint mobility • Digital blood flow	• Transient improvement in blood flow in 'few" patients • No improvement in cutaneous or visceral disease.
Lane (60)	10	48 hours (3 patients followed for 6 months)	• Change in digital temperature	• (one patient couldn't tolerate the temperature of the water & not included in analysis) • No significant benefit observed.
Dodman & Rowell (61)	21	24 weeks	• Digital temperature	• No difference in skin temperature between placebo & dextran groups.

[a]HMWD, High molecular weight dextran
[b]LMWD, Low molecular weight dextran

was not affected in any of the patients. The side effects of treatment were a generalized rash and fever in one patient who had a history of allergies to other agents. Another patient developed migraine headaches during the infusions.

Lane (66) treated 10 patients with SSc and severe RP with low molecular weight dextran infusions while measuring digital temperatures. Dextran infusion was administered to all patients under uniform conditions, in an attempt to eliminate atmospheric variables that might cause vascular spasm. There was no benefit observed in any of the patients either in the short term or during the 6 month follow-up.

In a double-blind, controlled, single case, crossover study, perfusions of normal saline, 6% dextran, and 10% low molecular weight dextran were infused once weekly (67). Using digital pulse recording as a parameter of response, the authors reported that 6% dextran resulted in a 400% increase in pulse amplitude, which was in-

creased to 430% over baseline by low molecular weight dextran.

Dodman and Rowel (68) performed a double-blind, placebo-controlled trial in 21 SSc patients with severe RP. Ten patients were randomized to receive 10% low molecular weight dextran in 5% dextrose, and 11 patients received 5% dextrose infusion alone at 8-week intervals for 3 doses. Response was measured by digital temperature at baseline, 24 hours, and 4 weeks after the infusions. Half the patients receiving dextran thought their circulation was improved, while 40% of the dextrose group also reported improvement. The subjective improvement did not translate into improvement in objective criteria, as there was no difference in skin temperature between the dextrose and dextran groups.

As one analyzes the various controlled and uncontrolled trials, it becomes clear that based on currently available data, low molecular weight dextran does not appear to have beneficial effects on cutaneous, visceral, or vascular manifestations of scleroderma.

Factor XIII (Fibrin Stabilizing Factor)

SSc skin changes result from an accumulation of immature collagen (69,70) as a result of fibroblastic dysregulation (71). Factor XIII has a stabilizing action on fibrin and a transamidination function (72,73), which plays a role in collagen synthesis (74). Activated Factor XIII stimulates the binding of fibronectin to collagen (75,76). Hypothetically, this could help remove polymerized collagen by the reticuloendothelial system. In fact, as a local cutaneous phenomenon, fibronectin levels are increased in SSc (77). Factor XIII may also increase macrophage activity and opposes the excess activity of fibroblasts, which may be pathogenetic in SSc (76).

In an uncontrolled study of 20 SSc patients treated with Factor XIII, seven patients reported definite benefit and five moderate benefit with improved joint mobility and suppleness of the skin (78).

Maekawa et al (79) reported 2 cases with generalized SSc treated with daily intravenous Factor XIII for 3 weeks. They found the lower esophageal sphincter pressure increased from 14 to 20 cm H_2O in the first patient, and a lesser improvement in the second patient.

Guillevin et al (80) performed a long term follow up of 86 patients with SSc who were treated with a variety of regimens of intravenous Factor XIII. All had cutaneous disease and some had visceral involvement. After a mean follow-up of 1.5 years, there was improvement or stabilization of the skin disease in 44 of 86 patients. No improvement was observed in visceral disease.

Guillevin et al (81,82) also conducted a multi-center, double-blind, crossover, controlled trial comparing Factor XIII with placebo in 25 patients, who had SSc of 2 to 8 years duration and varying degrees of cutaneous and visceral involvement. Patients received either 170 mg/day

(2 ampules) intravenously of Factor XIII or placebo continuously for 3 weeks. This was followed by a 6 week nontreatment period and a 3 week treatment crossover period. Measurements included the physician's assessment of improvement, the physician and the patient's global impression, a functional index using several measurements of activities of daily living, skin elasticity, range of motion of joints, opening angles of the mouth and spacing between finger prints. Only two measurements indicated a difference between the treatment and placebo: the physician and the patient's global assessment and the functional index.

These limited studies provide some encouraging data for the use of Factor XIII in SSc. However, larger, controlled studies with better patient selection are needed.

Cyclofenil

Cyclofenil has weak estrogen properties. The use of cyclofenil in SSc originated from reports that it suppressed cartilage collagen biosynthesis *in vitro* (83).

The use of cyclofenil in SSc first appeared as a case report (84) in which the patient had increased skin elasticity and improved lung volume. Cyclofenil was used as 300 mg/day for 6 months followed by 600 mg/day. A subsequent case report (85) involved a 48-year-old man with SSc of the lungs treated with cyclofenil for 1 year. Most parameters of lung function improved, including vital capacity and diffusion capacity. No comment was made about cutaneous disease.

These case reports generated interest in this treatment modality and were followed by an uncontrolled trial of 29 patients with SSc. In this trial, there was improvement of skin changes, RP, joint pain, and stiffness (86).

Blöm-Bülow et al performed a double-blind, placebo-controlled, crossover trial in 38 patients with an average 6 years of SSc (87). Patients received 6 months of placebo or cyclofenil 600 mg/day before crossing over. Twenty seven patients completed the study. There was improvement in some parameters of skin disease, such as grip strength and finger extension. Patients with disease for less than 5 years showed reduced joint pain and stiffness on drug vs placebo. Esophageal peristalsis was not better in the treatment group when compared to placebo.

Gibson and Grahame (88) performed a double-blind, placebo-controlled, crossover trial in which 11 patients with varying degrees of SSc were randomly assigned to cyclofenil 600 mg/day or placebo for 4 months before crossing over for an additional 4 months. During the first treatment period, four out of six patients on cyclofenil had to withdraw because of liver function test abnormalities, and one person died from accelerated hypertension. At the end of both treatment periods, results were difficult to interpret because of the small number of patients and the large number of dropouts. Among the parameters monitored, finger extension and gape (mouth opening) remained unchanged. Grip strength was slightly better in the treatment group—the only clinical measurement favoring the treatment group. Significant hepatotoxicity associated with the use of cyclofenil was observed in this trial.

Another comparative trial was conducted by Wollheim and Äkesson (89) in which cyclofenil was compared with D-penicillamine in a prospective open trial that lasted up to 2 years for some patients. No changes in pulmonary or esophageal function was seen in either group. Half of the patients in the cyclofenil group had to drop out because of toxicity.

The most common toxicity associated with cyclofenil appears to be hepatic enzyme elevation, which is reported in most studies. There has also been one case report of hemolytic anemia during cyclofenil treatment (90).

As one analyzes the data available on use of cyclofenil in SSc, it seems that, at best, it has modest effects on a few parameters of skin disease in a few patients. This is at the risk of significant toxicity in a substantial number of patients. Cyclofenil probably should not be recommended as a treatment option in SSc at this time.

Paraaminobenzioc Acid

The use of paraaminobenzoic acid (PABA) in the treatment of SSc was first advocated by Zarafonetis et al in 1950 (91). Their rationale for PABA in SSc came from earlier encouraging results of its use in patients with SLE (92). It was thought that the photosensitivity associated with use of sulphur compounds in SLE patients may be counteracted by PABA, which is an antagonist of sulphonamide. For similar reasons, PABA was used empirically in a patient with dermatomyositis, photosensitivity, and overlapping features with SSc. During treatment, her SSc regressed remarkably, encouraging the use of PABA in patients with SSc. These investigators reported improvement in skin tightening in three out of four patients within a few days of treatment. No objective parameters were used.

This was followed by a larger study (93) in which 60 consecutive patients were treated with PABA regardless of duration and severity of SSc. The author reported that 58 patients had "moderate to marked" cutaneous improvement. This was based on an increase in skin softness and elasticity, subjective improvement in skin texture, and weight gain. It was observed that treatment for longer than 3 months was more effective than treatment for less than 3 months.

In a larger retrospective review (94), Zarafonetis et al analyzed charts from 223 patients with SSc receiving PABA for varying periods of time. These patients were compared to 96 patients with SSc who had never received PABA. The authors reported that 64% of patients receiving PABA showed marked to moderate skin improvement. There was, however, no mention of the parameters used to assess response.

The same authors have also published survival data on 390 PABA and non-PABA treated patients with SSc, also in a retrospective analysis (95). The 5- and 10-year survival was 89% and 77% in the PABA treated patients, compared to 70% and 57% in non-PABA treated patients. Although patients in this study were younger then those used in other large studies, the authors still felt that the mortality difference was large enough to compensate for age (no statistical adjustments were made).

However, despite these encouraging reports, PABA does not fare as well when studied in controlled settings. The first double-blind, placebo-controlled trial was conducted by Bushnell (96) et al in 1966. Twelve patients with diffuse cutaneous SSc were randomized to PABA (N = 7) or placebo (N = 5) in a 6 month study. The PABA treated group had a qualitative increase in skin mobility compared to baseline with no change in the placebo group. Additionally, no changes were noted in the extent of visceral disease.

In a double-blind, controlled, crossover trial, Silber and Gitlin (97) studied 15 patients with SSc for 6 months. Although they felt that 87% of patients did not respond to therapy, the study was limited by the lack of objective measurements.

Clegg et al conducted the largest controlled trial of PABA in SSc to date (98). The study was a multicenter, prospective, randomized, 48-week, double-blind, placebo-controlled trial involving 146 patients with SSc of at least 3 months duration. Patients received PABA 12 gm daily, or an identical appearing placebo (containing potassium chloride 15%, potassium citrate 46% and lactose 44%), in 4 divided doses. Measurements included skin mobility (measured at 20 specified sites), skin thickening (specified sites graded from 0–3 for a maximum score of 45), maximal oral aperture, range of motion of both hands, and physician and patient global assessment of skin involvement (scale of 0–3).

Seventy-six of the 146 (52%) patients completed the trial. The withdrawals did not differ in demographic or clinical characteristics from "completers." Reasons for withdrawal were as follows: four patients from each group because of progression of SSc; eight in the PABA group and three in the placebo group because of intercurrent illnesses. Adverse events are listed in Table 27.6. There were no differences in any of the outcome variables between PABA and placebo treated groups. The results were analyzed to determine whether PABA may benefit minimally involved skin to a greater degree than more severely involved skin. This was done by examining total mobility scores of the most distal skin site that the investigator graded as uninvolved. No differences were found between the PABA and placebo groups. The authors concluded that PABA did not alter the skin changes of SSc in patients with relatively stable, long standing or lesser involved skin disease.

The studies of PABA in SSc are encouraging when performed in uncontrolled settings. Controlled trials, although few, are not supportive of any benefit. A long term controlled trial of 2 or more years would be needed to establish any benefit. At this time the data suggest that PABA is ineffective in SSc.

Relaxin

Relaxin is a polypeptide hormone derived from the ovaries of pregnant mammals. It acts on fibrocartilage to allow dilatation of the pelvis during delivery of the fetus(es). Relaxin was used in SSc in the 1950s when several authors reported

Table 27.6. Paraaminobenzoic Acid (PABA) Adverse Drug Reactions During Trials Leading to Withdrawal

Adverse Drug Reaction	PABA	Placebo
Nausea and dyspepsia	9	6
Vomiting	3	0
Anorexia	0	1
Diarrhea	7	0
Flatulence	0	1
Fever and Chills	4	3
Epistaxis	1	0
Rash	2	0
Pruritis	2	0
Headache	4	1
Thrombocytopenia	1	0
Metallic taste	0	1
Body odor	0	1
Total ADR[a]	33	14
Total withdrawals[a]	18	6

[a]Total ADR are greater than total withdrawals because of patients being withdrawn for more than one ADR.

benefit (99–101). However, relaxin fell into disfavor because of its high cost and questionable benefit. Although there is little information available on relaxin, there has been a renewed interest and recent active research on this agent. This interest is based on the presence of increased SSc skin fibroblasts collagen synthesis (102), combined with relaxin-induced decreased collagen expression on normal dermal fibroblasts. Relaxin is effective in suppressing collagen overexpression after cytokine stimulation with TGF-β or IL-1β (103).

As noted previously, Unemori et al (11) studied dermal fibroblasts treated with relaxin and IFN-γ from seven patients with SSc. The agents both reduced collagen expression and had an additive effect when used in combination prompting interest in further research.

Since the information on relaxin is preliminary, the agent cannot be recommended for SSc at this time.

N-Acetylcysteine

Limited data is available on the use of N-acetylcysteine for the treatment of SSc. N-acetylcysteine is thought to act by reducing disulfide bonds of susceptible proteins to sulfhydryl groups. Varying degrees of sulfhydryl deficiency have been reported in connective tissue diseases, including SSc (104). N-acetylcysteine has also been studied in RA with proposed benefit (105) (Barley JP, Vanal ME. Acetylcysteine in the treatment of rheumatoid arthritis: Unpublished study courtesy of Mead Johnson Research Center, 1970.)

Furst et al performed a double placebo, controlled trial of N-acetylcysteine on 22 patients with limited and diffuse cutaneous SSc (106). Treatment was initiated with 2 to 4, 500 mg capsules or equivalent appearing placebo each day, increased to a maximum of 20 capsules daily, administered over a 12 month period. Patients were allowed the highest tolerable or full dose. Examinations at baseline and at 6 and 12 months included radiographs (chest, hand, and feet x-rays, cine esophagram, upper gastrointestinal series, barium enema), esophageal manometry, cardiac function, pulmonary function tests, and electromyogram. The authors mentioned a possible selection bias for long standing established disease based on the knowledge that N-acetylcysteine is a benign drug. Clinical parameters monitored included oral aperture, hand spread, grip strength, ring size, and joint count.

Four patients in each group discontinued the drug: (a) N-acetylcysteine group—gastrointestinal distress (2), rash (1), and worsening disease (1); (b) placebo group—gastrointestinal distress (1), worsening disease (2), non compliance (1). The study was discontinued after 1 year because additional supplies of N-acetylcysteine and placebo were not available.

At the end of the study, there were no significant changes when comparing the two groups to their baseline values. The authors felt that the study provided valuable insight into the natural history of visceral involvement in SSc, but did not show any benefit of N-acetylcysteine in either cutaneous or visceral disease. The study supported the high frequency of an abnormal DLCO in patients with interstitial lung disease as a highly sensitive measure of pulmonary function change in these patients.

N-acetylcysteine does not appear to be of value in patients with SSc.

Ketotifen

Ketotifen acts both as a histamine antagonist and inhibitor of mast cell release of mediators (107, 108). Ketotifen inhibited fibrosis in the tight-skin mouse model of SSc (109). With recent emphasis on the role of the mast cell in SSc (110), there has been increasing interest in the use of ketotifen for human SSc.

Gruber and Kaufman were impressed with results of ketotifen in two patients with SSc refractory to D-penicillamine, prompting them to embark on a double-blind, 6-month, randomized, controlled trial of ketotifen in early diffuse cutaneous SSc (111). Patients received ketotifen 3 mg twice daily, or identical placebo tablets, and were evaluated at 6-week intervals. Measurements included global assessment, severity of pruritis, total skin score, weight of a 4 mm punch biopsy of the skin with hydroxyproline analysis, pulmonary function tests, and mast cell releasability after stimulation by intradermal skin testing.

There were no significant changes and no trends for change in either of the groups. There were no adverse effects from ketotifen and the two discontinuations were for worsening disease. One placebo-treated patient discontinued for somnolence from the medication.

At this time there is minimal information available on ketotifen in SSc. Unfortunately, what little information that is available points to lack of efficacy, and ketotifen cannot be recommended for treatment of SSc at this time.

References

1. Medsger T. Systemic sclerosis (scleroderma), localized forms of scleroderma and calcinosis. In: McCarty D, ed. Arthritis and allied conditions, 12th cd. Philadelphia: Lea and Febiger 1993; 1253–1292.

2. Wigley FM. Treatment of systemic sclerosis. Curr Opin Rheumatol 1992;4:878–886.

3. Seibold JR, Furst DE, Clements PJ. Why everything (or nothing) seems to work in the treatment of scleroderma. J Rheumatol 1992;19:673–676.

4. Jimenez S, Freundlich B, Rosenbloom J. Selective inhibition of human diploid fibroblast collagen synthesis by interferons. J Clin Invest 1984;74:1112–1116.

5. Rosenbloom J, Feldman C, Freundlich B, Jimeniz S. Inhibition of excessive scleroderma fibroblast collagen production by recombinant γ-IFN. Arthritis Rheum 1986;29:851–856.

6. Skurkovich S, Skurkovich B, Bellanti JA. A unifying model of the immunoregulatory role of the interferon system: Can interferon produce disease in humans?. Clin Immunol Immunopathol 1987;43:362–373.

7. Kahan A, Amor B, Menkes CJ, Strauch G. Recombinant IFN-γ in the treatment of systemic sclerosis. Am J Med 1989;87:273–277.

8. Hein R, Behr J, Hundgen M, Hunzelmann N, Meurer M, Braun-Falco O, Urbanski A, Krieg T. Treatment of scleroderma with IFN-γ. Br J Dermatol 1992;126:496–501.

9. Freundlich B, Jimenez S, Steen V, Medsger T Jr, Szkolnicki M, Jaffe H. Treatment of scleroderma with recombinant IFN-γ. Arthritis Rheum 1992; 35:1134–1142.

10. Barnett AJ, Miller MH, Littlejohn GO. A survival study of patients with scleroderma diagnosed over 30 years (1953–1983): The value of a simple cutaneous classification in the early stages of disease. J Rheumatol 1988;15:276–283.

11. Unemori E, Bauer E, Amento E. Relaxin alone and in conjunction with IFN-γ decreases collagen synthesis by cultered human scleroderma fibroblasts. J Invest Dermatol 1992;99:337–342.

12. Mahrle G, Schulze H-J. Recombinant interferon in dermatology. J Invest Dermatol 1990;95(suppl):132S-137S.

13. Rombaldi A, Young DC, Herman F, Canistra SA, Griffin JD. Interferon gamma induced expression of IL2 receptor gene in human monocytes. Eur J Immunol 1987;17:153–156.

14. Girard HT, Hjaltadittirs A, Fejes-Toth AN, Guyre PM. Glucocorticoids enhance the γ interferon augmentation of human monocyte IgG Fc receptor expression. J Immunol 1987;138:3235–3241.

15. Stevens W, Vancheeswaran R, Black CM, UK Systemic Sclerosis Study Group. Alpha interferon 2_ in the treatment of diffuse cutaneous systemic sclerosis: A pilot study. Br J Rheumatol 1992;31:683–689.

16. Uitto J, Bauer EA, Eisen AZ. Scleroderma: Increased biosynthesis of triple helical type I & III procollagens associated with unaltered expression of collagenase by skin fibroblasts in culture. J Clin Invest 1979;64:921–930.

17. Scherbel AL. Effect of percutaneous DMSO on cutaneous manifestations of scleroderma. Ann NY Acad Sci 1983;411:120–130.

18. Gries G, Bublitz G, Lindner J. The effect of DMSO on components of connective tissue. Ann NY Acad Sci 1967;141:630–637.

19. Roa C. Differential effects of detergents and DMSO on membrane PGE and disease receptors. Life Sci 1977;20:2013–2022.

20. Scherbel AL, McCormack LJ, Poppo MJ. Alteration of collagen in generalized scleroderma (progressive systemic sclerosis) after treatment with dimethyl sulfoxide: Preliminary report. Cleve Clin Q 1965;32:47–56.

21. Scherbel AL, McCormack LT, Layle JK. Further observations on the effects of DMSO in patients

with generalized scleroderma. Ann NY Acad Sci 1967;141:613–629.

22. Tuffanelli D. A clinical trial with DMSO in scleroderma. Arch Dermatol 1966;93:724–725.

23. Engel M. DMSO in the treatment of scleroderma. South Med J 1972;65:71–73.

24. Becker DP, Young HF, Nulsen FC, et al. Physiological effects of DMSO on peripheral nerves. Exp Neurol 1969;24:272–276.

25. Binnick S, Shore SS, Corman A, Fleischmajer R. Failure of DMSO in the treatment of scleroderma. Arch Dermatol 1977;113:1398–1402.

26. Williams HJ, Furst DE, Dahl SL, Steen VD, Marks C, Alpert ES, Henderson AM, et al. Double-blind, multicenter controlled trial comparing topical dimethyl sulfoxide, normal saline for treatment of hand ulcers in systemic sclerosis. Arthritis Rheum 1985;28:308–313.

27. Brown JH. Clinical experience with DMSO in acute musculoskelatal conditions comparing a noncontrolled series with a controlled double blind study. Ann NY Acad Sci 1967;141:496–505.

28. Casas J, Sabauste C, Alarcon G. A new promising treatment in systemic sclerosis: 5-FU. Ann Rheum Dis 1987;46:763–767.

29. Medsger TA, Steen VD, Zeigler G, Rodnan GP. The natural history of skin involvement in PSS. Arthritis Rheum 1980;23:720.

30. Malaviya A, Singh R, Dhar A, Gupta Y, Kumar A, Agarwal P, Mathur R, et al. 5-FU in progressive systemic sclerosis: Is it safe? Ann Rheum Dis 1988;47:964–967.

31. Casas J, Saway PA, Villarreal I, Nolte C, Menajovsky BL, Escudero EE, Blackburn WD, et al. 5-FU in the treatment of scleroderma, a randomized double-blind placebo controlled international collaborative study. Ann Rheum Dis 1990; 49:926–928.

32. Perez M, Edelson R, Laroche L, Berger C. Inhibition of antiskin allograft immunity by infusions with synergeic photoinactivated effector lymphocytes. J Invest Dermatol 1989;92:669–676.

33. Edelson R, Berger C, Gasparro F, Jegasothy B, Heald P, Wintroub B, Vonderheid E, et al. Treatment of cutaneous T cell lymphoma by extracorporeal photochemotherapy: Preliminary results. N Engl J Med 1987;316:297–303.

34. Malawista S, Trock SH, Edelson RL. Treatment of rheumatoid arthritis by ECPC: A pilot study. Arthritis Rheum 1991;34:646–654.

35. Rook AH, Jegasothy BV, Heald P, Nahass T, Ditre C, Witmer WK, Lazarus G, et al. Extracorporeal photochemotherapy for drug-resistant pemphigus vulgaris. Ann Intern Med 1990;112:303–305.

36. Rook AH, Heald PW, Nahass GT, Macey W, Witmer WK, Lazarus GS, Jeasothy BV. Treatment of autoimmune disease with ECPC: Pemphigus vulgaris—preliminary report. Yale J Biol Med 1989; 62:647–652.

37. Rook AH, Freundlich B, Jegasothy BV. Treatment of systemic sclerosis with extracorporeal photochemotherapy: Results of a multicenter trial. Arch Dermatol 1992;128:337–345.

38. Steen VD, Medsger TA Jr, Rodnan GP. D-penicillamine therapy in progressive systemic sclerosis: A retrospective analysis. Ann Intern Med 1982; 97:652–659.

39. Fries J, Seibold JR, Medsger TA Jr. Photopheresis for scleroderma? No! (Editorial) J Rheumatol 1992;19:1011–1013.

40. Kahaleh MB, Sherer GK, LeRoy EC. Endothelial injury in scleroderma. J Exp Med 1979;149:1326–1335.

41. Rodnan GP. The vascular hypothesis in scleroderma. In: Black CM, Myers AR, eds. Systemic sclerosis (scleroderma). New York: Gower Medical Publishing, 1985.

42. Cohen S, Johnson AR, Hurd E. Cytotoxicity of sera from patients with scleroderma: Effects on human endothelial cells and fibroblasts in culture. Arthritis Rheum 1983;26:170–178.

43. Holland CD, Jayson MIV. Venous blood fibrinolysis and fibrinolytic potential in primary Raynaud's and systemic sclerosis associated with Raynaud's phenomenon. In: Black CM, Myers AR, eds. Current topics in rheumatology: Systemic sclerosis (scleroderma). New York: Gower Medical Publishing, 1985;267–273.

44. Furey NL, Schmid FR, Kwaan HC, Friederici HH. Arterial thrombosis in scleroderma. Br J Dermatol 1975;93:683–693.

45. Baumgartner S, Deng JS, Grau R, Franks J, Steigerwald J, Tan EM. Evidence for low grade coagulation abnormalities in progressive systemic scleroderma. Arthritis Rheum 1980;23:652.

46. Fritzler J, Hart DA. Prolonged improvement of Raynaud's phenomenon and scleroderma after recombinant tissue plasminogen activator therapy. Arthritis Rheum 1990;33:274–276.

47. Lui CY, Wallen P. The binding of tissue plasminogen by fibrin. Circulation 1984;70:365.

48. The TIMI Study Group. The thrombolysis in myocardial infarction (TIMI) trial. New Engl J Med 1985;312:932–936.

49. Alper J, LeRoy EC. Scleroderma (systemic sclerosis). In: Katz WB, ed. Rheumatic diseases, diagnosis and management. New York: JB Lippincott, 1977;467–481.

50. Klimink P, Kay E, Illingworth K, Morris W, Taylor L, Gush R, Jayson M. Tissue plasminogen activator in the treatment of digital ischemia

in scleroderma: Further observations (abstract). Fibrinolysis 1988;2(suppl 1):158.

51. Kliminik P, Kay EA, Ilingworth KJ, Gush RJ, Taylor LJ, Baker RD, Perkins C, et al. A double-blind placebo controlled trial of recombinant tissue plasminogen activator in the treatment of digital ischemia in scleroderma. J Rheumatol 1992;19:716–720.

52. Halpern A, Kuhn PH, Shaftel HE, Samuels SS, Shaftel N, Selman D, Birch HG. Raynaud's disease, Raynaud's phenomenon and serotonin. Angiology 1960;11:151–167.

53. Winkelman RK, Goldyne ME, Linscheid B. Hypersensitivity of scleroderma cutaneous vascular smooth muscle to 5-hydroxytryptamine. Br J Dermatol 1976;95:51–56.

54. Boucek RJ, Speropoulos AJ, Noble NL. Serotonin and ribonucleic acid and collagen metabolism of fibroblasts in vitro. Proc Soc Exp Biol Med 1972;140:599–603.

55. Lysen JE, Awouters F, Kennis L, Laduron PM, Vandenberk J, Janssen PA. Receptor blinding profile of 41,468, a novel antagonist at 5-HT2 receptors. Life Sci 1981;28:1015–1022.

56. Seibold JR, Jageneau AHM. Treatment of Raynaud's phenomenon with ketanserin, a selective antagonist of the serotonin receptor. Arthritis Rheum 1984;27:139–146.

57. Altomare GF, Pigatto, PD, Polenghi MM. Ketanserin in the treatment of progressive scleroderma. Angiology 1988;39:583–586.

58. Ortonne JP, Torzuoli Ck, Dujardin P, Fraitag B. Ketanserin in the treatment of systemic sclerosis: A double-blind controlled trial. Br J Dermatol 1989;120:261–266.

59. Gelin LE, Ingelman B. Rheomacrodex—a new dextran solution for rheological treatment of impaired capillary flow. Acta Chir Scand 1961;122:294–302.

60. Gregerson ML, Peric B, Usami S, Chien S, Chang C, Sinclair DG. Studies on blood viscosity at low shear rates: Effects of low and high molecular dextrans. Fed Proc 1963;22:641.

61. Schenk WGI, Delin NA, Domanig E, Hahnloser P, Hoyt RK. Blood viscosity as a determinant of regional blood flow. Arch Surg 1964;89:783–796.

62. Holti G. The effect of intermittent low molecular weight dextran infusions upon the digital circulation in systemic sclerosis. Br J Dermatol 1965;77:560–568.

63. Cooper KE. Comparison of methods for gauging blood flow through the hand. Clin Sci 1949;8:217–234.

64. Kantor I. Scleroderma treated with dextran 40 (Rheomacrodex). Arch Dermatol 1966;94:675–677.

65. Kirk JA, Dixon AS. Failure of low molecular weight dextran infusions in scleroderma. Ann Rheum Dis 1969;28:49–54.

66. Lane P. Low molecular weight dextran infusions in systemic sclerosis with Raynaud's phenomenon: A report of nine cases. Br Med J 1970;4:657–659.

67. Fountain RB, Stevens A. Scleroderma treated with low molecular weight dextran. Br J Dermatol 1966;78:605–606.

68. Dodman B, Rowell NR. Low molecular weight dextran in systemic scleosis and Raynaud's phenomenon. Acta Derm Venereol 1982;62:440–442.

69. Fleischmajer R, Gay S, Meigel WN, Perlish JS. Collagen in the cellular and fibrotic stages of scleroderma. Arthritis Rheum 1978;21:418–428.

70. Keiser HR, Stein HD, Sjöerdsma A. Increased protocollagen proline hydroxylase activity in sclerodermatous skin. Arch Dermatol 1971;104:57–60.

71. Uitto J, Ohlenschlager K, Lorenzen I. Solubility of skin collagen in normal human subjects and in patients with generalised scleroderma. Clin Chem 1971;31:13–18.

72. Craig S, Kitchen S, Newcomb TF. Factor XIII. Medicine 1979;58:413–429.

73. Mosher D. Cross linking of plasma and cellular fibronectin by plasma transglutaminase. Ann NY Acad Sci 1978;312:38–42.

74. Wachtel E. Biocheonie und klinische Bedeutung des Gerinnungsfactor XIII Pharmazeut. Zeitung 1973;118:1571–1578.

75. Soria A, Soria C, Boulard C. Fibrin stabilizing factor (F XIII) and collagen polymerization. Experientia 1975;31:1355–1357.

76. Soria J, Soria C, Ryckewaert U, Naveau B, Lafay P, Ryckewaert A. Normal level of plasma fibronectin and fibrin stabilizing factor in scleroderma. Arthritis Rheum 1980;23:1334–1335.

77. Cooper SM, Keyser AJ, Bealey AD, Ruoslanti E, Nimni ME, Quismorio FP. Increase in fibronectin in the deep dermis of involved skin in PSS. Arthritis Rheum 1979;22:983–987.

78. Thivolet J, Perrot H, Meunier F. Action therapeutique du facteur XIII de la coagulation dans la sclerodermie. Nouv Presse Med 1975;4:2779–2882.

79. Maekawa Y, Nogita T, Yamada M. Favorable effects of plasma factor XIII on lower esophageal sphincter pressure of PSS. Arch Dermatol 1987;123:1440.

80. Guillevin L, Euller-Ziegler L, Chouvet B, De Gery A, Chassoux G, Lefay P, Zeigler G, et al. Traitement de la sclerodermie systemique par le facteur XIII chaz 86 malades suivis a long terme. Presse Med 1985;12:2327–2329.

81. Guillevin L, Chouvet B, Mery C, De Gery A, Thivolet J, Godeau P, Delbarre F. Treatment of progressive systemic sclerosis using Factor XIII. Pharmatherapeutica 1985;4:76–80.

82. Delbarre F, Godeau P, Thivulet J. Factor XIII treatment for scleroderma. Lancet 1981;2:204.

83. Herbai G. Separation of growth inhibiting potency from estrogenicity in different weak oestrogenic drugs of various chemical structure. Acta Endocrinol 1971;68:249–263.

84. Herbai G. Treatment of progressive systemic sclerosis with a synthetic weak estrogen: Cyclofenil (Sexovid). Report of a case. Acta Med Scand 1974;196:537–540.

85. Blöm-Bülow B, Friariksson H, Herbai G. Improvement of lung function in a scleroderma patient treated for 12 months with cyclofenil. Ups J Med Sci 1980;85:67–73.

86. Blöm-Bülow B. Cyclofenil in the treatment of scleroderma—a general view on the results after treating 29 cases. Z Rheumatol 1980;39:1–8.

87. Blöm-Bülow B, Oberg K, Wollheim F, Persson W, Janson B, Malmberg P, Bostrom H, et al. Cyclofenil vs placebo in PSS. A one year double-blind crossover study of 27 patients. Acta Med Scand 1981;210:419–28.

88. Gibson T, Grahame R. Cyclofenil treatment of scleroderma—a controlled study. Br J Rheumatol 1983;22:218–223.

89. Wollheim FA, Äkesson A. Treatment of scleroderma in 1988. Semin Arthritis Rheum 1989;15:181–188.

90. Wollheim FA, Ljunggren H, Blöm-Bülow B. Hemolytic anemia during cyclofenil treatment of scleroderma. Acta Med Scand 1981;210:429–430.

91. Zarafonetis CJD, Curtis AC, Gulick AE. Use of paraaminobenzoic acid in dermatomyositis and scleroderma. Arch Intern Med 1950;85:27–43.

92. Zarafonetis C, Curtis AC, Grekin RH. Effects of paraaminobenzoic acid in systemic lupus erythematosus; preliminary report. University Hospital Bulletin, Ann Arbor 1947;13:122–125.

93. Zarafonetis C. Treatment of scleroderma. Ann Intern Med 1959;50:343–365.

94. Zarafonetis CJD, Dabich L, Skovionski JJ. Retrospective studies in scleroderma, skin response to potassium paraaminobenzoate therapy. Clin Exp Rheumatol 1988;6:261–268.

95. Zarafonetis CJD, Dabec L, Negri D, Skovronski JT, DeVol EB, Wolfe R. Retrospective studies in scleroderma: Effect of potassium paraaminobenzoate on survival. J Clin Epidemiol 1988;41:193–205.

96. Bushnell WJ. Treatment of progressive systemic sclerosis: A comparision of paraaminobenzoate and placebo in a double-blind study. Arthritis Rheum 1966;9:495.

97. Silber W, Gitlin N. Progressive systemic sclerosis (diffuse scleroderma). A follow-up report of treatment with Potaba. S Afr Med J 1973;47:1001–1002.

98. Clegg D, Reading JC, Mayes MD, Seibold JR, Harris C, Wigley FM, Ward JR, et al. Comparison of aminobenzoate potassium and placebo in the treatment of sleroderma. J Rheumatol 1994;21:105–110.

99. Casten G, Boucek RJ. Use of relaxin in the treatment of scleroderma. JAMA 1958;166:319–324.

100. Graciansky P, Boulle S. Essais de traitement de la sclerodermie parla relaxine. Bull Soc Fr Dermatol 1961;68:83–86.

101. Reynolds H. Use of relaxin in management of ulceration and gangrene due to collagen disease. AMA Arch Dermatol 1959;80:407–409.

102. LeRoy EC. Increased collagen synthesis by scleroderma skin fibroblasts *in vitro*. J Clin Invest 1974;54:880–889.

103. Unemori EN, Amento EP. Relaxin modulates synthesis and secretion of procollagenase and collagen by human dermal fibroblasts. J Biol Chem 1990;265:10681–10685.

104. Lorber A, Bocy RA, Chang CC. Sulfhydryl deficiency in connective tissue disorders: Correlation with disease activity and protein alterations. Metabolism 1970;20:446–455.

105. Lorber A, Chang CC, Masuoka D, Mecham I. Effect of thiols in biological systems on protein sulfhydryl content. Biochem Pharmacol 1970;19:1551–1560.

106. Furst DE, Clements PJ, Harris R, Ross M, Levy J, Paulus HE. Measurement of clinical change in progressive systemic sclerosis: A 1 year double-blind placebo-controlled trial of N-acetylcysteine. Ann Rheum Dis 1979;38:356–361.

107. Craps LP, Ney UM. Ketotifen: Current views on its mechanism of action and their therapeutic implications. Respiration 1984;45:411–421.

108. Huston DP, Bressler RB, Kaliner M, Sowell LK, Baylor MW. Prevention of mast cell degranulation by ketotifen in patients with physical urticaria. Ann Intern Med 1986;104:507–510.

109. Walker M, Harley R, LeRoy EC Ketotifen prevents skin fibrosis in the TSK/+ mouse. J Rheumatol 1990;17:57–59.

110. Claman HN. On scleroderma: Mast cells, endothelial cells, and fibroblasts. JAMA 1989;262:1206–1209.

111. Gruber BL, Kaufman LD. A double-blind randomized controlled trial of ketotifen versus placebo in early diffuse scleroderma. Arthritis Rheum 1991;34:362–366.

28

Surgical Approach to Hand Involvement

IN ADDITION TO INVOLVEMENT OF THE SKIN, gastrointestinal tract, kidneys, lungs, and heart, systemic sclerosis (SSc) or scleroderma frequently affects the hands. Manifestations of SSc in the hand include Raynaud's phenomenon (RP), digital tip ischemia which may progress to ulceration or frank gangrene, severe contractures of the proximal interphalangeal (PIP) joints and metacarpophalangeal (MCP) joints, and intracutaneous and subcutaneous calcinosis.(1–3)

SSc may be sub-divided into diffuse and limited cutaneous variants. Either variant may be associated with the CREST syndrome, which consists of calcinosis, RP, esophageal dysfunction, sclerodactyly, and telangiectasia. Patients with the diffuse cutaneous variant of SSc tend to develop joint contractures, and patients with the limited cutaneous variant are more susceptible to ischemic problems, RP, and digital ulcerations; however, joint contractures may also be seen in the limited cutaneous variant, and ischemic problems may develop in patients with the diffuse cutaneous variant. In most patients with SSc who have early involvement of their hands, RP is usually the presenting symptom and is uniformly present in the limited cutaneous variant. In the early phases, the fingers are puffy or swollen and the skin feels thickened and tight. In the later stages, after the development of joint contractures, the fingers appear slender with thin, shiny, sclerotic skin. Severe joint contractures develop more often in the diffuse variant primarily because of the involvement of the joint capsule, collateral ligaments, and tendon sheaths. Tendon friction rubs are palpable over the flexor and extensor tendons of the fingers in the majority of patients with the diffuse cutaneous variant but in less than 3% of patients with the limited cutaneous variant. Calcinosis of the digits is more common in the limited cutaneous variant.

Involvement of the hands in SSc is functionally disabling and its medical and surgical treatment remains frustrating both for the rheumatologist and the hand surgeon. The role of reconstructive hand surgery in scleroderma has only been documented infrequently.(1–8) This chapter distills the experience of the collaborative effort between two rheumatologists (Thomas A. Medsger, MD and Virginia Steen, MD) and one hand surgeon (Neil Jones, MD) in 70 patients with SSc over the 10-year period from 1984 through 1994, and discusses the surgical management of digital ischemia, digital ulcerations, contractures of the PIP and MCP joints, calcinosis, and carpal tunnel syndrome in 127 hand surgery operations.

Raynaud's Phenomenon and Digital Ischemia

In 1865, Raynaud first described paroxysmal blanching and cyanosis of the digits followed by reactive hyperemia. These attacks are usually induced by cold exposure or emotional upset. It is well established that RP may antedate the other manifestations of SSc by several years.

An exaggerated sympathetic vasoconstrictive response to cold was initially proposed to explain the pathophysiology of RP in SSc. This theory provided the rationale for the medical management of RP by various drugs that reduce sympathetic tone and the surgical operations of cervical sympathectomy and digital artery sympathectomy. According to the alternative theory, RP is the result of a normal vasoconstrictive response to a cold stimulus acting upon structurally abnormal arteries in the hand. This concept is supported by angiographic and histological evidence of multiple small areas of narrowing and occlusion of the proper digital arteries in patients with SSc. The common digital arteries are less frequently involved, and the radial artery is relatively spared. However, narrowing or occlusion of the ulnar artery at the wrist has been reported in almost 50% of patients and total obstruction of the superficial palmar arch in 10% of patients.(9) Rodnan et al (10) examined the digital arteries obtained at post mortem from patients with SSc and RP: 80% had marked luminal narrowing of greater than 75% caused by severe intimal hyperplasia and fibrosis. Adventitial fibrosis and telangiectasia of the vasa vasorum in the adventitia were also noted. Since thickening of the intima produces a permanent increase in the wall-to-lumen ratio, and since blood flow is inversely proportional to the fourth power of the radius of the vessel lumen, intimal hyperplasia will obviously cause a significant reduction in blood flow to the fingers. Consequently, even a minimal increase in the vasoconstrictive response to a cold stimulus may produce further significant functional narrowing in an artery already partially occluded by structural changes. Kristensen (11) has confirmed that 70% of patients with SSc have reduced arterial perfusion pressure (less than 75%) of normal when evaluated by plethysmography. Because the pressure decrement was greatest between the wrist and the proximal phalanges, he postulated an increased resistance to flow within the palmar arch.

MEDICAL TREATMENT OF RAYNAUD'S PHENOMENON AND DIGITAL ISCHEMIA

For a more complete discussion of RP and its medical management, please refer to Chapter 17, Organ Involvement: Peripheral Vascular. Since surgical management of RP and digital ulceration requires optimal concurrent medical management, the hand surgeon should strongly emphasize to the patient the importance of stopping smoking and avoiding cold exposure by wearing gloves or mittens, hats, and scarves. Various drugs that reduce sympathetic activity have been reported to be of benefit in the control of RP and the healing of digital ulcers. Nifedipine 10 to 20 mg TID, a calcium channel blocking agent that induces vasodilatation (12), prazosin, a direct arterial smooth muscle relaxant, and the rheologic agent pentoxifylline, 400 mg TID, have been the most effective pharmacologic agents in our experience for the control of RP and in preventing progressive digital ulceration.

SURGICAL TREATMENT OF RAYNAUD'S PHENOMENON AND DIGITAL ISCHEMIA

There is now increasing interest in whether prophylactic surgical procedures, such as digital sympathectomy and microsurgical revascularization, can increase digital blood flow in patients with SSc. Such surgery might thereby reduce the frequency and severity of symptoms of RP, promote the healing of digital ulcers, and prevent the progression to frank gangrene. For many years, cervical sympathectomy was the only surgical option available for the treatment of RP. However, analysis of the long-term results of sympathectomy has been equivocal (13), probably because many sympathetic nerve fibers bypass the cervicothoracic trunk through alternative pathways, such as the sinovertebral nerve, the carotid plexus, and the nerve of Kuntz, to provide additional contributions to the sympathetic nerve supply of the upper limb. Because sympathetic nerve fibers leave the median and ulnar nerves at the level of the wrist to innervate the radial and ulnar arteries and superficial palmar arch and pass from the common digital and proper digital nerves to the corresponding common digital arteries and proper digital arteries, Flatt (14) introduced the concept of a distal sympathectomy at the level of the common digital and proper digital arteries. To interrupt these sympathetic nerve fibers passing into the adventitia, the hand surgeon separates the digital nerves from the proper digital arteries and strips the adventitia from the digital arteries under the operating microscope. Digital sympathectomy provided relief of pain and an increase in baseline temperature of 2°F in the finger of one patient with SSc, but was not followed by complete healing of the ulcer (14). Wilgis (15) emphasized the strict selection of patients by plethysmography and cold stress testing. Only those patients who demonstrated an improvement in their response to cold stress testing after local anesthetic block in the distal palm were considered to exhibit increased sympathetic tone and hence be potential candidates for digital sympathectomy. He also modified the technique by removing adventitia from a 2 cm segment of both the common digital artery and proper digital artery, and reported healing of digital ulcers in eight of nine patients with chronic digital ischemia.

INVESTIGATIONS

Under our protocol, patients with disabling symptoms of RP and digital ulcerations refractory to medical management are investigated by digital plethysmography (pulse volume recordings), cold stress testing, and intra-arterial digital subtraction angiography. Cold stress testing involves measurement of either digital temperatures, pulse volume recordings, or laser Doppler flow values in the digits before and during exposure of the hands in a cold environment and during subsequent rewarming. Angiography is performed through a femoral puncture and not by direct puncture of the brachial artery, so that the entire upper extremity can be visualized from the origin of the subclavian artery down to the hand.

To prevent vasospasm, angiography is performed under axillary block anesthesia and with intra-arterial injection of 25 mg tolazoline immediately before injection of the contrast medium. If the angiogram does not reveal any segmental occlusions of the radial or ulnar arteries or superficial palmar arch, but shows normal visualization of the digital vessels, and if pulse volume recordings after cold stress testing improve after local anesthetic block, then vasospasm is considered to be the major pathophysiological mechanism producing RP and digital ulcerations.

DIGITAL SYMPATHECTOMY

Our technique of digital sympathectomy (16) has evolved into a much more extensive technique than that originally described by Flatt (14), Wilgis (15), and Egloff (17). Patients with SSc seem to have a striking degree of proliferative fibrous tissue in their palms similar to that seen in Dupuytren's contracture. Not only does there appear to be a proliferation of fibrous tissue extending down on either side of the neurovascular bundles, but there is also increased peri-adventitial fibrosis around the common digital arteries and superficial palmar arch. Consequently, an inverted J-shaped incision is used to explore the palm. Fibrous septa passing down around each side of the neurovascular bundles are sharply divided to allow inspection of the entire superficial palmar arch and common digital arteries under the operating microscope to determine whether there are any segmental occlusions or areas of focal calcification that may be amenable to resection and reconstruction using interposition vein grafts. The adventitia is then stripped away from the superficial palmar arch, the radial digital artery to the index finger, the common digital arteries to the second, third, and fourth web spaces and their continuation as the radial and ulnar proper digital arteries and the ulnar digital artery to the little finger, out to the level of the web spaces. If necessary, the dissection can be extended farther out to the level of the proximal interphalangeal joint in an individual finger. On several occasions, common digital arteries that appeared totally occluded prior to resection of the adventitia subsequently became soft and patent (Fig. 28.1). This is analogous to the situation in microsurgery in which a vein graft eventually dilates after stripping off the adventitia with jeweler's forceps. We therefore believe that RP occurring in SSc may be caused by three different mechanisms:

(i) An exaggerated sympathetic vasoconstrictive response to cold.
(ii) Segmental occlusions of the common digital and proper digital arteries due to intimal proliferation.
(iii) External compression of the common digital arteries and proper digital arteries due to peri-adventitial fibrosis.

Consequently, digital sympathectomy may promote improved blood flow in the digital arteries not only by interrupting the sympathetic nerve control of the digital arteries, but more simply by removal of the external constrictive cuff of peri-adventitial fibrosis from around the arteries. We have therefore described digital sympathectomy as a "decompression arteriolysis," which is analogous to the epineurectomy of a peripheral nerve during surgical release of a compression neuropathy (16). O'Brien et al have similarly advocated a much more radical resection of the adventitia from the distal radial and ulnar arteries and superficial palmar arch (18).

Sixteen patients with SSc, involving 68 digits, have undergone digital sympathectomy. Although digital sympathectomy may promote healing of ulcers and improvement in symptoms of cold intolerance, it is our impression that patients still complain of pain and in long term follow-up, 20% of these patients have developed recurrent ulcerations within 2 years. Long term follow-up to document the incidence of recurrent digital ulceration will therefore be necessary to determine whether digital sympathectomy is in fact an effective treatment for patients with SSc, or whether it merely has a short-term effect as the occlusive disease in the digital arteries becomes the predominant component of the disease.

MICROSURGICAL REVASCULARIZATION

Even though the pathophysiological mechanism producing ischemia in SSc is assumed to be a combination of vasospasm and focal segmental occlusions within the proper digital arteries themselves, we now believe that the reason patients deteriorate so rapidly is because they suddenly develop a significant reduction in arterial inflow into the palmar arches due to more

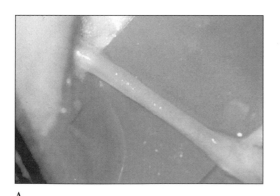 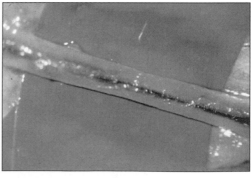

A   B

Figure 28.1. Digital artery seen through the operating microscope (*a*) before and (*b*) after removal of the adventitia during digital sympathectomy. Blood is seen filling the lumen of the artery in (*b*).

proximal occlusion of the inflow radial and ulnar arteries at the wrist, presumably due to the same intimal proliferation (16,19). This is manifest clinically by:

(i) Increasing severity of RP.
(ii) Progression or recurrence of digital ulcerations despite good medical management.
(iii) Progression to incapacitating ischemic pain.

If segmental occlusion of either the radial or ulnar artery or both arteries can be documented by angiography (Fig. 28.2), and if there is satisfactory evidence of distal "run-off" by visualization of the common digital arteries on angiography, SSc patients with unremitting rest pain, severe RP, or multiple recurrent digital ulcerations that cannot be controlled by medical therapy may be candidates for resection of the

occluded arterial segment and microsurgical reconstruction of the distal radial and ulnar arteries and the superficial palmar arch (Fig. 28.3) (16,19). If, at the time of exploration, the common digital arteries are found to be patent with satisfactory back flow, reconstruction of the superficial palmar arch, using a reversed interposition vein graft with end-to-end anastomosis to the distal radial or ulnar artery and end-to-side anastomoses to the common digital arteries, might be expected to increase the inflow perfusion pressure to the digits, even though multiple small areas of narrowing and occlusion of the proper digital arteries may still remain. Histolog-

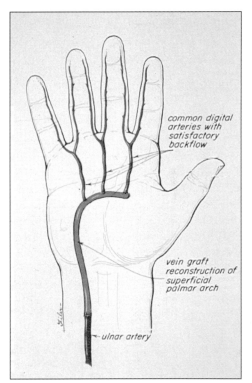

Figure 28.3. Diagrammatic representation of microsurgical revascularization of the hand for ischemia due to occlusion of the ulnar artery in SSc. The reversed interposition vein graft is anastomosed end-to-end to the distal ulnar artery and the common digital arteries to the second, third, and fourth web spaces are anastomosed end-to-side to the "new" superficial palmar arch.

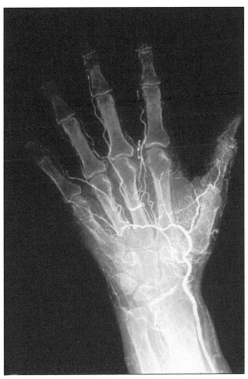

Figure 28.2. Angiogram of a patient with SSc showing occlusion of the distal ulnar artery.

ical examination of these inflow arteries at the level of the wrist in such patients has revealed virtual occlusion of the lumen (Fig. 28.4). This adds credence to the hypothesis that in the more advanced stages of SSc, intimal hyperplasia is responsible for the diminished blood flow in RP rather than pure sympathetic overactivity. Patients undergoing microsurgical revascularization are maintained post-operatively on a continuous intravenous infusion of low molecular weight dextran for 5 days. Patients have obtained subjective relief of their hand pain, improvement in the frequency and severity of RP, and healing of digital ulcers. Improved digital blood flow to the fingers has been confirmed objectively with pulse volume recordings taken immediately post-operatively, and this has been maintained at least 1 year later (16,19).

Although microsurgical revascularization might be assumed empirically to increase the inflow perfusion pressure to the digits, two alternative mechanisms may also play a role. First, it has been demonstrated that resection alone of a thrombosed segment of artery may reduce the sympathetic discharge from this thrombosed segment, thereby preventing vasoconstriction of the remaining collateral circulation. Second, the extensive dissection required to expose the superficial palmar arch and common digital arteries to allow resection of the occluded segment may, in itself, be a form of distal sympathectomy and may therefore alleviate some of the secondary vasospasm. Whatever the mechanism, microsurgical revascularization can only be expected to be a palliative intervention, because it is likely that any underlying arteriopathy will continue to progress not only in the remaining digital arteries, but also in the reconstructed vein grafts themselves. It therefore remains unknown as to whether these improvements in digital blood flow will be maintained long term. However, because our patients have remained asymptomatic in follow-up with confirmatory evidence of improved pulsatile digital blood flow by digital plethysmography, we have been encouraged that microsurgical revascularization may play a role in the salvage of SSc patients with RP and severe hand or digital ischemia.

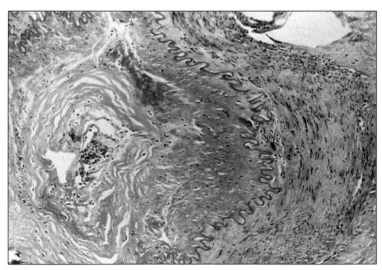

Figure 28.4. Histological cross-section of the resected ulnar artery reveals intimal hyperplasia and luminal occlusion.

DIGITAL ULCERATIONS

Progressive digital ischemia may result in ulcerations of the finger tips and eventually frank gangrene (Fig. 28.5a). With progression of the disease, small foci of ischemic necrosis or ulceration develop in the fingertips. These are extremely painful and tend to heal slowly leaving pitted depressed scars. Radiographs may reveal bony resorption of the tufts of the distal phalanges. Skin grafts have been described for coverage of digital ulcers in SSc (1), but a clinically normal skin graft placed on a sclerodermatous recipient bed becomes sclerodermatous itself (6). Gahhos et al (7) reported that partial fingertip amputations were the only definitive measure of relieving incapacitating pain.

In our experience, early digital ulcerations should be treated by meticulous local wound care including penetrating topical antibiotics, such as silver sulfadiazine, and short-term protective immobilization using finger splints and casts. Infection of these digital ulcers is usually caused by *Staphylococcus aureus* (>90%) or *Pseudomonas aeruginosa*. Digital ulcerations that progress to frank gangrene may be allowed to autoamputate, providing that infection has not supervened and that pain can be controlled without addiction to narcotics, because this treatment maximizes the length of the finger that may be salvaged. However, formal surgical amputation may be required should the patient develop osteomyelitis of the distal phalanx, infection of the distal interphalangeal (DIP) joint, or extensive gangrene with unremitting pain (Fig. 28.5b) (3). Amputations should not be performed under local anesthetic but under axillary block or intravenous regional block and with tourniquet control. After release of the tourniquet, the surgeon should look for signs of punctate bleeding at the edges of the dorsal and palmar skin flaps, and the stumps should be closed loosely without any tension whatsoever. In our experience of 51 digital amputations in 20 SSc patients, the amputation stumps have healed relatively normally as long as punctate bleeding has been seen at the edges of the skin flaps and the flaps have been approximated without tension, except in three patients on high doses of corticosteroids or with markedly decreased serum protein levels.

PIP and MCP Joint Contractures

Progressive flexion contractures of the PIP joints may develop, especially in patients with the diffuse cutaneous variant of SSc (Fig. 28.6A). This

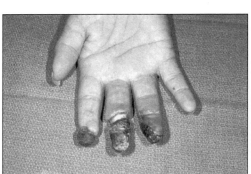
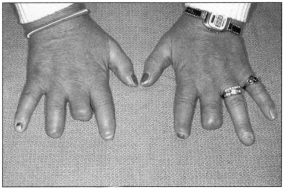

A   **B**

Figure 28.5. (*A*) Gangrene of the right index, middle, and ring fingers in a patient with limited cutaneous scleroderma (CREST syndrome). (*B*) After amputation of the right index, middle, and ring fingers, the patient had primary healing of the amputation stumps and resolution of her pain with improved hand function.

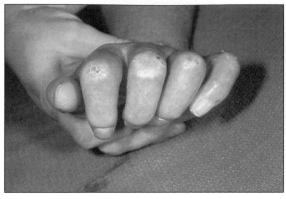
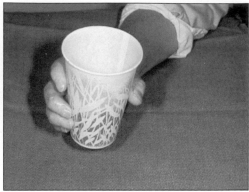

A   B

Figure 28.6. (*A*) 90° to 110° flexion contractures of the PIP joints of the left hand with ulcerations over the dorsal aspect of the PIP joints. (*B*) Three months post-operatively after arthrodesis of the PIP joints in 45° to 55° of flexion, there was complete healing of the dorsal ulcerations and improved grasp function of the left hand.

significantly interferes with the patient's hand function. Pathophysiologically, PIP joint flexion contractures are the result of sclerosis of all tissues—the skin, collateral ligaments, joint capsule, and flexor tendon sheaths. The central slip of the extensor tendon mechanism becomes attenuated, and the lateral bands are displaced palmarly. With increasing flexion contracture of the PIP joint, the dorsal skin overlying the PIP joint becomes stretched thin and atrophic. Dorsal ulceration is very common and may progress to pyogenic arthritis of the PIP joint or osteomyelitis of the head of the proximal phalanx or the base of the middle phalanx. These dorsal ulcers should not be confused with the ischemic ulcers at the tips of the fingers. Dorsal PIP joint ulcerations are the result of pressure on the sclerodermatous skin from the underlying head of the proximal phalanx and are therefore similar to pressure sores and are not caused primarily by digital ischemia.

The loose fascial tissue between the extensor tendon and the MCP joint capsule may also become involved by the process of fibrosis, and this eventually results in extension or hyperextension contractures at the MCP joints. There appear to be at least two subsets of hand deformities in patients with the diffuse variant of SSc: those with flexion contractures of the PIP joints, but who maintain satisfactory flexion and extension at the MCP joints; and those who not only develop flexion contractures at their PIP joints, but also develop hyperextension deformities at their MCP joints (3). Finally, SSc patients may also develop adduction contractures of the thumb-index finger web space, which significantly compromises both thumb-index finger tip pinch and grasp of large objects.

SURGICAL TREATMENT OF PIP AND MCP JOINT CONTRACTURES

Surgical treatment of PIP joint flexion contractures in SSc has included amputations, skin grafts to the dorsal ulcers, flexor tendon lengthening (2), arthrodesis (4), and arthroplasty (8). Statistically significant improvements in hand function have been documented even after a single physical therapy treatment with paraffin baths, friction massage, and active exercises (20). Arthrodeses of the PIP joints, combined with capsulotomies or arthroplasties of the MCP joints, have been proposed to improve the function of the hand in SSc (2–4). Silicone implant arthroplasties of the PIP joints have also been described, but the active range of motion postoperatively only averaged 30°: 20% were complicated by delayed healing and 10% of the implants required removal (8).

It is vitally important for the hand therapist, occupational therapist, or physical therapist working with these patients not to become fixated on the flexion contractures at the PIP joints, but to work prophylactically to maintain an active arc of flexion at the MCP joints and to work on stretching the skin of the thumb-index finger web space to prevent the future development of an adduction contracture.

In our experience, flexion contractures and dorsal ulcerations of the PIP joints should be treated by arthrodesis of the PIP joints in a position of 45° to 55° (3). Bony shortening of the head of the proximal phalanx and the base of the middle phalanx allows debridement of the dorsal ulcers and will allow primary healing of these dorsal ulcers. Arthrodesis is accomplished using a combination of Kirschner pins and intraosseous wires. Bony union is usually achieved within 8 to 12 weeks. PIP joint arthrodesis effectively improves the position of the fingers for both thumb-index finger pinch and gross grasp of large objects (Figs. 28.6 and 28.7). Ninety PIP joint flexion contractures in 23 patients have undergone PIP joint arthrodeses. The subset of patients who retain flexion at the MCP joints obtain far greater improvement in hand function compared with those patients who have an associated hyperextension contracture at the MCP joint (3).

Extension or hypertension contractures with restricted flexion at the MCP joints remains the unsolved problem in reconstructive hand surgery for SSc. Capsulotomies of the MCP joints, metacarpal head resections, and silastic arthroplasties have been performed in 38 digits in eight patients, but the resultant motion at the MCP joints has been disappointing, averaging only 20°. Potentially, flexion at the MCP joints might be improved with early motion after surgery using a continuous passive motion machine.

Calcinosis

The frequency of calcinosis of the fingers ranges from 15% in patients with the diffuse cutaneous variant to 44% in patients with the limited cutaneous variant. Most patients remain asymptomatic, but occasionally these deposits ulcerate through the skin and extrude calciferous material. In a few patients, skin breakdown may lead to secondary bacterial infection of the subcutaneous tissues with chronic draining sinus tracts. Calcinosis is more common on the palmar surface of the proximal, middle, and distal phalanges of the index and long fingers and the distal phalanx of the thumb, and may interfere with pinch or fingertip sensation. These deposits do not have a uniform consistency. Around the neurovascular bundles they appear as loculated masses of whitish-gray "toothpaste-like" material. In contrast, the spicules that erode into the dermis are very hard like chalk.

Surgical excision combined with pulsed-fluid irrigation and fragmentation of the calcific deposits with a dental burr have all been described (5,21–23). In our experience of 17 patients with 32 involved digits, it has been preferable to "debulk" rather than totally excise symptomatic deposits, by using a combination of excision under loupe magnification, curettage using fine cha-

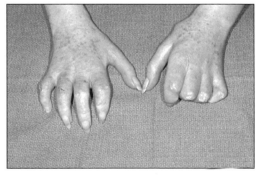

Figure 28.7. A similar patient with the diffuse cutaneous variant 6 months post-operatively after arthrodesis of the PIP joints of her right hand for dorsal ulcerations, showing complete healing and the comparison with the un-operated left hand.

lazion curettes, and saline irrigation (3). Viability of the skin flaps has not been compromised, and there have been no major problems with wound healing. In fact, paradoxically, these excisions of calcinosis have often been left open and treated with dressing changes and allowed to contract and heal by secondary intention with excellent results. "De-bulking" of calcinosis has resulted in subjective improvement both in pain relief and improved thumb-index finger pinch.

Carpal Tunnel Syndrome

With thickening of the skin and subcutaneous tissues in SSc, one might expect that SSc patients would be predisposed to develop symptoms of carpal tunnel syndrome as a result of thickening of the transverse carpal ligament or fibrosis around the flexor tendons in the carpal tunnel. Paradoxically, symptoms of numbness within the median nerve distribution in patients with SSc are relatively infrequent compared with patients with rheumatoid arthritis (24–28). Only six patients out of the total series of 70 patients with SSc have required a surgical carpal tunnel release. Interestingly, two patients developed carpal tunnel-like symptoms because of sclerodermatous involvement of the antebrachial fascia in the distal forearm proximal to the carpal tunnel. Carpal tunnel release has been effective in all symptomatic SSc patients in relieving their symptoms of numbness and paresthesiae.

Hand Surgery and Anesthesia in Systemic Sclerosis Patients

Surgical procedures involving the hands of SSc patients should be performed under general anesthesia or axillary block anesthesia (3). Axillary block is the method of choice in those patients with cardiac or pulmonary manifestations of SSc. Local anesthetic digital block should not be used because of the possibility of further ischemic embarrassment to the fingers. Intra-

venous regional anesthesia (Bier block) may be difficult, because the thickened skin over the dorsum of the hand may preclude intravenous access. All hand surgery procedures should be performed under tourniquet control after exsanguination of the extremity. The tourniquet should be deflated after amputations of gangrenous digits to assess the vascularity of the skin flaps. There has been only one complication associated with the use of the tourniquet in the 70 patients with SSc who have undergone 127 separate hand surgery procedures.

Conclusion

Reconstructive hand surgery for patients with SSc has only been reported infrequently, probably reflecting the fear that wound healing is compromised in these patients and that surgical intervention may precipitate further deterioration in the vascularity of the hand and fingers. However, based on our experience of 127 surgical procedures in 70 patients, we believe that a hand surgeon should collaborate closely with the rheumatologist in the management of SSc patients with RP, recurrent digital ulcerations and gangrene, progressive contractures of the PIP and MCP joints, and calcinosis, so that, hopefully, a gratifying improvement in hand function can be produced for the patient.

References

1. Gordon S. The hand in scleroderma. Plast Reconstr Surg 1959;23:240–244.
2. Entin M, Wilkinson RD. Scleroderma hand: A reappraisal. Orthop Clin North Am 1973;1031–1038.
3. Jones NF, Imbriglia JE, Steen VD, Medsger TA. Surgery for scleroderma of the hand. J Hand Surg 1987;12A:391.
4. Lipscomb PR, Simmons GW, Winkelmann RK. Surgery for sclerodactylia of the hand. J Bone Joint Surg Am 1969;51:112–117.
5. MacDowell F. Digital involvement of extremities in scleroderma. NY State J Med 1969;69:935–937.

6. Fries JF, Hoopes JE, Shulman LE. Reciprocal skin grafts in systemic sclerosis (scleroderma). Arthritis Rheum 1971;14:571–578.

7. Gahhos F, Ariyan S, Frazier WH, Cuono CB. Management of scleroderma finger ulcers. J Hand Surg 1984;9A:320–327.

8. Norris RW, Brown HG. The proximal interphalangeal joint in systemic sclerosis and its surgical management. Br J Plast Surg 1985;38:526–531.

9. Dabrich L, Bookstein JJ, Zweifler A, Zarafonetics CID. Digital arteries in patients with scleroderma. Arch Intern Med 1972;130:708–714.

10. Rodnan GP, Myerowitz RL, Justh GO. Morphological changes in the digital Raynaud phenomenon. Medicine 1980;59:393–408.

11. Kristensen JK. Local regulation of digital blood flow in generalized scleroderma. J Invest Dermatol 1979;72:235–240.

12. Winston EL, Pariser KM, Miller KB, Salem DN, Creager MA. Nifedipine as a therapeutic modality for Raynaud's phenomenon. Arthritis Rheum 1983;26:1177–1180.

13. Baddeley RM. The place of upper dorsal sympathectomy in the treatment of primary Raynaud's disease. Br J Surg 1965;52:426–430.

14. Flatt AE. Digital artery sympathectomy. J Hand Surg 1980;5:550–556.

15. Wilgis EFS. Evaluation and treatment of chronic digital ischemia. Ann Surg 1981;193:693–696.

16. Jones NF. Ischemia of the hand in systemic disease: The potential role of microsurgical revascularization and digital sympathectomy. Clin Plast Surg 1989;16:547–556.

17. Egloff DV, Mifsud RF, Verdan D. Superselective digital sympathectomy in Raynaud's phenomenon. Hand 1983;15:110–114.

18. O'Brien BM, Kumar PA, Mellow CG, Oliver TV. Radical microarteriolysis in the treatment of vasospastic disorders of the hand, especially scleroderma. J Hand Surg 1992;17B:447.

19. Jones NF, Raynor SC, Medsger TA. Microsurgical revascularization of the hand in scleroderma. Br J Plast Surg 1987;40:264–269.

20. Askew LJ, Beckett VL, An KN, Cho EYS. Objective evaluation of hand function in scleroderma patients to assess effectiveness of physical therapy. Br J Rheumatol 1983;22:224–232.

21. Berggren RB, Long PM, Trevaskis AE, Randall P. Calcinosis circumscripta: Report of a case involving the hands. Plast Reconstr Surg 1965;36:609–618.

22. Schlenker JD, Clark DD, Weckesser EC. Calcinosis circumscripta of the hand in scleroderma. J Bone Joint Surg Am 1973;55:1051–1056.

23. Mendelson BC, Linscheid RL, Dobyns JH, Muller SA. Surgical treatment of calcinosis cutis in the upper extremity. J Hand Surg 1977;2:318–324.

24. Quinones CA, Perry HO, Rushton JG. Carpal tunnel syndrome in dermatomyositis and scleroderma. Arch Dermatol 1966;94:20–25.

25. Lee P, Bruni J, Sukenik S. Neurological manifestations in systemic sclerosis (scleroderma). J Rheumatol 1984;11:480–483.

26. Sukenik S, Abarbanel JM, Buskila D, Potashnik G, Horowitz J. Impotence, carpal tunnel syndrome and peripheral neuropathy as presenting symptoms in progressive systemic sclerosis. J Rheumatol 1987;14(3):641–643.

27. Barr WG, Blair SJ. Carpal tunnel syndrome as the initial manifestation of scleroderma. J Hand Surg 1988;13A:378–380.

28. Machet L, Vaillant L, Machet MC, et al. Carpal tunnel syndrome and systemic sclerosis. Dermatology 1992;185:101–103.

JANET L. POOLE

29

Occupational and Physical Therapy

OCCUPATIONAL AND PHYSICAL THERAPY are health professions that provide evaluation and treatment of functional deficits and disruptions in lifestyle seen in patients who have systemic sclerosis (SSc), or scleroderma. Treatment consists of management of limited joint motion and strength, application of pain control modalities (such as heat), the provision of assistive devices/adapted equipment or alternate methods to accomplish daily tasks, and patient education. The following section describes specific therapeutic interventions used by occupational and physical therapists. Although specific data proving the efficacy of these interventions are often lacking, they represent the "state-of-the-art" and, at the very least, provide patients with some sense of control over their illness.

Range of Motion Exercises

Although SSc affects each person differently, certain joints, namely the hands and temporomandibular joints, seem more vulnerable for the development of limiting contractures. Range of motion exercises for these and other joints should be started early in the course of the disease before there is any observed loss of motion (1). The purpose of range of motion exercises is to prevent or slow down the development of joint contractures. Range of motion exercises should be performed frequently and beyond the point of initial resistance. Individuals are encouraged to maintain a position of stretch for 3 to 5 seconds, even if the skin blanches.

HAND EXERCISES

The hand has a tendency to develop a claw type of deformity with limitations in metacarpophalangeal (MCP) joint flexion, proximal interphalangeal (PIP) joint extension, and thumb flexion and abduction. Therefore, an exercise program should emphasize these motions (Table 29.1). Individuals should be encouraged to make a fist emphasizing flexion of the MCP joints. If necessary, the heel of one hand may have to press down on the dorsum of the proximal phalanges of the other hand. To encourage PIP extension, an individual can use the heel of one hand to press the fingers of the other hand flat down against a table, or place the hands and fingers flat against each other in a "prayer" position (Fig. 29.1). Another exercise for the PIP joint uses three points of pressure (Fig. 29.2). The first point of pressure is the pulp of the index finger on the volar surface of the middle phalanx of the contracted finger. The second point of pressure is the pulp of the third finger on the volar surface of the proximal phalanx of the contracted finger. The third point of pressure is the thumb against the dorsum of the contracted PIP joint. The thumb pushes against the joint while the index and middle fingers apply counter pressure to attempt to straighten the joint. To maintain thumb motion, individuals are encouraged to bend the thumb to touch the base of the little finger, and to place the

581

Table 29.1. Range of Motion/Stretching Exercises

A. Finger joints
    1. MCP flexion
        a. making a fist
        b. wearing a splint
    2. PIP extension
        a. pressing fingers flat against a table
        b. pressing fingers flat against each other
        c. using three points of pressure
        d. wearing a splint
    3. Thumb motion
        a. touching thumb to base of little finger
        b. pushing pulps of thumb and index away from
            each other
B. Temporomandibular joints
    1. exaggerated facial movements such as smiling,
        pursing lips
    2. manual stretching of mouth with fingers
    3. augmentation with tongue depressors
C. Other joints
    1. moving all joints through full range of motion
    2. retracting shoulders and neuromuscular facilita-
        tion patterns for chest expansion

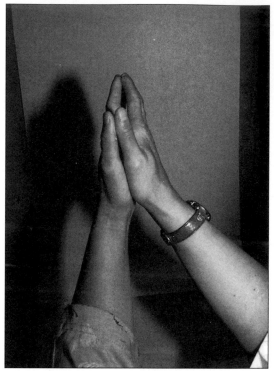

Figure 29.1. A self-administered exercise to encourage PIP joint extension. The individual presses the hands and fingers against each other in a "prayer" position.

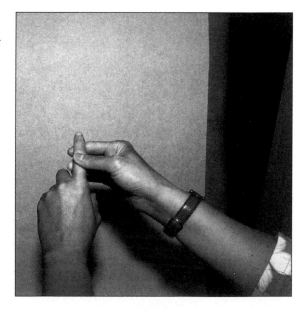

Figure 29.2. A self-administered exercise to encourage PIP joint extension. The individual places the pulp of the index finger on the volar surface of the middle phalanx, the pulp of the middle finger on the volar surface of the proximal phalanx, and the thumb against the dorsum of the contracted joint. The thumb then pushes against the joint, while the index and middle fingers apply counter pressure in an attempt to straighten the joint.

pulps of the thumb and index fingers of both hands together and push the thumbs away from the index fingers. Additional hand exercises are provided in Melvin (1). Individuals can be encouraged to monitor their own range of motion using a template. Cardboard or wood templates can be made by cutting a wedge to represent the maximum passive joint angle that can be achieved (2).

TEMPOROMANDIBULAR JOINTS

In SSc, the skin on the face becomes tight and shiny. In addition, alterations in the oral soft tissues lead to decreased oral opening, or microstomia. Three types of oral exercises are recommended for individuals with SSc to maintain mouth opening: exaggerated facial movements, manual stretching, and augmentation (3). Exaggerated facial movements include pursing the lips, puffing out the cheeks, and smiling in an exaggerated fashion. The hands can be used to stretch the oral tissues (Fig. 29.3). The right thumb is placed in the corner of the left side of the mouth, while the left thumb is placed in the corner of the right side of the mouth. The thumbs are then used to stretch the mouth laterally. Naylor, Douglass, and Mix (4) recommend

following the manual stretch exercises with oral augmentation. Oral augmentation consists of inserting tongue depressors between the teeth from the left premolar area to the right molar area (Fig. 29.4). The position is held for several seconds. Additional tongue depressors are added as motion increases. A study comparing the exaggerated facial movements to the manual stretch plus augmentation revealed that both methods increased maximum mouth opening without any temporomandibular joint dysfunction (4). Individuals with SSc can monitor their own mouth opening by using an index card to mark the distance between the upper and lower teeth. The card can be held up to the teeth while standing in front of a mirror. Exercises to stretch all facial tissue are described in Melvin (1).

OTHER JOINTS

In addition to the hand and temporomandibular joints, SSc affects other joints as well. Thus, it is recommended that individuals move all joints through full range of motion at least once a day and to concentrate on the joints that seem limited or tight. Fibrosis of the skin, along with fibrosis of intercostal muscles and internal organs, can result in decreased chest expansion. Exercises to

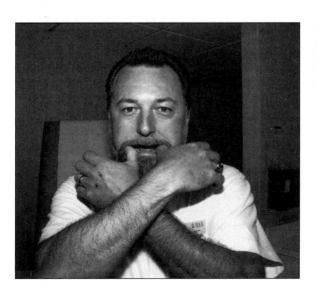

Figure 29.3. A self-administered exercise to stretch the oral aperture. The right thumb is placed in the corner of the left side of the mouth, while the left thumb is placed in the corner of the right side of the mouth. The thumbs are then used to stretch the mouth laterally.

Figure 29.4. Oral autmentation involves the insertion of a stack of tongue depressors between the teeth from the left premolar area to the right molar region. Additional tongue depressors can be added to the stack as motion increases.

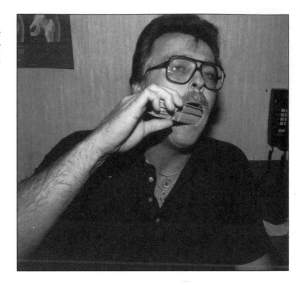

maintain motion in the chest consist of retracting the shoulders and neuromuscular facilitation patterns with an emphasis on full shoulder flexion and abduction. Good posture is also stressed.

SPLINTS

Splints are often used to maintain and/or increase range of motion. In SSc, splints have been advocated to maintain MCP flexion and/or PIP extension and to protect the skin (1). However, their use must be monitored carefully for resultant edema, decreased circulation, and skin vulnerability. Static splints, which restrict joint motion, should be used judiciously and removed on a regular basis for range of motion exercises. However, if the individual has carpal tunnel syndrome or a ruptured tendon imposed upon the SSc, then static splints would be appropriate. In some instances, static splints may be used to protect ulcers on the fingertips or dorsum of the PIP joints. Dynamic splints apply a constant force over a period of time to passively stretch a joint, and would seem to be potentially effective in elongating connective tissue. However, Seeger and Furst (5) found that over a 2-month time period, dynamic splints did not maintain or in-

crease the motion in the PIP joints in individuals with SSc. Furthermore, many of the subjects exhibited splint-exacerbated Raynaud's phenomenon (RP).

Strengthening

The proximal muscles of the pelvic girdle and shoulder are most commonly affected in SSc, and muscle mass may be lost in the vicinity of severely contracted joints (Table 29.2). Although isotonic exercise is preferred over isometric exercise, isometrics are appropriate when the individual has joint pain and/or limited joint motion. Resistance can be provided with elastic material such as theraband, theratubing, and dental dam. Exercise putty, which is available in several grades of resistance, can be used to provide resistance to the hand muscles. General conditioning exercise programs are recommended in moderation with periodic rests, because subjects with SSc have been shown to have limitations in physical capacity (6). A conditioning program should be established in collaboration with the individual's physician. Swimming in a very warm pool is an excellent aerobic conditioning exercise to maintain joint motion and endurance. Chlorine has a drying effect on the skin; therefore, the skin should be lathered with lanolin lotion after swimming.

Pain Control Modalities

Heat modalities, such as paraffin, hot packs, hydrotherapy, and fluidotherapy, may help relieve pain and inflammation, increase blood flow, and increase extensibility of collagen tissue (Table 29.3). Individuals with cardiac and respiratory instability and hypertension may not be able to tolerate the stress produced by generalized heat. Individuals with SSc should only use heat modalities under the direction of a therapist. Furthermore, care should be taken when using heat modalities in the presence of RP. A fall in local tissue temperature can occur when the heat is removed because of a transient vasoconstriction (7). Heat modalities in conjunction with friction massage and range of motion exercises were shown to increase hand function in individuals with SSc (8).

PARAFFIN BATH

A paraffin bath is a tank containing a mixture of paraffin and mineral oil. It delivers superficial conductive heat and helps soften the skin. The individual's hands are dipped in the paraffin until a glove of wax accumulates on the hand. This wax glove provides heat. The limb is wrapped in a plastic bag and then in an insulated fabric, and remains wrapped for approximately 20 minutes. Care must be taken in using paraffin because of the vascular component of SSc. For the individual with scleroderma, temperature of the bath should be within the range of 126° to 130°F (8). Some individuals who cannot tolerate this temperature range may tolerate a lower temperature. Paraffin is contraindicated for those with open sores; however, the patient can wear rubber gloves before placing the hands in the paraffin.

HOT PACKS

Hot packs, another method of superficial heat conduction, deliver moist heat to local areas. Hot packs are filled with a silica gel and are usually stored immersed in water at approximately 170°F, which is maintained by a thermostatically-controlled heater. Because each pack can retain heat for approximately 30 minutes, they are applied for 15 to 30 minutes. Hot packs must be padded with at least 6 to 8 layers of toweling (9). Electric moist heat pads are available for home use.

HYDROTHERAPY

Hydrotherapy, such as whirlpools, Hubbard tanks, therapeutic pools, warm water soaks, and hot showers, involves the use of water for therapeutic purposes. While in the water, range of motion exercises should be performed. There are many books available that describe specific exercises (10). Aquatic programs specially designed for individuals with arthritis are available at many YMCAs. Local Arthritis Foundation chapters can provide information on specific programs. Following hydrotherapy, a lanolin cream should be applied to the skin to prevent drying from chlorine (11).

Table 29.2. Strengthening Exercises

A. Isotonic exercises with or without resistance
B. General conditioning
C. Exercises in water

Table 29.3. Pain Control Modalities Used in Scleroderma

A. Heat
   1. paraffin bath
   2. hot packs
   3. hydrotherapy
   4. fluidotherapy
B. Massage
C. Biofeedback

FLUIDOTHERAPY

Fluidotherapy is a form of dry heat used to relieve pain through heat convection. The part to be treated is inserted into an airtight port in a container that holds preheated ground corn husk particles. A variable speed blower sets the materials in motion. The part is usually kept in the container for approximately 20 minutes. If the individual has open sores, the sore can be covered with an airtight dressing prior to treatment. Fluidotherapy is often contraindicated in SSc, because the patient's skin should be kept moist and well-lubricated.

MASSAGE

Massage is performed to increase circulation, increase tissue elasticity, and decrease edema. In SSc, a lanolin massage using deep kneading motion helps to preserve the integrity of the skin (8).

BIOFEEDBACK

Biofeedback has been used for temperature control to manage RP in SSc (12). This technique provides an individual with information about his or her physiological status, and can be used to influence autonomic activity. The tip of one or more fingers is attached to a temperature probe, which is connected to an electric thermometer. The probe detects the skin temperature, which is input into the thermometer. The individual concentrates on warming the hands by visualizing holding the hands over a warm fire, lying on a hot beach, etc. The information is transmitted to the cortex, to influence the limbic system, and the hypothalamus, to change the temperature of the hand (13). Finger tape temperature monitors are available for performing this technique at home.

Assistive/Adapted Devices

Assistive devices were specifically designed to aid in independent functioning, while adapted devices are commonly used tools that have been modified. Individuals with scleroderma often need devices to compensate for decreased strength, endurance, and joint limitations. However, since devices are expensive, it is important to issue devices only as necessary. Many local Arthritis Foundations, occupational therapy departments in hospitals, and hospital equipment and supply companies have access to this kind of equipment. The Arthritis Self Help Manual (14) lists many assistive and adaptive aids, and sources for purchase are listed in its Appendix.

Difficulty manipulating utensils when eating is a problem that is commonly reported by SSc patients (15, 16). Utensils are commercially available with built-up handles. Individuals can build up the handles of their own utensils by wrapping foam around the handle or purchasing tubular foam to slip over the utensil handle. Light-weight glasses with large handles, stemmed glasses, or hour-shaped glasses are easier to grasp when individuals have hand joint contractures.

The major difficulties with bathing include reaching different parts of the body and getting into and out of the bathtub. Long handled sponges help reach the back and lower extremities. For those individuals who do not have the stamina to stand when showering, numerous types of tub benches, grab bars, and hand held showers are available. A regular straight back chair can also be used in the bathtub. Soap-on-a-rope minimizes the need to manipulate the soap.

With regard to dressing, individuals with SSc have difficulty with reach and/or manipulation (16). Reachers, dressing sticks, long handled shoe horns, and sock aids compensate for a lack of reach. Button hooks can assist with buttoning, or an individual could choose to wear clothes without buttons. Slip-on shoes eliminate the need to tie shoes. However, if an individual requires more foot and/or ankle support than that which is provided by a slip-on shoe, Velcro fasteners, elastic shoelaces that stay tied, or various shoe lace locks are available.

In SSc, the likelihood of dental caries and

dental problems is increased, because patients may have Sjörgren's syndrome and microstomia. Good oral hygiene is often difficult because of the microstomia and limited hand dexterity. Electric toothbrushes, such as Interplak™, water jets, small children's toothbrushes with built-up handles, and a curved bristle toothbrush (17) can allow for more effective toothbrushing. Dental floss and toothpick holders that have large handles for easier manipulation, yet will fit into a small mouth, are commercially available. Finally, SSc patients will find it is easier to use a pump toothpaste dispenser.

Proximal weakness in the hip musculature in individuals with SSc makes it difficult for some individuals to rise from a bed, toilet, chair, or the bottom of a bathtub. A simple solution is to raise the height of the surface by placing blocks of wood under the legs of the furniture or by using chair leg extenders. In addition, a variety of raised toilet seats are commercially available, as are different types of tub benches.

Many household tasks require a degree of general strength and endurance that is limited in individuals with SSc. Opening jars, bottles, and milk cartons are commonly reported problems. Jar openers are available that can be mounted under a cupboard. Rubber grip mats, such as Dycem™, are inexpensive yet effective. Other approaches toward saving the patient's energy include use of lightweight utensils and cookware, and use of electrical appliances such as can openers, blenders, crock pots, and microwave ovens. Suctioned cutting boards that use a nail or other device to hold food, and ergonomically-designed knives make it easier and safer to chop food. Cleaning and laundry activities should be spread out during the course of a week. Family members should be encouraged to assist.

Patient Education

Patient education programs for individuals with SSc focus on joint protection, energy conservation, and precautions regarding RP.

JOINT PROTECTION

A small proportion of individuals with systemic sclerosis develop "true" arthritis (18). The purpose of joint protection is to minimize stress on the joints and reduce the possibility of infection. Individuals are encouraged to maintain their strength and range of motion, use larger joints, avoid static positioning of joints, respect pain, and avoid hitting the dorsum of the PIP joints, because that area is susceptible to skin breakdown. Protective splints of foam padding over the PIP joint may be necessary to prevent injury during household tasks. Many of the assistive devices and adapted equipment are prescribed to protect the joints. For example, raised toilet seats minimize stress to the hip and knees when arising from a sitting position, jar openers minimize torque on the hand joint, and a U-shaped or miracle vegetable peeler protects the PIP joints from injury. More detailed information about joint protection can be found in Melvin (1) and Cordery (19).

ENERGY CONSERVATION

Instruction in energy conservation is necessary because of the fatigue associated with cardiac and pulmonary involvement (6). In addition, fatigue and stress contribute to circulatory problems; therefore, the practice of energy conservation may minimize the occurrence of RP. Individuals are encouraged to plan activities to balance work and rest, pace their activities throughout the day or week, prioritize which activities are necessary, and to position their bodies in the best position for the task.

PRECAUTIONS FOR RAYNAUD'S PHENOMENON

Individuals with RP should be educated about minimizing an attack during daily living tasks. The hands should be insulated from cold during kitchen and laundry activities. Gloves or mittens should be worn when reaching into the refrigerator, freezer, freezer compartment in a grocery store, or a washing machine that had a cold water rinse. The skin should be protected from cuts, scratches, and abrasions, and it should be kept moist with lanolin cream. Gloves should be worn if strong detergents or irritating chemicals or cleansers are to be used. Individuals should be cautious when using sharp objects such as knives, scissors, and sewing needles. Gloves should be worn when working outside to protect the skin from sharp objects and bacteria.

Summary

In summary, occupational and physical therapy can be valuable resources in the management of functional deficits seen in patients with scleroderma. Assistive devices/adapted equipment, exercises, modalities, splints, and patient education can improve patients' abilities to perform daily tasks in the home, community, and work environments.

References

1. Melvin JL. Systemic sclerosis. In: Melvin JL, ed. Rheumatic disease in the adult and child: Occupational therapy and rehabilitation. Philadelphia: FA Davis Company, 1989.
2. Melvin JL, Brannan KL, LeRoy EC. Comprehensive care for the patient with systemic sclerosis (scleroderma). Clin Rheumatol Pract 1984;2:112–130.
3. Naylor WP. Oral management of the scleroderma patient. J Am Dent Assoc 1982;105:814–817.
4. Naylor WP, Douglass CW, Mix E. The nonsurgical treatment of microstomia in scleroderma: A pilot study. Oral Surg 1984;57:508–511.
5. Seeger MW, Furst DE. Effects of splinting in the treatment of hand contractures in progressive systemic sclerosis. Am J Occup Ther 1987;41:118–121.
6. Blöm-Bülow B, Jonson B, Bauer K. Factors limiting exercise performance in progressive systemic sclerosis. Semin Arthritis Rheum 1983;13:174–181.
7. Griffin JE, Karselis TC. The infrared energies. In:Griffin JE, Karselis TC, eds. Physical agents for physical therapists. Springfield, IL: Charles C Thomas, 1988.
8. Askew LJ, Beckett VL, An KN, Chao EYS. Objective evaluation of hand function in scleroderma patients to assess effectiveness of physical therapy. Br J Rheum 1983;22:224–232.
9. Hayes KW. Conductive heat. In: Hayes, KW. Manual for physical agents. Chicago: Northwestern University, 1984.
10. Stewart JB, Basmajian JF. Exercises in water. In: Basmajian JF, ed. Therapeutic exercise, 3rd ed. Baltimore: Williams and Wilkins, 1978.
11. Barnes LW. Physical therapy management of juvenile arthritis. In: Banwell BF, Gall V, eds. Physical therapy management of arthritis. New York: Churchill Livingstone, 1988.
12. Fredman RR, Ianni P, Wenig P. Behavioral treatment of Raynaud's phenomenon in scleroderma. J Behav Med 1984;7:343–353.
13. Currier DP. Electrophysiological testing and biofeedback. In: Griffin JE, Karselis TC, eds. Physical agents for physical therapists. Springfield, IL: Charles C Thomas, 1988.
14. Self-Help manual for patients with arthritis. Atlanta: The Arthritis Foundation, 1980.
15. Poole JL, Steen V. The use of the health assessment questionnaire to determine physical disability in systemic sclerosis. Arthritis Care Res 1991;4:27–31.
16. Poole JL, Williams CA, Bloch DA, Hollack B, Spitz P. Concurrent validity of the health assessment questionnaire in scleroderma. Arthritis Care Res 1995;8:189–193.
17. Williams NJ, Schuman NJ. The curved-bristle toothbrush: An aid for the handicapped population. J Dent Child 1988;55:291–293.
18. Rodnan GP, Medsger TA JR. The rheumatic manifestations of progressive systemic sclerosis (scleroderma). Clin Orthop 1968;57:81–93.
19. Cordery JC. Joint protection: A responsibility of the occupational therapist. Am J Occup Ther 1965;19:285–294.

Appendix
Resources for Devices and Modalities

EQUIPMENT FOR STRENGTHENING EXERCISES
(Theraband, Theraputty, Weights)

1. adaptAbility (catalog available for both health professionals and clients)
   PO Box 515
   Colchester, CT 06415-9978
2. Sammons
   PO Box 386
   Western Springs, IL 60558-1386
3. Enrichments
   PO Box 471
   Western Springs, IL 60558-0471
4. J.A. Preston Corp
   PO Box 89
   Jackson, MI 49204
5. The Hygenic Corporation (theraband, theratubing)
   1245 Home Ave.
   Akron, OH 44310-2575

AQUATIC PROGRAMS

1. YMCAs located through local Arthritis Foundation chapters

PARABATHS, HOT AND COLD WRAPS

1. adaptAbility
   PO Box 515
   Colchester, CT 06415-9978
2. Sammons
   PO Box 386
   Western Springs, IL 60558-1386

3. Flaghouse Rehab
   150 N. MacQuesten Parkway
   Mt. Vernon, NY 10550
4. J.A. Preston Corp
   PO Box 89
   Jackson, MI 49204

HYDROTHERAPY/AQUATIC EQUIPMENT

1. Flaghouse Rehab
   150 N. MacQuesten Parkway
   Mt. Vernon, NY 10550
2. J.A. Preston Corp
   PO Box 89
   Jackson, MI 49204
3. Aqua-Source International
   4538 NW 50th Street
   Oklahoma, OK 73122

BIOFEEDBACK

1. Lafayette Instrument
   PO Box 5729
   3700 Sagamore Parkway N.
   Lafayette, IN 47903
2. Complete Medical Products
   2052 N. Decatur Road
   Decatur, GA 30033

FLUIDOTHERAPY

1. Henley Healthcare
   104 Industrial Boulevard
   Sugar Land, TX 77478

ASSISTIVE DEVICES/ADAPTED
EQUIPMENT FOR EATING, DRESSING,
GRIPPING, BATHING, TOILETING,
HOMEMAKING, LEISURE, AND
AMBULATION

1. adaptAbility
   PO Box 515
   Colchester, CT 06415-9978
2. Sammons
   PO Box 386
   Western Springs, IL 60558-1386
3. Enrichments (for clients)
   PO Box 471
   Western Springs, IL 60558-0471
4. J.A. Preston Corp
   PO Box 89
   Jackson, MI 49204
5. Maddak, Inc.
   Pequannock, NJ 07440-1994
6. Cleo Living Aids
   3957 Mayfield Road
   Cleveland, OH 44121
7. North Coast Medical, INC
   187 Stauffer Boulevard
   San Jose, CA 95125
8. Lumex (benches and bars for tubs and toilets)
   100 Spence St.
   Bay Shore, NY 11706-2290
9. Self-Help Manual for Patients with Arthritis
   (illustrates and lists sources for equipment)
   Available from: The Arthritis Foundation
   3400 Peachtree Road NE
   Atlanta, GA 30326
10. Occupational and Physical Therapy Departments at local hospitals

ASSISTIVE DEVICES/ADAPTED
EQUIPMENT FOR ORAL HYGIENE

1. Sammons (toothbrushes and floss aids)
   PO Box 386
   Western Springs, IL 60558-1386
2. Maddak, Inc. (toothbrushes and floss aids)
   Pequannock, NJ 07440-1994
3. General Electric Co. (electric toothbrushes)
   Housewares Division
   2185 Boston Ave.
   Bridgeport, CT 06602
4. Teledyne Waterpik
   1730 East Prospect St.
   Ft. Collins, CO 80521

SPLINTS

1. Contact local occupational therapy departments

PATIENT EDUCATION MATERIALS

1. Arthritis Foundation
   3400 Peachtree Road, NE
   Atlanta, GA 30326
2. United Scleroderma Foundation, INC
   PO Box 350
   Watsonville, CA 95077
3. Scleroderma Federation
   1725 York Avenue, 29F
   New York, NY 10128
4. Occupational and Physical Therapy Departments at local hospitals

30

Treatment of Organ System Involvements

THE AUTHORS of Chapter 4 (*Localized Scleroderma*) and chapters in *Section III: Organ Involvement* present their specific approaches to treatment of organ involvement in systemic sclerosis.

Personal Management of Patients with Localized Scleroderma

Joan Guitart, Giuseppe Micali, Lawrence M. Solomon

The treatment of scleroderma in its localized forms has really not been very successful, no matter what has been tried. One of the reasons is the lack of controlled studies. This lack results from the difficulty in determining what parameters identify early morphea from fully developed morphea, as well as those which distinguish developing from resolving morphea. Under these circumstances, it is probably best to delay and observe most cases of morphea in the hope that spontaneous resolution will occur. This should be emphasized in the childhood types. Numerous treatments from potassium paraaminobenzoic acid (POTABA) through penicillamine and photopheresis have been suggested. There is a lack of convincing evidence for the efficacy of these approaches in resolving the lesions beyond that which occurs spontaneously.

If a localized patch of morphea appears to be progressing, it is not unreasonable to try small injections of triamcinolone acetonide 10 mg/cc at the periphery or an advancing edge of the lesion, because that is the site of active inflammation. A total of 5 mg of triamcinolone solution may be used in two or three sites. A useful device to initiate resolution has been used by one of the authors (Solomon LM, anecdotal information). This device consists of a small adhesive bandage with a tiny drop of potent steroid placed in the center of the bandage and applied to the middle of the lesion. Unfortunately, adhesive bandages will often tear superficial epidermis, and one must be careful not to use additional adhesives that are strongly adherent and may induce a small ulcer. The bandages are changed daily over a period of several weeks to a month. Appearance of a superficial ulcer in the middle of the lesion indicates the need to stop treatment. This treatment has a built-in control for efficacy, because one can evaluate the treated area against the rest of the lesions.

Physical therapy for individuals with large area involvement is necessary as an adjunct to help maintain appropriate motion and to avoid contractures. Joint contractures may occur in spite of all efforts, and limb shrinkage may also occur no matter what one does to avoid it. Under these circumstances, it may be appropriate to use surgical techniques to release contracted limbs None of the benefits attributed to liposuction autotransfer have been personally observed. A surgical approach is probably the best solution when large areas of morphea (linear, or otherwise) involve the joints.

Children and adults should engage in vigorous swimming every day. It appears to be the most beneficial form of exercise, allowing the limbs to extend themselves under the least weight-bearing load.

Morphea is a disease, or diseases, of mystery. It probably results from more than one cause, assumes multiple forms, and has an unpredictable outcome. Because of these variables, most patients must await resolution of the disorder without treatment.

Organ Involvement: Sjögren's Syndrome

Pierre Youinou, Yvon-Louis Pennec

Drugs available for treatment are far from "ideal" therapeutic agents because none of them are curative. Currently, the treatment is essentially symptomatic. Treatment of the ocular component is practically based upon the use of artifical tears (methylcellulose and polyvinyl alcohol solutions). Commercial tears are plentiful, differing in viscosity and preservatives. Clearly, the patient has to test several preparations to determine which is the best for her/him, because the acceptance of these artifical tears is widely variable. The patient's subjective response remains the one and only guideline. Tear substitutes have to be applied frequently (i.e., 4 to 6 times a day). Healon™ (1% hyaluronic acid solution in BSS, Pharmacia, France) may be of value to improve 80% of severe eye symptoms, but it is expensive ($200 per month, French). Ointments and oil-based drugs are contraindicated in dry eyes, except at night when the blink is suppressed. When tear substitutes do not provide satisfactory relief, efforts to preserve exiting tears may be of some benefit. The goggle-type treatments (i.e., swim goggles) lack social acceptability and are infrequently used in practice. Punctal occlusion with silicone plugs (and eventual cautery) is becoming a convenient form of treatment.

Treatment for dry mouth is aimed at relieving its symptoms, and simple advice to take frequent small drinks and mouthwashes may be sufficient for mild symptoms. In our experience, the topical application of artifical salivary compounds has no advantage when compared to water. Some patients favor the use of sweets to stimulate salivation; this practice should be discouraged because the risk of dental caries is increased in Sjögren's (sicca) sydrome. The use, however, of sugarless chewing gum and sugarless lemon drops may be encouraged. Regular dental assessment is strongly advised. Prevention of periodontal problems can be achieved by using detergent-free toothpastes and regular application of topical fluoride. In our experience, potassium iodine, parasympathetic agents (i.e., pilocarpine or neostigmine), bromhexine, and trithioparamethoxyphenylpropene do little to affect mouth dryness. In an open study, we found that diosamine (500 mg 2 times a day) reduces the complaint of dryness of the mouth and increases whole salivary flow in 60% of patients. In our hands, electrostimulation is not effective in stimulating production of saliva and reducing the symptoms.

For parotid gland enlargement, we first use non-steroidal anti-inflammatory drugs (NSAIDS) and, occasionally, low-dose corticosteroids when NSAIDS are ineffectual in relieving symptoms. Low-dose corticosteroids may also be useful in patients complaining of arthritis. We do not use anti-malarial or other immunosuppressive drugs, such as cyclophosphamide, gold, or penicillamine, for sicca symptoms or parotid enlargement. Our own belief is that these drugs are ineffective in patients with severe systemic disease.

Organ Involvement: Pulmonary

Carol M. Black, Ron M. du Bois

THE INITIAL EVALUATION

Our algorithm for evaluation and management of SSc patients with possible/verified lung involvement is illustrated in Figure 30.1. A full history and examination are central to an effective management strategy with particular regard to excluding factors, such as previous drug history, current infection, and occupational histories, which could confound the interpretation of the other investigations. Chest radiography is also used as an initial screen to detect diffuse lung disease and also to detect the possibility of secondary infection or aspiration because of esophageal abnormalities. Lung function tests can be discriminatory. A normal set of lung function tests, particularly on exercise, can exclude a diagnosis of

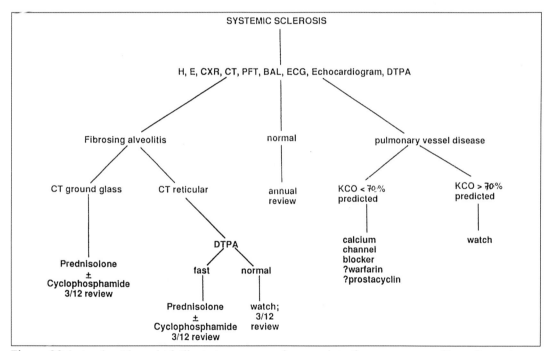

Figure 30.1. An algorithm which illustrates our general approach to the management of lung disease in systemic sclerosis.

H   = history
E   = examination
CxR   = chest radiography
PFT   = pulmonary function tests
BAL   = bronchoalveolar lavage
ECG   = electrocardiogram
DTPA   = clearance of [99]technetium-labelled diethyline triamine pentacetate
CT   = high resolution computed tomography
KCO   = gas transfer corrected for alveolar volume

diffuse lung disease. Lung function tests that show normal volumes but reduced gas transfer in the face of normal imaging are suggestive of pure vessel disease. The most common finding in patients with fibrosing alveolitis and scleroderma is a restrictive ventilatory defect indicating interstitial inflammation and fibrosis. Bronchoalveolar lavage (BAL) is useful in confirming the neutrophil alveolitis associated with fibrosing alveolitis. Occasionally, an excess of lymphocytes is found, and this may indicate (by comparison with data from cryptogenic fibrosing alveolitis) that corticosteroids alone may be effective therapy.

ECG and echocardiogram are performed to exclude primary cardiac disease, which can be part of the scleroderma process, and also to gauge the effect of the lung disease on right heart function.

If these preliminary investigations reveal lung disease, we use high resolution computed tomography (HRCT), diethyline triamine pentacetate (DTPA), and lung function studies (together with BAL, as outlined above) to guide our approach to treatment.

FIBROSING ALVEOLITIS

If the first line of investigations indicate that the patient has fibrosing alveolitis (see Fig. 30.1), and if the HRCT pattern suggests that there is ground glass opacification, patients are treated with low dosage prednisolone at 20 mg every other day together with cyclophosphamide up to 125 mg per day for 3 months, following which they are reviewed.

Major problems with cyclophosphamide therapy include bone marrow toxicity, hemorrhagic cystitis, hair loss, liver dysfunction, and anovulation, which can be irreversible. These are all *potential* problems from which many patients do not suffer. For a female of childbearing years, however, careful counseling is needed before cyclophosphamide therapy is contemplated. Azathioprine, in a dosage of up to 150 mg per day (at 2.5 mg per kg), and low dose prednisolone (20 mg on alternate days) is an alternative approach which can be considered (but has been used less extensively) following a 3 month induction phase with cyclophosphamide. Blood counts need to be monitored weekly for 4 weeks following the institution of immunosuppressive therapy, and then monthly thereafter, together with liver function tests. Patients are advised to report any hint of infection early so that appropriate investigations can be undertaken. This may include bronchoscopy and BAL to identify opportunistic infections if a patient presents with fever and no clear cause.

In the group of patients whose HRCT suggests a predominantly reticular pattern indicative of predominantly fibrotic disease, we use DTPA in its predictive role (Fig. 30.1). If DTPA is fast, the patient is in the group whose disease is more likely to progress. If DTPA is normal, an expectant policy can be followed. In the rapid clearance group, treatment is the same as for those in the "ground glass" group.

High dosage prednisolone (1 mg/kg/day) is often used as first line treatment in the isolated form of fibrosing alveolitis and is known to be particularly efficacious in treating patients with high numbers of lymphocytes in BAL fluid. This is not a recommended strategy in scleroderma, because patients with diffuse disease are more likely to undergo renal crisis on prednisolone. Similar comments apply to the use of cyclosporin A, for which there are observational data to suggest that it can benefit some patients with isolated fibrosing alveolitis and fibrosing alveolitis in scleroderma. In scleroderma, however, there is a risk of causing renal dysfunction in patients already at risk of this complication from the disease itself.

There is little evidence to support the role for therapy, such as penicillamine, to treat fibrosing lung disease. This, in common with all of the treatments used to treat fibrosing alveolitis in scleroderma, must become the subject of prospective controlled studies, which need to be multicenter and must be undertaken in the near future so that full outcome measures can be evaluated properly.

NO EVIDENCE OF LUNG DISEASE

If first line investigations are completely normal, patients should be reviewed every 6 months to detect the first hint of a disease process which may require further attention. All of the tests that are used for first line of investigation are repeated, except for HRCT, DTPA, and BAL, unless there are positive indications to undertake these. These indications would include evidence of deterioration from other indices when these tests can be helpful for the reasons outlined above.

If tests are normal at the second review, then further investigation is annual and includes HRCT and DTPA, but lavage is only repeated if there is doubt about disease activity. Annual review should continue for a minimum of 5 years, but could lengthen to biannual thereafter if there is no evidence of progression.

PULMONARY VESSEL DISEASE

If the first line of investigations suggests pulmonary vessel disease (normal imaging, relatively normal lung volumes with disproportionately reduced gas transfer measurement), guidelines are less clear because little is known about measures that can improve outcome (see Fig. 30.1). We know, however, that patients whose gas transfer is less than 50% normal have a much poorer prognosis than those whose gas transfer is above this cut off. If gas transfer is reduced to 25% of normal, the likelihood of surviving more than 1 year is low.

Therefore, we recommend the use of a cut off of gas transfer measurement corrected for alveolar volume (KCO) of 70% as being indicative of already established vessel disease, the progression of which needs to be arrested. If KCO is less than 70% predicted, we would recommend the introduction of a calcium channel blocker (see Fig. 30.1). Nifedipine has been shown to be of use in short-term studies, and there are suggestions from other studies that long-term benefit may accrue from its use. There have been no definitive studies which show that survival has been im-

proved. In addition, consideration needs to be given to the introduction of anticoagulants. In patients with primary pulmonary hypertension, a survival advantage is gained by those on anticoagulants. The pattern of disease in primary pulmonary hypertension is similar to that in scleroderma, and it is possible that warfarin may benefit patients in the same way. We would recommend that they be considered in individual patients but, again, the value and outcome measures of warfarin treatment need to be the subject of a controlled study. In a similar vein, the use of prostacyclin (iloprost) as a vasodilator is now well established in peripheral vessel disease in scleroderma. There are good theoretical reasons why it might benefit the pulmonary vasculature, and this therapy should be considered in selected patients. If KCO is greater than 70% predicted, we would counsel an expectant policy.

ASSESSMENT OF RESPONSE

This can be the most difficult aspect of management. Diseases that progress slowly are likely to improve slowly. Furthermore, diseases that cause irreversible fibrosis and injury can often not be improved by therapy, and the best that can be expected is an arrest of decline. If that decline has been gradual, it will take a period of many months to determine with any certainty that benefit has been obtained. The decision-making is made easier if there has been a period of observation which shows a definite decline prior to the institution of therapy, and of course the situation is obvious if significant improvement is obtained in pulmonary function indices (greater than 10%) following therapy.

There is a similar paucity of information about how long one should continue therapy, particularly with immunosuppression. It is our policy to continue for at least 1 year before making a decision about efficacy. If improvement has occurred, then therapy is continued until that improvement has plateaued. If disease becomes or remains stable, consideration is given to withdrawing treatment gradually, but there are no clear-cut algorithms for this. We adopt an individualized approach, which takes into account factors such as disease severity, patient age, and patient attitude to continuing treatment. In general, we continue treatment for roughly 3 years before contemplating a reduction. It must be emphasized, however, that there are no evaluative studies to provide unequivocal evidence that this is the most effective strategy.

With regard to prednisolone, it is our practice not to reduce dosage below 10 mg on alternate days particularly if there has been some improvement. In interstitial disease, observational evidence suggests that discontinuation of corticosteroids can provoke a rebound activation of pulmonary inflammation and fibrosis, which can then be very difficult to control. If patients fail to respond or continue to deteriorate on first-line treatment, consideration is given to a combination of the same low dose prednisolone regimen together with azathioprine at 2.5 mg/kg to a maximum of 150 mg/day.

There are no data about length of treatment with calcium channel blockers or anticoagulation. Once a decision has been made to start these therapies, it is generally for life.

Organ Involvement: Cardiac

William P. Follansbee

The treatment of cardiac involvement in SSc is currently symptomatic and largely empiric. Specific therapies have not yet been demonstrated to prevent or modify the course of myocardial fibrosis, the hallmark of myocardial involvement. As reviewed in the chapter on cardiac involvement, there is a substantial body of evidence to indicate that the coronary vascular system is centrally involved in the pathogenesis of myocardial fibrosis. There appears to be at least some component of small artery coronary vasospasm contributing to the vascular pathology. Based upon results of thallium perfusion studies in particular, there may be a role for vasodilator therapy in the treatment of myocardial disease. Calcium channel blockers, especially the dihydropyridines nifedipine and nicardipine, may be of benefit in preserving myocardial perfusion. Empiric treatment with these agents is reasonable, particularly in the individual patient who has demonstrated thallium perfusion defects which resolve with calcium channel blockade.

Angiotensin converting enzyme (ACE) inhibitors have well demonstrated efficacy in the treatment of SSc renal crisis, a complication with a clear vasospastic component which previously was virtually universally fatal. This writer has seen an individual patient who had advanced myocardial involvement, including repeated life-threatening episodes of acute pulmonary edema, who dramatically responded to ACE inhibition therapy with an increase in ejection fraction from 21% to 45% and complete resolution of symptoms. She did not have significant renal involvement or systemic hypertension, and had a completely normal coronary angiogram. The patient remained stable on ACE inhibition therapy over 6 years, except when she decreased her medication for financial reasons, at which time her ejection fraction again fell precipitously. The findings from this case suggested the presence of angiotensin-mediated coronary vasospasm with resulting ischemic biventricular myocardial dysfunction that resolved with ACE inhibition. Based upon this experience and the demonstrated efficacy of ACE inhibition in renal crisis, this author considers ACE inhibition to be the initial vasodilator of choice in the treatment of myocardial scleroderma.

The primary effect of nitrates on the coronary arteries is on the proximal R1 vessels, which do not appear to be predisposed to vasospasm in

SSc. Nitrates have very little effect on the small arteries (the R2 vessels). Acccordingly, there is unlikely to be a useful role for nitrate therapy in the treatment of these patients.

Beyond vasodilator therapy, the treatment of myocardial dysfunction in SSc is similar to other patients with congestive heart failure, and includes diuretics and probably digoxin therapy. Caution with both of these is warranted, however. Patients with myocardial involvement appear to be predisposed to development of renal failure; diuretics may exacerbate this risk. Diuretics can be used on a symptomatic basis, but it is essential that renal function be closely monitored. Similarly, patients with conduction system disease may be at risk of developing high grade heart block or other manifestations of digoxin toxicity. Monitoring of digoxin levels is also important in patients treated with this agent.

For SSc patients with evidence of skeletal and myocardial muscle disease, particularly those with elevated creatine phosphokinase (CPK), it is reasonable to treat with corticosteroids in sufficient dose to normalize the CPK. The efficacy of this therapy in preventing progression of myocardial involvement is unknown. Because of the suggestion that there may be a vasospastic component to the "myocarditis," aggressive treatment with vasodilators is also reasonable. Other than in patients with active "myocarditis," however, there is no likely role for corticosteroid treatment for any of the other cardiac manifestations of scleroderma, with the possible exception of short-term therapy of refractory pericarditis. Indeed, corticosteroids may predispose to the development of premature coronary atherosclerosis and renal crisis.

Pericardial effusion should be treated with diuretics only with considerable caution for two reasons. First, in the patient with a hemodynamically significant effusion, diuretics may result in a substantial decline in cardiac output, because it is heavily dependent upon ventricular filling pressures. Second, diuresis of patients with pericardial effusion may predispose to the development of renal failure. Non-steroidal anti-inflammatory agents may be tried in the patient with pericardial effusion or symptoms of acute pericarditis. Because of the potential risk of malignant arrhythmias, the patient with acute pericarditis is probably best followed on a cardiac monitor during initial treatment. For the patient with hemodynamically significant pericardial effusion, pericardiocentesis is the treatment of choice.

The treatment of arrhythmias in SSc, as in most other contexts, remains empiric. Treatment should be restricted to symptomatic arrhythmias. In patients with palpitations, particularly those with atrial ectopy or those with isolated premature ventricular contractions, treatment with beta blockade is often symptomatically beneficial and is usually surprisingly well tolerated. However, the potential for beta blockers to worsen Raynaud's phenomenon, pulmonary disease, or heart failure is significant, so these patients need to be followed particuarly closely. Nevertheless, this writer's experience has been that even patients with significant myocardial involvement often tolerate beta blockers very well with considerable symptomatic improvement. Criteria for use of type 1 (for example, quinidine or procainamide) or type 3 (such as encanide or flecanide) antiarrhythmic agents for treatment of arrhythmias in SSc patients are similar to those in other patient populations. The potential toxicity and proarrhythmic effect of these agents is significant, particularly in patients with myocardial dysfunction, so their use should be restricted to patients with either refractory supraventricular tachyarrhythmias or potentially life-threatening ventricular arrhythmias. Because of its pulmonary toxicity, amiodarone is not a desirable agent to use in treating SSc patients. For patients with high risk of malignant arrhythmias, invasive electrophysiology studies should be considered.

The indications for cardiac pacemaker in SSc patients are the same as in other patient groups.

Organ Involvement: Peripheral Vascular

Hildegard R. Maricq, Edwin A. Smith

Nearly all SSc patients have symptoms and physical problems due to Raynaud's phenomenon (RP) as a result of the underlying vascular abnormality of this connective tissue disease. These difficultires range from pain, numbness, and tingling associated with RP attacks to loss of digits, hands, or feet as a result of ischemic necrosis.

GENERAL SUGGESTIONS TO ALL PATIENTS WITH RAYNAUD'S PHENOMENON

Prevention of the normal vasoconstrictive response to body cooling is the first line of defense against RP. Avoidance of cool temperatures is obvious, and modifications of both behavior and environment are necessary, though they may be difficult. Although patients who have moved from cold to warmer areas claim a reduction in attack frequency, there is no need to recommend moving to areas with warmer climates. Indeed, air conditioning often constitutes as much of a stimulus for attacks as do cold outside temperatures. Patients with RP often have great difficulty in the spring and summer months as a result of the swings in ambient temperature associated with conditioned air, particularly in grocery stores where there are often open, chest-type freezers.

Care must be taken to retain core body heat. Thus, patients should be told to dress warmly overall rather than simply protecting extremities. A particularly troublesome period is just after exiting the bath or shower when evaporative cooling causes rapid heat loss. The avoidance of outdoors on extremely cold days is prudent, but if outdoor activities cannot be avoided, dressing in multiple layers with insulating clothing (wool, down, etc.) is advisable. Mittens provide better protection than do gloves, and battery operated, resistance heated gloves and socks are recommended.

Some drugs which can exacerbate RP are to be avoided. The β-blockers are able to worsen RP by causing unopposed α-adrenergic effects. Caffeine, nicotine, pseudoephedrine (and other vasoconstrictors commonly used to reduce nasal congestion), and cocaine can cause worsening of RP.

Behavioral therapy with finger temperature biofeedback may help reduce frequency or severity of attacks. Although this is felt to be more effective in primary than in secondary RP, definitive studies are lacking.

TREATMENT OF MILD SYMPTOMS

When symptoms are limited to numbness, some moderate pain, and/or tingling on cold exposure, no measures other than those mentioned above may be necessary. The use of calcium channel blockade is reasonable as the environment cools in the fall or travel to a cooler environment is anticipated. A delayed release or extended half-life calcium channel blocker is most useful. Only the form of nifedipine that requires frequent (q.i.d.) dosing has been subjected to formal trials in SSc patients, but many individuals taking this form have significant side-effects of light-headedness, headache, dizziness, or leg swelling. For that reason, the delayed release form of nifedipine (Procardia XL™ or Adalat CC™) is a more useful formulation of the drug. This can be given on a once-a-day basis, and should be started at 30mg/day. Titration of the dose by 30 mg intervals, as tolerated, may be necessary to bring the RP under acceptable control. A newer calcium channel blocker, amlodipine (Norvasc™), is very closely related to nifedipine chemically but has a prolonged biological half-life so that it can be administered on a daily basis. This medication is given at 5 or 10 mg per day. Other calcium channel blockers are not as effective. Some, but not all, calcium channel blockers (i.e., nifedipine but not diltiazen) in SSc patients are capable of inhibiting alimentary smooth muscle contractility and thereby increasing esophageal reflux and/or delaying peristalsis in the stomach or gut.

TREATMENT OF MODERATE SYMPTOMS

Other pharmacologic therapies can be added to calcium channel blockade when the frequency or severity of symptoms has not been brought under satisfactory control. Because platelet activation has been demonstrated to occur *in vivo* in SSc patients, platelet inhibition is used (although it has not been well studied) to treat RP. Patients are started on low dose aspirin, such as a baby aspirin, or an 81 mg extended-release aspirin, such as that prescribed to individuals with coronary disease for prevention of second myocardial infarctions. Dipyridamole (Persantine™) is initiated at 50 mg orally t.i.d. and titrated up to 100 mg q.i.d. as the patient is able to tolerate the symptoms of flushing and headache, which often accompany administration of this drug.

Other vasodilating drugs can be substituted for calcium channel blockers, or used in addition to the drugs mentioned above, when symptoms are more severe. The α-adrenergic blockers prazosin (Minipress™, 1 to 10 mg b.i.d.) or the longer-acting terazosin (Hytrin™, 1 to 20 mg q.d.) are often useful for additional or substitute therapy when calcium channel blockers alone have not been adequately effective.

TREATMENT OF SEVERE SYMPTOMS

When symptoms are incapacitating to the degree that individuals cannot live without great inconvenience, and particularly when there are digital ulcers which are or are likely to be infected or ischemic changes are threatening the viability of digits, all means in the armamentarium should be brought to bear. Patients should be restricted to warm environments, either at home or in the hospital, if the evidence of ischemia leading to gangrene warrants such treatment. Ambient temperature should be maintained at or above 85°F (29.4°C). Immersion of hands in water only as cool as room temperature should be avoided because of the great thermal conductivity of water. If the hands are wet, immediate drying should be undertaken to avoid cooling by evaporation of heat.

Additional pharmacological treatment is also undertaken. The addition of the drug pentoxyphylline (Trental™) (400 mg t.i.d.), which increases the deformability of erythrocytes, may help perfusion. Nitroglycerin paste should be applied at the bases of the most affected digits, along the radial and ulnar sides where the digital arteries lie. An amount of the paste that is small enough not to reduce the systemic pressure should be found. Patients can determine this amount by keeping the dose lower than that which induces vascular headache. Oral narcotic analgesics, such as acetaminophen with codeine or oxycodon or morphine or meperidine given parenterally, may alleviate the pain associated with severe attacks and have the additional benefit of being vasodilating. Because there is a risk of dependence, these drugs should be prescribed in only the most severe cases, but it is important to remember that pain is itself a vasoconstricting stimulus and should therefore be treated. The pain associated with ischemia and gangrene should not be underestimated, and the use of a patient controlled analgesic pump should be considered.

The use of stellate ganglion blockade to bring about temporary sympathectomy can greatly alleviate pain and induce vasodilation, as indicated by an immediate rise in finger temperature. A similar and longer lasting result can be obtained with the use of cervical epidural catheters through which is pumped a mixture of a narcotic analgesis, such as fentanyl, and a local anesthetic, such as bupivicaine. This can provide considerable relief of the acute pain associated with ischemia as well as considerable vasodilation.

When there is frank infection of a digital ulcer, the use of a local means of cleansing is imperative. The application of "wet-to-dry" gauze dressings can help to debride the most necrotic tissue. When this has been accomplished, the application of an antibacterial ointment, such as bacitracin, can be helpful. Sometimes the infection is so severe as to require systemic antibiotics, which should be selected to provide optimal treatment for *Staphylococcus aureas.* Oral dicloxacillin or cephalexin are both adequate and relatively inexpensive. Occasionally, the infection is so rapidly progressive or has advanced to the point of having associated osteomyelitis that therapy with parenteral nafcillin or a first generation cephalosporin is indicated.

Surgical therapy has been applied to the treatment of RP. While sympathectomy has been felt to reduce attack frequency and severity for a short time following the operation, there is often a recurrence of symptoms within 6 months. This is therefore not recommended. Selective sympathectomy of digital arteries, first performed by Flatt in 1980, has been advocated to treat RP. This surgical therapy has been applied to RP in scleroderma patients by Jones and O'Brien. In the latter series, digital sympathectomy in 11 scleroderma patients was reported to have resulted in relief of pain and ulceration. After a 1-year follow-up, mild recurrence of small ulcers was seen in four patients. In the authors' limited experience (two patients), the results have been disappointing and, therefore, we cannot recommend this expensive procedure. Jones et al feel, on the other hand, that this procedure may be beneficial. For further discussion by Jones of this procedure, see Chapter 28, *Surgical Approach to Hand Involvement.*

Amputation of a phalanx or digit is an alternative that can quickly relieve pain and is sometimes the most effective means of dealing with infection. Healing is always a problem in SSc patients even after amputation. The amputation may also result in the removal of more of the digit than may be salvaged by medical treatment, when effective.

Since drug treatments are often associated with side effects, other treatment forms have been proposed, such as hand warming procedures. Another non-drug therapy for RP, biofeedback treatment, is not believed to be effective in SSc even by those advocating it for primary RP.

In a few cases in which ulnar or radial artery occlusion was found associated with RP, microsurgical repair was found beneficial (see Chapter 28, *Surgical Approach to Hand Involvement*).

Organ Involvement: Skin

Philip J. Clements, Thomas A. Medsger, Jr.

DISEASE MODIFYING THERAPIES (DMARDS)

Currently, there are no therapies which have been shown conclusively to alter the natural history of SSc skin disease. While we patiently await the results of the needed randomized, blinded, controlled trials addressing this question, what do we recommend for the management of SSc skin disease? Both of the co-authors have presented data suggesting that one or more currently available medications might be efficacious: D-penicillamine (TAM, Jr) and cyclosporin A (PJC). Other possible beneficial agents have also been proposed.

We have adopted the following basic approach:

1. *Determine if DMARD treatment should be initiated.* The best patient candidates are those in whom there is potential reversibility of skin sclerosis, i.e., early diffuse disease before the peak of skin thickening or late diffuse disease with recent progression of skin thickening (see Fig. 3.2), and those in whom there is the potential, and the need, to prevent or to ameliorate visceral disease and to improve survival.

2. *Educate the patient and family.* The patient and family should understand which subtype and stage of disease is present and what the risks

are for the skin and other organ systems, and for morbidity and mortality if untreated.

3. *Be aggressive if treatment is indicated. Choose one of four options.*

   a) Encourage the patient to enter into an ongoing placebo-controlled experimental trial if one is available and the patient satisfies eligibility criteria.

   b) If the pace of skin thickening is average or slow, begin D-penicillamine:

     i) 250 mg/day on an empty stomach;

     ii) Increase the dose by 250 mg/day every 6 weeks (if disease pace is more rapid) or every 12 weeks (if the disease pace is slower) to a maximum of 1000 to 1500 mg/day;

     iii) When maximum skin improvement has been reached, reduce the dose by 250 mg/day every 6 months to a maintenance dose of 250 mg/day;

     iv) Continue 250 mg/day for a minimum of 5 years after initial onset of skin thickening before considering discontinuation.

   c) If the pace of skin thickening is rapid, begin cyclosporin A or both cyclosporin A and D-penicillamine with the intention of discontinuing cyclosporin A if the pace slows or the peak of skin thickening is reached and passed. Cyclosporin is prescribed only if blood pressure and renal function are normal, and the patient should not be taking NSAIDs or diuretic drugs. The starting dose is 2.0 mg/kg/day, increasing by 0.5 to 1.0 mg/kg/day every 4 weeks to a maximum of 4.5 to 5.0 mg/kg/day, given in two doses/day 12 hours apart. If the serum creatinine increases by 30% or more over the baseline pre-therapy value, or if the blood pressure increases by >20 mm Hg systolic, the dose should be reduced to 1.0 mg/kg/day or cyclosporin A discontinued until these values return to normal or near normal.

   d) Choose another DMARD treatment, outside a formal protocol. Several possibilities include:

     i) Methotrexate, beginning at 7.5 mg/week and increasing to 15 to 20 mg/week as tolerated;

     ii) Apheresis, preferably lymphoplasmapheresis, 3 times/week for 2 weeks, 2 times/week for 2 weeks, and then once per week for 10 weeks (total 20 weeks).

4. *Follow the patient closely.* A physical examination, including skin score or equivalent, should be performed every 6 to 12 weeks. Laboratory toxicity monitoring should be completed, as appropriate, for the DMARD being used. Studies to evaluate SSc disease status should be done if indicated by clinical symptoms. Even if there are no complaints or physical findings, the predicted forced vital capacity (FVC) should be performed every 6 months for the first 2 years, and the left ventricular ejection fraction (EF) annually for the first 2 years.

LOCAL THERAPY FOR SKIN INVOLVEMENT

Dryness

Whether sclerodermatous skin is edematous, indurated, or atrophic, it is dry because normal sebaceous glands are "choked out" by excessive connective tissue. Excessive bathing and hand-washing should be discouraged. Preparations with high concentrations of glycerine and lanolin are reported by patients to be most effective in relieving dryness, provided they are thoroughly rubbed into affected skin to maximize penetration. These preparations include: Vaseline Intensive Care Lotion™, Neutrogena Norwegian Formula™, Carmol-10™, Nivea™, Vaseline Petroleum Jelly™, vitamin-E based skin care products (which are all oily from the vitamin E), Alpha-Keri™ Lotion and Bath Oil, etc. These preparations should be applied several times a day and particularly after bathing or after spa/swimming.

Pruritus

Early in diffuse cutaneous SSc, the involved skin is often intensely pruritic. The use of oatmeal-based cleanser bars/bath flakes (i.e., Aveeno™) can reduce loss of natural skin oils which occur with use of regular soap (leading to dryness and itching) and leave a soothing invisible anti-pruritic oatmeal layer on the skin. Systemic anti-pruritics can be tried (i.e., diphenhydramine, hydroxyzine, Temaril™, Periactin™). In some instances, a 2-week course of systemic oral corticosteroids or a brief (14-day) course of topical fluoride-based steroid, Temavate™, applied twice daily in the early edematous/indurative phase of skin thickening may break the itch cycle. Pruritus virtually always ceases later in the disease, and, in fact, its disappearance is a good prognostic sign that skin involvement in a given area will not progress further.

Ulcerations

Digital tip ulcerations, paronychiae, and periungual skin cracks are the results of vascular ischemia. It is important to make sure that large arteries are intact (i.e. ulnar artery in the forearm and hand). If not, consideration must be given to microsurgical bypass procedures. If no evidence of arterial disease is present, therapeutic measures should be directed at improving local circulation, including increased trunk clothing, higher ambient temperatures, and vasodilators (see Chapter 17, *Organ Involvement: Peripheral Vascular*). Other extremity ulcers tend to occur over pressure points (elbow) or trauma sites (proximal interphalangeal, or PIP, joints) and are less clearly related to ischemia, but the use of vasodilating therapy is still reasonable. Often it is difficult to distinguish between ischemia and bacterial infection of ulcerations in SSc patients. Ischemic lesions tend to be painful without drainage, while infected areas are more likely to have purulent drainage and surrounding hyperemia. If ulcers

appear infected, use of antibiotics directed at staphylococcus, by far the most frequent infectious agent encountered, is warranted. *Streptococci* and *Pseudomonas* are occasionally at fault. Intravenous antibiotic administration is most effective, but if oral agents are prescribed, a prolonged course (2 or more weeks) is desirable, because of disease-related ischemia resulting in limited tissue penetration. If ulcers are located on the distal lower extremities, elevation is important to reduce the adverse effects of edema and venous stasis. The application of Duoderm pads on ulcers located on relatively flat surfaces, or Duoderm granules in other ulcers, may speed their healing. Patients prefer open wounds to be covered with some antibiotic ointment, which reduces pain, while physicians believe that healing is more rapid if ulcers are left open to the air.

Calcinosis

Most calcifications in SSc are hidden in soft tissues and do not represent a cause of morbidity. Soft-tissue calcifications that become red, warm, and painful and are oozing may be infected, but more frequently are actively inflamed from the soft tissue reaction to subcutaneous hydroxyapatite crystal deposition. Colchicine (0.6 mg once or twice a day) may be employed, not because of any postulated DMARD activity, but because it may quiet crystal-induced inflammation. Antibiotics directed against *Staphylococcus* and *Streptococcus* may be employed at the same time, because it is often not possible to prove/disprove infection or crystal-induced inflammation. The calcium-channel blocker diltiazem has been suggested as a vasodilating agent which may also retard soft tissue calcification. Other calcifications are so massive, or are constantly oozing, or are located in a particularly strategic site (i.e., the thumb, the finger(s), the ulnar surface of the forearm) that a surgeon should be called in to "debulk" the area and allow it to heal. The calcifications may return, but most patients enjoy some period of time away from the "mess and aggravation" of calcifications.

Organ Involvement: Musculoskeletal

Ken Blocka

Many patients with scleroderma exhibit a spectrum of musculoskeletal symptoms during the course of their illness. Symptoms may arise from the articulations themselves, from the adjacent non-articular supporting structures such as tendons and bursae, or from the surrounding skeletal muscles. Rarely the predominant source of morbidity, musculoskeletal involvement may nonetheless significantly contribute to the symptom complex of patients with systemic sclerosis (SSc), especially in the early stage of illness. While there are no specific treatments for SSc, the recognition and skillful management of the musculoskeletal manifestations can contribute greatly to the patient's sense of well-being. While recognizing that these symptoms may often present concurrently, this discussion will consider the musculoskeletal management of SSc under the separate headings of articular, non-articular, and muscular components.

ARTICULAR SYMPTOMS

The majority of patients report non-specific arthralgias and stiffness. Occasionally, patients, especially those with disease overlap, may present with a frank symmetrical polyarthritis indistinguishable from that of rheumatoid arthritis. Most patients will respond to simple analgesics and/or non-steroidal anti-inflammatory drug therapy. Patients with more resistant signs of joint inflammation will often do well with low dose oral corticosteroids (i.e., prednisone less than 10 mg per day). Caution should be exercised with both non-steroidal anti-inflammatory drugs and corticosteroids, because of the high prevalence of gastroesophageal motility disorders in SSc patients. It is rarely necessary to resort to second line therapy with agents such as methotrexate or azathioprine. There are no controlled studies supporting the efficacy of these drugs, nor is there any evidence that they will, in

any way, retard or prevent the digital resorptive or articular erosive changes associated with this disorder.

Isolated patients may present with an acute monarthritis, which mandates a diagnostic synovial fluid aspiration in order to distinguish between infection and crystal-induced synovitis. Scleroderma patients are at increased risk for septic arthritis because of skin ulceration and secondary infection at sites of subcutaneous calcinosis. As well, rare cases of crystal-induced synovitis have also been reported as a result of intra-articular calcium hydroxyapatite deposition. The latter patients generally respond to short courses of high dose non-steroidal anti-inflammatory drugs, oral colchicine, or corticosteroids.

The most important and practical rheumatologic concern relates to the development of slowly progressive joint contractures caused by a combination of skin, capsular, and tendon fibrosis. Early aggressive physiotherapy to maximize joint flexibility and movement is rewarding, especially in the early phases of the disease, but is unlikely to forestall the eventual development of contractures. The results of serial dynamic splinting have been uniformly disappointing. For advanced states of contracture, PIP fusions may restore a more functional and cosmetically acceptable hand, providing there is some preservation of metacarpophalangeal (MCP) mobility. PIP arthroplasties and thumb to index finger mobilization procedures may also play a role in selected patients.

NON-ARTICULAR SYMPTOMS

Tendinitis and Bursitis

Palpable and/or audible tendon friction rubs caused by fibrinous adhesions within tendon sheaths and/or juxta articular bursae are often a distinctive finding in patients with SSc. Although frequently asymptomatic, this form of tendon involvement may be surprisingly painful. Diagnostic confusion may occur in patients in whom subscapular bursitis may mimic a pleural friction rub, or in whom trochanteric bursitis may suggest primary hip disease. Most symptomatic patients with this dry, leathery form of tendon or bursal crepitus will respond to physical modalities such as heat, ultrasound, simple analgesics, or non-steroidal anti-inflammatory drug treatment.

A minority of patients may present with more florid bursal inflammation with signs of redness, heat, and swelling. Radiographically apparent intra-bursal calcification may or may not be present. As the underlying etiology may include cellulitis, acute calcific periarthritis, or septic bursitis, a soft tissue aspiration with analysis of contents for cell count, crystals, and culture is always prudent. Culture-positive aspirates (almost always *Staphylococcus aureus*) should be treated with appropriate antibiotics. Sterile bursal effusions with or without evidence of crystal deposition (usually calcium hydroxyapatite) respond best to intra-bursal corticosteroid injections. It has also been suggested in isolated reports that focal inflammatory reactions associated with calcinosis may respond to short courses of oral colchicine or diltiazem.

ENTRAPMENT NEUROPATHIES

Scleroderma patients may infrequently develop signs of median nerve entrapment, especially in the early acute edematous phase of the disease. Symptoms generally respond to conservative measures, such as wrist splints and/or a short course of corticosteroids, with surgery rarely becoming necessary. Entrapment neuropathies at other sites are distinctly less common.

MUSCULAR PROBLEMS

While most scleroderma patients will complain of muscular weakness attributable to joint and skin contractures and the debilitating effect of the underlying condition, it is now recognized that a disease-related myopathy may also be present in many of these patients. The muscle weakness, however, is usually slight and rarely associated with significant CPK elevations (usually less than 3–4 times the upper limit of normal). The EMG may show polyphasic potentials, but without the insertional irritability and fibrillation typical of classic myositis. Muscle biopsies typically show perimysial and perivascular fibrosis with little or no evidence of muscular nerosis or inflammation. Patients with this benign non-progressive form of myopathy may benefit from regular strengthening and flexibility exercises but do not require specific medical therapy (i.e., corticosteroids). In fact, the muscular symptoms are typically *unresponsive* to medical measures. These observations may serve to differentiate this condition from the more serious inflammatory myopathy described in the following paragraph.

A much smaller subgroup of SSc patients (less than 10%) present with more pronounced proximal limb girdle weakness. The CPK's are significantly elevated (at least 3–4 times normal), and the EMG and muscle biopsy show abnormalities more typical for classic inflammatory polymyopathy. These patients are felt to suffer from a true polymyositis, either as a complication of the scleroderma or by virtue of disease overlap. In contrast to the first group, this category of patients generally responds both clinically and biochemically to corticosteroids and/or immunosuppressive therapy. It should be noted that several authorities have expressed concerns about the potential role of high dose corticosteroids in precipitating renal failure in scleroderma. Under the circumstances, the early initiation of cotherapy with steroid sparing agents, such as methotrexate and/or azathioprine, would seem advisable.

Organ Involvement: Renal

Virginia D. Steen

Patients with systemic sclerosis who develop new hypertension (diastolic pressure >110 mm Hg) should be considered to have SRC until proven otherwise (Fig. 30.2). Peripheral renin activity and complete laboratory evaluation should be obtained without waiting for results and the patient should immediately receive a short-acting ACE inhibitor, preferably captopril, beginning at a dose of 6.25 to 12.5mg every 8 hours. Blood pressure should be monitored closely striving to obtain a blood pressure in the normal range (e.g., 120–140/70–90 mm Hg) within 72 hours. The dose of ACE inhibitor should be increased every 8 to 12 hours, as necessary, until the blood pressure remains in the normal range. If blood pressure control is not achieved with 75 mg to 100 mg

captopril every 6 hours, additional drugs, such as calcium channel blockers, hydralazine or minoxidil, should be added but the ACE inhibitor should not be discontinued. Higher doses of captopril should be used cautiously with close observations for allergic reactions. Because of the rapidity and effectiveness of ACE inhibition on this severe hypertension, nitroprusside is rarely needed.

It is not unusual for renal insufficiency to progress despite control of blood pressure. The serum creatinine initially will increase by 0.5mg/dl to 1mg/dl daily. When the blood pressure is controlled, the serum creatinine may continue to rise but the rate of increase usually is slower. In many instances, the serum creatinine peaks after 7 to 14 days, reverses, and then slowly returns toward normal.

In some cases, ACE inhibitors have themselves been implicated as a cause of renal dysfunction. However, in the setting of renal crisis we have not detected any instances in which the ACE inhibitor clearly caused reversible renal dysfunction. Although "allergic" interstitial nephritis with eosinophilia also occurs with ACE inhibition, we have not seen this complication in our patient population. In over 60 SRC cases treated with these drugs, none of them have improved with the discontinuation of the ACE inhibitor. Thus, regardless of deteriorating renal function, an ACE inhibitor should be continued as part of the antihypertensive regimen. Even patients on dialysis should continue to receive small amounts of an ACE inhibitor even though blood pressure may be normal. Holding the dose prior to dialysis may avoid hypotension during dialysis. Conversion to a long-acting ACE inhibitor for compliance or toxicity can be safely accomplished. There are case reports of long-acting rather than short-acting ACE inhibitors successfully used as primary therapy of SRC, but our anecdotal experience suggests that early use of

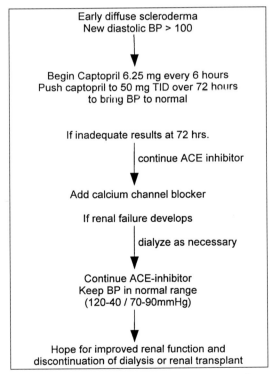

Figure 30.2. Approach to the management of patients with systemic sclerosis who develop hypertension.

the shorter acting drugs is associated with increased flexibility and an improved outcome.

Complications related to SRC (i.e., hypertensive encephalopathy, microangiopathic hemolytic anemia, or heart failure) will usually improve with the control of the blood pressure. Retinal hemorrhage, headache, confusion, and even seizures were not uncommon prior to ACE inhibitors but are now rarely a problem. Microangiopathic hemolytic anemia with thrombocytopenia usually resolves with control of the blood pressure, although in one of our patients it continued relentlessly for 4 weeks until the time of her death. Congestive heart failure, both from primary scleroderma cardiac fibrosis as well as the effects of the hypertension, is a risk factor for a poor outcome. Treatment may be difficult, but controlling the blood pressure and using cardiac medication usually controls the heart failure.

Skin thickening may either improve or worsen after SRC. A number of patients have been reported whose skin thickening has promptly and impressively improved after surviving SRC, but this response is not limited to patients receiving ACE inhibitors. In the one third of patients who experience worsening of their skin thickening after SRC, other possible disease-modifying drugs may be necessary. If the latter is used, it is best that a long-acting ACE inhibitor (rather than captopril, which like D-penicillamine has a sulfhydryl group, and both drugs share similar toxicities) be employed. In many patients, additional therapy may not be indicated.

Prevention of SRC with ACE inhibitors is an attractive idea that has not been formally tested. However, the use of ACE inhibitors has the potential undesirable effects of hypotension, hyperkalemia, leukopenia, etc. We have followed five systemic sclerosis patients receiving ACE inhibitors for RP or essential hypertension who subsequently developed classic SRC. Thus, prophylactic ACE inhibitor therapy may not be completely effective, but further study is definitely necessary.

Organ Involvement: Nervous System

Ariane L. Herrick, Malcolm I. V. Jayson

Nervous system involvement is rare in SSc. As a result, the experience of treating the different neurological manifestations that have been reported in SSc is very limited. No firm guidelines can be offered. In cases where there is likely to be an inflammatory component to the problem, steroids or immunosuppressants may be justified.

Organ Involvement: Gastrointestinal and Hepatic

Geoffrey C. Jiranek, James E. Bredfeldt

GASTROINTESTINAL

Patients with gastrointestinal reflux should be instructed that reflux is a chronic problem that demands chronic treatment. Patients should sleep with the head of the bed elevated at least 4 to 6 inches. Food should be avoided for at least 3 hours before recumbency. The intake of coffee, chocolate, peppermint, onions, garlic, and fat should be minimized. H2 blocker therapy is given for mild disease in 2 divided daily doses (ranitidine 150 mg b.i.d., nizatidine 150 mg b.i.d., or famotidine 20 mg b.i.d.). More severe disease is best managed by omeprazole 20 mg (occasionally 40 mg) per day. There is no benefit from combining H2 blocker with omeprazole therapy. The risk of gastric carcinoid tumors and gastric adenocarcinoma from long-term use of omeprazole is probably very small. Omeprazole can increase the tendency for bacterial overgrowth if there is concomitant small bowel dysmotility. Cisapride (10–20 mg q.i.d.) can be combined with either an H2 blocker or omeprazole if acid reduction therapy alone is not satisfactory. Cisapride by itself has been disappointing for severe reflux in SSc because of unresponsive esophageal motor dysfunction. Surgical antireflux procedures seldom lead to relief from reflux without causing severe dysphagia and are best avoided except in extraordinary circumstances.

Dysphagia from an esophageal stricture is best managed by endoscopic dilatation and aggressive antireflux therapy, as discussed in the previous paragraph. Neuromuscular dysphagia is difficult to treat, but is generally mild and responds best to eating soft food in the upright posture.

Gastroparesis should be treated with cisapride (10–20 mg q.i.d.) before meals and at bedtime. If cisapride fails, erythromycin (250–500 mg t.i.d.) can be tried.

Malabsorption in SSc patients resulting from small bowel overgrowth is treated by tetracycline (250 mg q.i.d. for 10 days). Organisms can develop a resistance to tetracycline. Therefore, if tetracycline fails, metronidazole (250 mg t.i.d.) plus cephalexin (250 mg q.i.d.) can be used for 10 days. Cyclic therapy with treatment every 6 weeks is required in some patients. Standard prokinetic medications, such as metaclopramide, cisapride, and erythromycin, have been disappointing and rarely improve small bowel dysmotility.

Octreotide (50 mcg subcutaneously at bedtime) is worth trying for symptoms of small bowel dysmotility and for antibiotic-resistant bacterial overgrowth. Patients with malabsorption often benefit from monthly injections of vitamin B12 and oral supplementation of calcium, iron, and vitamins. Total parenteral nutrition is required in rare refractory cases of malabsorption and pseudo-obstruction.

Constipation is initially treated with fiber supplementation. When increasing fiber is no longer tolerated, then an osmotic agent, such as milk of magnesia 15-45 cc per day can be used provided there is no renal failure. For severe refractory constipation, stimulant laxatives, such as bisacodyl (Ducolax™ 30 mg) tablets, are often useful.

Pneumatosis cystoides intestinalis and *pneumatosis cytoides coli* with or without pneumoperitoneum should not be treated with laparotomy if signs of peritonitis are absent. Most patients do not require any specific therapy. For rare symptomatic patients, reduction of oral carbohydrate intake and oxygen therapy are useful.

HEPATIC

Because many of the patients with PBC (primary biliary cirrhosis) have a concomitant autoimmune disease, a team approach to the overall management of the patient is required. My initial approach to treating the individual patient with PBC depends upon several factors, including symptoms requiring direct intervention, the clinical stage, and the findings of the liver histology. I encourage calcium supplementation, sometimes with the addition of 1-25 dihydroxyvitamin D_3 when serum vitamin D levels are low or borderline, in an attempt to forestall the development of osteopenia.

I recommend the use of ursodiol, 10 to 12 mg/kg/day, particularly in patients with early stage disease, since ursodiol appears to be a safe medication and may provide therapeutic benefit over the long term. Whenever it is feasible, I encourage patients to enroll in prospective, double-blind trials. Since PBC is a relatively rare liver disease, it will only be through these trials that we will develop an understanding of the proper treatment for this potentially disabling disorder.

In patients with histologic stage 3 or 4 disease, attention should be paid toward the development of portal hypertension complications and the progression of jaundice, as a liver transplantation may be indicated. Because survival is altered after an episode of bleeding from esophageal varices, I recommend that patients be evaluated for esophageal varices by either endoscopy or barium esophagography, looking for large-size varices that might place the patient at high risk for subsequent variceal hemorrhage. In this context, I recommend that prophylactic treatment against variceal bleeding be instituted using a non-selective beta antagonist such as propranolol or nadolol. Ascites should be vigorously treated with diuretics, as its presence indicates a risk for spontaneous bacterial peritonitis, a potentially life-threatening infection. The presence of portal-systemic encephalopathy indicates the urgent need for a referral for a liver transplantation so that irreversible neurologic injury does not occur.

Bleeding from gastrointestinal telangiectasias in patients with SSc are best managed with endoscopic thermal hemostasis with a heater probe, a bipolar electrocautery probe, or an Nd-YAG laser.

Organ Involvement: Sexual Function and Pregnancy

Steven R. Weiner

Males with systemic sclerosis should be provided with the opportunity of discussing issues regarding sexuality and impotence in addition to all aspects of SSc involvement. Genetic counseling should be given when it is known. Erectile impotence may have a devastating impact on a patient who does not know ahead of time that it can occur. Patients should be advised that urologists have a variety of treatment options to ameliorate impotence. Also, effects of medication on spermatogenesis as well as erectile potency should be discussed in plain language.

Women with systemic sclerosis must also be provided with a forum to discuss issues of sexuality, genetic information, and medication and disease effects on both sexual function (i.e., vaginal dryness/dyspareunia) and conception. Systemic sclerosis gynecologic concerns and concerns about the breast should not be neglected.

Medication use during pregnancy and during breast feeding is listed in Chapter 23 and Table 23.4 in particular. Pregnancy management issues are listed in Table 23.5 and discussed in the text. As Steen et al suggest, certain women with systemic sclerosis should avoid conception, making discussion of contraception imperative. For those electing pregnancy it is best to consider all scleroderma pregnancies as high risk and to involve high risk obstetricians, anesthesiologists, and perinatologists with relevant experience. A team approach with significant rheumatologic input is ideal. As noted in Table 23.5, patients must be seen frequently. Delivery is often premature and Caesarean section options should be available. At delivery, the room, intravenous fluids, and most especially the patient must be kept warm. Positioning for delivery in the near-squatting position is preferred to prevent gastroesophageal reflux. Epidurals are preferred for pain control as they induce peripheral vasodilation. Long before delivery time, management of possible problems of vascular access and oral/nasal aperture narrowing (as a problem for intubation) must all be planned for, and pulmonary/cardiac/renal status must be assessed and specialty consultation considered. Since sclerodermatous skin involvement may limit hip movement or narrow the vaginal introitus, a larger vaginal opening (episiotomy) must also be considered to allow for passage of the fetal head. While in most cases systemic sclerosis does not worsen, the marked stresses of the postpartum period require frequent maternal as well as newborn follow-up.

Organ Involvement: Psychosocial Aspects

Robert P. Roca, Fredrick M. Wigley

It is impossible to shield the patient from the truth about scleroderma: the physical signs are readily visible and the symptoms undeniable. Fortunately, most patients don't want to stay in the dark and are in fact relieved to discover an explanation for their symptoms. While patients are in some ways unique in their informational needs and their readiness for education, several general points can be made. The explanation of the nature and prognosis of the illness is best done in stages over a series of visits. It is often necessary to cover the same ground repeatedly over time to ensure that it is properly understood. It is important to address every symptom and respond to every question that the patient raises. It is important to explain the differences between chronic and acute illness and to emphasize that the chronic nature of scleroderma does not preclude long periods of stability and even improvement; such concepts provide the basis for hope and optimism.

Simplified explanations of the clinical manifestations of the disease (e.g., "the skin is tight because collagen is overproduced in the skin") help demystify the illness and reassure patients that their physician is knowledgeable about scleroderma. It is helpful to individualize the patient's clinical status and the possible disease course (e.g., "The course of this disorder is highly variable; every patient is different and we need to focus on you and how you are doing"). Patients should also have an accurate appraisal of the severity of their illness. Patients with limited cutaneous SSc (CREST variant) should understand that their prognosis is quite good and that severe disability from "incurable scleroderma" is unlikely. On the other hand, patients with severe disease need to understand the adjustments in lifestyle that may be necessary to optimize their quality of life.

The key element in the psychosocial management of scleroderma is a comfortable physician-patient relationship. The development of such a relationship takes time, and the physician must allow for office visits of sufficient duration and frequency, particularly early in the course of the illness. It is also important that the physician

afford the patient ready access in the event of questions and problems. Open conversation with the spouse or other family members—in the patient's presence—further facilitates communication and helps family members understand both the plan of treatment and the patient's needs at home. It may even be appropriate to communicate with the patient's employer to ensure that the patient's functional limitations are understood. As noted above, counseling about sexual relationships should not be overlooked. Literature published by scleroderma organizations can be useful for some patients.

Treatment should focus primarily on two goals: enhancing the patient's social support system and reducing the patient's symptoms. The importance of social support cannot be overemphasized; recently, a 35-year-old patient with severe restrictive lung disease requiring continuous oxygen informed us that she was able to cope and enjoy her life principally because her husband was understanding and supportive. This is consistent with empirical data showing that social support correlates with good psychosocial adjustment and protects against depression.

Although there is no cure for scleroderma, there are a number of pharmacologic and non-pharmacologic measures that reduce symptoms and improve patients' quality of life; these are discussed in detail throughout this book. The patient needs to understand which symptoms can be controlled with appropriate treatment and which cannot. It is often helpful to have patients seen by a scleroderma expert early in the course of the disease so that they know that every treatment method is being considered and that their physician is well-informed. A team approach is often necessary, but one physician needs to "quarterback" the plan in consultation with the patient. It is critical that all clinicians convey to patients that they understand the situation and that they will work collaboratively toward improvement.

V

Resources

MILDRED GOEKE STERZ

31

The Role of the Nurse in the Management of Patients with Systemic Sclerosis: Advice Specific to Nursing Personnel

AMONG THE VALUABLE RESOURCES available to patients with scleroderma are nurses. The roles of the nurse in the care of patients with scleroderma are several: sometimes as empathetic caregivers; sometimes as referral liaison for medical and ancillary care needs; sometimes as a health educator; and sometimes as a link between the physician, family, and patient. Independently, the nurse has the responsibility of establishing rapport with the patient, which can be very helpful in maintaining the patient's quality of life. The needs of patients with scleroderma can cover a wide spectrum. Some patients will proceed with their lifestyle in minimally compromised ways, some, who have given birth after diagnosis, may be very busy with child care, or some patients may have prepared for their demise secondary to a very acute, volatile process. The nurse is a professional who supports complete care for her/his patients. The nurse's role can be very fulfilling when performed with the sincerity and sensitivity inherent to the profession, and especially when coupled with specific knowledge of the disease process and the resources available to patients, family, and health care professionals. The discussion that follows is based in large part on my sixteen years of personal caring for several hundred patients with SSc, many of whom were participating in clinical trials.

Nursing Skills

The responsibilities of the nurse can be divided into those dealing with the psycho-social aspects of care and those dealing with the physical needs of the patient. Nursing care of a patient diagnosed with scleroderma begins with the patient's first visit to the physician's office. The moment the nurse is introduced to the patient and family, a sense of respect for the patient should be conveyed. These patients have often been referred to a rheumatologist by a general practitioner or dermatologist who has informed them that they may have a rare condition for which there is little known treatment and which can be fatal. Such patients are often very ill and are looking for any sign of comfort and reassurance that they can find. A relationship that imparts support and education, and that reinforces information presented by the physician will be invaluable during the course of their evaluation, status assessment, and treatment. This approach will lay the foundation for trust, will help the patient adjust to the disease, and will enhance the quality of life for the patient and family.

Being told that they have scleroderma is often very traumatic for the patient. It is not a disease that is well known, nor one that is in vogue. Patients are truly at odds with the disease and, therefore, its many stages will introduce new challenges for all involved. Close observation of the patient and a close working relationship with the physician will allow the nurse to support the patient. Take the time to visit with the patient while administering care. Get to know the person: their personality, profession, lifestyle, and interests. Take time to notice their personal appearance at the initial and successive visits and how it changes over time. Also observe whether they come alone or with relatives and how they interact with each other. Information about the patient's family and friends is critical to establishing the foundation on which to build a sensitive, resourceful therapeutic relationship.

The nurse can help the patient understand that despite what may seem like obvious disease, both clinically and from records that accompany the patient, each patient must be evaluated carefully before the diagnosis is confirmed by the rheumatologist or "sclerodermatist." This evaluation usually requires repeat history, physical examination, and additional laboratory studies, including venipuncture, which can be painful when the skin is very hard and the vessels are constricted. The nurse can facilitate the evaluation by helping patients get to various departments of a clinic or hospital for other studies. The purpose of this assistance is to minimize the tiring, uncomfortable, and anxiety-provoking nature of these tests with support and confirmation.

As in all diseases, individuals do not necessarily progess, either physically or psychologically, from one phase of this illness to another according to the text. The patient will decide for her/himself the best way to cope with the many stages of this disease. As a nurse, you cannot force the process, but you can help patients to understand and live better with the disease. Patients are incredibly strong.

Nursing Review of Systems

Even though scleroderma is a multisystem disease, no two patients will have exactly the same complaints or involvement. The physician is ultimately responsible for the diagnosis and management of the various involvements. The nurse, however, is in the unique position of being able to pick up on nuances that may be missed or slighted, and is often aware of psycho-social issues not obvious to the physician. Consequently, it is important for the nurse to help guide the patient's education and understanding and to offer insights into better self-management.

The following paragraphs briefly address some of the more frequent organ system involvements likely to be encountered by patients with scleroderma. Knowledge of these problem areas will help the nurse to uncover potential problems that may not be obvious to others or to the family. These knowing foresights will increase the patient's trust that the medical team really "knows what is going on" and will facilitate instruction and management of and by the patient.

GENERAL

Patients with scleroderma may experience a variety of non-specific symptoms, including fatigue, lack of energy, generalized weakness, weight loss, and vague aching of muscles, joints, or bones. Such patients should be evaluated by their physician. The nurse's role is to teach patients how to sort through and develop treatment strategies for these symptoms. Discussion about their daily routine and responsibilities may reveal ways to reorganize their day, to include rest periods, to develop alternative ways of doing things, and even to obtain outside help with certain tasks.

RAYNAUD'S PHENOMENON

The most common physical symptom to appear initially in scleroderma patients is Raynaud's phenomenon of the hands: color changes induced by cold, often accompanied by numbness, tingling, and pain. Less commonly, Raynaud's phenomenon may involve the toes, ears, nose, and tip of the tongue. Patients should be taught the importance of maintaining warmth in the core of their body by covering the torso with layered clothing of natural fibers such as wool, cotton, or down, in addition to keeping their hands and feet warm with gloves and socks. Disposable warm packs may hold warmth for up to 12 hours. When there is a choice about ambient temperature, it should be stressed that warmer temperatures are better for the patient's circulation. Whenever possible, they should avoid outdoor cold weather, excessive air conditioning, or reaching into a refrigerator or freezer. In any event, the patient should dress warmly before being exposed to cold temperatures. The nose and ears also can be covered and the mouth should be closed when the patient is out in the cold. In addition, rubbing or massaging the hands and feet may help. Electric heaters, blankets, or comforters can supplement the heat in the home of the patient. Sometimes local utilities will offer reduced rates or increased baseline allowances for households of patients with scleroderma, since the increased need for warmth can create an increased financial hardship because of increased utility expenses. Avoiding emotional upset as much as possible is helpful, but not always possible. Relaxation techniques, whether self taught or learned through training courses, have effectively reduced stress for some patients. Biofeedback has been used to control finger temperature. Since smoking is thought to aggravate Raynaud's phenomenon, it should be discouraged.

Medications can help to decrease the severity of Raynaud's phenomena and in healing obvious ulcers (discussed in Chapter 17). Patients should clearly understand that they need to take their medication as directed and should continue to follow the practices described above for optimum benefit.

SKIN

Swelling or puffiness of the hands or feet may be early symptoms of scleroderma. This may be especially noticeable when the patient awakens in the morning. The skin is quite full in appearance and the skin creases disappear. The skin may feel tight and it may be difficult to make a fist. Sores or ulcerations on the finger tips and the knuckles are a common symptom of scleroderma. They may be very slow to heal, in part because of poor circulation and tight skin. These sores or ulcerations may also occur on the elbows, toes, or other sites of the body where the skin is tightly stretched or exposed to trauma. If an ulcerated area becomes painful, analgesics or a topical anesthetic such as Xylocaine™ may be helpful. The affected area should be kept warm to increase blood flow and kept very clean to prevent infection. If infection develops (especially if the surrounding areas become red and warm or the ulcer exudes yellow/green purulent material) it is prudent to soak the affected area in warm water, then apply an antiseptic such as peroxide or Betadine™, or use a topical antibiotic such as Neosporin™ or Neosporin-Plus™. Should these remedies prove unsuccessful the patient may need to take oral or parenteral antibiotics, and should take them for longer than the customary period because of decreased circulation.

The term *scleroderma* comes from the hardening and thickening of the skin. The myriad skin changes that occur in scleroderma cannot be prevented, but there are certain ways to lessen the severity of complications. Although there are no proven treatments to alter the course of this disease, there are several treatments which can lessen some of the symptoms.

Deposits of calcium under the skin, referred to as calcinosis, can be very painful. These deposits may occur in the form of hard lumps or nodules, and may break through the skin producing white chunks or liquid material, which may be associated with local infection. The area should be protected from bumping and injury, usually by an adhesive bandage or light dressing. Warm water soaks may be helpful.

Telangiectasias are a group of small blood vessels near the surface of the skin that are visible as small, red or purple, cherry-like spots, usually on the fingers, palms, face, and lips. Special cosmetics may be used to mask the spots or reduce their visibility. One very popular brand of cosmetics is Dermablend™, which is waterproof and has not had fragrance added. Dermatologists, plastic surgeons, and other patients can suggest other

and Friday). This is particularly important during the first few years of scleroderma. Symptoms of headache, visual disturbances, shortness of breath, chest pain or discomfort, or mental confusion, may be signs of hypertension and/or kidney failure. Patients should be instructed to report abnormal signs and symptoms and high blood pressure to their physician as soon as possible.

Renal crisis (kidney failure) can be suspected by the appearance of new-onset hypertension, and may be confirmed by an elevated or rising serum creatinine. The importance of the rapport between clinician and nurse is stressed in this case because renal crisis is the most threatening (but potentially correctable) complication of scleroderma. It should be made very clear to the patient that if this complication is diagnosed and treated early (within the first days or weeks), it is often possible with medication (i.e., angiotensin converting enzyme [ACE] inhibitors) to forestall kidney failure and to control the hypertension.

LUNG

Lung problems occur frequently in scleroderma. Air pollutants may aggravate breathing problems and should be avoided. Smoking should be absolutely forbidden. Patients should know that medications can sometimes be prescribed to make their breathing easier. Reflux occurs frequently, but respiratory problems related to reflux are uncommon. Nevertheless coughing at night, breathing problems worsening at night, wheezing, and hoarseness may be clues to reflux problems. Patients with underlying lung disease from scleroderma should be given a "pneumonia shot" (Pneumovax™) and yearly flu shots to prevent infections which could lead to serious respiratory complications.

NUTRITION

Nutrition may be discussed in the office where the nurse can provide tips on nutritional supplements (such as Ensure™) and small frequent feedings. Sometimes warming the food will help soothe feelings of being cold and of body aches.

Summary

Not every patient will experience the same symptoms, nor the same degree of involvement. Nonetheless, all are patients with a disease for which there has been no cure found to date. Many treatments are discussed throughout this book for modifying many symptoms. The availability of these treatments for symptoms of scleroderma is an important point that must be presented to the patient and the family. This is also where nursing input can be very important. Patient education and psycho-social support to help patients know themselves and understand their disease cannot be stressed enough. In addition, the patient must know the warning signs for the problems inherent to scleroderma and know that the nurse is a person who will listen and address their questions.

It is important to adopt a positive attitude toward patients with scleroderma, in large part because of the availability of many constructive suggestions and treatments for scleroderma's complications. Health practitioners must instill a sense of hope in both patients and their families. It will become clear during the course of scleroderma that its progression will be quite slow in many patients, and that effective treatment is now available for many of the complications that arise. Therefore, the importance of an open and supportive relationship among the patient, physician, and the nurse cannot be stressed enough. Since the patient may need additional support at any time, it will be this rapport that will result in additional needs to be addressed by the family, the patient, the nurse, and the physician. Education of the family and patient remains of the foremost importance in helping them to maintain as normal a lifestyle as possible.

Suggested Reading

Alper J, LeRoy EC. Scleroderma (systemic sclerosis). In: Katz WA, ed. Philadelphia, JB Lippincott Co, 1988, pp 467–481.

Coppok JS, Bacon PA. Outcome, assessment and activity. In: Jayson MIV, Black CM, eds. Systemic sclerosis: scleroderma. New York, John Wiley Sons, 1988, pp 279–288.

Liang M. Psychosical management of rheumatic disease. In: Kelley WN, Harris ED, Ruddy S, Sledge CB, eds. Textbook of rheumatology. 4th ed. Philadelphia, WB Saunders, 1993, pp 535–544.

Seibold J. Scleroderma. In: Kelley WN, Harris ED, Ruddy S, Sledge CB, eds. Textbook of rheumatology, 4th ed., 1993, pp 1113–1143.

Seibold J, Furst D, Clements PJ. Why everything (or nothing) seems to work in the treatment of scleroderma. J Rheumatol 1992;19:673–676.

MARIE A. COYLE
DIANE WILLIAMS

32

Scleroderma Patient Support Groups and Organizations

SELF-HELP GROUPS have been described as those in which people with a common need or illness meet to share thoughts and feelings with others, and sometimes solve related problems. Self-help groups, also called mutual aid or support groups, have proliferated in recent years. There are an estimated 500,000 such organizations in the United States, and groups now exist for virtually every problem. The need is apparent as groups develop quite naturally. Members seek to become more knowledgeable about their own disease, and to find the companionship and support of others who share their concerns and fears.

Scleroderma patient organizations began forming in the early 1970s, with groups in Pennsylvania, Massachusetts, and California. Through the years, their ranks have enlarged to include groups in other states as well as Canada, England, Germany, the Netherlands, Australia, and New Zealand. Initially, many of the groups were "coffee-klatch" gatherings, but they soon blossomed into well-organized self-help groups dedicated to assisting other patients, particularly the newly-diagnosed. Many of the group leaders had gone through the initial period following diagnosis dealing with feelings of isolation and anxiety. Helping other people overcome these frightening feelings became a common goal of the groups.

Persons with scleroderma and their families often have special needs, which arise not only from living with an unpredictable and difficult chronic illness on a day-to-day basis, but also because scleroderma is relatively uncommon. Oftentimes, both patients and family members feel locked into an overwhelming, all-encompassing situation which intrudes upon, and dramatically changes, many areas of their lives. Certainly when first diagnosed, scleroderma is viewed as a tragedy by all concerned which can leave patients frightened, confused, or embittered. Thus, the groundwork is laid for anxiety and depression, leading to feelings of hopelessness and powerlessness. It is at this point that a self-help group, in conjunction with the care offered by health professionals, can provide the educational and emotional support necessary to help patients adjust to their situation. As well-informed consumers, patients are better equipped to work hand-in-hand with health-care providers and assume an active role in their treatment plan. This enhanced sense of control is an important contributing factor to emotional recovery and the ability to cope successfully. While the advent of a chronic illness in a person's life is something over which one has little control, how individuals identify and respond to the special challenges can have either positive or negative effects. It is the mission of all self-help groups to lessen the negative impact of the circumstance or illness and to help patients maintain a positive focus.

Currently, there are two principal organizations in the United States for scleroderma patients and their families: the Scleroderma Federation and the United Scleroderma Foundation, Inc. It is expected that these organizations will merge in the not-too-distant future. This chapter describes each of these principal self-help organizations. The addresses and telephone numbers for the Scleroderma Federation, United Scleroderma Foundation, and related organizations in Canada and Europe are provided in Appendix I.

Scleroderma Federation (Marie A. Coyle, President)

The Scleroderma Federation (SF) was established in 1980. At the time, the leaders of several autonomous groups servicing Chicago, New England, New Jersey, New York, and Washington met to explore the possibility of working collectively. SF was born out of that meeting. Today, it numbers 17 independent groups scattered across the United States and Canada, who operate autonomously but in accordance with SF guidelines. Most SF affiliates are located in major urban areas and several have memberships numbering in the thousands.

All SF groups share the same literature, newsletter, etc., and have established a national office to service their own needs as groups, and the needs of patients in areas of the country not serviced by local support groups.

The SF is generally a volunteer effort. There are no salaries paid to either group leaders or board members. The only salaries paid are for minimal administrative/secretarial assistance. Because expenses have been kept to a minimum, most of the funding raised above operating expenses is distributed to research through a successful collaborative grant funding program.

MISSION

The mission of SF is to promote the welfare of scleroderma patients and their families by providing educational and emotional support; to promote and support medical research designed to identify the cause, discover the cure, improve methods of treatment and prevent the occurrence of scleroderma; and to enhance the public's awareness of the disease.

OFFICE

The major thrust of the national SF office staff is to service patient needs. It is SF policy to service all inquiries on the day that they are received. The SF Help Line (1-800-422-1113) is handled by patient volunteers who are professionally trained to serve as peer counselors. In addition, the national office provides a physician referral service, provides for the needs of its affiliate groups, participates in national publicity, raises funds for research, and administers the SF grant award program.

COLLABORATIVE FUNDING PROGRAM

In an effort to contribute more meaningful sums to scleroderma research, the SF was instrumental in developing a collaborative funding program. Initially, groups were giving whatever funds they raised to doctors of their choice without benefit of written proposals or peer review. Once organized, all SF groups began voluntarily contributing the funds raised in their areas to a collective endeavor to increase the total amount of money that could be provided for research each year. In order to distribute the funding wisely, the SF sought direction from its Medical Advisory Board and other prominent members of the scleroderma community. Their expertise and guidance resulted in the formation of the National Grant Review Board, which is composed of the top physicians and scientists currently involved in scleroderma research. The Board Chairperson serves for 2 years, and reviewers are rotated as necessary. The Board meets annually in conjunction with the American College of Rheumatology Meeting. At that time, Board members hold final discussions and scoring of grants, which are reviewed in advance of the meeting.

Currently, the SF donates approximately $500,000 a year to research through its funding program and the effort of all its affiliates.

MEETINGS

The SF provides a variety of meetings for its members. The meetings may take the form of informational gatherings, emotional support groups, medical information meetings, all-day patient education seminars, and workshops. The frequency of these meetings varies from location to location, and with need. Most SF-affiliated groups strive for at least 4 meetings a year with an all-day patient seminar or workshop once or twice a year.

Informal meetings can consist of as few as three or four people getting together to discuss their particular problems of the moment. Emotional support group meetings require the services of a facilitator to ensure that the meetings move smoothly, that everyone has an opportunity to fully express his/her feelings, that no one monopolizes the meeting, etc. Family members are often included in these meetings, and it is important that a professional be utilized as a facilitator because very sensitive feelings may emerge. "Exit interviews" are often necessary to ensure that someone who may have become upset during a meeting has come to terms with the problem and is feeling better. Follow-up calls the next day are sometimes employed if a group leader senses that a particular person may need to express further emotions on a particular issue.

CONTINUING MEDICAL EDUCATION MEETINGS

One of SF's goals is to sponsor continuing medical education meetings. Two such accredited meetings have been conducted thus far. The first was directed at physicians and other health professionals, while the second was aimed at medical specialists other than rheumatologists.

PUBLIC AWARENESS AND EDUCATION

The SF and members of its affiliates have concentrated much time and effort in making the general public aware of scleroderma. To this end, there have been advertisements and features in magazines and newspapers, television appearances, and speaking engagements before service organizations and other local groups. Additionally, each year, the SF has petitioned for the designation of "Scleroderma Awareness Month" during the month when fund-raising events are held and enhanced publicity efforts and other special events are scheduled.

SF SERVICES

Quarterly Newsletter

The BEACON is a quarterly publication with information of special interest to persons with scleroderma and their families. A recent reader survey lists the following as the four most helpful and informative features:

Health Information Exchange. Written by a health professional, this column is devoted to answering specific questions sent in by patients.

Sharing. Stories submitted by patients describing their personal experiences with scleroderma and sharing their own coping techniques.

Living with Scleroderma. A popular feature written by Mark Flapan, Ph.D., devoted to dealing with the emotional issues involved in living with a chronic disease. Readers identify strongly with Dr. Flapan because he also suffers from scleroderma.

Ask the Pharmacist. A registered pharmacist answers specific inquiries dealing with medications, vitamins, etc.

Other features in *The BEACON* include research updates, reports on special treatments and/or drugs, information on group activities, and many other informative articles related to scleroderma's symptoms and treatments. Readers use the *People Needing People* column and *Bits & Pieces* feature to communicate with others about product information, assistive aids, suggested reading titles, and other useful information. A newsletter such as "The BEACON" is especially helpful to people living in areas where there are not support groups or large medical centers.

Physician Referrals

Another important service is to provide a list of physician referrals based on recommendations by the SF's Medical and Scientific Advisory Board, the American College of Rheumatology, and other directories.

Peer Counseling

Peer counseling may be arranged by calling the SF patient Help Line at 1-800-422-1113.

Library Resources

SF maintains a modest library of medical journal, newspaper, and magazine articles relating to scleroderma. Files are also maintained on controversial, unorthodox, or experimental treatments, e.g., bee venom, hyperbaric oxygen, DMSO, blue algae, maleleuca oil, evening primrose oil, plasmapheresis, photopheresis, etc. Audio and video tapes, professionally-developed advertisements, and public service announcements are also available for patient and professional use. Table 32.1 lists some of the materials that are available from SF at no cost or for a modest fee.

For a fairly comprehensive listing of products and services that can be of benefit to the scleroderma patient please see Appendix II at the end of this chapter.

United Scleroderma Foundation, Inc. (Diane Williams, Founder)

The United Scleroderma Foundation (USF) was established with the goals of providing educational and emotional support for scleroderma

Table 32.1. Literature for Scleroderma Patients

Scleroderma Federation Literature[a]

1. If You Have Scleroderma . . . You Need Not Feel Alone.
2. About Scleroderma.
3. About Localized Scleroderma.
4. *Understanding and Managing Scleroderma* (a 36-page booklet). $5.00
5. Medical List Update (currently available drugs used to treat common symptoms).
6. *Helpful Hints for Living with Scleroderma* (60-page booklet) $7.00
7. *Shared Favorites Cookbook* (450 recipes) $10.00

United Scleroderma Foundation Literature[b]

1. USF Informational Brochure
2. SD Out of Hiding
3. Let's Come to Terms
4. Questions and Answers
5. Raynaud's in SD
6. Localized SD
7. The Crest Syndrome
8. SD and the GI Tract
9. SD and Oral Health
10. Sexuality and SD
11. Facing Emotions
12. SD Handbook
13. SD Digest II ($10.50)

[a] Literature is provided to patients at no cost unless price is stated. Bulk amounts to health professionals are sold at cost. Proceeds of all literature sales are donated to scleroderma research.
[b] At no cost unless listed. Nominal fee for literature ordered in bulk amounts.

patients and their families, increasing awareness of this disease, raising research dollars to determine its cause, improving treatment, and finding a cure.

OFFICE

The USF staff devotes much of its time to providing patients with hope by responding to telephone calls and letters, researching answers to individual questions, and counseling grieving patients and families. This supportive counseling helps the patients and their families to realize that they are not alone, that someone understands, and that with education and treatment they can still live productive and fruitful lives.

USF SERVICES

Chapter/Support Group

As of 1994, the USF had over 55 chapters and support groups throughout the United States and in Canada. USF provides patients, their families, and others with chapter and physician referrals, and encourages patients to contact each other through these chapters and support groups.

USF groups are composed of volunteers who extend the organization's services to people in their communities. Complementary USF informational brochures are provided for distribution to patients and physicians, at health fairs, and chapter meetings. In turn, chapters contribute a portion of their income to help support USF research and educational programs. All groups hold regular meetings, promote public awareness, and provide a great deal of emotional support to patients and their families.

Annual Conference

USF hosts an annual convention which is a three-day educational and social event. Attendees learn about USF's accomplishments during the past year and goals for the future. Patient information workshops deal with subjects such as coping with a chronic illness, physical and occupational therapy, health insurance, and disability benefits. A medical workshop featuring doctors from various medical research centers provides presentations and an overview of scleroderma, internal and external involvement, treatments, and a question and answer session.

Educational Material

The United Scleroderma Foundation provides patients and health professionals with current information on various aspects of the disease through its educational brochures (Table 32.1). Annual membership entitles USF members to brochures, handbooks, fact sheets, and a quarterly newsletter.

USF provides patients and health professionals with other information including centers of research, treatment information on prescription drugs, and various resource articles related to available treatment. Much of the literature is provided in four languages.

Quarterly Newsletter

The USF newsletter "Scleroderma Spectrum" has several features of interest to scleroderma patients including: *Current News* on health reform and other congressional activity; *Medical Updates*, written by health professionals; *Mail Bag*, featuring letters from patients; *Coping with Illness* has articles about the emotional aspects of living with a chronic illness; *Ask the Doctor* features patient letters and responses from a medical professional; and *Kids Korner* devotes space to articles and correspondence related to juvenile scleroderma. The "Spectrum" shares with the membership news on activities involving office activities, fund raising, and public relations.

Medical Workshops

USF organizes and sponsors workshops throughout the United States to bring experts in the field of scleroderma together with patients and health care professionals. USF welcomes input from health care professionals and patients on workshop locations, and encourages joint sponsorship with those in the medical field.

Physician Referrals

The USF provides physician referrals and maintains a list of qualified physicians.

Advocacy

Since 1979, USF has actively funded grants for basic and clinical research at major research centers worldwide. USF also provides summer fellowships and fosters an interest in postgraduate education.

The USF also issues appeals to its membership to contact legislators regarding patient care, health reform, and government funding of research. USF is a member of the Coalition of Patient Advocates for Skin Disease and Research and has helped to create interest in funding for several skin disease research centers in the United States. It works with the professional community in Washington, DC, to appeal for increased funding. Members of the USF testify before both the US House of Representatives and Senate and participate in rallies. USF attends conferences of the National Organization for Rare Disorders, the American Autoimmune Related Diseases Association, Inc., and Independent Sector.

Public Awareness and Personal Resources

Since 1982, USF has actively sought White House recognition of June as "Scleroderma Awareness Month." During that month, the organization strives to educate the public through a professionally produced television public service announcement, newspaper articles about patient lifestyles, chapter activities, radio news releases, etc. These promotional materials are available to patients and organizations on request. The campaign to create awareness continues throughout the year. USF also provides a slide presentation that can be used to explain the disease to service groups and to increase public awareness. The organization feels that its educational campaigns via magazine and newspaper articles, local and national television talk shows, and various local and syndicated radio segments have successfully increased public awareness.

In addition, when a patient is newly diagnosed or has a question that is troubling her/him, a help line (1-800-722-HOPE[4673]) is available.

For a fairly comprehensive listing of products and services that can be of benefit to the scleroderma patient please see Appendix II at the end of this chapter.

Library Resources

For patient questions, USF has a library that includes medical journal articles, patient-oriented newspaper and magazine stories, a listing and description of USF research grant awards, information on how to form a chapter, and the booklets listed in Table 32.1. The library also provides information on unproven and unconventional therapies such as "wheat grass," bee venom, DMSO, hyperbaric oxygen, plasmapheresis, and photophoresis.

Appendix I
Scleroderma Foundation Offices

UNITED SCLERODERMA FOUNDATION, INC.
PO Box 399
Watsonville, CA 95077
Tel: (408) 728-2202
Fax: (408) 728-3328
Help Line: 1-800-722-HOPE (4673)

SCLERODERMA FEDERATION
Peabody Office Building
One Newbury Street
Peabody, MA 01960
Tel: (508) 535-6600
Fax: (508) 535-6696
Help Line: (800) 422-1113

CANADA

The Saskatchewan Scleroderma Support
  Group
PO Box 553
Tisdale, Sask. Canada S0E 1T0
Tel: 306-873-2791

The Scleroderma Association for British
  Columbians
895 W. 10th Ave.
Vancouver, BC, Canada V5Z 1L7
Tel: 604-940-9343

The Okanagan Scleroderma Support Group
RR 4, Box 21, Site 22
Westbank, BC V0H 2AU

The Scleroderma Society of Quebec
10 Charles De Lonqueil
Ste. Julie, PQ J0L 2S0
Tel: 514-649-5334

The Ottawa Scleroderma Support Group
455 Blake Blvd.
Ottawa, Ontario, Canada K1K 1A9
Tel: 613-745-7829

Northern Ontario Scleroderma Association
159 Fifth Ave. W
North Bay, Ontario T1B 3N4
No Telephone Listing

The Scleroderma Society of Ontario
c/o Arthritis Society
250 Bloor Street, Ste. 401
Toronto, Ontario, Canada M4W 3P2
Tel: 416-967-1414

Scleroderma Foundation of Victoria, Inc.
c/o Health Promotions Centre
Alfred Hospital
Commercial Road
Prahan, Vic 3181

The Scleroderma Association of Atlantic Canada
Tel: 902-423-3942

The Edmonton Chapter of the United Sclero-
derma Foundation
POB 37 Edmonton Main
Edmonton, Alberta T5J 2G9
Tel: 403-434-3517

The Winnipeg Scleroderma Association
325 Sherbrook St.
Winnipeg, Manitoba R3A AM5
No telephone listing

GREATER EUROPE

The Scleroderma Society
16 Cherry Orchard Gardens
West Molesey, Surrey Great Britain KT8 1QY

Scleroderma Group
Attn: Babro Anderstrom, Sec.
Hembygdsgatan #6D
Klippan, Lu, Sweden S26436

Association des Sclerodermiques de France
9, Avenue de la Mare aux Canes
02400 Chateau-Thierry, France
Tel: 011-26-04-82-19

Nationale Vereriging
Met Lupus Sclerodermie
on MCTD
The Netherlands
Tel: 011-3-46-552401

Selbsthilfegruppe Sklerodermie
in Deutschland
Siege, Germany
Tel: 011-2-71-85519

Scleroderma Israeli Association
Attn: Liora Levy
16 Migdal Shorsham St.
Tel Aviv, Israel 69015

AUSTRALIA/NEW ZEALAND

Scleroderma Group of Arthritis Foundation of
New Zealand, Inc.
Wellington, New Zealand
Tel: 011-4-72-1427

Scleroderma/Lupus Support Society, Inc.
Warners Bay, NSW, Australia
Tel: 011-49-236-146

The Scleroderma Association
Chatswood, NSW, Australia
Tel: 011-2-411-3459

The Lupus/Scleroderma Group
Ashford, SA, Australia
Tel: 011-8-297-2488

Scleroderma Foundation of Victoria, Inc.
Victoria, NSW, Australia
Tel: 011-49-529-5230

Appendix II
Products and Services

PRODUCTS AND SERVICES
(Telephones/Faxes listed where available)

Abbey Medical Catalog Sales
13782 Crenshaw Blvd.
Gardena, CA 90249
800-262-1294 (toll free in CA)
800-421-5126 (toll free in other states)
Assistive and other aids for home use

R.G. Abernathy, Inc.
Route 1, Box 1
Creston, NC
800-334-0128
Custom shoes

Able Data
National Rehabilitation Information Center
4407 Eighth Street NE
Washington, DC 20017
(202) 635-6090
(202) 635-5884 (TTP)
Computerized national data base for rehabilitation products

Accent on Living Magazine
Gillum Road and High Drive
PO Box 700
Bloomington, IL 61702
Supplier to the disabled and chronically ill; write for catalog

Access Travel: A Guide to Accessibility of Airport Terminals
US General Services Administration
Washington, DC 20405
A guide to accessibility of airport terminals

Aids for Arthritis
3 Little Knoll Court
Medford, NJ 08055
(609)654-6918
Aids/gadgets for those with limited hand movement

Air Travelers Fly Rights
Office of Consumer Affairs
Civil Aeronautics Board
Washington, DC 20428
Write for information

All Ways Medical, Inc.
786 East 7th Street
St. Paul, MN 55106
(612) 771-0046
Can call collect. Three- and four-wheel scooters, electric and manual wheelchairs, and all other adaptive equipment.

Amigo Sales, Inc.
6693 Dixie Highway
Bridgeport, MI 48603
Electric go-carts/scooters

Arthritis Foundation
Self-Help Manual
4311 Wilshire Blvd.
Los Angeles, Ca 90010
Send name and address along with a check or
    money order for $3.65

Battle Creek Equipment
307 W. Jackson Street
Battle Creek, MI 49017-2385
800-253-0854
Request catalog of equipment from exercise
    bikes to an automatic moist heat pack

Birkenstock Shoes
46 Valli Drive
Vorata, Ca 94947
Sandals

Bruce Medical Supply
411 Waverly Oaks Rd.
Waltham, MA 02154
Medical and assistive aids

Cleo Living Aids
3957 Mayfield Road
Cleveland, OH 44121
Write for catalog on daily living aids including
    bath and shower devices

Comfortably Yours
52 West Hunter Avenue
Maywood, NJ 07607
Write for catalog on aids for easier living

Consumer Product Information Service
Public Documents Distribution Center
Pueblo, CO 81009
Write for catalog on information available

Dr. Leonard's Health Care Catalog
74 20th Street
Brooklyn, NY 11232
Healthcare, household, and grooming products

Eddie Bauer
Fifth & Union
PO Box 3700
Seattle, WA 98130-0006
800-426-6253
Warm clothing

Enrichments: Helping Hands for Special
    Needs
PO Box 579
145 Tower Drive
Hinsdale, IL 60921
Aids - clothing for daily living

Fashion-Able, Inc.
Rock Hill, NJ 08553
Write for adaptive clothing catalog, mail order
    clothes for women

Fashion Ease
Division of M&M Health Care Apparel Co.
1541 60th St.
Brooklyn, NY 11219
718-853-6376
Easy access clothing

Fred Simmons, Inc.
Medical Supplies
POB 386
Western Springs, IL 60558
800-323-5547
Professional healthcare catalog

Gander Mountain, Inc.
Outdoor Sportsmen Supplies
PO Box 248, Hwy. W
Wilmot, WI 53192
800-558-9410
Warm clothing

Grass Roots Promotions
322 W. Roosevelt St., Dept. W
Freeport, IL 61032

Gresham Driving Aids
PO Box 405
30800 Wixom
Wixom, MI 48096
Driving aids & equipment

Hammacher Schlemmer
145 E. 57th St.
New York, NY 10022
Catalog for gadgets and aids for kitchen products

Hapad, Inc.
PO Box 6
5301 Enterprise Blvd.
Bethel Park, PA 15102
Felt pads to help relieve pressure points on
    painful feet

Helping Hand for Independent Living
PO Box 19083
Washington, DC 20036-9083
Write for $3.00 catalog of products for people
    with special needs

Help Yourself Aids
PO Box 192
Hinsdale, IL 60521
Eating, dressing, wheelchair, household, com-
    munication aids

Hide & Chic Hats by Marebar
Marebar Inc.
PO Box 547
Marlton, NJ 08053
Hats designed for people experiencing hair loss
    as a result of chemotherapy and other med-
    ical problems

Independent Living Aids, Inc.
1500 New Horizons Blvd.
Amityville, NY 11701
800-262-7827
Fashions for the physically challenged

L.L. Bean
Outdoor Sporting Specialties
Freeport, ME 04033
800-221-4221
Warm clothing

Miles Kimball
Kimball Building
41 W. 8th Ave.
Oshkosh, WI 54901
Catalog of gadgets and practical devices

Maddak, Inc.
Paquannock, NJ 07440
Write for catalog of home health care equip-
    ment, "Special products for people with spe-
    cial needs"

Medic Alert Foundation International
PO Box 1009
Turlock, CA 95380
Free bracelet with membership

Medmek Limited
PO Box 18
Romsey, Hampshire
England SO5 9ZY
Electrically heated gloves and socks

Jerry Miller I.D. Shoes
Marble Street
Whitman, MA 02382
Custom molded shoes

National Safety Council
444 N. Michigan Ave.
Chicago, IL 60611
(312) 527-4800
National Safety Council Medical Information
    Card

Nova Design
279-B Great Valley Parkway
Malven, PA 19355
Therapeutic heat products